# BLOOD CONSERVATION
# IN THE SURGICAL PATIENT

# BLOOD CONSERVATION IN THE SURGICAL PATIENT

Editor

## M. Ramez Salem, M.D.

Chairman
Department of Anesthesiology
Illinois Masonic Medical Center
Chicago, Illinois

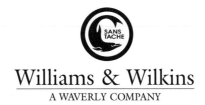

Williams & Wilkins
A WAVERLY COMPANY

BALTIMORE • PHILADELPHIA • LONDON • PARIS • BANGKOK
BUENOS AIRES • HONG KONG • MUNICH • SYDNEY • TOKYO • WROCLAW

1996

*Executive Editor:* Carroll Cann
*Developmental Editor:* Tanya Lazar
*Production Coordinator:* Peter J. Carley
*Book Project Editor:* Susan Rockwell
*Copy Editors:* Pam Goehrig and Annette Kugel
*Designer:* Maria Karkucinski
*Typesetter:* Maryland Composition
*Printer:* Maple Press
*Binder:* Maple Press

351 West Camden Street
Baltimore, Maryland 21201–2436 USA

Rose Tree Corporate Center
1400 North Providence Road
Building II, Suite 5025
Media, Pennsylvania 19063-2043 USA

Accurate indications, adverse reactions, and dosage schedules for drugs are provided in this book, but it is possible that they may change. The reader is urged to review the package information data of the manufacturers of the medications mentioned.

*Printed in the United States of America*

**Library of Congress Cataloging in Publication Data**

Blood conservation in the surgical patient / [edited by] M. Ramez Salem.
    p.  cm.
    Includes index.
    ISBN 0-683-07531-4
    1. Blood—Transfusion.  2. Blood—Transfusion, Autologous.
3. Hemostasis, Surgical.  I. Salem, M. Ramez (Mohammed Ramez), 1936—
    [DNLM: 1. Blood Transfusion.  2. Blood Preservation.  3. Disease
Transmission—prevention & control.  4. Hemostasis, Surgical.
5. Intraoperative Care.  WB 356 B6538  1996]
RM171.B587  1996
615′.39—dc20
DNLM/DLC
for Library of Congress

*The Publishers have made every effort to trace the copyright holders for borrowed material. If they have inadvertently overlooked any, they will be pleased to make the necessary arrangements at the first opportunity.*

95 96 97 98 99
1 2 3 4 5 6 7 8 9 10

Reprints of chapters may be purchased from Williams & Wilkins in quantities of 100 or more. Call Isabella Wise, Special Sales Department, (800) 358-3583.

*In memory of*
*my beloved parents*
*Dr. and Mrs. Salem*

# Foreword

## PART I

I am very pleased to have been asked to write an introduction for the new textbook *Blood Conservation in the Surgical Patient,* edited by M. Ramez Salem, M.D., Chairman of the Department of Anesthesiology at Illinois Masonic Medical Center. Although I am an internist, I am also a specialist in the field of Infectious Diseases, and traditionally, blood and blood products have been the route of transmission of a variety of infectious agents from donor to recipient. Historically, the field began by simply trying to work through ways to conserve and handle blood and blood products to replace missing blood components (predominantly red blood cells to maintain oxygenation); however, the field is now enormously complex with a variety of different components available for transfusion, a variety of different clinical indications for each transfusable component, and an enormously complex array of circumstances during which blood and blood products should or should not be given.

While this book focuses on the "surgical patient," the data provided and principles espoused are important for health at all levels and in all specialties. From the premedical student through the medical student, resident and practicing physician, and for all variety of non-physician health care professionals, the topics outlined have extraordinary relevance. Medicine has just entered the new era haunted by the evolution and expression of the human immunodeficiency virus and its ultimate product, the syndrome of AIDS. AIDS alone makes extraordinarily relevant the need to review and re-think blood conservation techniques in surgery and trauma patients. We all must re-look at every earlier transfusion practice, at every usable blood component (and more are being made available at a rapid rate) and at all the techniques involved in manipulating patients during repair of trauma and the performance of elective surgery considering the impact of the HIV whether present in the patient, the health providers, or in the transfusion products.

Finally, even as HIV is becoming better understood, other retroviruses such as HTLV-2 are becoming a concern as well as a variety of other more traditional viruses about which little thought has been given in the past. Thus, it is highly appropriate to bring together acknowledged experts in the variety of fields concerned with blood conservation and transfusion in surgery in order to construct the superb textbook which follows this introduction.

Finally, my own sensitivity has recently been raised to new heights with regard to the issues of blood conservation and transfusion as I personally have undergone hip-replacement, struggling with educating myself about the need for autologous blood donation, indications for blood transfusions and the physiologic effects in the postoperative period of blood loss and anemia. I certainly would have welcomed a book as extensive as the present textbook to have answered a variety of questions which, though addressed effectively by my personal caregivers, took far longer and was more time consuming than had I a reference available such as the present textbook. I certainly am in a better position now to answer questions raised by my patients, residents and students, and I will personally add the present textbook to my library as one of the "core textbooks" required by the active internist.

My final point is that more and more frequently our patients, as enlightened consumers, ask us for "literature" regarding their illness or the therapeutic approaches recommended. This textbook will serve too as an excellent reference for the educational process demanded more frequently by patients and requiring focused literature summarizing the issue-at-hand by physicians and other health providers.

In summary, *Blood Conservation in the Surgical Patient* is a timely contribution to the field and excellent in its scientific and clinical content.

*John N. Sheagren, M.D.*

# Foreword

## PART II

Blood conservation in the surgical patient must rank high among those activities most needed today to benefit the entire population, not only of this country but of the world.

We live, unfortunately, in an age when the spread of blood-borne infections is of concern not only to the medical community, but to anyone who reads a newspaper or watches television. Although hospitals are the setting for only a minute portion of AIDS and hepatitis transmission, we in health care have a dual need to be scrupulous in our practices and our safeguards. First as physicians and health care workers, we have a personal and professional commitment to "do no harm." We have chosen our life's work to help, not to hurt. Second, patients who monitor their own lifestyles carefully to guard against infection (and even those who don't) have every right to assume that the institutions and personnel they seek out for care will not expose them to avoidable risks.

We also have two kinds of responsibility. We must first observe all known precautions in our routine activities, for the benefit of our patients and our own colleagues, whose risk of exposure is far greater than those they treat. We must also pursue diligently every available means of improving these techniques and precautions, and share our knowledge with others.

The detailed and meticulous review of this subject presented here is the result of years of careful, painstaking research and experience, with greatly intensified activity in the past 2 years. Each individual involved is clearly expert in his or her area, and together they represent a remarkable multidisciplinary team of researchers and clinicians. This textbook will undoubtedly be a benchmark achievement in this area. It certainly will become required reading for everyone who deals with the use of blood in the surgical patient.

We at Illinois Masonic Medical Center are proud of the efforts of these colleagues. They have worked on this critical problem both diligently and creatively. In an era of diminished staff and budgetary resources, a work such as this requires twice the dedication that it might have in an earlier period. We are all fortunate that the men and women whose work you hold possess that measure of dedication.

*Edwin Feldman, M.D.*

# Preface

It has been estimated that over 23 million blood components are transfused each year in the United States. The potential benefits gained from blood transfusion are improved tissue oxygenation, correction of coagulopathy, and overall improved outcome. Balanced against these benefits are the adverse effects and spiraling costs associated with transfusion, which averages $155.00 per transfused unit of whole blood (or red blood cells) or an annual cost of 2 billion dollars in the United States. Because almost 25% of this annual cost has been deemed unnecessarily due to inappropriate use of blood transfusion, various national medical organizations have issued stricter recommendations for blood component use and launched comprehensive educational programs for physicians and dissemination of practice guidelines. In 1994, the American Society of Anesthesiologists convened the Task Force on Blood Component Therapy to develop evidence-based guidelines on the proper indications for perioperative and peripartum administration of blood components. Regarding the effectiveness of red blood cell transfusion, the Task Force concluded that:

(1) transfusion is rarely indicated when the hemoglobin concentration is greater than 10 g/dL and is almost always indicated when it is less than 6 g/dL; (2) the determination of whether intermediate hemoglobin concentrations (6–10 g/dL) justify or require red blood cell transfusion should be based on the patient's risk of developing complications of inadequate oxygenation; (3) the use of a single hemoglobin "trigger" for all patients, and other approaches that fail to consider all important physiological and surgical factors affecting oxygenation, are not recommended; (4) where appropriate, preoperative autologous blood donation, acute normovolemic hemodilution, intraoperative and postoperative blood recovery, and measures to decrease blood loss (deliberate hypotension and pharmacologic agents) should be employed; and (5) the indications for transfusion of autologous red blood cells may be more liberal than for allogeneic red blood cells because of the lower risks associated with the former.

Blood conservation strategies are by no means new, some having been in clinical use since the 1940s by surgeons who realized that their surgical results were being compromised by the inability to control bleeding. Multiple factors have lead to renewed interest in these previously established blood conservation measures as well as in the development of new strategies in the last two decades.

Blood has long been regarded as a natural scarce human resource, always in great demand. Although tremendous efforts have been made to ensure optimum blood supply, blood banks frequently cannot always cope with the increased demand. New and more sophisticated surgical procedures (e.g., liver transplantation, trauma surgery) requiring unprecedented amounts of blood have increased the demand for blood and blood components.

The need for surgery on patients who refuse blood transfusions because of religious beliefs has stimulated hemorheologic studies. Tissue oxygenation is well maintained at lower hemoglobin concentrations during acute normovolemic hemodilution, without an increase in morbidity or mortality. This technique, used alone or in combination with other measures of blood conservation has been advocated to minimize blood loss during certain major surgical procedures, and thus, can reduce or even eliminate exposure to allogeneic blood. From the many studies of physiologic, and chronic types of anemia, it became evident that hemoglobin concentration *per se* is neither an adequate descriptor of the severity of anemia, nor is it reflective of the adaptive factors that preserve oxygen delivery to the tissues. The concept of "designation of anemia on functional basis" was thus introduced. The understanding of the compensatory mechanisms associated with anemia led to acceptance of lower perioperative hemoglobin values than the previously held 10 g/dL.

Although the overall risk of acquiring the human immunodeficiency virus is less than 1 in 200,000 per transfused unit of blood, the fear of the risk of transmission of the disease has led to major changes in transfusion practices. More sensitive tests for detection of antibodies have been developed to identify infectious donors. Physician's interest in blood conservation grew and some measures became rapidly an accepted standard. Contributing to the widespread acceptance of blood conservation measures such as preoperative autologous blood donation were hospital and physician concerns about litigation. In some states, hastily conceived legislation required that in addition to the risks and benefits of blood transfusion, alternatives to allogeneic blood be presented to patients (the California Statute CB-37, Paul Gann Blood Safety Act, 1990).

Advances in genetic engineering paved the way to the synthesis of recombinant human erythropoietin. Its usefulness in the management of certain anemias and the procurement of larger amounts of blood donated preoperatively became apparent. Great progress has also been made to develop a hemoglobin-based red blood cell substitute. The issues delaying clinical applications were primarily related to safety and limitations. Through polymerization, many of the problems have been overcome. Enthusiastic clinical trials have already begun. It is expected that hemoglobin solutions would be available for clinical use in the near future.

Clinicians resorted to combining blood conservation techniques to achieve a greater reduction of blood loss during certain major surgical procedures. When these techniques are combined (deliberate hypotensions and acute normovolemic hemodilution) critical reduction in oxygen delivery to vital organs may ensue. Advances in monitoring permitted accurate measurements of indices of oxygen delivery and oxygen utilization thus enhancing the safety of the combined techniques.

*Blood Conservation in the Surgical Patient* attempts to cover the historical, physiological, and pharmacological basis of blood conservation and blend them with clinical and techni-

cal aspects. Because of the multidisciplinary nature of blood conservation strategies, contributors have been selected from various specialties. These contributors include clinicians, scientists, and technologists who are involved in practicing these measures and/or involved in studying research aspects of blood conservation. The book is intended to serve as a comprehensive base for blood conservation techniques. The targeted audience are medical students, residents in various anesthesia and surgical specialties, clinicians in various subspecialties, scientists, and technologists who are interested in learning and practicing these techniques.

To all who have assisted in the preparation of this book, I am most appreciative of their efforts. I thank all the contributors for taking time from their busy daily schedules to prepare these chapters. Certain people, who without them the book would have never been written deserve special gratitude. To Mr. Carroll Cann and Ms. Tanya Lazar of Williams & Wilkins, I express my deep appreciation for their dedication, patience, encouragement, and professionalism. My sincerest gratitude goes to Mr. Ninos Joseph and Ms. Grace deKelaita for their relentless dedication, hard work, and long hours, which made this book possible. To our secretarial staff and the Illinois Masonic Medical Center Audiovisual Department, I wish a special thanks for all their efforts. Finally, I thank my own resident and attending staff at the Illinois Masonic Medical Center and Shriner Hospital for Crippled Children, Chicago Unit, who I have been privileged to work with for the last 14 years and have inspired me to edit this book.

I would like to remind our readers that transfusion medicine and blood conservation are rapidly evolving fields. As this book is being published, continued scientific advances and newer developments are expected. Feedback from the reader is sincerely appreciated.

# Contributors ⅄

**Lisa M. Bibb, M.D.**
Attending Pathologist
Ingalls Memorial Hospital
Harvey, Illinois

**Rinaldo F. Canalis, M.D.**
Chief
Division of Head and Neck Surgery
Harbor-UCLA Medical Center
Torrance, California
Professor of Surgery
University of California, Los Angeles
Los Angeles, California

**Juan R. Chediak, M.D.**
Attending Physician
Departments of Pathology and Medicine
Illinois Masonic Medical Center
Chicago, Illinois
Assistant Professor of Medicine
Rush University School of Medicine
Chicago, Illinois

**George J. Crystal, Ph.D.**
Director
Research Laboratory
Department of Anesthesiology
Illinois Masonic Medical Center
Chicago, Illinois
Associate Professor of Anesthesiology and
    Physiology
University of Illinois College of Medicine
Chicago, Illinois

**Edward A. Czinn, M.D.**
Attending Anesthesiologist
Illinois Masonic Medical Center
Chicago, Illinois
Clinical Assistant Professor of Anesthesiology
University of Illinois College of Medicine
Chicago, Illinois

**Peter J. Davis, M.D.**
Director of Pediatric Anesthesia
Children's Hospital of Pittsburgh
Pittsburgh, Pennsylvania
Associate Professor of Anesthesiology and
    Pediatrics
University of Pittsburgh School of Medicine
Pittsburgh, Pennsylvania

**Fawzy G. Estafanous, M.D.**
Chairman
Division of Anesthesiology
Cleveland Clinic Foundation
Cleveland, Ohio

**Nabil R. Fahmy, M.D.**
Anesthetist
Massachusetts General Hospital
Boston, Massachusetts
Associate Professor of Anaesthesia
Harvard Medical School
Cambridge, Massachusetts

**Richard J. Fantus, M.D.**
Director of Trauma Services
Director, Surgical Intensive Care
Illinois Masonic Medical Center
Chicago, Illinois
Assistant Professor of Surgery
University of Illinois College of Medicine
Chicago, Illinois

**Edwin Feldman, M.D.**
Senior Vice President, Medical Affairs
Illinois Masonic Medical Center
Chicago, Illinois
Associate Dean
Rush University School of Medicine
Chicago, Illinois

**Michael Friedman, M.D.**
Head, Section of Otolaryngology
Department of Surgery
Illinois Masonic Medical Center
Chicago, Illinois
Associate Professor of Otolaryngology and
    Bronchoesophagology
Rush Medical College
Rush University
Chicago, Illinois

**Steven A. Gould, M.D.**
President
Northfield Laboratories, Inc.
Evanston, Illinois
Professor of Surgery
University of Illinois College of Medicine
Chicago, Illinois

**Hanafy A. Hanafy, M.D.**
Resident Physician
Department of Surgery
University of Illinois Hospital
Chicago, Illinois

**Renée S. Hartz, M.D.**
Division Chief
Department of Cardiothoracic Surgery
Department of Surgery
University of Illinois Hospital
Chicago, Illinois

Professor of Surgery and Chief of Division of
  Cardiothoracic Surgery
University of Illinois College of Medicine
Chicago, Illinois

**Harold J. Heyman, M.D.**

Attending Anesthesiologist
Illinois Masonic Medical Center
Chicago, Illinois
Clinical Associate Professor of Anesthesiology
University of Illinois College of Medicine
Chicago, Illinois

**Ninos J. Joseph, B.S.**

Research Associate
Department of Anesthesiology
Illinois Masonic Medical Center
Chicago, Illinois

**Judith Kamaryt, RN, CCP**

Perfusionist
Section of Cardiovascular Surgery
Department of Surgery
Illinois Masonic Medical Center
Chicago, Illinois

**Arthur J. Klowden, M.D.**

Attending Anesthesiologist
Illinois Masonic Medical Center
Chicago, Illinois
Clinical Assistant Professor of Anesthesiology
University of Illinois College of Medicine
Chicago, Illinois

**Frank J. Konicek, M.D.**

Section Chief
Section of Gastroenterology
Department of Medicine
Illinois Masonic Medical Center
Chicago, Illinois
Clinical Associate Professor of Medicine
Loyola University—Stritch School of Medicine
Maywood, Illinois

**David J. Lang, D.O.**

Attending Anesthesiologist
Illinois Masonic Medical Center
Chicago, Illinois
Assistant Clinical Professor of Anesthesiology
Illinois Masonic Medical Center
Chicago, Illinois

**John L. Lubicky, M.D.**

Chief of Staff
Shriners Hospitals for Crippled Children
Chicago Unit
Chicago, Illinois
Professor of Orthopaedic Surgery
Rush Medical College
Rush University
Chicago, Illinois

**Sheldon B. Maltz, M.D.**

Attending Surgeon: Trauma Services
Department of Surgery
Illinois Masonic Medical Center
Chicago, Illinois
Clinical Assistant Professor of Surgery
University of Illinois College of Medicine
Chicago, Illinois

**Steven Manley, M.D.**

Attending Anesthesiologist
Illinois Masonic Medical Center
Chicago, Illinois
Clinical Assistant Professor of Anesthesiology
University of Illinois School of Medicine
Chicago, Illinois

**Louise Mastrianno, MT (ASCP), SBB**

Supervisor
Blood Bank
Illinois Masonic Medical Center
Chicago, Illinois

**Michele M. Mellett, M.D.**

Attending Surgeon: Trauma Services
Department of Surgery
Illinois Masonic Medical Center
Chicago, Illinois
Clinical Assistant Professor of Surgery
University of Illinois College of Medicine
Chicago, Illinois

**Gerald S. Moss, M.D.**

Dean
University of Illinois College of Medicine
Chicago, Illinois
Dean of College of Medicine
University of Illinois College of Medicine
Chicago, Illinois

**Usharani Nimmagadda, M.D.**

Attending Anesthesiologist
Illinois Masonic Medical Center
Chicago, Illinois
Clinical Assistant Professor of Anesthesiology
University of Illinois College of Medicine
Chicago, Illinois

**Sharon Noble, M.D.**

Chief Resident
Metropolitan Group Hospital's Residency in
  General Surgery
Chicago, Illinois

**Robert Paulissian, M.D.**

Attending Anesthesiologist
Illinois Masonic Medical Center
Chicago, Illinois
Clinical Associate Professor of Anesthesiology
University of Illinois College of Medicine
Chicago, Illinois

**Jose L. Salazar, M.D.**

Chairman
Department of Neurosurgery
Department of Surgery
Illinois Masonic Medical Center
Chicago, Illinois
Associate Professor of Neurosurgical Surgery
University of Illinois College of Medicine
Chicago, Illinois

**M. Ramez Salem, M.D.**

Chairman
Department of Anesthesiology
Illinois Masonic Medical Center
Chicago, Illinois
Clinical Professor of Anesthesiology
University of Illinois College of Medicine
Chicago, Illinois

**Paul D. Schanbacher, M.D.**

Attending Anesthesiologist
Illinois Masonic Medical Center
Chicago, Illinois

**Victor Scott, M.D.**

Attending Anesthesiologist
Presbyterian-University Hospital
Pittsburgh, Pennsylvania
Assistant Professor of Anesthesiology
University of Pittsburgh School of Medicine
Pittsburgh, Pennsylvania

**Hansa L. Sehgal**

Associate Director of Research and
    Development
Northfield Laboratories, Inc.
Evanston, Illinois

**Lakshman L. Sehgal, Ph.D.**

Vice President, Research and Development
Northfield Laboratories, Inc.

Evanston, Illinois
Research Assistant Professor of Surgery
University of Illinois College of Medicine
Chicago, Illinois

**John N. Sheagren, M.D.**

Chairman
Department of Internal Medicine
Illinois Masonic Medical Center
Chicago, Illinois
Professor of Medicine
Rush University School of Medicine
Chicago, Illinois

**Salwa A. Shenaq, M.D.**

Service Chief
Cardiovascular Anesthesia
The Methodist Hospital
Houston, Texas
Associate Professor of Anesthesiology
Baylor College of Medicine
Houston, Texas

**Fernando Viñuela, M.D.**

Chief, Therapeutic Neuroradiology
Department of Radiology
UCLA Medical Center
Los Angeles, California
Professor of Radiology
UCLA School of Medicine
Los Angeles, California

**Raymond L. Warpeha, M.D.**

Chief
Division of Plastic Surgery and Reconstructive
    Surgery
Department of Surgery
Loyola University Medical Center
Stritch School of Medicine
Maywood, Illinois
Professor of Surgery
Loyola University Stritch School of Medicine
Maywood, Illinois

# Contents

# 1
# PRINCIPLES OF BLOOD TRANSFUSION

*Lisa M. Bibb, Usharani Nimmagadda, and Louise Mastrianno*

## HISTORICAL PERSPECTIVES

## HOMOLOGOUS TRANSFUSIONS

In the mid-17th century, France and England were competing in the areas of political expansion, military supremacy, and scientific achievement, including medical science. Between 1656 and 1668, scientists in France and England performed the first blood transfusions in humans, including animal-to-animal and animal-to-man transfusions. Also, during this time, the first transfusion reaction was recorded.[1] Initially, in the 1650s, there were animal experiments involving intravenous injection of various substances, e.g., opium, milk, dye, wine, and emetics. In 1665, John Wilkins, an Oxford scientist, reported to the Royal Society of England that he and his colleagues had succeeded in transfusing about 2 ounces of blood, using a syringe from one dog to another, without any harmful effects.[2] The first public demonstration of transfusion in an experimental animal was presented to the Royal Society by Richard Lower, an English physician at Oxford. Lower[3,4] subsequently performed a series of experiments on dogs, involving direct vein-to-vein and artery-to-vein transfusions, which were then published in the *Philosophical Transactions.*

At the same time in France, Jean Baptiste Denis, physician-in-ordinary to King Louis XIV, and Paul Emmerez, a surgeon, also began performing animal transfusion experiments at the Academie de Sciences. They reported transfusion of calves' blood into dogs in *Philosophical Transactions.*[5] The first blood transfusion to a man was performed by Denis, assisted by Emmerez, on June 25, 1667. The procedure was published as a letter in *Philosophical Transactions.*[6]

Interestingly, blood transfusions in humans during the 17th century were used for altering mental aberrations, rather than for replacement of blood loss. This first transfusion in a human involved a 15-year-old boy, who had been repeatedly phlebotomized for a condition described as a "comtacious and violent fever."[7] This procedure, performed by Denis, involved removal of approximately 3 ounces of the patient's blood with subsequent infusion of 9 ounces of lamb's blood. Following the procedure, the patient reportedly slept well that night.

Lower and King in 1667,[8] transfused a 32-year-old man with approximately 12 ounces of sheep's blood without any serious sequelae. The patient was again transfused uneventfully in the presence of the Royal Society.

Denis continued his human transfusions, his most famous case being that of a 34-year-old man with mania, who was transfused with calves' blood on three separate occasions during late 1667 and early 1668. The day following the second transfusion, the patient "made a great glass of urine with a color as black as if it had been mixed with a soot of a chimney."[7] This was presumably the first recorded hemolytic transfusion reaction in man. During the third attempted transfusion 2 months later, the patient developed seizures, went into shock, and expired the next day. Denis was brought to trial for murder, but was exonerated of any wrongdoing. The Faculty of Medicine at Paris determined that blood transfusions were scientifically unsound and dangerous. The Parliament of Paris passed a law in 1678 making blood transfusion illegal. In 1679, the Pope banned blood transfusions in almost all parts of Europe following two more transfusion-related deaths in Rome. The Royal Society in London also outlawed the procedure.

Only sporadic attempts at transfusion of animal blood to humans occurred during the remainder of the 17th and throughout the 18th centuries. James Blundell, an English obstetrician, performed the first allogeneic transfusion in a human in December 1818. This case involved infusion of approximately 14 ounces of blood into a 35-year-old male with gastric cancer. The patient died 56 hours later.[9] Blundell recommended that only human-to-human transfusions were acceptable, and was the first to use transfusions to replace blood loss, rather than to heal psychic or emotional problems. He developed several different transfusion devices and performed the first successful allogeneic transfusion in 1828.[10] He subsequently transfused several women with postpartum hemorrhage, resulting in an apparent 50% success rate.

During the 1800s, direct vessel anastomoses between donor and recipient were used, making blood transfusions highly impractical. Direct transfusions were performed because of the absence of refrigeration, preservation, and anticoagulation techniques.[11] A simple multiple syringe method with rapid injection of blood, proposed by Edward Lindeman in 1913, put an end to direct vessel anastomosis transfusion.[12]

During the 19th and early 20th centuries, efforts were directed towards improvement of mechanical transfusion devices for both direct and indirect transfusions. The devices used for direct transfusions included a hand-operated pump and direction-control valve interposed between donor and recipient veins, and devices using rubber tubing and stopcocks. Indirect transfusion devices involved withdrawal of blood to be transfused into a collection device, which was then immediately transfused to the recipient, with or without an anticoagulant. Transfusion was probably not practiced in the United States before 1830. Although never published, George McClellan reportedly transfused a patient with cholera in 1832. During the entire Civil War, only four transfusions were recorded.[13]

Plasma was first used as a volume expander during World War I.[11] Strumia popularized the clinical use of plasma and transfused it routinely in place of whole blood in patients with hemorrhagic anemia in 1931.[14] During World War II, lyophilized pooled plasma that was reconstituted on the battlefield was used.[11] An estimated 13 million units of banked blood were used during World War II. In the United States, the organized collection of blood for use in transfusion of civilians began in 1947.

## BLOOD PRESERVATION AND BLOOD BANKING
### Blood Banking

Robertson is credited with developing the first blood bank for storage of human blood at United States Army casualty clearing stations in France during World War I.[15] Wooden ice boxes were used to store anticoagulated blood for up to 26 days. The first blood bank in the United States was established at Cook County Hospital, Chicago, Illinois by Dr. Bernard Fantus in 1937.[16,17] The availability of preservative solutions and electrical refrigeration permitted the development of blood storage facilities. Blood banking, by providing long-term preservation of blood, made available an unlimited supply of blood within the time required for cross matching, resulting in a dramatic increase in the use of allogeneic blood.

### Cryopreservation

Glycerol techniques were applied to the freezing of red blood cells (RBCs) in the 1950s.[18] Deglycerolized frozen RBCs were first successfully transfused in 1951.[19] Frozen RBCs became clinically useful in the 1960s, after the development of effective techniques for removing glycerol, including the use of several mechanical devices.

### Blood Storage Containers

Glass bottles, steel needles, rubber seals, and tubing were first used for collecting preserved blood. This equipment was reused after sterilization and needles were resharpened.[20] However, pyrogenic reactions in blood recipients due to bacterial contamination were common. Baxter Laboratories developed commercially prepared gravity collection bottles in 1936 and vacuum collection bottles in 1939. Air embolism in blood donors was a complication noted with use of these types of bottles.[20] Embolism was also observed in recipients when air was pumped into glass bottles to hasten transfusion.[21]

Beginning in the 1950s, sterile plastic blood containers with attached tubing and satellite containers were used. The use of plastic bags eliminated problems with turbulence, foaming, and pyrogenic reactions. In the 1960s, plastic bags also made it possible to centrifuge whole blood and divide it into multiple components, including platelet concentrates.[22] Component therapy provided more specific replacement of the blood component(s) that the patient required.

### Anticoagulants

In 1860, Neudorfer developed one of the first anticoagulant additives—sodium bicarbonate.[23] Braxton-Hicks performed six unsuccessful transfusions using sodium phosphate as an anticoagulant.[24] In 1914 and 1915, use of sodium citrate as an anticoagulant was proposed independently by four different investigators. Albert Hustin, a Belgian, was apparently the first to use a solution of citrate, salt, and glucose in 1914. Richard Weil, a pathologist at German Hospital in New York, noted that citrated blood could be stored in a refrigerator for several days before use.[25] In 1916, Rous and Turner developed a solution of salt, isocitrate, and glucose anticoagulant-preservative solution which although cumbersome, was the only such solution available for almost 25 years.[26] The Rous-Turner solution permitted the first transfusions of preserved blood during World War I. The Rous-Turner solution was also used during most of World War II. Until the 1940s, sodium citrate solutions, usually supplemented with glucose, served as the usual blood preservative.[27]

Loutit and Mollison[28] introduced acid-citrate-dextrose (ACD) as a preservative in 1943, permitting storage of blood for 21 days. Many modifications of ACD were subsequently introduced. ACD remained the mainstay of RBC preservation until approximately 1970.

The only significant change in blood preservatives since ACD was a 20% reduction in citrate, an addition of phosphate, and a significant increase in pH from 5.0 to 5.7, resulting in the development of citrate-phosphate-dextrose (CPD). CPD replaced ACD as the predominant RBC preservative in the United States.

Nakao and associates[29] discovered the role of adenine in RBC preservation. The addition of adenine to ACD resulted in decreased glycolysis with decreased glucose consumption and lactate formation, better preservation of glycolytic capacity, and higher ATP levels.

Citrate-phosphate-dextrose-adenine-formula 1 (CPDA-1) was approved in the United States in 1977 for blood preservation, extending the shelf-life from 21 days (for ACD and CPD) to 35 days. Claes Hogman introduced the first additive solution, saline-adenine-glucose (SAG) in 1978,[30] which was later modified by the addition of mannitol (SAGMAN). This extended the shelf-life to 42 days.[31]

## Components

Experiments with hemophilic dogs by Brinkhous and coworkers led to widespread use of fresh frozen plasma (FFP) for treatment of hemophilia A in humans.[32] Judith Pool introduced cryoprecipitate in 1964.[33] By 1970, cryoprecipitate and factor VIII concentrate replaced FFP in the management of hemophilia A.[11] After the introduction of commercial human factor VIII concentrate, it was soon realized that these concentrates carried a substantial risk of transfusion-transmitted infection, such as hepatitis and acquired immunodeficiency syndrome (AIDS).[34,35]

Factor IX complex concentrates became widely available in the United States by the early 1970s. These concentrates, which contain several clotting factors that fractionate together (factors II, VII, IX, and X), were recognized to cause thrombotic complications. Pure factor IX concentrates, which are far less thrombogenic, were developed in the 1980s.

Duke reported the efficacy of transfusing platelets in patients with bleeding disorders in 1910.[36] During the 1960s, the value of platelet transfusion to support thrombocytopenic leukemic patients was established.[22] The first blood cell separators were described in the late 1960s,[37] subsequently leading to automated apheresis for preparation of blood components from a single individual.

## BLOOD GROUPS, ANTIGLOBULIN TESTING, CROSS MATCH

In a review of all published transfusions in 1849, Routh found 18 out of 48 transfusions resulted in a fatal outcome.[38] In the late 1800s, the increasing numbers of adverse reactions due to unrecognized immune destruction of RBCs led to discouragement of blood transfusions. As a result, saline infusion as a blood substitute was advocated in 1884 by Bull.[39] Troublesome and, at times, serious transfusion reactions stimulated further investigations. Karl Landsteiner discovered the A and B antigens and their corresponding antibodies in 1901.[40] Landsteiner subsequently divided human blood into three groups: A, B and C, (C was subsequently renamed O) on the basis of serologic reactions of RBCs with these agglutinins. Thus, the modern era of blood transfusions began. DeCastello and Sturli[41] completed the ABO system by their discovery of group AB in 1902. Jansky of Czechoslovakia[42] and Moss[43] of the United States described four blood groups using roman numeral designations. The discovery of the ABO blood types made it possible to be selective in choosing blood for transfusion. Landsteiner indicated the importance of these blood groups in predicting successful outcome of transfusions.

In 1908, Reubin Ottenberg,[44] a pathology intern at German Hospital in New York, was the first to perform ABO typing of a patient and donor before blood transfusion, and the first to use compatibility testing. Moss[43] developed conventional in vitro agglutination testing and cross matching. By 1917, typing serum simplified donor selection and most laboratories continued to use major and minor cross matches to detect irregular antibodies. In 1927, the American Association of Immunologists sponsored the present classification of blood groups (A, B, AB, and O) suggested by Landsteiner. New blood groups, beginning with N, M and P, were discovered in 1927. The New York Blood Transfusion Betterment Association introduced the first commercially available blood grouping reagents in 1936.[20] Landsteiner and Weiner[45] discovered the Rh system in 1940. The advent of antiglobulin testing based on the work of Coombs and associates[46] and the use of high protein medium and enzyme techniques have greatly expanded knowledge of blood group serology. These methods, which enhance agglutination in serologic testing, led to the rapid development of blood banking during the third quarter of the 20th century. Introduction of newer reagents, such as low-ionic strength saline solution and polyethylene glycol (PEG), and the recognition that the antiglobulin phase of the cross match can be eliminated when the indirect antiglobulin test is negative, have led to abbreviation of the cross match procedure.

## BLOOD SHORTAGES
### Impact of Transfusion-Transmitted Infectious Diseases

Transfusion-transmitted infections consist of an increasing number of viral, *Treponemal* and protozoan diseases.[47] Approximately 2 to 10% of the whole blood units donated are discarded, due to "false-positive" infectious disease screening test results.[48]

### SYPHILIS

Syphilis was the first disease known to be transmitted by blood transfusion and was first described as a transfusion-transmitted infection in 1915.[49] This was before there was refrigerated storage of blood. Syphilis then disappeared as a major risk of blood transfusion in the 1940s, with the widespread use of penicillin and refrigerated storage of blood. *Treponema pallidum* becomes nonviable in blood stored at 4° C for longer than 72 hours. In the United States, federal regulations have required that a serologic test for syphilis antibodies be performed on all units of blood since the 1930s. Almost no cases of transfusion-transmitted syphilis have been reported over the past 40 years, although most cases are probably not clinically recognized. There is still a risk of syphilis transmission by fresh blood or components stored at room temperature (e.g., platelet concentrates).[50] In recent years, there has been an increasing prevalence of syphilis infection in the United States.[51] Screening for syphilis also identifies donors who are at high risk for other sexually transmitted diseases (e.g., human immunodeficiency virus (HIV)). Therefore, screening of all donated blood units for syphilis will continue.

### HEPATITIS B VIRUS

Hepatitis was the first known blood-borne viral disease. Hepatitis due to parenteral exposure to blood, was first reported in 1885, when an epidemic of jaundice occurred in German shipyard workers given a smallpox vaccine prepared from human lymph.[52] Beeson (1943)[53] first recognized the connection between blood transfusion and the development of hepatitis. The long latency period in the development of posttransfusion hepatitis delayed its recognition for several decades. At the time of Beeson's discovery, the sole means for preventing the transmission of hepatitis was taking a careful history from each prospective donor and deferring those with a history of clinical hepatitis. Early screening tests used for hepatitis included bilirubin, thymol turbidity, and cephalin flocculation.

In addition, transferase tests were introduced in 1955. The Australian antigen, which is now known as hepatitis B surface antigen (HBsAg), was discovered by Blumberg in 1967.[54] Federal regulations required first generation immunodiffusion tests for detecting HBsAg for donor testing in 1971.[50] It then became mandatory to use an improved sensitivity third generation test in 1975.[55] The current transmission rate of hepatitis B virus (HBV) is 1 in 200,000 units of blood transfused.[56] Ten to 20% of the posttransfusion hepatitis cases are caused by HBV.[57] Hepatitis B virus transmission has been markedly reduced by HBsAg testing, elimination of paid donors, and donor deferral mechanisms. The blood products drawn from paid donors carry up to seven times the risk of hepatitis transmission as those from volunteers.[58] Institution of the National Blood Policy in 1974 essentially eliminated the use of paid donors, except for the collection of plasma for the pharmaceutical industry.[20] Currently, donors are carefully questioned regarding risk factors for HBV infection.

## HEPATITIS C VIRUS

After initiation of donor screening for HBsAg, it soon became apparent that 80 to 90% of posttransfusion hepatitis was of the non-A, non-B type. Non-A, non-B hepatitis (NANBH) was the term first used in 1975 to describe the absence of serologic markers for hepatitis A or B in cases of transfusion-associated hepatitis. Seventy to 90% of NANBH cases are estimated to be actually caused by hepatitis C virus (HCV). The remaining cases are due to other agents (e.g., Epstein-Barr virus and Cytomegalovirus), or are not detectable by first generation tests. Hepatitis C virus is a major infectious complication following transfusion of blood and blood products. Studies conducted before 1980 indicated that the risk of posttransfusion hepatitis in transfusion recipients was 7 to 12%.[59]

Surrogate tests that are nonspecific indicators of NANBH include alanine aminotransferase (ALT) and hepatitis B core antibody (HBcAb). Alanine aminotransferase testing of donor units began in 1986 and HBcAb testing began in June of 1987. It is estimated that these surrogate tests have detected approximately 50% of hepatitis C virus antibody-positive donors.[60] After institution of ALT and HBcAb screening tests, the incidence of NANBH infections may have decreased to 1 in 100 or less, per unit. There was a decline in the number of transfusion-associated hepatitis cases between 1981 and 1987, due to changes in donor selection criteria to decrease the risk of HIV infection, initiation of surrogate testing, and viral inactivation of pooled plasma products.

Numerous efforts to isolate the virus(es) responsible for NANBH were unsuccessful. Cloning of the HCV and development of an assay to detect an antibody against a major gene product of that agent[61,62] have been major breakthroughs in the long search for the causative agent for NANBH. In May of 1990, a specific test for antiHCV using an enzyme immunoassay format (EIA-1) was required for routine screening of all blood donors. Between 0.2 to 1.2% of random blood donors are found to be reactive for anti-HCV.[62] Donahue[63] demonstrated an 84% reduction in the risk of HCV seroconversion per unit transfused using EIA-1, as compared to the period when donors were screened only with the surrogate tests.

A more sensitive and specific multi-antigen second generation test (EIA-2) was licensed by the United States Food and Drug Administration (USFDA) in March of 1992. The prevention rate of HCV transmission with routine use of EIA-2 for donor screening could increase over 90%.[64] Kleinman[65] estimates a reduction in per unit risk from 1 in 1,000 for EIA-1 to 1 in 2,000 for EIA-2.

## HUMAN IMMUNODEFICIENCY VIRUS, TYPE 1

In 1981, the first report of cases of what is now recognized as AIDS occurring in homosexual men, appeared in the literature.[66] The first case of possible transfusion-associated AIDS in a neonate was reported in 1982.[67] Evidence of antibodies to human immunodeficiency virus-1 in hemophiliacs transfused with factor VIII concentrates, began to appear in 1982 and 1983.[68-70] In 1983, the Institut Pasteur in Paris, headed by Luc Montagnier, identified the AIDS virus, which it named the lymphadenopathy associated virus (LAV).[71] Currently, this virus is called the human immunodeficiency virus, Type 1 (HIV-1). AIDS was not recognized as a transfusion-transmitted disease until January of 1984.[72]

Beginning in 1983, the medical history questionnaire for potential blood donors incorporated questions regarding high-risk behavior for AIDS and symptoms suggestive of AIDS. This questionnaire has been repeatedly modified up to the present time.[73] Routine screening of donated blood for the antibody for human immunodeficiency virus, Type I (anti-HIV-1) using an enzyme-linked immunosorbent assay (ELISA), began in 1985. In 1986, the confidential unit exclusion procedure was introduced to allow a donor to indicate that his or her blood should not be transfused. The combination of careful donor screening and antibody testing has drastically reduced transfusion-associated AIDS.

Public opinion data have indicated that many people think that AIDS can be contracted from a blood donation, which has adversely affected the blood supply.[74] The United States Centers for Disease Control and

Prevention (CDCP) indicated an incidence of HIV-1 seropositivity in blood donors of 0.25% in 1985.[75] A CDCP report which includes data collected through mid-1988, indicated an incidence of 0.01%.[76] The CDCP received 222,418 reports of AIDS cases through June 1992. Of these, 4619 (2.0%) were transfusion-associated.[77] Most of these transfusions occurred before routine testing for anti-HIV-1 began. Fewer than five transfusion recipients per year are estimated to have been infected by HIV-1 between 1986 and 1992 in the United States, during which time approximately 3.5 million people received transfusions annually.[77] Cumming and coworkers (1989)[78] showed that the frequency of confirmed positive donors for anti-HIV-1 is only about 1 in 50 (2%) of the prevalence expected in a random population sample. Currently, the transmission rate of HIV-1 infection through a blood transfusion is estimated at 1:225,000 units.[79] The absence of a single antigen-positive, seronegative donor among over 1 million blood donors has led to the USFDA decision not to recommend HIV-1 antigen testing as a screening test.[80,81]

## HUMAN T-CELL LYMPHOTROPHIC VIRUS, TYPES I/II

Human T-cell lymphotrophic virus, Type I (HTLV-I) is an oncogenic retrovirus associated with adult T-cell leukemia/lymphoma, tropical spastic paraparesis (TSP) in the Caribbean, and HTLV-I-associated myelopathy (HAM) in Japan. HTLV-I was the first human retrovirus to be identified. It was first isolated in 1978 and first reported in 1980.[82]

Approximately 90% of patients infected with HTLV-I never experience an adverse effect. This virus has been transmitted through blood transfusions in Japan,[83] with a seropositivity rate of 1 in 20 potential donors noted.[84] Seropositivity in the United States has been noted in intravenous drug abusers, thalassemic and sickle cell patients in New York, patients with adult T-cell leukemia, and healthy individuals. Studies in the United States have identified 2.5 per 10,000 confirmed positive donors.[85] This seroprevalence rate initiated donor screening for the antibody for HTLV-I (anti-HTLV-I) using an ELISA method, beginning in 1988.[86] A closely related virus, HTLV-II, is awaiting confirmation as an etio-

logic agent for certain neurologic disorders. The screening test for anti-HTLV-I is also effective in detecting anti-HTLV-II due to cross-reactivity. The current estimated infection rate for HTLV I/II is less than 1 in 50,000 units.[87,88]

## HUMAN IMMUNODEFICIENCY VIRUS, TYPE 2

Human immunodeficiency virus, Type 2 (HIV-2) also referred to as leukemia-associated virus, Type II (LAV-II) is a human retrovirus capable of causing AIDS, which is closely related to HIV-1. The first reports of HIV-2 seropositive persons appeared in 1986 when the virus was isolated from West African AIDS patients. This virus is endemic in West Africa and is also present in Europe and South America. HIV-2 has been associated with a case of transfusion-transmitted disease.[89] The first documented case of AIDS due to HIV-2 in the United States, was reported by the CDCP in 1988.[90] The patient, who was diagnosed in December 1987, acquired the infection in Africa. As of July 1991, 31 cases of HIV-2 infection in the United States have been reported to the CDCP. In April 1988, donor exclusion criteria included persons who have immigrated from sub-Saharan Africa since 1977, or who have had sexual contact with such persons. After surveying over 26 million blood donors in the United States, only one HIV-2 infected donor has been found. Therefore, the USFDA is currently requiring donor screening, using either a combination enzyme immunoassay for antibodies to HIV-1/2, or separate HIV-1 and HIV-2 tests.

## IDIOPATHIC CD4+ T-LYMPHOCYTOPENIA

In July 1992, an unusual AIDS-like syndrome was first described in five HIV-seronegative patients from the New York City area.[91] The new entity, termed "idiopathic CD4+ T-lymphocytopenia" (ICL), was defined by the CDCP as a reproducible depletion of CD4+ lymphocytes below $300/mm^3$ in the absence of known causes of immunodeficiency.[92] The possibility of a new virus that could be transmitted by blood transfusions raised great public concern.

Forty-seven such cases were compiled by

the CDCP between 1985 and September 1992.[93] Sixty-two percent of these cases were found to have no identifiable risk factors for AIDS.[94] Twenty-three contacts, including six persons who had donated blood to these patients, were immunologically normal.[94]

Idiopathic CD4+ T-lymphocytopenia, which is a rare syndrome, is epidemiologically, clinically, and immunologically distinct from HIV infection. There is lack of case-clustering or direct transmission data, to suggest an infectious agent or an environmental cause. To date, no microbiologic agent has been proven to be the cause. Idiopathic CD4+ T-lymphocytopenia differs from HIV infection clinically in its apparent lack of progression over time. CD4+ T-cell counts remain stable or even spontaneously revert to normal.

Idiopathic CD4+ T-lymphocytopenia has not been shown to be transmissible in blood components. None of the 4018 persons enrolled in the Transfusion Safety Study since 1985 has illnesses meeting the criteria for ICL.[95] A survey of 1771 healthy blood donors at several large blood centers has also shown no cases meeting the criteria for ICL.[94]

Because of the heterogeneity of the syndrome, it is highly likely that there is no common cause for ICL. Further epidemiologic studies are ongoing. It is felt that current donor screening and tests should protect the blood supply.

## Impact of New Medical/Surgical Techniques and Impact of AIDS

Advances in medical care, such as sophisticated open heart surgery procedures, bone marrow transplantation, liver transplantation, and more aggressive chemotherapy programs for cancer patients, have contributed to increased blood component usage.[22] The emergence of cardiac surgical procedures caused a serious nationwide depletion of the blood supply in the early 1970s. For example, the percentage of all blood donated at the Milwaukee Blood Center that was used for open heart surgery, increased from 6.6% in 1967 to 26.1% in 1971.[96] In 1991, coronary artery bypass grafting (CABG) procedures were reportedly performed on 265,000 patients in the United States.[97] A review by Surgenor and coworkers[98] of 3216 CABG procedures performed in eleven hospitals, revealed an average RBC product use of 3.46 units per patient. The average transfusion volume for open heart surgical patients has declined, due to advances such as nonblood-containing bypass priming solutions, use of different types of oxygenators, blood conservation techniques, and revised attitudes regarding postoperative HCT.[99] The annual number of CABG procedures has declined with the advent of percutaneous angioplasty. However, CABG is still one of the most commonly performed surgical operations, and accounts for approximately 10% of all RBC units transfused in the United States.

Liver transplantations are being performed in increasing numbers and require extensive blood component support, both intraoperatively and postoperatively. Farrar and associates (1988)[100] showed the following mean intraoperative blood component usage (in units) in adult liver transplantations: packed RBCs—22.0, FFP—38.2, platelet concentrates—26.1, and cryoprecipitate—12.2. They noted that between 1983 and 1987, there has been a reduction in blood component use, due to improved surgical techniques and management of coagulopathies, more judicious selection of patients, and the use of intraoperative blood salvage.

Another recent medical procedure requiring extensive blood component usage is bone marrow transplantation. It is estimated that there are approximately 5000 bone marrow transplants being performed per year worldwide. The number of bone marrow transplants performed in the United States is projected to be 8000 procedures per year by the mid-1990s, representing a two-fold increase over procedures performed in 1987. Jansen[101] showed that these patients require an average of 18 units (range, 6 to 30) of RBC products and 144 units (range, 44 to 1843) of platelet concentrates.

Therapeutic plasmapheresis is increasing at an annual rate of about 10% in the United States. Replacement fluids for these procedures are often blood products. As more patients are treated for AIDS, it is likely that blood transfusions will increase.[102] Fischl and colleagues[103] estimate that the demand on the national blood supply to support patients with AIDS being treated with azidothymidine (AZT), could increase by 1 million units per year in the early years of the next decade.

The risk of transfusion-transmitted infectious disease has led to a search for pharmacologic agents that improve hemostasis and, thereby, reduce or even eliminate the need for blood products in certain patients. The impact of recombinant human erythropoietin on RBC transfusion therapy is being established. Erythropoietin may be administered preoperatively, during, or following surgery for management of perioperative blood loss. It has been demonstrated to reduce transfusions in anemic patients with end-stage renal disease.[104] Erythropoietin may dramatically reduce nonsurgical transfusion requirements in patients with chronic anemia associated with such diseases as cancer, myelodysplasic syndromes, liver disease, rheumatoid arthritis, and AIDS. Erythropoietin is also a consideration for miscellaneous anemias, including anemia of prematurity, sickle cell disease, and β-thalassemia intermedia. Drugs such as desmopressin acetate and aprotinin have been shown in certain patient groups to reduce surgical blood loss.[73] Recombinant hematopoietic growth factors and transfusions of peripheral blood cell progenitors are now being used to treat cytopenias of various etiologies, including those related to chemotherapy and bone marrow transplantation.[105]

## Changing Patterns of Blood Transfusions

Currently, the blood supply of the United States is marginal. While more than 50% of Americans are eligible, less than 10% actually donate blood.[48] An annual total of 13 million donations in this country are processed to give about 20 million transfused products.[87] The United States must import packed RBCs from Western Europe to augment its blood supply. Between 1982 and 1989, 200,000 to 300,000 units of packed RBCs were imported per year. Two national surveys[106,107] revealed a peak supply of allogeneic blood of 13.4 million units in 1986, which did not grow between 1986 and 1989. Increasing constraints on the blood supply include an increasing frequency of blood intensive procedures, aging of the United States population, and decreased blood donations due to restrictions on donor eligibility (because of risk factors), and an increasing number of screening tests.[74] In the past 20 years, seven infectious disease

markers have been implemented in donor screening.[87] More Americans may have access to health care in the future under a Federal health care plan, which will also impact the blood supply.

Blood wastage is another constraint on the blood supply. Clark and Ayoub (1989)[108] noted a projected 3.08% (412 out of 13,368 units) wastage rate of blood components, prior to corrective action in their institution. Their study revealed that physicians are responsible for most wastage, principally by failing to administer thawed or pooled blood products.

Surgenor and associates[106] noted that transfusion of whole blood and RBCs reached a peak of 12.2 million in 1986, which has leveled off to 12.0 million units in 1989. Transfusions of plasma are declining from a peak of 2.3 million units in 1984. In contrast to the RBC and plasma transfusion rates, the platelet transfusion rate continues to grow. Total platelet transfusions in 1989 (7.3 million) increased 13.7% over the total in 1987.[107] The proportion of platelets transfused as single donor platelets grew from 11% in 1980 to 29% in 1989.[106,107]

## Blood Utilization Monitors

Excessive use of blood components has been a long-standing concern. Widespread deficiencies in physician knowledge of transfusion risks and indications exist.[109] The National Institutes of Health (NIH) held consensus development conferences which defined appropriate indications for transfusion of FFP,[110] platelet concentrates,[111] and RBCs in the perioperative period.[112] Peer review of transfusion practices has been required by the Joint Commission on Accreditation of Health Care Organizations (JCAHCO) since 1985.[113,114] The intent is to reduce inappropriate transfusion of homologous blood, evaluate performance of individual physicians, and modify their transfusion practices through education, when necessary.[50] Blood utilization reviews may also be effective in reducing the blood shortage and contributing to cost containment. Transfusion utilization audits can be prospective, concurrent, or retrospective.[115] Audit criteria to evaluate appropriate use of blood components are developed by a representative group of physicians of a hospital (usually the transfusion committee), using pertinent published criteria, such as the NIH consensus conferences' recommendations. Such reviews have been effective in reducing inappropriate use of blood components.[116]

Monitoring of the crossmatched-to-transfused ratio (C/T) for the hospital overall and the various medical departments, is also required. The purpose of this monitor is to reduce the blood outdate rate, due to excessive cross matching. This, in turn, also reduces blood bank technologist time. An acceptable range for an overall C/T ratio for an acute care facility is 1.5 to 2.5.[117]

Friedman and colleagues[118] introduced a "maximum surgical blood order schedule" (MSBOS) in an attempt to decrease RBC outdating by avoiding excessive cross matching. Based on transfusion experience in surgery, individual hospitals can form a list of common surgical procedures and their maximum allowable preoperative blood order. When an MSBOS is implemented, only the indicated amount of blood on the schedule is cross matched for a surgical procedure, regardless of the number of units of blood ordered by the surgeon. This, of course, may be circumvented under extenuating circumstances. The concept of a "type and screen" order was developed for procedures highly unlikely to require blood.[119]

Factors that have prevented serious blood shortages in the face of decreasing blood collections, include a decline in total transfusions and increased use of autologous blood. Some hospitals have reported up to a 10% reduction in homologous blood use, due to autologous blood programs.[120] Also, component therapy has had a favorable effect on the national blood supply by allowing 1 unit of blood to be used for several patients. Between 1973 and 1989, there has been a disappearance of the use of whole blood.

## Autologous Donations

Autologous transfusion has been practiced for more than 150 years.[74] Predeposit autologous blood donation was first used, in the usual sense by Grant, in a polycythemic patient undergoing a craniotomy for a cerebellar tumor.[121] The blood was collected preoperatively, using 0.2% sodium citrate as the anticoagulant, and refrigerated for 24 hours prior to

the surgery. Fantus described the use of this procedure at the Cook County Hospital Blood Bank.[16] He also described the feasibility of autologous blood donation in pregnancy at that time.

Blood banks were developed in the 1930s, making allogeneic blood convenient to use. Therefore, there were few reports of autologous transfusions between 1930 and 1960, due to the predominant use of allogeneic transfusions. Milles and coworkers[122] performed early pioneering studies in predeposit autologous blood donation in the early 1960s. They demonstrated the use of autologous transfusion for patients undergoing a variety of elective surgical procedures, including thoracic, gynecologic, urologic, and cardiovascular. They also studied various physiologic effects of autologous donation, including electrocardiographic changes and effects on hematologic parameters and intravascular volume. During the late 1960s and early 1970s, there were reports in the literature on the use of preoperative autologous donation for various surgical procedures, such as cardiovascular procedures[123-126] and elective head and neck surgery.[127]

Concerns about the quality of the blood supply caused a resurgence of interest in autologous transfusion. Up until 1981, preoperative autologous donations were limited primarily to patients undergoing orthopedic or plastic surgery, or to those with anticipated transfusion-related complications. A survey conducted by the American Association of Blood Banks (AABB) showed a 17-fold increase in the number of preoperative autologous blood donations between 1982 and 1988 (18,737 versus 338,000).[128] Preoperative autologous deposits represented 4.6% of the total blood supply in 1989.[107] A study conducted by Renner[129] also showed an increase in transfusions of predeposit autologous blood between 1990 and 1992 (2.6% versus 3.9%). Intraoperative autologous transfusion has increased by 152% (from 25,000 patients to 63,000) between 1985 and 1989.[106-107] There is growing concern over unwarranted collections of autologous blood for low-risk surgical procedures. Slightly over one-half of autologous units were transfused to their intended recipients in 1989.[107] Better guidelines for autologous transfusions are needed. In addition to avoiding risks associated with allogeneic blood transfusions, all types of autologous transfusions, including cell salvage techniques, help conserve the blood supply.

## Directed (Designated) Donations

Technically, some of the earliest blood transfusions performed during the 17th century represented directed (recipient-designated) donations involving direct transfusion of blood from artery to vein.[47] During the early 1900s, donors were procured individually for each patient, usually from among the patient's relatives and friends, from a panel of paid donors (often hospital personnel), or from medical students. Pressure to eliminate directed donations developed in the 1950s and 1960s, with the racial integration of the blood supply.[130]

Public pressure on blood centers and hospitals to obtain directed donations began early in 1983, after the first case of possible transfusion-associated AIDS was reported. Direct donation services are being offered by increasing numbers of blood centers and hospital transfusion services throughout the United States. Although there was initial concern that directed donor programs may jeopardize the voluntary blood supply, they actually may have recruited new voluntary repeat donors.[47] In 1989, directed donations represented 2.5% of the total blood supply.[107]

## BLOOD DONORS SCREENING

Blood centers and transfusion services depend on voluntary donors to provide the blood necessary to meet the needs of the patients they serve. Voluntary donors may donate every 8 weeks.[131] Donor selection is based on a limited physical examination and a medical history containing specific questions that will determine whether giving blood will harm the donor, or if transfusion of the unit will harm the recipient.

The donor screening begins with a private interview, during which the prospective donor is questioned about risk factors and behaviors associated with AIDS transmission, and signs and symptoms suggestive of AIDS. The donor is then asked to read educational material concerning AIDS, and the testing performed by the blood bank on donated units.

The prospective donor should appear to be in good health. The physical examination consists of height, weight, temperature, hemoglobin (HGB) level, blood pressure, and pulse. Donors must weigh at least 110 pounds to withstand the donation of 450 mL of blood. The donor's oral temperature is not to exceed 99.5° C. The minimum HGB level for both men and women is 12.5 g/dL. The pulse should be regular and between 50 and 100 beats per minute, and the blood pressure between 90 and 180 mm Hg, systolic and between 50 to 100 mm Hg, diastolic.[131]

Upon the successful completion of the donor screening process, the unit of blood is collected by a trained member of the blood bank staff, working under the direction of a qualified, licensed physician. Blood must be removed by aseptic methods, using a sterile closed system and a single venipuncture.

## PREOPERATIVE AUTOLOGOUS BLOOD DONATION

Autologous blood transfusion involves collection of blood from a donor/patient for subsequent transfusion to that same person, usually after a period of storage. Preoperative donation is the simplest and most common form of autologous blood used.[128] Preoperative autologous blood donation is discussed in detail in Chapter 6, including indications, contraindications, donor criteria, and techniques. (See Chapter 6: Preoperative Autologous Blood Donation)

## DIRECTED (DESIGNATED) DONORS

A directed donor is a patient-selected donor. Blood from a directed donor is considered allogeneic blood with all the inherent risks. Several large studies have shown no differences between directed donations and first-time voluntary donations, with regard to the incidence of serologic markers for transfusion-transmitted diseases.[130,132-134] Directed donations should be reserved for patients who are medically ineligible for autologous donation.

Directed donors are screened in the same manner as random donors and must be ABO and Rh compatible with the intended recipient. A directed donor may donate more frequently, up to every 3 days, as long as the minimum HGB value is maintained. Because of the time required to process a unit of blood (48 to 72 hours minimum), directed donor units cannot be used in an emergency situation.[130] A directed donor may provide apheresis-harvested platelets, granulocytes, FFP, or cryoprecipitate in addition to RBC products. All cellular blood components from a directed donor who is a blood relative of the patient, must be irradiated with 1500 to 2000 rads to prevent graft-versus-host disease (GVHD). This occurs due to human leukocyte antigen (HLA) similarities between the donor and recipient, allowing engraftment of viable donor lymphocytes.

Medically accepted indications for directed donation include: (1) situations involving donor-specific transfusions and renal transplantation to enhance graft survival; (2) serologically compatible relatives of a patient immunized to a high frequency RBC antigen; (3) platelets or granulocytes from a related HLA-matched donor for an alloimmunized recipient; use of an allogeneic marrow donor as a compatible source of platelets and/or granulocytes; and maternal platelets for a neonate with alloimmune thrombocytopenia.[47]

A directed donation to a woman of child-bearing age from her husband or his close relatives, is contraindicated due to risk of alloimmunization to paternal RBC, white blood cell, or platelet antigens.[47] Transfusion from a potential bone marrow donor to the recipient, prior to bone marrow transplantation, is also contraindicated.[130] Directed donations, at the very least, help provide a positive psychological benefit to the patient. However, in 1989, only 28% of all directed donor units were actually transfused to their intended recipients.[107] This overcollection of directed donations has raised concern over lack of indications and cost-effectiveness.

## LIMITED DONOR EXPOSURE

Limited-exposure donation involves satisfying a patient's total blood needs by either one, or a very small group of dedicated donors. Limited donor exposure programs decrease overall allogeneic-donor exposure for the patient.[135,136] These programs are easily applied to pediatric patients, often using a parent as the donor. An example of such a program is the preparation of cryoprecipitate from plasma, collected from desmopressin acetate stimulated donors by automated plasmapheresis. This allows a dedicated donor to meet the total factor VIII needs of a patient with hemophilia.[137,138] Other applications of limited-exposure donor programs include children with chronic hematologic disorders, and pediatric patients undergoing elective cardiac or orthopedic procedures.[136] Administration of erythropoietin may allow collection of more RBCs. Other products that may be collected include apheresis platelets, granulocytes, FFP, and fibrin glue.[135]

## BLOOD BANKING TECHNIQUES

## PROCESSING DONOR UNITS

Blood and blood products are considered to be drugs by the USFDA. Therefore, all collection and processing protocols must conform to the manufacturing policies mandated by the USFDA and the AABB. Donor processing must include the following: (1) a serologic profile consisting of ABO and Rh typing; (2) antibody screening; (3) a disease testing profile consisting of HBsAg, HBcAb, anti-HCV, anti-HIV-1/2, anti-HTLV-I/II, and ALT; and (4) a serologic test for syphilis.[131,139] Currently in the blood banking community, there is some controversy within various autologous donor programs, over how much donor processing is sufficient for autologous units. The USFDA guidelines stipulate that if an autologous unit is drawn outside the facility performing the transfusion, minimum testing required is ABO and Rh typing, HBsAg testing, anti-HIV-1 testing, and a serologic test for syphilis. If the unit is drawn at the same facility as the transfusion, the disease testing can be waived.[139] A sound argument can be made for treating all autologous units in the same manner as homologous units. Complete testing of all units enables the institution to avoid breaks in standard operating procedure, a risk reduction measure that acknowledges the fact that variations of normal routines lead to errors.

## COMPONENT PREPARATION

The basic goal underlying preparation of blood components is to achieve the maximum utilization of each specific blood fraction from a unit of whole blood. These fractions are ob-

## BOX 1

## General Guidelines for Donor Processing

1. Unique identification numbers placed on blood bag, processing tubes and donor records must be rechecked prior to processing.
2. All reagents used for required testing must meet or exceed appropriate FDA regulations.
3. The results of all tests must be recorded immediately after observation and interpretations recorded upon completion of testing.
4. ABO group must be determined with anti-A, anti-B, A1 and B cells. All ABO discrepancies must be resolved prior to release.
5. Rh type must be determined with anti-D. Units found to be D negative in direct agglutination techniques must be tested to detect the $D^u$ antigen. $D^u$ positive units are labelled as Rh positive.
6. All disease testing must be performed by a method approved by the FDA and must be performed according to the manufacturer's specifications.
7. Each unit must be appropriately labelled including the anticoagulant, proper name of the product, volume of the unit, required storage conditions, name and address of the collection facility, reference to Circular of Information, expiration date and donor status (i.e. volunteer, autologous, or paid). In addition, autologous units should have an additional tag with the donor/patient name, identification number (hospital number, social security number or date of birth), the ABO group and the date of expiration.
8. The record system must be such that any unit of blood or component can be traced from its source to its disposition. All records must be retrievable.

therapeutically useful quantities of platelets from a single donor during one visit to the donor center.

## Packed Red Blood Cells

Packed RBCs are one of the most commonly transfused components in the blood bank. Packed RBCs are prepared by centrifugation or gravitational sedimentation of the RBCs from the plasma. The usual 300 mL unit has a HCT of 65 to 80%. RBCs must be maintained within a 1° to 10° C range during processing, and must be stored within a temperature range of 1°to 6° C. RBCs that are prepared in a closed system retain the same expiration date of the original unit. If the unit was prepared from a single donor bag (one without integral satellite packs), the unit must be used within 24 hours.[140]

## Fresh Frozen Plasma

Fresh Frozen Plasma (FFP) is the liquid portion of a single unit of whole blood that contains the intrinsic and extrinsic coagulation factors. The plasma is removed aseptically from the RBCs and frozen solid within 6 hours of the drawing time to protect labile factors. This component generally contains between 180 to 300 mL of anticoagulated plasma. One unit of FFP contains about 200 units of factor VIII, plus the other labile coagulation factor V. All stable coagulation factors are present (2 to 4 mg/mL of fibrinogen and 1 unit/mL of other coagulation factors).

Fresh Frozen Plasma maintained at -30° C has a shelf-life of 1 year. After thawing, FFP should be used as soon as possible, but no more than 24 hours after thawing in a waterbath at 37° C. It cannot be refrozen.[140]

## Cryoprecipitated AHF (Cryoprecipitate)

Cryoprecipitate is the cold insoluble fraction of plasma proteins recovered when FFP is thawed at 1° to 6° C until the ice crystals have melted. The cold insoluble precipitate is refrozen. On the average, each bag of cryoprecipitate contains 80 or more factor VIII (FVIII:C) units, and at least 150 mg of fibrinogen in less than 15 mL of plasma. Cryoprecipitate must be stored at -18° C and can be stored for up to 1 year. Before administration, the

tained by various manipulations of whole blood. By using these techniques, the blood bank can provide packed RBCs, platelet concentrate, FFP, and cryoprecipitate.

Components can be prepared from whole blood donations or by automated apheresis techniques. Apheresis is a procedure in which blood is removed from a donor and separated into specific blood components, some of which are retained, and the remaining fractions returned to the donor. Using automated technology, it has become feasible to collect cryoprecipitate must be thawed in a 37° C water bath and aseptically pooled into one dose.[140]

## Fibrin Glue

Fibrin glue has been advocated by many surgeons as the material that best approaches the ideal sealant. As a naturally occurring and partially human derived product, the material seems to have no tissue toxicity, promotes a firm seal in seconds to minutes, is reabsorbed in days to weeks following application, and appears to promote local tissue growth and repair.[141] This product is not commercially available in the United States. However, an acceptable substitute can be prepared in the operating room by combining cryoprecipitate with reconstituted thrombin (reconstitute bovine thrombin to 1000 units/mL with 40 mMol calcium chloride).[142]

## Platelet Concentrate

Platelet concentrates prepared from freshly drawn units of whole blood generally contain $5.5 \times 10^{10}$ platelets, suspended in 40 to 70 mL of plasma. They are stored at room temperature and have a shelf-life of 5 days.[140] Due to these limitations, harvesting therapeutic dosages of autologous platelet concentrates is not feasible. If autologous platelet concentrates are desired, apheresis techniques should be taken into consideration.

## Fresh Red Blood Cells/ Deglycerolized Red Blood Cells

The ability to cryopreserve RBCs became clinically available in the late 1960s. A cryoprotective agent (usually glycerol) is added to minimize cold injury to the cells. The glycerolized RBCs are then frozen at −65° C or colder and can be stored for up to 10 years. Prior to transfusion, the units are thawed at 37° C and the glycerol removed by equilibration with a hypertonic solution, followed by washing with solutions progressively less hypertonic, and final resuspension in an isotonic electrolyte solution. After deglycerolization, the unit must be stored at 1° to 6° C with a maximum shelf-life of 24 hours.[140]

Providing deglycerolized RBCs for transfusion is costly, in terms of supplies and is labor intensive, as well. For most patients in autologous donor programs, this process is unnecessary. Sufficient amounts of blood can be collected in the 35-day standard expiration period to satisfy most surgical needs. However, in those patients who have been immunized to high frequency antigens, or who have multiple antibodies which make finding compatible blood difficult, stockpiling of frozen blood units may be of value.

All blood bank refrigerators and freezers have specific temperature requirements established by the USFDA and the AABB to assure that all products are stored in a manner which will provide the most efficacious product. All blood bank storage conditions are continually monitored, and the accuracy of the thermometers and chronographs are checked on a regular basis against thermometers certified by the National Bureau of Standards.

## VIRAL INACTIVATION TECHNIQUES

Manufactured products such as factors VIII and IX concentrates are derived from large pools (5000 to 20,000 mL) of plasma that can become contaminated if even one infected donor unit is present. Therefore, the product can only be made safe by sterilization of the final product. With the advent of AIDS, the efforts of manufacturers of coagulation factor concentrates to inactivate HBV, HCV, and HIV began. Human immunodeficiency virus, Type 1 infection has occurred in 80 to 90% of patients with severe hemophilia A. Retrospective analysis of stored serum samples has shown that seroconversion to HIV-1 occurred as early as 1978 in some hemophiliacs.[143]

Prior to use of virus-inactivating steps in the manufacturing process of coagulation factor concentrates, clinical studies have revealed a transmission rate of NANBH of 30 to 100%. In the 1980s, viral inactivation processes and production of anti-hemophilic factor concentrates by recombinant DNA techniques were developed. Techniques for viral inactivation of plasma derivatives include both physical and chemical inactivation procedures which do not denature the plasma proteins.

Albumin and purified protein fraction are exposed to high temperatures (60° C for 10 hours) and are essentially noninfective for hepatitis or HIV.[50] These products have been considered free of infectious risks for over 30 years. The fractionation process itself for albumin production removes much of the virus from the starting plasma pool. Heating of albumin is done in the presence of a specific ligand such as caprylate or tryptophanate, which increases the temperature threshold of protein denaturization.

The first dry-heated clotting factor concentrate became available in the United States in 1983. This procedure involved heat-treating lyophilized clotting factor concentrates for 32 to 72 hours at 60° to 68° C. Unfortunately, this first dry-heated product was found to be highly infectious for NANBH[144] and sporadic reports of HIV transmission appeared.[145,146] After 1987, the dry-heated concentrates were replaced by pasteurized preparations. Pasteurization involves heating in a stabilized aqueous solution at 60° C for 10 hours. This technique has been reported to prevent transmission of HBV, NANBH, HIV-1, and HIV-2.[147-149] A third method for viral elimination involves affinity chromatography with a mouse monoclonal antibody to either factor VIII or von Willebrand factor attached to a solid-phase agarose support.[150] Other techniques developed include wet vapor-heating treatment of anti-hemophilic factor concentrates, and extreme dry heating at 80° C for 72 hours.

Chemical solvent-detergent methods, which were first licensed in 1985 have been used to inactivate viruses by disrupting their lipid-envelope.[151-153] Lipid-coated viruses include HBV, HCV and HIV. Solvent-detergent methods eliminate HIV transmission and essentially eliminate the various forms of hepatitis. However, protein-coated viruses such as B19 parvovirus and hepatitis A virus (HAV) are not inactivated by solvent detergent treatment.[154] Most manufacturers now offer solvent-detergent-extracted factor VIII preparations. The methods used for viral inactivation of factor IX concentrates are similar to those for antihemophilic factor concentrates. Factor IX concentrates are now heat- or solvent-detergent treated.

All manufactured coagulation factor concentrates now available in the United States are virus-inactivated. Viral-inactivation procedures have greatly improved the safety of commercially prepared clotting factor concentrates since 1985. The half-life, recovery, and efficacy of virally-inactivated factor VIII preparations are essentially unchanged from the parent product.[155] Clinical trials evaluating a synthetic factor VIII product prepared by recombinant DNA technology, have demonstrated it to be safe and effective, with no risk of viral transmission.[156-158] The USFDA approved two such products (Recombinate™ Baxter Health Care Corp. and Kogenate™ Miles, Inc.) in November 1992 and February 1993, respectively.

Currently awaiting USFDA licensure is a solvent-detergent treated fresh frozen plasma (SD-FFP). This is a mass-produced pooled plasma derivative which maintains excellent hemostatic properties and has shown no evidence of HIV, HBV, or HCV transmission. A SD-cryoprecipitate should ultimately be anticipated, as well.

Presently, the ability to inactivate infectious viruses in cellular products is limited, and has become an area of active research.[159] Cellular components cannot be sterilized without destroying viable cells, and cells harbor and protect viruses against inactivation. Leukoreduction of cellular blood components may prevent the transmission of some infections that are leukocyte-associated such as Cytomegalovirus.[160] One of the most popular devices used is a bedside filter for either RBCs or platelets.

## BLOOD STORAGE

Liquid RBC products are stored in monitored refrigerators at 1° to 6° C to slow glycolytic activity. Anticoagulant-preservative solutions prevent clotting and provide nutrients for continued metabolism of blood cells during storage. All such solutions used today employ citrate as the anticoagulant, which binds ionized calcium, thereby preventing several calcium-dependent steps in the coagulation cascade. Citrate also retards glycolysis. For all anticoagulant-preservative solutions, the shelf-life of the blood is determined by a standard of 70% survival of donor RBCs in the recipient 24 hours posttransfusion.[50]

### Biochemical and Biophysical Changes

As stored RBCs metabolize glucose to lactic and pyruvic acid, hydrogen ions accumulate and the pH falls. The pH of packed RBCs

**Table 1–1.    Biochemical changes of red blood cell stored in CPDA-1**

| Days in storage | 0 | 35 |
|---|---|---|
| % viable cells (24 hours post transfusion) | 100 | 71 |
| pH (measured at 37° C) | 7.55 | 6.71 |
| ATP (% of initial value) | 100 | 45 (± 12) |
| 2,3-DPG (% of initial value) | 100 | <10 |
| Plasma K$^+$ (mMol/L) | 5.1 | 78.5 |
| Plasma Na$^+$ (mMol/L) | 169 | 111 |
| Plasma HGB (mg/L) | 78 | 6580 |

Modified from Walker RH: Technical manual. 10th ed. Arlington, Va: American Association of Blood Banks; 1990.

stored in CPDA-1 for 35 days is 6.71 (Table 1–1). RBC degradation leads to release of potassium and ammonia in the plasma. The plasma load of potassium in stored packed RBCs increases during storage, achieving a concentration of 78.5 mMol/L when stored for 35 days in CPDA-1. The increase in potassium is due to paralysis of the RBC membrane sodium-potassium pump at cold temperatures with resultant leakage of potassium from cells.

Red Blood Cell 2, 3—diphosphoglycerate (2,3-DPG) levels of stored blood decline during storage due to decreasing pH.[27] Because 2,3-DPG promotes release of oxygen from HGB to the tissues, stored blood exhibits increased HGB oxygen affinity. Levels of adenine triphosphate (ATP) also decline during blood storage.[27] Following transfusion, donor RBCs regenerate ATP and 2,3-DPG levels fairly rapidly. Severely depleted RBCs regenerate one-half of their 2,3-DPG levels within 3 to 8 hours and normal levels are restored within 24 hours.

Stored RBCs progressively lose membrane lipids, undergo echinocytic morphologic changes, and develop increased osmotic fragility and increased rigidity.[27] Therefore, plasma-free HGB increases during storage of blood. Stored RBCs also progressively lose membrane-associated complement regulators, leading to deposition of complement components on their membranes and subsequent reduction in viability.[161]

During refrigerated storage in the liquid state, depletion of the labile coagulation factors

V and VIII occurs in a biphasic pattern with a half-life of approximately 24 hours. Other coagulation factors are remarkably stable during liquid storage.[110]

Since granulocytes and platelets have a very brief viability at 4° C, liquid stored blood is a poor source of these components. Blood collection processing and storage cause platelet activation, leading to irreversible loss of discoid shape and subsequent reduction in in vivo viability.[162] Also leading to compromised in vivo recovery and survival, is storage-induced depletion of platelet glutathione, resulting in oxidative stress. Microaggregates consisting of platelets, lymphocytes, and fibrin strands accumulate in refrigerated blood. The clinical significance of these microaggregates has not be established.

## Anticoagulants

Acid-citrate-dextrose and CPD permit liquid storage of blood up to 21 days at 1° to 6° C. CPDA-1 permits storage up to 35 days (Table 1–2). The low pH of anticoagulant-preservative solutions prevents the rise in pH that occurs with cooling. Dextrose supports continuing ATP generation by glycolytic pathways. The levels of 2,3-DPG are better maintained in CPD than ACD, due to the higher pH.[27] After 2 weeks of storage, the levels of 2,3-DPG are 80% of normal in CPD and only 10% of normal in ACD. The phosphates in CPD and CPDA-1 allow for better maintenance of 2,3-DPG and ATP concentrations.[27] By contributing to the adenosine phosphate pool, phosphates improve RBC viability. The adenine in CPDA-1 provides a substrate from

**Table 1–2.    Anticoagulants for blood collection**

| Constituent | ACD Formula A | CPD | CPDA |
|---|---|---|---|
| Trisodium citrate (gm) | 22.0 | 26.3 | 26.3 |
| Citric acid (gm) | 8.0 | 3.27 | 3.27 |
| Dextrose (gm) | 24.5 | 25.5 | 31.9 |
| NaH$_2$PO$_4$ (gm) | — | 2.22 | 2.22 |
| Adenine (gm) | — | — | 0.275 |
| Water added (mL) | 1000 | 1000 | 1000 |
| Volume (mL)/100 mL blood | 15 | 14 | 14 |

Modified from Lee CL, Henry JB: Blood banking and hemotherapy. In: Henry JB, ed. Todd, Sanford, Davidson Clinical Diagnosis and Management by Laboratory Methods. Philadelphia, Pa: WB Saunders; 1984.

**Table 1–3.  Biochemical changes of red blood cells stored in additive systems (AS)***

| Variable | AS-3† | | AS-1‡ |
|---|---|---|---|
| Days of storage | 42 | 49 | 49 |
| % viable cells (24 hours posttransfusion) | 83 ± 10 | 72 ± 9 | 76 (64–85) |
| ATP (% of initial value) | 58 | 45 | 64 |
| 2,3-DPG (% of initial value) | <10 | <15 | <5 |
| Plasma K$^+$ (mMol/L) | NA | NA | 6.5 |
| pH | 6.5 | 6.4 | 6.6 |
| Glucose (mMol/L) | 28 | 27 | 31 |
| % Hemolysis | 0.8 | 0.9 | 0.5 |

* Modified from Walker RH: Technical manual. 10th ed. Arlington, Va: American Association of Blood Banks; 1990.
† Modified from Simon TL, Marcus CS, Nelson EJ: Effects of AS-3 nutrient-additive solution on 42 and 49 days of storage of RBCs. Transfusion 1987; 27:178.
‡ Based on manufacturer's submission to FDA (1983).

which RBCs synthesize ATP resulting in improved viability.

More recently developed artificial additive solutions have extended the shelf-life of liquid refrigerated blood to 42 days (Table 1–3). Artificial additive solutions are fortified electrolyte solutions added, via a satellite bag, to centrifuged, concentrated RBCs with the plasma removed, which were originally collected in ACD or a modification of CPD. Examples of such solutions are SAG and SAGMAN and its modifications. Currently approved artificial additive solutions include Adsol (AS-1), Fenwal Laboratories, Roundlake, IL; Nutricel (AS-3), Cutter Biologicals, Berkeley, CA; and Optisol, Terumo Corporation, Elkton, MD. Additive systems enhance RBC survival and function, and preserve 2,3-DPG levels. This

is due to increased concentrations of dextrose and adenine, and the addition of mannitol, which diminishes RBC lysis (Table 1–4). Additive systems also decrease microaggregate formation.

## Cryopreservation

Glycerol is a penetrating (intracellular) cryoprotective agent which prevents injury to RBCs caused by freezing and thawing. RBCs should be frozen within 6 days of collection. There are three basic methods for freezing RBCs. All methods involve careful mixing and the slow, step-wise addition of glycerol to avoid excessive hemolysis. The "high glycerol method" is the most commonly used technique for freezing RBCs in the United States. The final frozen product contains approximately 40% glycerol in saline weight/volume. The cells are stored at −65° C or lower in an electric freezer. The "low glycerol method" involves a final concentration of approximately 20% glycerol in saline weight/volume. Using this method, cells are stored at −120° C or lower in liquid nitrogen. The third method is the "agglomeration" procedure devised by Huggins, which uses a high concentration of glycerol (approximately 40%) in glucose-fructose rather than saline.[163] The cells prepared using this procedure, may be stored in an electric freezer.

Frozen RBCs are thawed at 37° C and deglycerolized before issue. Deglycerolization of thawed hypertonic RBCs involves step-wise washing with solutions, which are progressively less hypertonic, and final suspension in an isotonic electrolyte solution containing glucose. The postwashing storage of frozen RBCs at 1° to 6° C is limited to 24 hours[131]

**Table 1–4.  Formulation of anticoagulant-preservative solutions present in blood collection sets**

| Constituent | CPDA-1 | Adsol | Optisol | Nutricel |
|---|---|---|---|---|
| Volume (mL) | 63 | 100 | 100 | 100 |
| Sodium chloride (mg) | None | 900 | 877 | 410 |
| Dextrose (mg) | 2000 | 2200 | 900 | 1100 |
| Adenine (mg) | 17.3 | 27 | 30 | 30 |
| Mannitol (mg) | None | 750 | 525 | None |
| Tri-sodium citrate (mg) | 1660 | None | None | 588 |
| Citric acid (mg) | 206 | None | None | 42 |
| Sodium phosphate (monobasic) (mg) | 140 | None | None | 276 |

Modified from Luban NLC, Strauss RG, Hume HA: Commentary on the safety of RBCs preserved in extended-storage media for neonatal transfusions, Transfusion 1991; 31:229.

because deglycerolization and resuspension occur in an open system with risk of bacterial contamination. Standards of at least 80% recovery of RBCs and at least 70% viability of transfused RBCs after 24 hours must be met.

Red blood cells from patients with hereditary spherocytosis, sickle cell trait, or glucose-6-phosphate-dehydrogenase deficiency may have unsatisfactory post-freeze-thaw recoveries.[47] Pretesting for HGB S in patients at risk is recommended, since special deglycerolization washing protocols to prevent agglomeration and excessive hemolysis are required for RBCs containing HGB S.

Platelets may be stored frozen using 4 to 6% dimethyl sulfoxide (DMSO) alone, or in combination with other agents as the cryoprotective agent. Freezing of platelets results in poor recovery of functional platelets, reported at 30 to 70% of control.[50] This is because platelets have low tolerance to osmotic stress. Following infusion of DMSO-stored platelets, patients develop an unpleasant garlic-like odor and symptoms of dizziness, nausea, and vomiting. Therefore, routine freezing of allogeneic platelets has not been considered practical. The only plausible use for frozen platelets at this time, is storage of autologous platelets for patients with expected episodic needs for platelets (e.g., cancer patients going in and out of remission and alloimmunized patients).

## BLOOD GROUPS AND COMPATIBILITY TESTING

Originally, there were only A and B, now there are well over 640 known antigens that can be detected on human RBCs. Safe blood transfusion is the most important application of blood group technology, however RBC polymorphism has made important contributions to anthropology, forensics, genetics, paternity testing, and immunology.

The first blood group to be discovered, the ABO system, still remains the most significant for transfusion practice. It is the only system in which reciprocal antibodies are consistently and predictably present in sera of normal people whose RBCs lack the corresponding antigen. Prevention of life threatening ABO incompatibility between a recipient and donor is the foundation on which all other pretransfusion testing is based. By 1951, nine major blood group systems had been categorized. In

order of discovery they are, ABO, MNSs, P, Rh, Lutheran, Kell, Lewis, Duffy and Kidd.

Antibodies defining blood group antigens are divided into two categories: alloantibodies and autoantibodies. Alloantibodies are either immune (requiring stimulation by RBC exposure, i.e,, pregnancy or transfusion), or naturally occurring (no RBC exposure) against antigens which the individual lacks. Autoantibodies react with antigens of the same individual who formed the antibody (i.e., antibodies against self), and are generally directed against high incidence antigens. Clinical importance is determined by whether the antibody can destroy RBCs in vivo, whether the antibody can cross the placenta, (thereby causing hemolytic disease of the newborn), and by the relative frequency of the antigen. Therefore, the ABO antibodies which cause immediate intravascular destruction are clearly the most important, followed by the Rh antibodies which are readily formed by immune stimulation and can cause severe "hemolytic disease of the newborn" or immune destruction of transfused RBCs.

## Pretransfusion Testing

The most crucial part of a RBC transfusion is the pretransfusion testing. The purpose of pretransfusion testing is to select, for each recipient, the blood, which when transfused, will have acceptable survival and will not cause significant destruction of the patient's RBCs. Despite advances in blood group serology, pretransfusion testing will not detect all unexpected RBC antibodies in the recipient serum, and also, will not guarantee normal survival of transfused RBCs. Minimum pretransfusion testing requirements established by the AABB for autologous transfusion, mandate that a new specimen be obtained and a type and Rh performed; antibody screening and compatibility testing are optional.

## INDICATIONS FOR BLOOD TRANSFUSION

Blood transfusion should not be instituted because of a single laboratory value of low HGB concentration or HCT value. Since the physician's clinical goal is to maintain oxygen delivery sufficient to meet the tissue demands, factors that contribute to the oxygen supply

## BOX 2

## Blood Bank Procedures Utilized in Pretransfusion Testing

1. Positive identification of recipient and recipient specimen. The collection of a properly labelled sample from the correct patient for pretransfusion testing is critical to safe blood transfusion. Transfusing the right blood to the wrong patient can cause life threatening ABO incompatible transfusion reactions. It is imperative that the same techniques of pretransfusion identification of recipient and recipient specimen be identical for both autologous and allogeneic transfusions.

2. Review of blood bank records for results of previous testing allows the technologist to review ABO & Rh typing as well as any abnormal serologic testing results. In addition to checking previous immunohematologic testing, there must be a mechanism in place to allow the transfusion service technologist to easily discern when a transfusion candidate has autologous blood available. Every effort must be made to assure that each autologous unit will be made available for the patient.

3. ABO & Rh typing. To determine the ABO & Rh type of the recipient, patient's RBCs are tested with anti-A, anti-B and anti-D and patient serum is tested with A1 and B cells. Donor ABO & Rh type also must be confirmed prior to transfusion.

4. Antibody Screening. The antibody screen is used to detect the presence of circulating irregular antibodies which could cause premature destruction of transfused RBCs. Patient serum is mixed with group O cells known to carry specific blood group antigens (the presence of D, C, E, c, e, M, N, S, s, P, Le, Le, K, k, Fy$^a$, Fy$^b$, Jk$^a$, Jk$^b$ antigens are the minimum requirement).[131] The test system is incubated at 37° C. and carried through the antihuman globulin phase. When the screening is positive, the specificity of the antibody must be determined by expanded serologic testing. When clinically significant irregular antibodies are shown to be present, blood for transfusion must be shown to be negative for all corresponding antigens (Table 1–5).

*continues*

5. Compatibility testing. Compatibility testing consists of combining recipient serum with donor cells obtained from an originally attached donor segment. The method used must demonstrate ABO incompatibility and detect clinically significant unexpected antibodies and must include an antihuman globulin test (Coomb's test). However, if the antibody screening is negative and the clerical record check does not demonstrate a history of a clinically significant antibody, the antihuman globulin phase may be eliminated. When clinically significant antibodies are present, the AHG phase must be performed.[131]

Table 1–5. **Summary of most commonly encountered red blood cell antibodies**

| Antibody | System | Transfusion reaction | Approximate percent compatible blood |
|---|---|---|---|
| D | Rh-Hr | Probable | 15 |
| C | | Probable | 30 |
| E | | Probable | 70 |
| c | | Probable | 20 |
| e | | Probable | 3 |
| f | | Probable | 33 |
| C$^w$ | | Probable | 98 |
| V | | Probable | 100C 82B |
| G | | Probable | 15 |
| Kell | Kell | Probable | 90C 97B |
| k | | Probable | 0.2C < 0.1B |
| Kp$^a$ | | Probable | 98C > 99B |
| Kp$^b$ | | Probable | < 0.1C < 0.1B |
| Js$^a$ | | None reported | > 99C 80B |
| Js$^b$ | | None reported | 0C < 0.1B |
| Fy$^a$ | Duffy | Probable | 33C 89B |
| Fy$^b$ | | Probable | 20C 77B |
| Jk$^a$ | Kidd | Probable | 25C 9B |
| Jk$^b$ | | Probable | 25C 57B |
| Xg$^a$ | Xg | Probable | 36M 13F |
| Le$^a$ | Lewis | Probable | 78C 82B |
| Le$^b$ | | Probable | 28C 40B |
| S | MNS | Probable | 45C 69B |
| s | | Probable | 11C 3B |
| U | | Probable | 0C < 1B |
| M | | Unlikely | 22C 30B |
| N | | Unlikely | 28C 26B |
| P$_1$ | P | Unlikely | 21C 5B |

Modified from Ortho Antibody Index, OrthoDiagnostic Systems, Raritan, NY, 1989.

and factors that alter the tissue demands, should be taken into consideration, and the overall condition of the patient should be assessed before starting a blood transfusion. Although, the higher HGB values of 12.5 to 16 g/dL have shown to improve survival of patients with acute respiratory failure[164] and septic shock,[165] in the majority of patients with normal cerebral blood flow and normal cardiac, pulmonary, renal, and hepatic functions, a HGB value of 7 to 8 g/dL is adequate. When HCT values are used for transfusion of blood, it should be kept in mind, that in situations such as dehydration and stress polycythemia, HCT will be higher, and with states of hydremia (as in the last trimester of pregnancy or with excessive crystalloid administration), HCT will be lower.

## TRANSFUSION FOR SURGICAL PATIENTS

For elective surgical procedures, the lowest value of HGB at which physicians transfuse their patients, varies. Until the early 1960s, a HGB value of 10 g/dL and a HCT of 30% was the lower preoperative value used by anesthesiologists and surgeons to administer blood. The experience over the years has shown that values much lower than these do not increase the morbidity and mortality in healthy surgical patients. A prospective study of 282 patients with preoperative HGB levels less than 10 g/dL, receiving 384 anesthetics, indicated that many patients can undergo anesthesia and surgery safely with lower preoperative HGB values.[166] However, critically ill patients may not tolerate these low HGB levels. A HGB level of 11 g/dL has been shown to improve survival in the postoperative period in critically ill patients.[167] For these patients, preoperative transfusions may be necessary. In addition to introducing the MSBOS as described earlier, Friedman and associates (1980)[168] also suggested that female surgical patients, who normally have lower HGB levels, may be able to accept lower perioperative HGBs than men.

For patients with low HGB values, a decision to transfuse preoperatively or to proceed with surgery without transfusion, depends on many important factors including: the age of the patient; duration of the anemia; degree of anemia; intravascular volume status; presence of coexisting diseases; and the extent of the proposed operation. If a decision is made to proceed without transfusion, additional precautions aimed at minimizing the morbidity and mortality during the perioperative period should be taken. These include maintaining adequate cardiac output, preventing leftward shift of the oxyhemoglobin dissociation curve, increasing oxygen-carrying capacity, and minimizing oxygen consumption.

Perioperative transfusion practices by anesthesiologists and surgeons have changed in recent years. Except with massive blood losses, HGB and HCT values should be checked whenever possible. For elective surgical procedures, complete cross matching should be done prior to the administration of blood. If only a type and screen was done prior to surgery, and a need for blood transfusion arises, cross matching can be completed within 20 to 30 minutes. For emergency surgical procedures where rapid and massive blood transfusions are required, depending upon the amount of time available, either a partially cross matched type specific blood, or uncross matched packed cells may have to be administered. Type O Rh-negative packed cells, instead of whole blood, will reduce the incidence of formation of high titres of hemolytic IgG, IgM, anti-A, and anti-B antibodies.

Although many anesthesiologists tend to use crystalloids up to 10% of blood loss, albumin between 10 and 20% of blood loss, and blood transfusion only after more than 20% blood loss, it is prudent to calculate the maximal allowable blood loss (MABL) prior to the start of any major surgical procedure. The easiest method of calculating the MABL is by the formula:[169,170]

$$MABL = EBV \times$$

$$\frac{preoperative\ HCT\ -\ lowest\ acceptable\ HCT}{preoperative\ HCT}$$

When EBV = estimated blood volume in mL; HCT in %

In a healthy patient, blood loss up to the MABL could be replaced entirely by crystalloid solutions. Blood loss in excess of the MABL, should be replaced with packed RBCs. The volume of packed RBCs required to return the HCT to an acceptable value, can be calculated using the following formula:[171]

$$Packed\ RBC\ (mL) =$$

$$\frac{[TBL - MABL\ (mL)] \times Desired\ HCT\ (\%)}{RBC\ HCT\ (\%)}$$

When TBL = total blood loss; RBC HCT = HCT of packed RBCs

## TRANSFUSION FOR VARIOUS ANEMIAS

Treatment of patients with chronic anemias varies widely. Controlling or eliminating the underlying cause of anemia is the most important aspect of the treatment. When this is not possible, substances that improve hematopoiesis, such as folic acid, iron, vitamin $B_{12}$, and erythropoietin should be administered. Transfusion of blood itself is the last mode of treatment and depends on the type and degree of anemia, overall condition of the patient, and the adequacy of the compensatory mechanisms. (See Chapter 5: Perioperative Hemoglobin Requirements).

With chronic anemia, the intracellular RBC 2,3-DPG increases and causes a shift of the oxyhemoglobin dissociation curve to the right. With this shift, at a given level of oxygen tension, more oxygen can be removed from the HGB. The most important cardiac compensation is the increase in cardiac output. Both the stroke volume and the heart rate increase.[172] With severe anemia, ventricular function and coronary blood flow decrease, leading to congestive heart failure. Blood transfusion could be life-saving, but it should be administered carefully, since blood volume can rise rapidly, leading to pulmonary edema.[173] Respiratory compensations include increase in the minute ventilation, with increase in both tidal volume and respiratory rate. With severe anemia, even the increased minute volume will be unable to meet the tissue oxygen demands and blood transfusion could be lifesaving.

## TRANSFUSION FOR NEONATES AND CHILDREN

The blood volume of a premature infant is higher than that of the newborn infant which, in its turn, is greater than that of an older child or an adult in proportion to the body weight. A premature infant's blood volume could be as high as 108 mL/kg, whereas a neonate has a blood volume of about 90 mL/kg. The placenta at term contains about 75 to 150 mL of blood, and if clamping of the umbilical card is delayed at birth, as much as 100 mL of blood can be transfused to the newborn.[174] Infants and children have blood volumes of 75 to 80 mL/kg, while a teenager's blood volume is about 65 to 75 mL/kg.

The same guidelines previously described for adult surgical patients can be applied to pediatric patients. Accurate measurement of blood loss in children is difficult, and the use of calibrated miniaturized suction bottles, weighing the sponges before and after the use and visual estimation, provide rough estimates. Serial HCT measurements taken from a central venous or arterial catheter provide more accurate estimates of blood loss.[175] With larger blood losses, even though fresh whole blood is helpful in supplying platelets and coagulation factors, component therapy is usually the rule.

The major problem in supplying blood for children is the wastage, if only a portion of an adult unit is given. The development of the "multiple blood pack" has reduced the wastage of the blood with pediatric transfusions. One unit of blood is collected into a triple or quadruple blood pack, which can be separated into 3 or 4 smaller units. More than one child can be cross matched with the same donor and each unit can be utilized more efficiently.

The most common indication of blood transfusion for the neonate is "hemolytic disease of the newborn." For these infants, exchange transfusion is considered if the HGB level is below 12 g/dL and the bilirubin level is more than 15 mg/dL, or if the neonate has jaundice or fetal hydrops. (See Chapter 5: Preoperative Hemoglobin Requirements)

## WHOLE BLOOD AND COMPONENT THERAPY

Transfusion practices have changed significantly over the last 15 to 20 years, since blood component therapy has replaced the use of whole blood. Although the use of whole blood has potential indications,[176] at the present time, few blood banks maintain whole blood stores. Over a 16-year period at the University of Pennsylvania, packed RBC has almost replaced whole blood (Fig. 1–1).[177] Coupled with this increase in packed RBCs, exponential increases in other blood components (platelets and FFP) were also seen in this

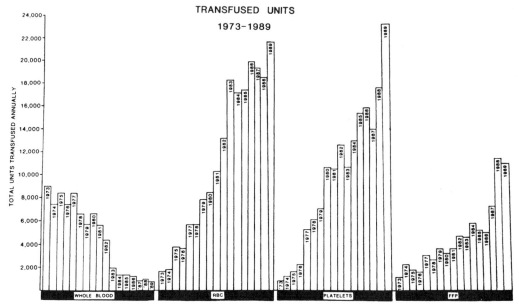

**Fig. 1–1.**  Blood transfusion practices over a 16-year period at the Hospital of the University of Pennsylvania. These practices mirror the nationwide move toward the disappearance of whole blood, the increased use of blood products with twice as much RBC transfused in 1989 as whole blood and RBC combined in 1973, and the exponential increase in the use of platelets and FFP. From Ellison N, Silberstein LE: A commentary on three consensus development conferences on transfusion medicine, Anesthesiol Clin N Am 1990; 8:609, with permission.

institution. Although blood component usage is increasing, the annual RBC transfusion rate, which peaked in 1982, has remained stable until 1988.[178] It should be noted that 1982 was the year in which the first transfusion-transmitted HIV infection was reported.[179]

The NIH developed guidelines for the use of FFP, platelet transfusion therapy, and perioperative RBC transfusion[110-112] because of major concerns regarding their inappropriate and unnecessary use. In addition to the three most commonly used blood products (packed RBCs, FFP, and platelets) there are other

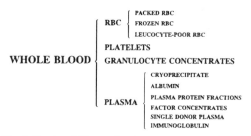

**Fig. 1–2.**  In addition to the three most commonly used blood products (packed RBCs, FFP and platelets there are other blood components that are available, either processed by the blood bank or commercially prepared.

blood components that are available, either processed by the blood bank or commercially prepared (Fig. 1–2).

## RED BLOOD CELL TRANSFUSION
### Packed Red Cell Transfusion

The use of packed RBCs has several advantages, as compared to whole blood, which are listed in Table 1–6. Compared to whole blood, packed RBCs have the same quantity of RBC in a reduced plasma volume, resulting in a HCT of approximately 70% (Table 1–7). Highly viscous, packed RBCs require dilution prior to administration. Although various solutions have been used for dilution of packed RBCs (Table 1–8), the AABB recommends only 0.9% saline be used with blood and blood products.[131] Solutions that are hypotonic (5% dextrose in water, hypotonic saline solutions, etc.) with respect to plasma, will cause the cells to swell, resulting in hemolysis. Solutions containing calcium (Ringer's solutions) are also undesirable since calcium interferes with citrate anticoagulants and may promote clotting. Packed RBCs containing Adsol (adenine-saline-dextrose, Fenwal Laboratories, Deerfield,

**Table 1–6.  Advantages and disadvantages of packed red blood cells over whole blood**

| | Advantages | Disadvantages |
|---|---|---|
| RBCs | Smaller volume | With several units of transfusion patient may develop factor deficiencies and hypoalbuminemia |
| | Higher HCT | Viscosity is higher and needs reconstitution |
| | One unit of donor blood can be used for several patients | |
| | Higher cancer survival (Blumberg, 1986) | |
| | Less incidence of hepatitis? | |
| | Reduced amount of potassium? | |
| Whole blood | Provides coagulation factors (except labile factors V & VIII) and proteins | Larger volume |
| | Beneficial during massive transfusions especially after 2000 to 2500 mL blood loss | May not be tolerated by older and cardiac patients |
| | No need for reconstitution | One unit is used for one patient |
| | | Higher plasma related complications? |

**Table 1–7.  Composition of packed red blood cells and whole blood**

| Value | Packed RBCs | Whole blood |
|---|---|---|
| Volume (mL) | 300 | 517 |
| HCT (%) | 70 | 40 |
| Total protein (gm) | 36 | 48.8 |
| Albumin (gm) | 4 | 12.5 |
| Globulin (gm) | 2 | 6.25 |
| Plasma potassium (mMol) | 4 | 15 |
| Plasma sodium (mMol) | 15 | 45 |

Modified from Miller RD: Transfusion therapy. In: Miller RD, ed. Anesthesia. 3rd ed. New York: Churchill Livingstone; 1990: 1467–1499.

**Table 1–8.  Compatibility of blood with intravenous solutions**

| | Hemolysis at 30 min | |
|---|---|---|
| Blood to intravenous solution: 1:1 ratio | Room temperature | 37°C |
| 5% dextrose in water | 1+ | 4+ |
| Plasmanate* | 1+ | 3+ |
| 5% dextrose in 0.2% saline | 0 | 3+ |
| 5% dextrose in 0.4% saline | 0 | 0 |
| 5% dextrose in 0.9% saline | 0 | 0 |
| 0.9% saline | 0 | 0 |
| Normosol-R, pH 4† | 0 | 0 |
| Lactated Ringer's solution | 0‡ | 0‡ |

* Cutter Laboratories, Inc., Berkeley, California.
† Abbott Laboratories, Chicago, Illinois.
‡ Clotted.
Modified from Miller RD: Transfusion therapy. In: Miller RD, ed. Anesthesia. 3rd ed. New York: Churchill Livingstone; 1990: 1467–1499.

IL) or Nutricel (Cutter Biological, Berkeley, CA) solutions, with 100 mL added as a preservative, can often be transfused without dilution. These are prepared by centrifuging donor blood and replacing most of the plasma with additive solution.

The blood should be kept in the refrigerator until use and should always be warmed to body temperature before infusion into the patient. It should be administered through a standard 170 $\mu$m filter, and during massive blood transfusions, through a 40 $\mu$m filter, particularly if the blood is older than 10 days.

## Frozen Red Blood Cell Transfusion

The storage of allogeneic and autologous blood has been greatly improved by freezing to a temperature below −80° C. More than 80% of the RBCs stored in this way, even after 10 years, function normally after transfusion.[180] Advantages of frozen RBCs are listed in Table 1–9. Unfortunately, at this time, frozen RBCs are not readily available because of the increased cost and time involved in storage, and the deglycerolization required prior to infusion. Other drawbacks include a 30-minute-reconstitution time and that once thawed, the RBCs must be transfused within a day (a delay may permit bacterial growth). In the mid-1970s, Cook County Hospital in

**Table 1–9. Advantages of frozen red blood cells**

Rare types of blood can be stored for many years. This is especially useful for patients who have multiple antibodies or patients who have been immunized to high frequency antigens.

For patients requiring massive transfusions, frozen RBCs would be safer because they are low in fibrin and leucocyte aggregates and also they provide better tissue oxygenation, because normal levels of 2,3-DPG and ATP are retained.

The freezing and washing process reduces sites with histocompatible antigens and so they are safer for patients who are susceptible to febrile nonhemolytic reactions as well as allergic reactions.

Chicago used 16,300 units during a 28-month period, and found that despite the cost and the time involved in processing these units, they are worthwhile and definitely improve transfusion services.[181] Initially, it was thought that frozen cells might reduce the incidence of hepatitis, but this has not been substantiated. Haugen (1979)[182] found that frozen RBCs do not reduce the incidence of posttransfusion NANBH virus or the HBV.

## PLATELETS

As for the recommendations of NIH in 1989,[183] platelets should be transfused to control or prevent bleeding associated with deficiencies in platelet number or function. For the clinically stable patient with an intact vascular system and normal platelet function, prophylactic platelet transfusions may be indicated for platelet counts of less than 10,000 to 20,000/$\mu$L. Platelet transfusions at higher platelet counts may be required for patients with systemic bleeding, and for patients at higher risk of bleeding because of additional coagulation defects, sepsis, or platelet dysfunction related to medication or disease. Platelets should not be transfused in the following situations: (1) to patients with immune thrombocytopenic purpura (unless there is life-threatening bleeding); (2) prophylactically with massive blood transfusions; and (3) prophylactically after CPB.

One unit of platelet concentrate should increase the platelet count in the average adult recipient by 5000 to 10,000/$\mu$L 1 hour after transfusion. Before transfusing the platelets, ABO and Rh compatibility should be tested.

Microaggregate filters should not be used with platelet transfusions because they tend to remove significant numbers of platelets. Filters with a pore size of 170 $\mu$m are acceptable. A large intravenous catheter should be used to prevent damage to platelets during transfusion. Following platelet infusion, the bag and the administration tubing should be rinsed with 0.9% saline to recover any platelets adhering to the bag and tubing walls.

## GRANULOCYTE CONCENTRATES

Granulocytes are transfused to patients who are severely leukopenic (leucocyte count less than 500/mm$^3$) and who have fever and septicemia. They should be ABO, Rh compatible, and administered very slowly through a filter. Rapid infusion may cause pulmonary complications.

## FRESH FROZEN PLASMA

The NIH has issued a statement regarding the indications and contraindications of FFP.[183] FFP should be given to increase the level of clotting factors in patients with a demonstrated deficiency. If prothrombin time and activated partial thromboplastin time are less than 1.5 times normal, FFP transfusion is rarely indicated. Patients with rare conditions such as antithrombin III deficiency and thrombotic thrombocytopenic purpura, may benefit from FFP transfusion. If patients on warfarin sodium become deficient in vitamin K-dependent coagulation factors II, VII, IX and X, and bleed or require emergency surgery, FFP transfusion may be necessary.

Fresh frozen plasma should not be transfused: (1) for volume expansion; (2) as a nutritional supplement; (3) prophylactically with massive blood transfusion; and (4) prophylactically following CPB. Fresh frozen plasma should be given through a large bore catheter and standard 170 $\mu$m filter, immediately after thawing, and definitely within 24 hours.[131]

## CRYOPRECIPITATE

In addition to significant levels of fibrinogen and factor VIII, cryoprecipitate contains vWf and fibronectin. For fibrinogen deficiencies, cryoprecipitate is preferable over the commercial fibrinogen preparation because of the lesser incidence of hepatitis. Currently, commercially prepared factor VIII preparations are used more often than the cryoprecipitate prepared from FFP for the treatment of hemophilia. The recent development of factor VIII with recombinant DNA techniques has practically eliminated the transmission of hepatitis.[184] Before administration, the cryoprecipitate must be thawed in a 37° C water bath and aseptically pooled into one dose. The thawed product should be stored at room temperature and administered rapidly through a filter. The infusion should be completed within 6 hours of thawing.[140]

## ALBUMIN AND PLASMA PROTEIN FRACTIONS

Five or 25% solution of albumin and $\alpha$- and $\beta$-globulins are available as commercial preparations and can be administered to patients without typing or cross matching. They should be administered to patients with documented hypoproteinemia, or with conditions where hypoproteinemia is common, such as peritonitis and burns. Unlike albumin, plasma protein fraction infusion may decrease systemic vascular resistance (Bland and others, 1973) and cause hypotension.

## FACTOR IX COMPLEX

A factor IX level of less than 5% of normal will give rise to spontaneous hemorrhage, while levels greater than 20% of normal will lead to satisfactory hemostasis, even after trauma or surgery. Administration of factor IX complex not only raises the level of factor IX, but also the other vitamin K-dependent factors II, VII and X. It is used for factor IX deficiency (hemophilia B, Christmas disease) to prevent or control bleeding episodes, and for reversal of coumarin anticoagulant-induced hemorrhage. There are other commercial preparations that are available. Two such preparations are Konyne (Cutter Laboratories) and Proplex (Travenol Laboratories). Proplex T contains more factor VII than Proplex SX-T and is used for prevention or control of bleeding episodes in patients with factor VII deficiency.

## IMMUNE GLOBULINS

Immune globulin (intravenous) is indicated for patients with primary defective antibody synthesis, such as an agammaglobulinemia or hypogammaglobulinemia. It primarily contains immunoglobulin G (IgG), is prepared from a large pool of at least 1000 donors, and represents the expected diversity of antibodies in that population. Severe anaphylactic or anaphylactoid reactions can occur with these preparations.

(D) immune globulin (intramuscular) is used to suppress the immune response in nonsensitized (D) negative individuals who are exposed to (D) positive blood as a result of fetomaternal hemorrhage or a platelet transfusion. The reactions after (D) immune globulin are rare.

## COMPLICATIONS OF BLOOD TRANSFUSION AND THEIR MANAGEMENT

Although improved blood banking procedures over the last few years have reduced the incidence of transfusion reactions, many complications continue to occur after blood administration. Some of these complications are preventable, but some cannot be prevented, despite careful screening by the personnel involved with the blood administration. Because of this, blood should be administered only when it is absolutely necessary and autotransfusions and other blood conservation techniques should be employed whenever possible.

Blood transfusion reactions can be classified as immunologic reactions, nonimmunologic reactions, and transmission of infections (Table 1–10). Both immunologic and nonimmunologic reactions can occur as immediate or delayed reactions. These reactions may also be classified according to their clinical significance. Immediate transfusion reactions usually occur during, or shortly after a blood transfusion, and become apparent within minutes to hours, usually within 24 hours. De-

Table 1–10.  **Blood transfusion reactions**

| Immunologic | Immediate |
| | Delayed |
| Nonimmunologic | Immediate |
| | Delayed |
| Transmission of diseases | |

**Table 1–11.** Immunologic responses to blood transfusion

| Type of response | Antibodies | Direct Coombs Test | Hemolysis |
|---|---|---|---|
| Nonresponsive | – | – | – |
| Seroconversion | + | – | – |
| RBC sensitization | + | + | – |
| Hemolysis | + | + | + |

layed transfusion reactions typically occur 5 to 7 days after the transfusion,[186] but may occur within several days or even months later.

## IMMUNOLOGIC TRANSFUSION REACTIONS (Table 1–11)

Immunologic responses to blood transfusion may manifest as seroconversion, RBC sensitization, or intravascular or extravascular hemolysis. In rare cases, cellular components from the donor's blood can mount an immunologic response against the recipient. This is called transfusion-associated GVHD. Seroconversion refers to the presence of antibodies after transfusion or pregnancy without positive direct antihuman globulin test or hemolysis. Red blood cell sensitization refers to the presence of alloantibodies detected by direct antihuman globulin test without any hemolysis. Intravascular hemolysis usually occurs immediately after the transfusion, and results in membrane lysis with release of free HGB and complement activation. Extravascular hemolysis is a delayed reaction and occurs when the macrophages of the reticuloendothelial system ingest the nonviable erythrocytes that are coated with IgG antibodies or complement component $C3_b$.

## Acute Immunologic Transfusion Reactions (Table 1–12)

In addition to intravascular hemolysis, other acute immunologic reactions include nonhemolytic febrile reactions, noncardiogenic pulmonary edema, and allergic reactions.

### INTRAVASCULAR HEMOLYSIS

The USFDA report on transfusion mortality between 1976 and 1985 showed that hemolytic reactions were responsible for the deaths in 58% of the patients.[187] Of these 58%, 71% were from ABO incompatibility and 26% from nonABO incompatibility. The frequency with which hemolytic transfusion reactions occurred varied anywhere from 1 in 4000[188] to 1 in 6000[189] transfusions. More recent evidence indicates that the incidence is much lower and is estimated to be 1:19,000 to 33,000 transfusions.[190,191] The incidence of a fatal hemolytic reaction in 1989 was estimated to be 1 in 100,000.[192] In 1994, it is estimated in the range of 1:500,000 to 1:800,000.[191] The most common cause of incompatible transfusion reaction is wrong identification of the patient and occurs more often in the operating room, either because the wrist bands are removed, or because the patient is anesthetized and unable to identify himself. Other mishaps are caused by blood bank technologists, due to improper identification of the patient, errors during testing of the blood, and/or mislabeling of the cross matched blood.

The most common presenting symptom of an acute hemolytic reaction is fever or fever with chills.[193] Other symptoms may include nausea, chest pain, flank pain, a vague sense of uneasiness, and dyspnea. Signs of hemolytic reaction may include flushing, hypotension, generalized oozing, or frank bleeding, secondary to disseminated intravascular coagulation (DIC), and oliguria or anuria, secondary to shock. In some cases red or dark colored urine caused by hemoglobinuria may be the first sign of a hemolytic reaction.

In the anesthetized patient, the early symptoms or signs of hemolytic reaction may not

**Table 1–12.** Acute immunologic transfusion reactions

| Type of reaction | Cause of reaction |
|---|---|
| Intravascular hemolysis | RBC incompatibility |
| Nonhemolytic febrile reactions | Antibodies to donor leukocyte antigens |
| Noncardiogenic pulmonary edema | Patient's leukocytes reacting to donor antibodies |
| Urticarial rash | Antibodies to donor plasma proteins |
| Anaphylaxis | Antibodies to IgA of donor |

be apparent, and patients may receive additional units of incompatible blood before a diagnosis is made. A high index of suspicion in any patient who develops hypotension, oozing from the surgical or intravenous sites, or dark colored urine should lead to an early diagnosis. Intravascular hemolysis can occur even after as little as 10 mL of blood or blood product has been transfused.

The most serious consequences of a hemolytic reaction are acute renal failure and DIC. Renal failure occurs either because of physical tubular obstruction by the acid hematin precipitate that is formed from the free HGB, or due to renal ischemia, secondary to decreased renal cortical blood flow from severe hypotension. One suggested mechanism for the hypotension during hemolytic transfusion reaction is activation of the kallikrein system.[194] Disseminated intravascular coagulation occurs from the erythrocytin that is released from the severed RBC stroma, which activates the intrinsic coagulation cascade leading to fibrin formation. Several coagulation factors and platelets are consumed in the process (See Chapter 2: Coagulation and Hemostasis).

Blood transfusion should be discontinued as soon as a hemolytic reaction is suspected, and the blood bag and administration set should be removed and replaced with fresh tubing and crystalloid solution (Table 1–13). The remaining blood should be sent back to the blood bank, along with a blood specimen from the patient for retyping, and repeat compatibility and direct antihuman globulin test. In addition, other measurements, such as serum potassium, haptoglobin, HGB, bilirubin, platelet count, activated partial thromboplastin time, and serum fibrinogen, may need to be obtained. A hemolytic transfusion reaction is confirmed when the direct antiglobulin test shows that antibodies are attached to the transfused donor RBCs[193] and/or when plasma free HGB levels are high.

Hypotension should be aggressively treated with intravenous fluids and low-dose (5 $\mu$g/kg/min) dopamine. A central venous pressure or pulmonary artery catheter may be needed to monitor fluid administration. Urine output should be maintained above 75 to 100 mL/hour, not only with intravenous fluids, but also with diuretics. Although mannitol was commonly used for posthemolytic oliguria at one time,[195] loop diuretics such as furo-

**Table 1–13.  Treatment of hemolytic transfusion reaction**

1. Stop the transfusion
2. Send the remaining donor blood and recipient blood and urine samples to the blood bank and laboratory
3. Treat hypotension aggressively
4. Maintain urine output between 75 and 100 mL/hr
5. Alkalinize the urine
6. Insert arterial line and central venous or pulmonary artery catheter to monitor the effectiveness of treatment methods

semide are preferable, since they not only increase urine flow, but also cause a redistribution of renal blood flow with an increase in renal cortical perfusion.[196] Alkalinizing urine with small doses of sodium bicarbonate may reduce the amount of acid hematin in the renal tubules.

Hyperkalemia could be a life-threatening factor during massive hemolysis and should be immediately and aggressively treated. In some cases, even acute dialysis may be necessary to reduce the high potassium levels. The use of extracorporeal circulation to facilitate exchange transfusion with compatible blood has been successfully tried in a patient with severe hemolytic reaction.[197] When DIC is suspected, a hematologist should follow the clinical course and the laboratory values.

## OTHER ACUTE IMMUNOLOGIC REACTIONS

The most common adverse reactions to transfused blood are febrile reactions without hemolysis. The incidence varies between 0.49%[198] and 1%[199] of transfusions. These reactions are more common in pregnant patients or patients who have been repeatedly transfused. They occur due to a reaction between recipient white cell antibodies with the donor's granulocytes. Fever, chills, headache, myalgia, and nausea are the most common symptoms. Blood transfusion should be stopped and a hemolytic reaction should be ruled out before the administration of antipyretics. The fever may be mild or severe, and may not occur until the transfusion is completed. If the patient requires further transfusions, use of special filters that selectively remove leukocytes, or the administration of leukocyte-poor blood will eliminate most of the febrile reactions. Use of frozen-thawed RBCs is another effective way of eliminating febrile reactions.

Noncardiogenic pulmonary edema is a rare transfusion reaction, and is caused by leukocyte antibodies in the donor's blood which react with the recipient's leukocyte antigens. The donors have developed these antibodies by prior transfusions or pregnancy. This reaction can occur with small amounts of transfusion and manifests as pulmonary edema without signs of congestive heart failure.[200] Prehilar nodule formation and lung infiltrates with overt pulmonary edema have been reported.[201] In severe cases chills, fever, cyanosis, and hypotension can occur. Treatment is usually symptomatic with the administration of oxygen and diuretics. Epinephrine and corticosteroids are used, if needed. The symptoms usually resolve within 12 to 24 hours and the chest x-ray improves within a few days.

Urticarial rash without other symptoms is a common, but mild allergic reaction between foreign protein in the donor's plasma, or sometimes in the blood bag, and antibodies in the recipient's plasma. Temporarily discontinuing the transfusion and administrating an antihistamine is usually sufficient.

The more serious form of allergic reactions to plasma are either an anaphylactic reaction which is mediated by IgE antibody, or an anaphylactoid reaction which is not mediated by IgE antibody (Table 1–14). Anaphylactic reactions are due to the activation of mast cells, which in their turn, release several mediators such as histamine, leukotrienes, prostaglandins, etc, causing severe reactions. Profound hypotension, bronchospasm, generalized urticaria or angioneurotic edema, and respiratory and cardiac arrest can occur very rapidly. Immediate and aggressive treatment with epi-

nephrine, large amounts of intravenous fluids, antihistamines, and aminophylline are essential to prevent the high incidence of mortality. For patients with a history of previous serious allergic reaction, pretreatment with steroids, antihistamines, and ephedrine could be beneficial, and reduces the incidence of serious reaction.[202]

## Delayed Immunologic Transfusion Reactions

### DELAYED HEMOLYTIC REACTIONS

Unlike an acute hemolytic reaction, in some patients the transfused donor cells survive initially, but hemolyze after several days to months.[203,204] In most cases, this reaction occurs in patients who were previously sensitized to RBC antigens by previous blood transfusion or pregnancy.[205] The patient has no detectable antibody at the time of transfusion, and RBC destruction occurs only when the level of antibody is increased after a secondary stimulus (anamnestic response). The antibodies most commonly involved in delayed reactions are those in Rh and Kidd systems, rather than the ABO system. The delayed hemolytic reactions are much less severe than acute hemolytic reactions, and may manifest only as a decreased HCT. This should be kept in mind in postoperative patients and in patients with chronic hemolytic anemia. Other symptoms may include mild forms of jaundice, hemoglobinuria, and impairment of renal function. In most patients, observation, adequate hydration, and administration of antigen-negative blood, if necessary, is all that is needed.

### GRAFT-VERSUS-HOST DISEASE

Graft-Versus-Host-Disease can result from the transfusion of immunocompetent lymphocytes into patients with primary or secondary immunodeficiency syndromes, or in immunocompetent patients receiving non-irradiated cellular components from first or second degree relatives (Table 1–15).

The diagnosis of posttransfusion GVHD is made after excluding a drug reaction or the underlying disease. A history of transfusion within 4 to 30 days, and a fulminant illness with severe maculopapular skin rash, liver and gastrointestinal manifestations, and the pres-

**Table 1–14.    Treatment of anaphylactic reaction**

1. Stop the transfusion
2. Administer epinephrine
3. Maintain oxygenation
4. Administer antihistamines
    H₁-antagonists— Diphenhydramine
                              Chlorpheniramine
    H₂-antagonists— Cimetidine
                              Ranitidine
5. Treat bronchospasm with aminophylline
6. Administer corticosteroids

**Table 1–15.   Patients at risk of graft-versus-host disease**

| High risk | Possible risk | Negligible risk |
|---|---|---|
| Allogenic or autologous bone marrow transplantation<br>Severe combined immunodeficiency syndrome | Intrauterine transfusion<br>Neonatal exchange transfusion<br>Acute leukemia and lymphoma during radiation or chemotherapy<br>Neuroblastoma during chemotherapy<br>Wiscott-Aldrich syndrome | Aplastic anemia<br>Patient with AIDS<br>Solid tumors<br>Granulocyte dysfunction syndromes |

From Petz LD, Swisher SN: Clinical practice of transfusion medicine. 2nd ed. New York: Churchill Livingstone, with permission; 1989.

ence of bone marrow hypoplasia and pancytopenia indicates GVHD. Skin biopsy will reveal diffuse lymphocytic infiltrates. Definitive diagnosis is made by the identification of mixed chimerism with mononuclear cells coming from the donor and the recipient.

Treatment of established GVHD includes supportive therapy and administration of methylprednisolone and anti-thymocyte globulin. Prevention of the disease can be accomplished by exposing the blood to radiation before transfusion.[206] The recommended irradiation dosages vary widely (1500 to 5000 rads), but one recent report suggests at least 3000 to 4000 rads may be needed.[207] When blood is removed from the radiation source, it is no longer radioactive and can be handled like any other blood product.

## IMMUNOSUPPRESSION

In 1973, cadaver renal allograft survival was shown to be prolonged in patients who had received pretransplant transfusions.[208] Subsequent studies have confirmed this observation in both cadaver and living-donor related grafts.[209-211] Later, with the use of cyclosporine A, a potent immunosuppressive drug, no differences were found between transfused and non-transfused renal transplant patients.[212]

In 1981, Yantt[213] noted a similarity between tumor and histocompatibility antigens and hypothesized that nonspecific immune suppression induced by blood transfusion might favor tumor growth. The following year, it was reported that colon cancer patients who received blood transfusions intraoperatively had earlier recurrence of their cancers and poorer outcomes compared to those who did not receive blood transfusions.[214] Later, the effect of intraoperative blood transfusions on other malignancies have also been reported.[215,216] In one study of patients with rectal cancer, the 10-year-survival rate was 82% in patients with no blood transfusion, 53% in patients who had received 1 to 5 units of blood, 31% in patients with 6 to 10 units, and 14% in patients with more than 10 units of blood.[217]

A relationship between intraoperative blood transfusions and the development of bacterial infections in open heart surgery patients[218] and trauma patients[219] has been documented. This relationship was also found in patients with colon cancer[220] and with Crohn's disease.[221]

The exact mechanism of immunosuppression by blood transfusions has not been identified. Increased synthesis of prostaglandin E,[222] fibrin degradation products in FFP,[223] and decreased interleukin 2 generation[224] have all been implicated. Some investigators have found that the administration of packed RBCs is associated with better survival rate, compared to whole blood administration in cancer patients.[225] They suggested that plasma in the whole blood contains an unidentified immunosuppressive factor that decreases survival of patients.

## POSTTRANSFUSION PURPURA

Posttransfusion purpura is a rare complication of platelet administration which usually occurs 1 week after transfusion. This disorder develops in $PL^{A1}$ antigen-negative patients when they receive $PL^{A1}$ antigen-positive platelets. The $PL^{A1}$ antibody destroys platelets and leads to thrombocytopenia.[226] Most often the condition is self-limiting with spontaneous remission within 4 to 6 weeks; but occasionally, it can be fatal. In severe cases, plasmapheresis may be needed.

# NONIMMUNOLOGIC TRANSFUSION REACTIONS

Many of the nonimmunologic transfusion reactions are due to the administration of large quantities of blood. These include hypothermia, hypocalcemia and hyperkalemia, acid-base abnormalities, coagulation abnormalities, congestive heart failure, possible postoperative respiratory failure, hypoxemia from carboxyhemoglobin and methemoglobin, and iron overload from chronic transfusions. Many of these complications occur due to the physical and chemical changes that a unit of blood undergoes during storage. Other non-immunologic transfusion reactions include hemolysis without symptoms, air embolus, and marked fever with shock.

## Hypothermia

The rapid infusion of intravenous fluids and blood products is often needed for patients in hypovolemic shock following trauma, during major vessel surgery, orthotopic liver transplantation, and other situations involving massive hemorrhage. The massive transfusion of refrigerated blood products (stored at 1° to 6° C) or even room temperature fluids without (or with improper) warming, may lead to or exacerbate hypothermia. This can result in serious complications such as increase in oxygen consumption, derangements in metabolism, abnormal hemostasis, and ventricular arrhythmias. Hypothermia can be prevented with pretransfusion warming of the fluids and blood products to 37° to 38° C before infusion into the patient.[227] Of the various technologies employed to warm blood—warm water bath, microwave, radiofrequency, dry heat, and countercurrent heat exchangers—dry heat and countercurrent are the most commonly employed in the United States.[228]

While conventional means of fluid and blood administration (gravity or pressure infusion through standard intravenous administration set and dry-heat blood warmers) are usually sufficient at slow and moderate infusion rates (< 50 mL/min), they may be inadequate to cope with massive transfusions. Use of low-capacity blood warmers for massive transfusion demands use of multiple blood warmers through several infusion sites and additional personnel. Dry heat blood warmers rely upon the rather inefficient heat exchange through narrow-bore polyethylene plastic tubing.[229,230]

In recent years, significant advances in rapid infusion devices have been made. Devices such as the H250 and H500 (Level 1 Technologies, Rockland, MA) and the R.I.S. Rapid Infusion System (Haemonetics Corp, Braintree, MA) are capable of infusing and warming intravenous fluids and blood products (including highly viscous undiluted packed RBCs) at rates of 250 mL/min to over 1000 mL/min.[228,230] Rapid infusion rates are accomplished by means of occlusive roller pumps, large bore intravenous administration sets, high-flow transfusion filters, and large bore intravenous cannulae.[231,232] Heat transfer is accomplished through countercurrent heat exchangers, using highly efficient copper or aluminum metal tubes.[228,230]

## Hypocalcemia and Hyperkalemia

When large quantities of CPD-stored blood is infused, citrate binds ionized calcium and can cause hypocalcemia. The hemodynamic effects of citrate toxicity include narrow pulse pressure, hypotension, and increased central venous and left ventricular end-diastolic pressures.[233] In addition, hypocalcemia is manifested as a prolonged Q-T interval on the electrocardiogram. Fortunately, the hypocalcemic effects are transient and do not require any treatment because citrate is metabolized, and endogenous calcium stores are mobilized very rapidly to replete the serum calcium.[234,235] The effects of citrate intoxication are more noticeable in patients with low-flow states[236] and when large quantities of blood are administered very rapidly.[237,238] In addition, patients with liver disease or those undergoing orthotopic liver transplantation may readily develop hypocalcemia,[239] and require close monitoring of ionized calcium levels. Hypothermia and hypocapnia should be avoided in these patients since both can decrease ionized calcium levels.

Although the potassium content of stored blood could be as high as 78 mMol/L at 35 days of storage, hyperkalemia rarely occurs, even with the administration of large quantities of blood. Actually, hypokalemia can be more of a problem during massive blood transfusion, since citrate, when converted to bicarbonate, makes the blood alkalotic and hypokalemia ensues.[240] Hyperkalemia can usually be diagnosed in an electrocardiogram by tall, peaked T waves. In contrast, hypokalemia is manifested by decreased T waves, widening of QRS complexes, and increases in U waves.

The rarity of hypocalcemia and hyperkalemia, and the possibility of hypokalemia, even with massive blood transfusions, makes routine administration of calcium unnecessary. Calcium administration is warranted only when electrocardiographic changes or clinical signs indicate hypocalcemia or hyperkalemia. Calcium chloride (10%), providing 3 times more calcium than an equal volume of 10% calcium gluconate (chloride has a molecular weight of 147 daltons compared to 448 daltons for gluconate), should be administered slowly to prevent irritation at the infusion site. Acute increases in potassium can also be treated with insulin and glucose infusion (1 unit/2 gm glucose). Hypokalemia can also occur with massive blood transfusions and can be corrected with an intravenous solution containing potassium to be given at a rate of no more than 0.5 mMol/kg/hour, while monitoring the electrocardiogram and/or serum potassium levels.

## Acid-Base Abnormalities

When CPD solution with a pH of 5.5 is added to freshly drawn blood, the accumulation of lactic and pyruvic acids from RBC metabolism and the very high $PCO_2$ in the plastic bags that do not provide an escape mechanism for the carbon dioxide, further decreases the pH of stored blood. When large quantities of this blood are transfused, acidosis can occur in the recipient. Routine administration of sodium bicarbonate to treat this acidosis is not recommended since citrate in the blood generates bicarbonate and compensates for the acidosis. Excessive amounts of sodium bicarbonate can be more harmful to the patient since it may interfere with coagulation and can result in leftward shifting of the oxyhemoglobin dissociation curve. Therefore, sodium bicarbonate should be administered only when blood gas analysis indicates metabolic acidosis.

## Coagulation Abnormalities

After massive blood transfusions, a bleeding tendency often develops. The causes of this bleeding are dilutional thrombocytopenia, factor V and VIII deficiency, and occasionally, DIC. Platelets have only 50 to 70%

of their original activity after 6 hours of storage in CPD solution at 4° C. After 24 hours, it is 10%, and at 48 hours, 5% of normal. The infusion of this blood will result in dilution of the available platelet pool, and can lead to hemorrhagic diathesis. Although bleeding can occur when the platelet count decreases to 50,000 to 75,000/mm$^3$, platelets should not be administered based on the laboratory value of platelet count alone. Only when there is clinical evidence of bleeding with low platelet count, should platelets be administered.

Factors V and VIII are unstable in stored blood and decrease significantly with storage. However, only 5 to 20% of factor V and 30% of factor VIII are needed for hemostasis during surgery. Administration of FFP is not indicated routinely during transfusion of large quantities of blood. When the partial thromboplastin time is more than 1.5 times normal, and there is clinical evidence of bleeding, FFP should be administered.

Disseminated intravascular coagulation has been reported after multiple transfusions of stored blood for the treatment of hemorrhagic shock. The acidotic, hypoxic tissues with stagnant blood flow release tissue thromboplastin, triggering the coagulation process. Many coagulation factors and platelets are consumed during the process, leading to hemorrhagic diathesis. Blood flow to vital organs is interrupted because of deposition of fibrin in the microcirculation of these organs. In order to lyse these fibrin deposits, the fibrinolytic system is activated and plasminogen is converted to plasmin which lyses clots and fibrin and increases bleeding. Disseminated intravascular coagulation is usually diagnosed when there is clinical evidence of bleeding, thrombocytopenia and hypofibrinogenemia (< 150 mg/mL) are present, and lysis of clot occurs within 2 hours. The treatment of DIC involves administration of heparin and then replacing the consumed factors.

## Congestive Heart Failure

Patients with expanded plasma volumes and cardiac disease may not tolerate rapid transfusions and may develop congestive heart failure. Similarly, small children and elderly patients are prone to develop heart failure when blood is administered too rapidly. Unless these patients are bleeding profusely, the calculated volume of packed RBCs, diluted in a minimal amount of saline, should be administered slowly. For correction of low HGB value, packed RBCs can be given at a rate of 1 mL/kg/hour. If congestive heart failure develops during transfusion, the transfusion is slowed to a minimum, the patient placed in a semi-sitting position, and oxygen and diuretics may be administered. If frank pulmonary edema develops, the patient may need to be artificially ventilated, and in severe cases, phlebotomy may be necessary.

## Postoperative Respiratory Failure

As early as 1938, the need to filter the blood was realized when it was noticed that clots and debris form during storage of blood.[17] From the 1940s to 1960s, it was believed that the standard 170 to 230 $\mu$m filters were sufficient to prevent the entry of the majority of clots and debris. In the 1960s, with the development of open heart surgical procedures and resuscitation of patients with major trauma, blood transfusions were commonly used and occlusion of end-organ capillaries with microaggregate debris and postoperative respiratory insufficiency became a major concern. To remove this microaggregate debris, the use of filters with smaller pore sizes was popularized. However, since these filters are expensive and tend to slow the rate of infusion, their routine use has been questioned. Some controversy has developed concerning the role of microaggregate debris in the development of respiratory insufficiency and the necessity of fine filtration of blood products, particularly during massive transfusions.[241-243] Based on current literature, the routine use of microfilters for blood transfusion is not necessary, except in certain situations including transfusions for neonates with pulmonary dysfunction,[244] massive blood transfusions,[245] or with blood older than 10 days.[246]

There are two types of microfilters that are available: screen and depth filters. The screen filters just intercept the debris, whereas the depth filters not only intercept, but also allow the debris to adhere to or absorb onto the filter medium. The pore sizes of screen filters are 20 $\mu$m to 40 $\mu$m and depth filters can remove particles above 10 $\mu$m size.

## Hypoxia and Impairment of Cardiovascular Function from Carboxyhemoglobin and Methemoglobin in Banked Blood

Both carboxyhemoglobin and methemoglobin reduce the amount of HGB available for oxygen transport and can cause hypoxia. Carboxyhemoglobin also shifts the oxyhemoglobin dissociation curve to the left and inhibits the release of oxygen at the tissue level.[247] A 2% level of carboxyhemoglobin can aggravate angina pectoris in patients with coronary artery disease.[248] Methemoglobin levels increase in stored blood as storage is prolonged[249] because the decreased ATP levels and pH result in inhibition of reduction enzymes.[250] Stored blood may contain as much as 13.8% abnormal hemoglobins, and when transfused to critically ill patients, can cause hypoxia and impairment of cardiovascular function.[251] Since carboxyhemoglobin levels in smokers' blood is increased, Uchida and associates (1990) have suggested that blood donors refrain from smoking for 12 hours to reduce the carboxyhemoglobin level in their blood.

## Iron Overload (Hemosiderosis)

Patients with congenital hemolytic anemias or long-standing aplastic anemia require chronic transfusion therapy. Each unit of blood contains approximately 250 mg of iron. When total body iron reaches 400 to 1000 mg/kg body weight, signs of clinical toxicity develop.[252] The organs that are most commonly affected are the liver, heart, pancreas, and other endocrine organs. Iron chelation therapy with deferoxamine[253,254] has been used successfully in some patients with hemosiderosis, but this treatment is a slow, tedious process and patient compliance is poor. Keeping the transfusions to a minimum and using young RBCs (neocytes) in high-risk patients is advised.

## TRANSMISSION OF DISEASES

Many viral, bacterial, and parasitic diseases can be transmitted from the donor to the recipient during transfusion. Over the last few years, careful screening of donors, use of fully assembled and sterilized plastic blood collec-

**Table 1–16.   Diseases transmitted by blood transfusions**

Viral diseases
  Hepatitis
  AIDS
  Herpes viruses
  HTLV-I/II
  Cytomegalovirus disease
  Epstein-Barr Virus diseases
  Parvovirus disease
Bacterial diseases
  Salmonellosis
  Other enteric bacterial infections
  Endotoxin shock by Yersinia *enterocolitica*
  Syphilis
  Brucellosis
Parasitic diseases
  Malaria
  Toxoplasmosis
  Babesiosis
  Filariasis
  Trypanosomiasis
  Leishmaniasis

tion equipment, and modern blood testing methods have eliminated or decreased the incidence of transmission of many of these diseases (Table 1–16).

## Viral Diseases

Transmission of viral diseases, especially hepatitis and AIDS, are the most feared complications of blood transfusion. Other viral diseases such as HTLV-I and HTLV-II, herpes viruses, and parvoviruses have all been reported following transfusions of blood or blood products.

### HEPATITIS

The USFDA drug bulletin of July 1989 states that the incidence of posttransfusion hepatitis was 1:100 per unit of blood given.[192] This incidence is much lower now,[56] Hepatitis is transmitted by A (HAV), B (HBV), non-A non-B (HCV), and δ (HDV) viruses. Hepatitis A virus infection is transmitted by fecal to oral or enteric route, and is usually not transmitted by transfusions. Occasional outbreaks of this disease through blood products have been reported,[255] but this is very rare.

The average incubation period for transfusion-transmitted HBV is about 11 to 12 weeks. Clinical manifestations may range anywhere from asymptomatic to severe fulminant disease with a fatal outcome. Usually the severe form of the disease develops in elderly patients, while infants and children develop asymptomatic acute and chronic infections. Chronic hepatitis can progress to cirrhosis and hepatocellular carcinoma. With hepatitis B infection, icteric cases are high, and jaundice can occur in as much as 60% of cases. Many organs other than the liver may be involved. Despite highly sensitive screening methods some cases of hepatitis B continue to occur, either because the blood donor is in the incubation period of acute hepatitis B, or is a carrier of low-level HBV at the time of donation.

As previously mentioned, the majority of posttransfusion hepatitis infections are caused by the HCV. The testing of blood for ALT and the HBcAb reduced the incidence by half. Recently, investigators at Chiron Corporation have synthesized an antigen (C100-3) specific for HCV.[61] This seems to be a reliable marker and anti-HCV have been found in many patients with NANBH following transfusions.[60] Unfortunately, this test does not detect the acute phase of hepatitis C at this time. Usually, the incubation period for hepatitis C is shorter, and clinical manifestations are less severe than hepatitis B. Less than 30% of patients develop jaundice, but as with hepatitis B, the disease can progress to cirrhosis and hepatocellular carcinoma.

Hepatitis δ is a blood-borne disease and the infection occurs more often in intravenous drug users, hemophiliacs, and thalassemics who have frequent exposure to blood-contaminated needles and multiple transfusions of blood products. HDV relies on the HBV for replication and expression, and the infection can occur only as a coinfection of HBV, or as a superimposed infection of an HBV carrier. When the incidence of hepatitis B after transfusion of HBsAg-negative blood was estimated to be about 1 in 100, the calculated risk of coinfection with HDV among HBsAg-negative recipients was approximately 1 in 3000.[256] This number should be lower now because of the lower incidence of hepatitis B. When HDV coinfection occurs with HBV, a fulminant form of hepatitis is more likely to occur than self-limited acute hepatitis. When superimposed infection of HBV carriers occurs with HDV, it is more likely that the mild, chronic hepatitis B will be transformed into chronic active hepatitis and cirrhosis.

At this time, the treatment measures for hepatitis include, immunoprophylaxis using immunoglobulin and vaccines, antiviral agents such as interferon-$\alpha$ , and in seriously ill patients, steroids. A single 5 mL dose of hepatitis B immune globulin has been found to be of benefit following accidental exposure of medical personnel to HBsAg-positive materials such as blood, plasma, or serum.[257] Intradermal recombinant hepatitis B vaccine given in quantities up to four doses, has been shown to produce seropositivity for HBsAg in 90% of the susceptible individuals who are vaccinated.[258] Administration of immune globulin, along with hepatitis B vaccine, provides faster protective levels of HBcAb than when the vaccine is administered alone.[259]

Antiviral agents such as vidarabine and interferon-$\alpha$ have been tried in patients with chronic hepatitis to inhibit viral replication, thus limiting the risks of cirrhosis and hepatocellular carcinoma. Interferon-$\alpha$ has a wide spectrum of antiviral activity and is known to inhibit the replication of all forms of hepatitis when administered for at least 6 months. Relapses occur in many patients when the treatment is stopped and thus, the treatment may have to be extended up to 12 to 18 months.[260] In some patients, prior administration of steroids such as prednisolone may be needed before starting the antiviral agents.

## ACQUIRED IMMUNODEFICIENCY SYNDROME

### Human Immunodeficiency Virus, Type 1

At this time, the most common virus causing AIDS in the United States is HIV-1. Most of the transfusion-associated cases of AIDS occurred prior to the routine testing of donors for the anti-HIV-1 using ELISA in conjunction with the western blot test. Unfortunately, even with these tests, some donors may not demonstrate antibodies in the early stages of infection. This interval is about 6 to 8 weeks and is known as the "window period."[261] Some investigators were able to detect HIV-1 DNA in high risk individuals before they were seroconverted, by using polymerase chain reaction.[262] In 1989, the incidence of transfusion-transmitted AIDS was 1:40,000

to 1:100,000.[183] Now, the incidence is estimated to be 1:225,000.[79,263]

The clinical manifestations of acute and chronic HIV infections are varied. The acute infection is usually transient and may resemble infectious mononucleosis. At a later time, the patient may develop AIDS-related complex (ARC) or lymphadenopathy syndrome, which may persist for days to months, and can progress to full-blown AIDS. When AIDS develops fully, the virus destroys the helper T cells and causes severe immunodeficiency. The patient then develops Kaposi's sarcoma, non-Hodgkin's lymphoma, and opportunistic infections, and dies within a few months to a few years.

Currently, treatment of AIDS consists of treating the symptoms, the opportunistic infections, and malignancies as they arise. Antiviral agents, such as AZT and interferon-$\alpha$ , have shown some promise in patients with Kaposi's sarcoma.[264]

### Human Immunodeficiency Virus, Type 2

Since the first documented case of AIDS due to HIV-2 was reported,[90] a single case of transfusion-related HIV-2 infection has been substantiated.[89] However, the USFDA now recommends that either a combination HIV-1/HIV-2 screening assay or individual HIV-1 and HIV-2 assays be performed.

### HUMAN T-CELL LYMPHOTROPIC VIRUS, TYPES I AND II

The human T-cell lymphotropic virus, type 1 is associated with adult T-cell leukemia and lymphoma, HTLV-I-associated myelopathy, and tropical spastic paraparesis.[265] In Japan, 1 in 20 potential donors are seropositive,[84] but in the United States, estimates suggest that less than 25 in 100,000 donors are seropositive, and most of them are intravenous drug users.[266] Even though none of the recipients of blood or blood products has developed the diseases associated with the virus so far, the USFDA has recommended screening all donors for HTLV-I and HTLV-II. This is because the incubation period is very long (several years to decades) and some of the recipients might not yet have developed the diseases associated with HTLV-I. Once developed, adult T-cell leukemia is a serious disease and survival time is less than 1 year.[267] An association of HTLV-II with hairy-cell leukemia is now considered coincidental. Epidemiological studies have failed to provide evidence of an association of HTLV-II with any hematologic or other malignant diseases.

## HERPES VIRUSES

Herpes simplex and Herpes zoster/varicella are not transmitted by blood. The two herpes viruses that are of concern are Cytomegalovirus and Epstein-Barr virus. Both these viruses produce asymptomatic chronic infection in many healthy adults. But in immunocompromised patients such as immature infants and recipients of bone marrow and organ transplants, they produce infectious mononucleosis-like illness several weeks following transfusion. Also, these viruses were reported to be responsible for postperfusion syndrome following open heart surgery.[268] Because of the immaturity of their immunologic system, preterm infants are susceptible to Cytomegalovirus infection. In 1987, the AABB recommended that seronegative infants weighing less than 1200 gm at birth, should only receive Cytomegalovirus-negative blood.[269] Seronegative blood should be used for seronegative transplant recipients who receive seronegative organs or bone marrow. Seropositive recipients should not receive seronegative marrow, since this could result in fatal Cytomegalovirus infection. If they receive seropositive marrow, the transfused antibodies prevent fulminant reactivation of the virus.[270]

The use of immune Cytomegalovirus globulin for bone marrow recipients[271] and for renal transplant patients[272] has been shown to reduce the incidence of clinically evident disease. Transfusion-related Epstein-Barr virus infection is very low, and routine serological screening for Epstein-Barr virus is not warranted. But, since both viruses are harbored in white blood cells, administration of leuko-depleted products to susceptible patients has been recommended. Many antiviral drugs, such as ganciclovir and foscarnet, have been tried with somewhat promising results in the treatment of active Cytomegalovirus infection.

## PARVOVIRUSES

It is estimated that about 1 in 10,000 to 20,000 donors harbor serum parvovirus-like virus. The virus precipitates with coagulation factor VIII and clotting factors obtained from large pools of donor plasma which can transmit the virus.[273] The infection following transfusion is usually mild and is of little significance.

## Bacterial Diseases

In recent years, improved collection and administration methods and storage in plastic bags decreased the incidence of bacterial contamination of blood. Out of 77 fatal transfusion reactions that were reported to the USFDA between 1976 and 1979, only two were caused by bacterial contamination.[274] Usually, severe reactions are caused by gram-negative organisms. Although most bacteria cannot survive storage at 4° C for prolonged periods, in recent years, endotoxin shock has been reported from contamination of blood with Yersinia *enterocolitica*.[275] These organisms proliferate under conditions of cold storage and iron enrichment from RBCs after a lag phase of 10 to 20 days. It has been suggested that blood stored for more than 25 days should be screened for endotoxin or the microorganism.

Since 1984, the storage time of platelets at room temperature has been extended from 5 to 7 days. This extended shelf-life at room temperature resulted in rapid proliferation of bacteria and severe transfusion reactions.[276] Although Salmonella and Staphylococci are most often associated with platelet contamination, other organisms, such as Escherichia *coli*, have also been implicated. Because of this risk of bacterial contamination, the USFDA recommended limiting the platelet storage to 5 days in 1986. Recently, Johns Hopkins oncology center studied the incidence of platelet-induced sepsis over a 42-month period.[277] The center found, that when compared with 4-day storage, platelets stored for 5 days produced a five-fold increase in the incidence of sepsis, indicating that platelets should be infused within 4 days of storage, whenever possible.

As previously mentioned, Trepenoma *pallidum*, the cause of syphilis, does not survive more than 3 days of storage at 4° C and thus, transmission of the disease through blood transfusion has been extremely rare. Measuring Treponemal antibodies is more sensitive

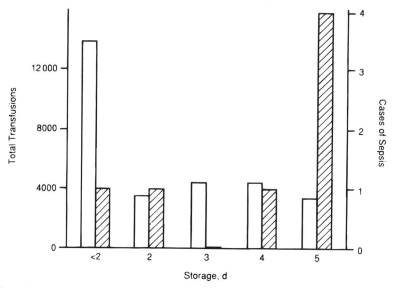

**Fig. 1–3.** Relationship of transfusion-associated sepsis to platelet storage time. Total platelet transfusions are shown in open bars with left scale. Numbers of cases of transfusion-associated sepsis are shown in cross-hatched bars with right-hand scale. From Morrow JF, Braine HG, Kickler TS, et al: Septic reactions to platelet transfusions, JAMA 1991; 266:555, with permission.

than serological testing. Brucellosis is another very rare bacterial infection that can be transmitted through blood transfusion.[278]

## Parasitic Diseases

### MALARIA

Malarial infection is endemic in Asia, Africa, and Central and South America. The incubation periods of Plasmodium *vivax* from southeast Asia and Plasmodium *falciparum* from West Africa are between 1 week and 1 month, but those of Plasmodium *ovale* and Plasmodium *malariae* are longer. Although, the disease is eradicated in the United States, many cases continue to occur because of the blood donors who come to United States from endemic areas. Normally, donors who resided in an endemic area for many years are not allowed to donate blood for 3 years, and those who temporarily visited an endemic area, are not allowed to donate blood for 6 months when they come to the United States, despite negative antibody testing. Most forms of malaria are mild and require a 3-day course of chloroquine, but sometimes *falciparum* malariae can lead to a rapid, lethal course, and requires more aggressive treatment. From 1972 to 1981 in the United States, there were

26 patients who developed malarial infections secondary to blood transfusions, four of whom died.[279] More sensitive serological tests, such as indirect immunofluorescence and ELISA, are now available for malarial testing.

### TOXOPLASMOSIS

*Toxoplasma gondii* is present in 20 to 80% of the general population and it can survive in vitro in stored blood at 4° C for many weeks. The infection, usually transmitted after the administration of leukocyte concentrates, especially in immunocompromised patients, clinically presents as fever, rash, and lymphadenopathy.[280] With severe forms of infection, many organs can be affected. Since granulocytes are rarely transfused, toxoplasmosis, secondary to transfusion, has not been reported in recent years.

### BABESIOSIS

*Babesia microti* is a parasite of rodents and is transmitted to humans by northern deer ticks. Transfusion-related babesiosis has been reported in endemic areas, such as the northeastern part of the United States.[281] The infection is usually mild and self-limited, but in patients who are asplenic or immunocompromised, the disease may result in hemolysis and renal failure, and occasionally, death.[282] Chloroquine or pentamidine and clindamycin are effective in most cases. Reported treatments even include exchange transfusion.[283]

## FILARIASIS

In nonendemic areas, only a mild allergic type of reaction develops when microfilaria are transmitted through blood transfusions, because the organisms need an insect vector for the second passage to humans to reach an adult stage.

## TRYPANOSOMIASIS

In Central and South America, the disease is transmitted by *Trypanosoma cruzi* and is called Chagas' disease. The parasites can survive many days in stored blood and can be transmitted to the recipient, resulting in significant illness.[284] To reduce the incidence of transmission, in addition to serological tests to screen the donors, sometimes gentian violet is added to blood to kill the organisms. African trypanosomiasis, or sleeping sickness, is not a transfusion problem because most carriers of the organism will have symptoms and thus, are disqualified as donors.

## LEISHMANIASIS

Leishmania parasites may circulate in polymorphonuclear leukocytes and monocytes, and can theoretically be transmitted by blood transfusions. One case of Kala-azar (visceral leishmaniosis) transmitted by *Leishmania donovani*, has been reported in a child following blood transfusion.[285] Additionally, there are only four other cases of transfusion-related Kala-azar reported in the literature. Recently, several members of the United States Armed Forces who participated in Operation Desert Shield/Storm, have been found to have acquired visceral and cutaneous leishmaniasis during their stay in the Persian Gulf. Because of this, in November 1991, the AABB issued a memorandum[286] suggesting that individuals who have traveled to the Persian Gulf area (after August 1990) should be deferred as donors of blood components until January 1993. Since no transfusion-related cases of leishmaniasis were ever diagnosed in Operation Desert Shield/Storm veterans, in January 1993, the AABB decided not to renew this recommendation.

## REFERENCES

1. Myhre BA. The first recorded blood transfusions: 1656 to 1668. *Transfusion*. 1990;30:358.
2. Frank RG Jr. *Harvey and the Oxford Physiologists: scientific ideals and social interaction.* Berkeley, Calif: University of California Press; 1981.
3. Lower R. The success of the experiment of transfusing the blood of one live animal into another. *Philos Trans R Soc Lond.* 1666;1:153.
4. Lower R. The method observed in transfusing the blood out of one animal into another. *Philos Trans R Soc Lond.* 1666; 1:353.
5. Denis JB. An extract of a letter of M. Denis prof. of philosophy and mathematics to M.*** touching the transfusion of blood, of April 2, 1667. *Philos Trans R Soc Lond.* 1667; 2:453.
6. Denis JB. A letter concerning a new way of curing sundry diseases by transfusion of blood, written to Monsieur de Montmor, Counsellor to the French King, and Master of Requests. *Philos Trans R Soc Lond.* 1667;2(27A):489.
7. Denis JB. An extract of a letter, written by J. Dennis, Doctor of Physick, and Professor of Philosophy and the Mathematicks at Paris, touching a late cure of an inveterate phrensy by the transfusion of blood. *Philos Trans R Soc Lond.* 1667;2:617.
8. Lower R, King E. An account of the experiment of transfusion, practiced upon a man in London. *Philos Trans R Soc Lond.* 1667;2:557.
9. Blundell J. Some account of a case of obstinate vomiting in which an attempt was made to prolong life by the injection of blood into the veins. *Med Chir Trans.* 1819;10:296.
10. Blundell J. Observations on transfusion of blood. *Lancet.* 1828;II:321.
11. Oberman HA. Appropriate use of plasma and plasma derivatives. In: Summers SH, Agranenko VA, eds. *Transfusion therapy: guidelines for practice.* Arlington, Va: American Association of Blood Banks; 1990.
12. Lindeman E. Simple syringe transfusion with special cannulas. *Am J Dis Child.* 1913;6:28.
13. Schmidt PJ. Transfusion in America in the eighteenth and nineteenth centuries. *N Engl J Med.* 1968;279:1319.
14. Strumia M. The development of plasma preparations for transfusions. *Ann Intern Med.* 1941;80:80.
15. Robertson OH. Transfusion of preserved red blood cells. *Br Med J.* 1918;1:691.
16. Fantus B. Therapeutics: the therapy of Cook Count Hospital. *JAMA.* 1937;109:128.
17. Fantus B, Schirmer EH. Blood preservation technic. *JAMA.* 1938;111:317.
18. Smith AU. Prevention of hemolysis during freezing and thawing of red blood cells. *Lancet.* II:910, 1950.
19. Mollison PL, Sloviter HA. Successful transfusion of previously frozen human red cells. *Lancet.* 1951;II:862.
20. Greenwalt TJ. An autobiographical perspective of blood banking. *Transfusion.* 1989;29:248.
21. Oberman HA. The history of transfusion medicine. In: Petz LD, Swisher SN, eds. *Clinical Practice of*

*Transfusion Medicine,* 2nd ed. New York, NY: Churchill Livingstone; 1989.

22. Slichter SJ. Mechanisms and management of platelet refractoriness. In: Nance SJ, ed. *Transfusion Medicine in the 1990's.* Arlington, Va: American Association of Blood Banks; 1990.

23. Neudorfer J. Über transfusionen bei anaemischen. *Oesterr Ztschr F Prakt Heild.* 1860;6:124.

24. Braxton-Hicks J. On transfusion and new mode of management. *Br Med J.* 1868;3:151.

25. Weil R. Sodium citrate in the transfusion of blood. *JAMA.* 1915;64:425.

26. Rous P, Turner P. The preservation of living red blood cells *in vitro.* II. The transfusion of kept cells. *J Exp Med.* 1916;23:239.

27. Beutler E. Erythrocyte metabolism and its relation to the liquid preservation of blood. In: Petz LD, Swisher SN, eds. *Clinical Practice of Transfusion Medicine.* 2nd ed. New York, NY: Churchill Livingstone; 1989.

28. Loutit JF, Mollison PL. Advantages of a disodium-citrate-glucose mixture as a blood preservative. *Br Med J.* 1943; 2:744.

29. Nakoa K, Wada T, Kamiyama T, et al. A direct relationship between adenosine triphosphate-level and *in vivo* viability of erythrocytes. *Nature.* 1962;194: 877.

30. Hogman CF, Hedlund K, Zetterstrom H. Clinical usefulness of red cells stored in protein-poor mediums. *N Engl J Med.* 1978; 299:1377.

31. Hogman CF, Akerblom O, Hedlund K, et al. Red cell suspensions in SAGM medium. Further experience of *in vivo* survival of red cells, clinical usefulness and plasma-saving effects. *Vox Sang.* 1983;45: 217.

32. Graham J, Buckwalter J, Hartley L, et al. Canine hemophilia: observations on the course, the clotting anomaly, and the effect of blood transfusions. *J Exp Med.* 1949;90:97.

33. Pool JG, Hershgold EJ, Pappenhagen AR. High-potency antihaemophilic factor concentrate prepared from cryoglobulin precipitate (Letter). *Nature.* 1964;203:312.

34. Aronson DL, Menaché D. Prevention of infectious disease transmission by blood and blood products. *Prog Hematol.* 1987;15:221.

35. Epstein JS. Current safety of clotting factor concentrates. *Arch Pathol Lab Med.* 1990;114:335.

36. Duke WW. The relation of blood platelets to hemorrhagic disease: description of a method for determining the bleeding time and coagulation time and report of three cases of hemorrhagic disease relieved by transfusion. *JAMA.* 1910; 55:1185.

37. Jones AL. Continuous-flow blood cell separation. *Transfusion.* 1968;8:94.

38. Routh C. Remarks statistical and general on transfusion of blood. *Med Times.* 1849;20:114.

39. Bull WT. On the intravenous injection of saline solutions as a substitute for blood. *Med Rec.* 1884; 25:6.

40. Landsteiner K. Über agglutinationserscheinungen normalen meuschlichen blutes. *Wein Klin Wochenschr.* 1901;14:1132.

41. DeCastello A, Sturli A. Über die isoagglutinine in serum gesunder und kranker menschen. *Munchen Med Wochenschr.* 1902; 49:1090.

42. Jansky J. *Kinicky Sbornik.* 1907;8:85.

43. Moss WL. *Trans Assoc Amer Physicians* 1909;24: 419.

44. Ottenberg R. Transfusion and arterial anastomosis. *Ann Surg.* 1908;47:486.

45. Landsteiner K, Weiner AS. An agglutinable factor in human blood recognized by immune serum for Rhesus blood. *Proc Soc Exp Biol.* 1940;43:223.

46. Coombs RRA, Mourant AE, Race RR. A new test for the detection of weak and "incomplete" Rh agglutinins. *Br J Exp Pathol.* 1945;26:225.

47. Sandler SG, Naiman JL, Fletcher JL. Alternative approaches to transfusion: autologous blood and directed blood donations. *Prog Hematol.* 1987;15: 183.

48. Simon TL. Public awareness and the safety of the nation's blood supply. *New Briefs.* American Association of Blood Banks; 1990;13:4.

49. De Schryner A, Meheus A. Syphilis and blood transfusion: a global perspective. *Transfusion.* 1990;30: 844.

50. Petz LD, Swisher SN. *Clinical Practice of Transfusion Medicine.* 2nd ed. New York, NY: Churchill Livingstone; 1989.

51. Centers for Disease Control: summary of notifiable diseases—United States 1987. *MMWR.* 1988;36: 39.

52. Lürman A. Eine icterusepidemie. *Berlin Klin Wochenschr.* 1885;22:20.

53. Beeson PB. Jaundice occurring one to four months after transfusion of blood or plasma: report of seven cases. *JAMA.* 1943;121:1332.

54. Blumberg BS, Gerstley BJS, Hungerford DA, et al. A serum antigen (Australia antigen) in Down's syndrome, leukemia, and hepatitis. *Ann Intern Med.* 1967;66:924.

55. Hoofnagle JH. Posttransfusion hepatitis B. *Transfusion.* 1990;30:384.

56. Hasley PB, Lave JR, Kapoor WN. The necessary and unnecessary transfusion: a critical review of reported appropriateness rates and criteria for red cell transfusions. *Transfusion.* 1994;34:110.

57. Polesky HF, Hanson MR. Transfusion-associated hepatitis C virus (non-A, non-B) infection. *Arch Pathol Lab Med.* 1989; 113:232.

58. Goldfield M, Black HC, Bill J, et al. The consequences of administering blood pretested for HBsAg by third-generation techniques: a progress report. *Am J Med Sci.* 1975;270:335.

59. Dienstag JL. Non-A, non-B hepatitis: recognition, epidemiology, and clinical features. *Gastroenterology.* 1983; 85:439.

60. Alter HJ, Purcell RH, Shih JW, et al. Detection of antibody to hepatitis C virus in prospectively followed transfusion recipients with acute and chronic non-A, non-B hepatitis. *N Engl J Med.* 1989;321: 1494.

61. Choo QL, Kuo G, Weiner AJ, et al. Isolation of a cDNA clone derived from a blood-borne non-A, non-B viral hepatitis genome. *Science.* 1989;244: 359.

62. Kuo G, Choo Q-L, Alter HJ, et al. An assay for circulating antibodies to a major etiologic virus of human non-A, non-B hepatitis. *Science.* 1989;244: 362.

63. Donahue JG, Muñoz A, Ness PM, et al. The declining risk of post-transfusion hepatitis C virus infection. *N Engl J Med.* 1992;327:369.

64. Aach RD, Stevens CE, Hollinger FB, et al. Hepatitis C virus infection in post-transfusion hepatitis. *N Engl J Med.* 1991; 325:1325.

65. Kleinman S, Alter HJ, Busch M, et al. Increased

detection of hepatitis C virus (HCV)-infected blood donors by a multiple-antigen HCV enzyme immunoassay. *Transfusion.* 1992;32:805.

66. Centers for Disease Control. Kaposi's sarcoma and *Pneumocystisis* pneumonia among homosexual men—New York and California. *MMWR.* 1981; 30:305.

67. Centers for Disease Control. Possible transfusion-associated acquired immune deficiency syndrome (AIDS)—California. *MMWR.* 1982;31:652.

68. Centers for Disease Control. Pneumocystitis carinici pneumonia among persons with hemophilia A. *MMWR.* 1982; 31:365.

69. Essex M, McLane MF, Lee TH, et al. Antibodies to human T-cell leukemia virus membrane antigens (HTLV-MA) in hemophiliacs. *Science.* 1983;221:1061.

70. Evatt BL, Stein SF, Francis DP, et al. Antibodies to human T cell leukemia virus-associated membrane antigens in haemophiliacs: evidence for infection before 1980. *Lancet.* 1983;II:698.

71. Montagnier L, Gruest J, Chamaret S. Adaptation of lymphadenopathy associated virus (LAV) to replication in EBV-transformed B lymphoblastoid cell lines. *Science.* 1984; 225:63.

72. Curran JW, Lawrence DN, Jaffee H, et al. Acquired immunodeficiency syndrome (AIDS) associated with transfusion. *N Engl J Med.* 1984;310:69.

73. Barnes A. Transfusion practice in the private hospital. *Arch Pathol Lab Med.* 1989;113:296.

74. Maffei LM, Thurer RL. Autologous blood transfusion: current issues. Arlington, Va: American Association of Blood Banks; 1988.

75. Centers for Disease Control. Update: public health service workshop on human T-lymphotropic virus type III antibody testing—United States. *MMWR.* 1985;34:477.

76. Centers for Disease Control. AIDS and human immunodeficiency virus infection in the United States: 1988 update. *MMWR.* 1989;4(suppl):38:1.

77. Selik RM, Ward JW, Buehler JW. Trends in transfusion-associated acquired immune deficiency syndrome in the United States, 1982 through 1991. *Transfusion.* 1993;33:890.

78. Cumming PD, Wallace EL, Schorr JB, et al. Exposure of patients to human immunodeficiency virus through the transfusion of blood components that test antibody-negative. *N Engl J Med.* 1989;321:941.

79. Petersen LR, Satten G, Dodd R, et al. Current estimates of the infections window period and risk of HIV infection from seronegative blood donations. In: *Programs and Abstracts of the Fifth National Forum on AIDS, Hepatitis, and Other Blood-borne Diseases.* Atlanta, GA: 1992:37.

80. Backer U, Weinauer F, Gathof G. HIV antigen screening in blood donors (Letter). *Lancet.* 1987; II:1213.

81. Menitove JE. Current risk of transfusion-associated human immunodeficiency virus infection. *Arch Pathol Lab Med.* 1990; 114:330.

82. Poiesz BJ, Ruscetti FW, Gazder AF, et al. Detection and isolation of type C retrovirus particles from fresh and cultured lymphocytes of a patient with cutaneous T-cell lymphoma. *Proc Natl Acad Sci USA.* 1980;77:7415.

83. Okochi K, Sato H, Hinuma Y. A retrospective study on transmission of adult T cell leukemia virus by blood transfusion: seroconversion in recipients. *Vox Sang.* 1984; 46:245.

84. Bove JR, Sandler SG. HTLV-1 and blood transfusion. *Transfusion.* 1988;28:93.

85. Williams AE, Fang CT, Slamon DJ, et al. Seroprevalence and epidemiological correlates of HTLV-1 infection in U.S. blood donors. *Science.* 1988;240:643.

86. Centers for Disease Control. Licensure of screening tests for antibody to human T-lymphotropic virus type 1. *MMWR.* 1988;37:736.

87. Dodd RY. Will blood products be free of infectious agents? In: Nance SJ, ed. *Transfusion Medicine in the 1990's.* Arlington, Va: American Association of Blood Banks; 1990.

88. Nelson K, Donahue J, Muñoz A, et al. Risk of transfusion-transmitted HIV-1 and HTLV-I/II. *Transfusion.* 1991; 31(suppl):47S.

89. Horsburgh CR, Holmberg SD. The global distribution of human immunodeficiency virus type 2 (HIV-2) infection. *Transfusion.* 1988;28:192.

90. Centers for Disease Control. AIDS due to HIV-2 infection—New Jersey. *MMWR.* 1988;37:33.

91. Laurence J, Siegal FP, Schattner E, et al. Acquired immunodeficiency without evidence of infection with human immunodeficiency virus types 1 and 2. *Lancet.* 1992;340:273.

92. MMWR-Morbidity Mortality Weekly Review. Unexplained CD4 T-Lymphocyte depletion in persons without evident HIV infection—United States. *MMWR.* 1992;41:541.

93. Busch MP, Holland PV. Idiopathic CD4+ T-Lymphocytopenia (ICL) and safety of blood transfusion: what do we know and what should we do? *Transfusion.* 1992;32:800.

94. Smith DK, Neal JJ, Holmberg SD, et al. Unexplained opportunistic infections and CD4+ T-Lymphocytopenia without HIV infection: an investigation of cases in the United States. *N Engl J Med.* 1993;328:373.

95. Aledort LM, Operskalski EA, Dietrich SL, et al. Low CD4+ counts in a study of transfusion safety. *N Engl J Med.* 1993;328:441.

96. Roche JK, Stengle JM. Open heart surgery and the demand for blood. *JAMA.* 1973;225:1516.

97. Graves EJ. 1991 Summary: National hospital discharge survey. *Vital Health Stat.* 1993;227:1.

98. Surgenor DM, Wallace EL, Churchill WH, et al. Red cell transfusions in coronary artery bypass surgery (DRGs 106 and 107). *Transfusion.* 1992;32:458.

99. Umlas J. Transfusion of patients undergoing cardiopulmonary bypass. *Human Pathol.* 1983;14:271.

100. Farrar RP, Hanto DW, Flye MW, et al. Blood component use in orthotopic liver transplantation. *Transfusion.* 1988;28:474.

101. Jansen J. Processing of bone marrow for allogeneic transplantation. In: Sacher RA, McCarthy LJ, Smit Sibinga CT, eds. *Processing of Bone Marrow for Transplantation.* Arlington, Va: American Association of Blood Banks; 1990.

102. Jacobson MA, Peiperl L, Volberding PA, et al. Red cell transfusion therapy for anemia in patients with AIDS and ARC: incidence, associated factors, and outcome. *Transfusion.* 1990;30:133.

103. Fischl M, Galpin JE, Levine JD, et al. Recombinant human erythropoietin for patients with AIDS

treated with zidovudine. *N Engl J Med*. 1990;322:
1488.

104. Eschbach JW, Abdulhadi MH, Browne JK, et al.
Recombinant human erythropoietin in anemic patients with end-stage renal disease: results of a phase
III multicenter clinical trial. *Ann Intern Med*. 1989;
111:992.

105. Goodnough LT, Anderson KC, Lane TA, et al. Indications and guidelines for the use of hematopoietic growth factors. *Transfusion*. 1993;33:944.

106. Surgenor DM, Wallace EL, Hao SH, et al. Collection and transfusion of blood in the United States,
1982-1988 [See comments]. *N Engl J Med*. 1990;
322:1646.

107. Wallace EL, Surgenor DM, Hao HS, et al. Collection and transfusion of blood and blood components in the United States, 1989. *Transfusion*.
1993;33:139.

108. Clark JA, Ayoub MM. Blood and component wastage report: a quality assurance function of the hospital transfusion committee. *Transfusion*. 1989;29:
139.

109. Salem-Schatz SR, Avorn J, Soumerai SB. Influence
of clinical knowledge, organizational context, and
practice style on transfusion decision making.
*JAMA*. 1990;264:476.

110. National Institutes of Health, Consensus Development Panel. Fresh frozen plasma: indications and
risks. *JAMA*. 1985; 253:551.

111. National Institutes of Health, Consensus Development Panel. Platelet transfusion therapy. *JAMA*.
1987;257:1777.

112. National Institutes of Health, Consensus Development Panel. Perioperative red blood cell transfusion. *JAMA*. 1988; 260:2700.

113. Joint Commission of Accreditation of Hospitals.
*Accreditation manual for hospitals*. Chicago, Ill:
Joint Commission of Accreditation of Hospitals;
1985.

114. Joint Commission of Accreditation of Hospitals.
*Medical staff monitoring functions: blood usage re-
view*. Chicago, Ill: Joint Commission of Accreditation of Hospitals; 1987.

115. Campbell JA. Appropriateness of blood product ordering: quality assurance techniques. *Lab Med*.
1989;20:15.

116. Toy PTCY. Effectiveness of transfusion audits and
practice guidelines. *Arch Pathol Lab Med*. 1994;
118:435.

117. Oberman HA. *General principles of blood transfusion*. Chicago, Ill: American Medical Association;
1985.

118. Friedman BA, Oberman HA, Chadwick AR, et al.
The maximum surgical blood order schedule and
surgical blood use in the United States. *Transfusion*. 1976;16:380.

119. Boral LI, Henry JB. The type and screen: a safe
alternative and supplement in selected surgical procedures. *Transfusion*. 1977;17:163.

120. Yomtovian R, Ceynar J, Kepner J. Autologous
blood donors: motivations and attitudes. *Transfusion*. 1986;26:599. Abstract.

121. Grant F. Autotransfusion. *Ann Surg*. 1921;74:253.

122. Milles G, Langston HT, Dalessandro W. *Autologous
Transfusion*. Springfield, Ill: Charles C. Thomas
Co; 1971.

123. Cuello L, Vazquez E, Perez V, et al. Autologous
blood transfusion in cardiovascular surgery. *Bol
Assoc Med P Rico*. 1966;58:93.

124. Cuello L, Vazquez E, Perez V, et al. Autologous
blood transfusion in cardiovascular surgery. *Transfusion*. 1967; 7:309.

125. Cuello L, Vazquez E, Rios R, et al. Autologous
transfusion in thoracic and cardiovascular surgery.
*Surgery*. 1967; 62:814.

126. Newmann MM, Hamstra R, Block M. Use of
banked autologous blood in elective surgery.
*JAMA*. 1971;218:861.

127. Sands CJ, Wood RP II, Schoonhoven PV. Autologous transfusions in head and neck surgery. *Arch
Otolaryngol*. 1968;88:103.

128. Check WA. Autologous blood use growing. *CAP
Today*. 1990; 4:1.

129. Renner SW, Howanitz PJ, Bachner P. Preoperative
autologous blood donation in 612 hospitals: a college of American pathologists' Q-probes study of
quality issues in transfusion medicine. *Arch Pathol
Lab Med*. 1992;116:613.

130. Page PL. Controversies in transfusion medicine: directed blood donations. *Transfusion*. 1989;29:65.

131. Widman F. *Standards for blood banks and transfusion services*. 14th ed. Arlington, Va: American Association of Blood Banks; 1991.

132. Cordell RR, Yalon VA, Cigahn-Haskell C, et al.
Experience with 11,916 designated donors. *Transfusion*. 1986;26:484.

133. Fischer A, Pura L, Smith L, et al. Safety and effectiveness of directed blood donation in a large teaching hospital. *Transfusion*. 1986;26:600. Abstract.

134. Shah VP, Molstad JR, Segall SL, et al. A hospital
donor room's three-year experience with directed
donations *Transfusion*. 1986;26:599. Abstract.

135. Brecher ME, Taswell HF, Clare DE, et al. Minimal-
exposure transfusion and the committed donor.
*Transfusion*. 1990; 30:599.

136. Strauss RG. Directed and limited-exposure blood
donations for infants and children. *Transfusion*.
1990;30:68.

137. McLeod BC, Sassetti RJ, Cole ER, et al. A high-
potency single-donor cryoprecipitate of known factor VIII content dispensed in vials. *Ann Intern
Med*. 1987;106:35.

138. McLeod BC, Sassetti RJ, Cole ER, et al. Long-term
frequent plasma exchange donation of cryoprecipitate. *Transfusion*. 1988;28:307.

139. Giles KH. Code of federal regulations: food and
drugs, Title 21. Washington DC: Office of the Federal Register, National Archives and Records Administration; 1991.

140. Walker RH. *Technical manual*. 10th ed. Arlington,
Va: American Association of Blood Banks; 1990.

141. Gibbee JW, Ness PM. Fibrin glue: the perfect operative sealant. *Transfusion*. 1990;30:741.

142. Lupinetti FM, Stoney WS, Alford WC Jr, et al.
Cryoprecipitated-topical thrombin glue: initial ex-
perience in patients undergoing cardiac operations.
*J Thorac Cardiovasc Surg*. 1985;90:502.

143. Marengo-Rowe AJ. Advances in hemostatic and
thrombolytic therapy. In: Nance SJ, ed. *Transfusion
Medicine in the 1990's*. Arlington, Va: American Association of Blood Banks; 1990.

144. Colombo M, Mannucci PM, Carnelli V, et al.
Transmission of non-A, non B hepatitis by heat-
treated factor VIII concentrate. *Lancet*. 1985;II:1.

145. White GC II, Matthews TJ, Weinhold KJ, et al.
HTLV-III seroconversion associated with heat-
treated factor VIII concentrate. *Lancet*. 1986;I:
611.

146. van den Berg W, ten Cate JW, Breederveld C, et al. Seroconversion to HTLV-III in haemophiliac given heat-treated factor VIII concentrate. *Lancet.* 1986;I:803.

147. Schimpf K, Mannucci PM, Kreuz W, et al. Absence of hepatitis after treatment with a pasteurized factor VIII concentrate in patients with hemophilia and no previous transfusion. *N Engl J Med.* 1987;316:918.

148. Goedert JJ, Kessler CM, Aledort LM, et al. A prospective study of human immunodeficiency virus type 1 infection and the development of AIDS in subjects with hemophilia. *N Engl J Med.* 1989;321:1141.

149. Schimpf K, Brackmann HH, Kreuz W, et al. Absence of anti-human immunodeficiency virus types 1 and 2 seroconversion after the treatment of hemophilia A or von Willebrand's disease with pasteurized factor VIII concentrate. *N Engl J Med.* 1989;321:1148.

150. Zimmerman TS. Purification of factor VIII:C by monoclonal antibody affinity chromatography. *Semin Hematol.* 1988; 25:25.

151. Prince AM, Horowitz B, Brotman B, et al. Inactivation of hepatitis B and Hutchinson strain non-A, non-B hepatitis viruses by exposure to tween 80 and ether. *Vox Sang.* 1984; 46:36.

152. Horowitz B, Wiebe ME, Lippin A, et al. Inactivation of viruses in labile blood derivatives. I. Disruption of lipid enveloped viruses by tri(n-butyl) phosphate detergent combinations. *Transfusion.* 1985;25:516.

153. Piet MPJ, Chin S, Prince AM, et al. Inactivation of viruses in plasma on treatment with tri(n-butyl) phosphate (TNBP) detergent mixtures. *Thromb Haematol.* 1987;58:370. Abstract.

154. Manucci PM. Outbreak of hepatitis A among Italian patients with haemophilia. *Lancet.* 1992;339:819.

155. Aronson DL. The development of technology and capacity for the production of factor VIII for the treatment of hemophilia A. *Transfusion.* 1990;30:748.

156. Addiego JE Jr, and Kogenate Study Group. Use of recombinant factor VIII (Kogenate) for successful hemostasis of 39 surgical procedures in 34 patients. *Transfusion.* 1993; 33:875.

157. Bray GL, High K, Liu-Maruya S, et al. Results of a clinical trial using recombinant factor VIII in previously untreated patients with hemophilia A. *Transfusion.* 1993;33:876.

158. Kasper CK, and the Kogenate Study Group. Safety and efficacy of recombinant factor VIII (Kogenate). *Transfusion.* 1993; 33:875.

159. Horowitz B, Williams B, Rywkin S, et al. Inactivation of viruses in blood with albumin phthalocyanine derivatives. *Transfusion.* 1991;31:102.

160. Sayers MH, Anderson KC, Goodnough LT, et al. Reducing the risk for transfusion-transmitted cytomegalovirus infection. *Ann Intern Med.* 1992;116:55.

161. Long KE, Yomtovian R, Kida M, et al. Time-dependant loss of surface complement regulatory activity during storage of donor blood. *Transfusion.* 1993;33:294.

162. Rao GHR, Escolar G, White JG. Biochemistry, physiology, and function of platelets stored as concentrates. *Transfusion.* 1993;33:767.

163. Huggins, CE. Practical preservation of blood by freezing. In: *Red Cell Freezing: A Technical Workshop.* Washington, DC: American Association of Blood Banks; 1973:31.

164. Asmundson T, Kilburn KH. Survival of acute respiratory failure: a study of 239 episodes. *Ann Intern Med.* 1969; 70:471.

165. Wilson RF, Walt AF. Blood replacement. In: Walt AF, Wilson RF, eds. *Management of Trauma: Practices and Pitfalls.* Philadelphia, Pa: Lea & Febiger; 1975:131.

166. Stehling LS. Surgery without transfusion: the anesthesiologist's view point. Presented at the NIH Consensus Conference on Perioperative RBC Transfusion; June 1988; Bethesda, Md.

167. Czer LSC, Shoemaker WP. Optimal hematocrit value in critically ill postoperative patients. *Surg Gynecol Obstet.* 1978;147:363.

168. Friedman BA, Burns TL, Schork MA. An analysis of blood transfusion of surgical patients by sex: a quest for the transfusion trigger. *Transfusion.* 1980; 20:179.

169. Bourke DL, Smith TC. Estimating allowable hemodilution. *Anesthesiology.* 1974;41:609.

170. Kallos T, Smith TC. Replacement of intraoperative blood loss. *Anesthesiology.* 1974;41:293.

171. Furman EB. Intraoperative fluid therapy. *Int Anesthesiol Clin.* 1975;13:133.

172. Varat MA, Adolph RJ, Fowler NO. Cardiovascular effects of anemia. *Am Heart J.* 1972;83:415.

173. Graettinger JS, Parsons RL, Campbell JA. A correlation of clinical and hemodynamic studies in patients with mild and severe anemia with and without congestive heart failure. *Ann Intern Med.* 1963;58:617.

174. Colozzi AE. Clamping of the umbilical cord: its effect on the placental transfusion. *N Engl J Med.* 1954;250:629.

175. Furman EB. Pediatric anesthesia: fluid balance. Presented at the ASA Refresher Course Lectures, 1977.

176. Manno CS, Wood K, Kim HC, et al. The hemostatic benefit of frozen whole blood after open heart surgery in children. *Blood.* 1989;74:100A.

177. Ellison N, Silberstein LE. A commentary on three consensus development conferences on transfusion medicine. *Anesthesiol Clin North Am.* 1990;8:609.

178. Surgenor DM, Wallace EL, Hale SG, et al. Changing patterns of blood transfusions in four sets of United States hospitals, 1980 to 1985. *Transfusion.* 1988;28:513.

179. Busch MP. Retroviruses and blood transfusions: the lessons learned and the challenge yet ahead, In: Nance SJ, ed. *Blood Safety: Current Challenges.* Bethesda, Md: American Association of Blood Banks; 1992.

180. Chaplin H Jr, Beutler E, Collins JA, et al. Current status of red-cell preservation and availability in relation to the developing national blood policy. *N Engl J Med.* 1974; 291:68.

181. Telischi M, Hoiberg R, Rao KPP, et al. The use of frozen thawed erythrocytes in blood banking. *Am J Clin Pathol.* 1977;68:250.

182. Haugen RK. Hepatitis after the transfusion of frozen red cells and washed red cells. *N Engl J Med.* 1979;301:393.

183. National Institutes of Health. National Blood Resource Education Program. Transfusion alert: use of autologous blood. NIH Publication No. 89-2974a, May 1989.

184. White GC II, McMillan CW, Kindon HS, et al.

Use of recombinant antihemophilic factor in the treatment of two patients with classic hemophilia. *N Engl J Med.* 1989; 320:166.

185. Bland JHL, Laver MB, Lowenstein E. Vasodilator effect of commercial 5% plasma protein fraction solutions. *JAMA.* 1973;224:1721.

186. Mollison PL, Engelfriet CP, Contreras M. Blood transfusion in clinical medicine. 8th ed. Oxford, England: Blackwell Scientific Publications; 1987.

187. Edinger SE. A closer look at fatal transfusion reactions. *Med Lab Observ.* 1985;17:41.

188. Seyfried H, Walewska J. Immune hemolytic transfusion reactions. *World J Surg.* 1987;11:25.

189. Moore SB, Taswell HS, Pineda AA, et al. Delayed hemolytic reaction. *Am J Clin Pathol.* 1980;74:94.

190. Linden JV, Paul B, Dressler KP. A report of 104 transfusion errors in New York state. *Transfusion.* 1992;32:601.

191. Linden JV, Kaplan HS. Transfusion errors: causes and effects. *Transfus Med Rev.* 1994;8:169.

192. Food and Drug Administration Bulletin. Information of importance to physicians and other health professionals. *FDA Bulletin.* 1989;19.

193. Pineda AA, Brzica SM Jr, Taswell HF. Hemolytic transfusion reaction: recent experience in a large blood bank. *Mayo Clin Proc.* 1978;53:378.

194. Lopas H. Immune hemolytic transfusion reactions in monkeys. Activation of the kallikrein system. *Am J Physiol.* 1973; 225:372.

195. Barry KG, Malloy JP. Oliguric renal failure: evaluation and therapy by the intravenous infusion of mannitol. *JAMA.* 1962;179:510.

196. Birtch AG, Zakheim RM, Jones LG, et al. Redistribution of renal blood flow produced by furosemide and ethacrynic acid. *Circ Rev.* 1967;21:869.

197. Seager OA, Nesmith MA, Begelman KA, et al. Massive acute hemodilution for incompatible blood reaction. *JAMA.* 1974; 229:788.

198. Goldfinger D, Lowe C. Prevention of adverse reactions to blood transfusion by the administration of saline washed red blood cells. *Transfusion.* 1981; 21:277.

199. Ahrons S, Kissmeyer-Nielsen F. Serological investigations of 1,358 transfusion reactions in 74,000 transfusions. *Dan Med Bull.* 1968;15:259.

200. Thompson JA, Severson CD, Parmely MJ, et al. Pulmonary hypersensitivity reactions induced by transfusion of non-HLA leukoagglutinins. *N Engl J Med.* 1971;284:1120.

201. Popovsky MA, Abel MD, Moore SB. Transfusion-related acute lung injury associated with passive transfer of anti-leukocyte antibodies. *Am Rev Resp Dis.* 1983;128:185.

202. Greenberger PA. Plasma anaphylaxis and immediate type reactions. In: Rossi EC, Simon TL, Moss GS, eds. *Principles of Transfusion Medicine.* Baltimore, Md: Williams & Wilkins; 1991.

203. Solanki D, McCurdy PR. Delayed hemolytic transfusion reactions: an often-missed entity. *JAMA.* 1978;239:729.

204. Hewitt PE, McIntyre EA, Devenish A, et al. A prospective study of the incidence of delayed hemolytic transfusion reactions following perioperative blood transfusion. *Br J Haemat.* 1988;69:541.

205. Greenwalt TJ. Pathogenesis and management of hemolytic transfusion reactions. *Semin Hematol.* 1981;18:84.

206. Luban NLC, Ness PM. Irradiation of blood products: invited comment. *Transfusion.* 1985;25:301.

207. Drobyski W, Thibodeau S, Truitt RL, et al. Third party mediated graft rejection and graft-versus-host disease after T-cell depleted bone marrow transplantation, as demonstrated by hypervariable DNA probes and HLA-DR polymorphism. *Blood.* 1989; 74:2285.

208. Opelz G, Sengar DPS, Mickey MR, et al. The effect of blood transfusions on subsequent kidney transplants. *Transplant Proc.* 1973;5:253.

209. Blamey RW, Knapp MS, Burden RP, et al. Blood transfusion and renal allograft survival. *Br Med J.* 1978;1:138.

210. Terasaki PI, Perdue S, Ayoub G, et al. Reduction of accelerated failures by transfusion. *Transplant Proc.* 1982; 14:251.

211. van Rood JJ. Pretransplant blood transfusion: sure! But how and why? *Transplant Proc.* 1983;15:915.

212. Opelz G. Improved kidney graft survival in non-transfused recipients. *Transplant Proc.* 1987;19: 149.

213. Yantt CL. Red blood cells for cancer patients. *Lancet.* 1981;II:363.

214. Burrows L, Tartter P. Effect of blood transfusion on colonic malignancy recurrence rate. *Lancet.* 1982;II:662.

215. Heal JM, Chuang C, Blumberg N. Perioperative blood transfusions and prostate cancer recurrence and survival. *Am J Surg.* 1988;156:374.

216. Stephenson KR, Steenberg SM, Hughes KS, et al. Perioperative blood transfusions are associated with decreased time to recurrence and decreased survival after resection of liver metastasis. *Ann Surg.* 1988; 208:679.

217. Arnoux R, Corman J, Peloquin A, et al. Adverse effect of blood transfusions on patient survival after resection of rectal cancer. *Can J Surg.* 1988;31: 121.

218. Ottino G, De Paulis R, Pansini S, et al. Major sternal wound infection after open heart surgery: a multivariate analysis of risk factors in 2,579 consecutive operative procedures. *Ann Thorac Surg.* 1987;44: 173.

219. Dellinger EP, Oreskovich MR, Wertz MJ, et al. Risk of infection following laparotomy for penetrating abdominal injury. *Arch Surg.* 1984;119:20.

220. Tartter PI. Blood transfusion and infectious complications following colorectal cancer surgery. *Br J Surg.* 1988; 75:789.

221. Tartter PI, Driefuss RM, Malon AM, et al. Relationship of postoperative septic complications and blood transfusions in patients with Crohn's disease. *Am J Surg.* 1988;155:43.

222. Waymack JP, Gallon L, Barcelli V, et al. Effect of blood transfusion on immune function. *Arch Surg.* 1987;122:56.

223. Donnell CA, Daniel SJ, Ferrara JJ. Fibrinogen degradation products in fresh frozen plasma. *Am Surg.* 1987;55:505.

224. Stephan RN, Kisala JM, Dean RE, et al. Effect of blood transfusion on antigen presentation function and on interleukin 2 generation. *Arch Surg.* 1988; 123:235.

225. Blumberg N, Heal JM, Murphy P, et al. Association between transfusion of whole blood and recurrence of cancer. *Br Med J.* 1986;293:530.

226. Shulman NR, Aster RW, Leitner A, et al. Immuno reactions involving platelets. V. Post-transfusion purpura due to a complement-fixing antibody against a genetically controlled platelet antigen: a

proposed mechanism for thrombocytopenia and its relevance in "autoimmunity." *J Clin Invest.* 1961; 40:1597.

227. Harrison GG, Bird AR, Jacobs P, et al. Method for the safe and rapid pretransfusion warming of stored blood: an in vitro and in vivo evaluation of a radio-frequency (RF) instrument. *J Clin Apheresis.* 1992; 7:12.

228. Yhl L, Pacini D, Kruskall MS. A comparative study of blood warmer performance. *Anesthesiology.* 1992;77:1022.

229. Durham CM, Belzberg H, Lyles R, et al. The rapid infusion system: a superior method for the resuscitation of hypovolemic trauma patients. *Resuscitation.* 1991;21:207.

230. Rothen HU, Lauber R, Mosimann M. An evaluation of the rapid infusion system. *Anaesthesia.* 1992;47:597.

231. Iverson KV, Knauf MA. Confirmation of high blood flow rates through $150\mu$ filter/high-flow tubing. *J Emerg Med.* 1990; 8:689.

232. Landow L, Shahnarian A Efficacy of large-bore intravenous fluid administration sets designed for rapid volume resuscitation. *Crit Care Med.* 1990; 18,540.

233. Bunker JP, Bendixen HH, Murphy BS. Hemodynamic effects of intravenously administered sodium citrate. *N Engl J Med.* 1962;266:372.

234. Howland WS, Jacobs RG, Goulet AH. An evaluation of calcium administration during rapid blood replacement. *Anesth Analg.* 1960;39:557.

235. Bunker JP. Metabolic effects of blood transfusion. *Anesthesiology.* 1966;27:446.

236. Urban P, Scheidegger D, Buchmann B, et al. Cardiac arrest and blood ionized calcium levels. *Ann Intern Med.* 1988; 109:110.

237. Denlinger JK, Narhwold ML, Gibbs PS, et al. Hypocalcemia during rapid blood transfusion in anaesthetized man. *Br J Anaesth.* 1976;48:995.

238. Dzik WH, Kirkley SA. Citrate toxicity during massive blood transfusion. *Transfusion Med Rev.* 1988; 2:76.

239. Marquez J, Martin D, Virji MA, et al. Cardiovascular depression secondary to ionic hypocalcemia during hepatic transplantation in humans. *Anesthesiology.* 1986;65:457.

240. Carmichael D, Hosty T, Kastl D, et al. Hypokalemia and massive transfusion. *South Med J.* 1984;77:315.

241. Collins JA, James PM, Bredenberg CE, et al. The relationship between transfusion and hypoxemia in combat casualties. *Ann Surg.* 1978;188:513.

242. Snyder EL, Hezzey A, Barash PG, et al. Microaggregate blood filtration in patients with compromised pulmonary function. *Transfusion.* 1982;22: 21.

243. Snyder EL, Bookbinder M. Role of microaggregate blood filtration in clinical medicine. *Transfusion.* 1983;23:460.

244. Sinko GE. Microaggregate filters and neonatal patients. Transfusion 1983;23:537.

245. Solis RT, Walker BD. Does a relationship exist between massive blood transfusion and the adult respiratory distress syndrome? If so, what are the best preventive measures? *Vox Sang.* 1977;32:319.

246. Arrington P, McNamara JJ. Mechanisms of microaggregate formation in stored blood. *Ann Surg.* 1970;171:329.

247. Roughton FJW, Darling RC. The effect of carbon monoxide on the oxyhemoglobin dissociation curve. *Am J Physiol.* 1944; 141:17.

248. Aronow WS. Aggravation of angina pectoris by 2% carboxyhemoglobin. *Am J Med.* 1977;63:904.

249. Tomoda A, Tanishima K, Tanimoto K, et al. Metform hemoglobin in long term stored blood. *Vox Sang.* 1980; 38:205.

250. Zeller WP, Eyzaguirre M, Hannigan J, et al. Fast hemoglobins and red blood cell metabolites in citrate phosphate dextrose adenosine stored blood. *Ann Clin Lab Sci.* 1985;15:61.

251. Uchida J, Tashiro C, Hee Koo Y, et al. Carboxyhemoglobin and methemoglobin levels in banked blood. *J Clin Anesth.* 1990;2:86.

252. Gordeuk VR, Bacon BR, Brittenham GM. Iron overload: causes and consequences. *Ann Rev Nutr.* 1987;7:485.

253. Cohen A, Martin M, Schwartz E. Depletion of excessive liver iron stores with deferoxamine. *Br J Haematol.* 1984;58:369.

254. Wolfe L, Oliveri N, Salan D, et al. Prevention of cardiac disease by subcutaneous deforoxamine in patients with thalassemia major. *N Engl J Med.* 1985;312:1600.

255. Rosenberg SA, Lotze MT, Muul LM. et al. A progress report on the treatment of 157 patients with advanced cancer using lymphokine-activated killer cells and interleukin-2 or high dose interleukin-2 alone. *N Engl J Med.* 1987;316:889.

256. Rosina F, Saracco G, Rizzetto M. Risk of post-transfusion infection with the hepatitis delta virus: a multicenter study. *N Engl J Med.* 1985;312:1488.

257. Grady GF, Lee VA, Prince AM, et al. Hepatitis B immune globulin for accidental exposures among medical personnel: final report of a multicenter controlled trial. *J Infect Dis.* 1978;138:625.

258. Lancaster D, Elam S, Kaiser AB. Immunogenicity of the intradermal route of hepatitis B vaccination with the use of recombinant hepatitis B vaccine. *Am J Infect Control.* 1989;17:126.

259. Szmuness W, Stevens CE, Olesko WR, et al. Passive-active immunization against hepatitis B: immunogenicity studies in adult Americans. *Lancet.* 1981;I:575.

260. Kiotz F, Debonne JM. Prognosis and treatment of chronic viral hepatitis. *Med Trop.* 1991;51:15.

261. Horsburgh CR, Ow C-Y, Jason J, et al. Duration of human immunodeficiency Virus infection before detection of antibody. *Lancet.* 1989;II:637.

262. Hewlet IK, Gregg RA, Ou C-Y, et al. Detection in plasma of HIV-1 specific DNA and RNA by polymerase chain reaction before and after seroconversion. *J Clin Immunoassay.* 1988; 11:161.

263. Petersen LR, Satten G, Dodd R, et al. Duration of time from onset of human immunodeficiency virus type 1 infectiveness to development of detectable antibody: the HIV Seroconversion Study Group. *Transfusion.* 1994;34:283.

264. Krown SE. Interferon and other biologic agents for the treatment of Kaposi's sarcoma. *Hematol/Oncol Clin N Am.* 1991;5:311.

265. Rosenblatt JD, Chen ISY, Wachsman W. Infection with HTLV-1 and HTLV-II: evolving concepts. *Semin Hematol.* 1988; 25:230.

266. Perez G, Ortiz-Interian C, Lee H, et al. Human immunodeficiency virus and human T-cell leukemia virus type I in patients undergoing maintenance hemodialysis in Miami. *Am J Kidney Dis.* 1989;14: 39.

267. Gibbs WN, Lofters WS, Campbell M. Non-Hodgkin's lymphoma in Jamaica and its relation to adult T-cell leukemia-lymphoma. *Ann Intern Med.* 1987;106:361.

268. Henle W, Henle G, Scriba M, et al. Antibody responses to the Epstein-Barr virus and cytomegalovirus after open heart and other surgery. *N Engl J Med.* 1979;282:1068.

269. Holland PV, Schmidt PA. *Standards for Blood Banks and Transfusion Services.* 12th ed. Arlington, Va: American Association of Blood Banks; 1987.

270. Grob JP, Grundy JE, Prentice HG, et al. Immune donors can protect marrow-transplant recipients from severe cytomegalovirus infections. *Lancet.* 1987;I:774.

271. Meyers JD, Leszczynski J, Zaia JA, et al. Prevention of cytomegalovirus infection by cytomegalovirus immune globulin after marrow transplantation. *Ann Intern Med.* 1983;98:442.

272. Snydman DR, Werner BG, Heinze-Lacey B, et al. Use of cytomegalovirus immune globulin to prevent cytomegalovirus disease in renal transplant recipients. *N Engl J Med.* 1987; 317:1049.

273. Mortimer PP, Luban NLC, Kelleher JF, et al. Transmission of serum parvovirus—like virus by clotting factor concentrates. *Lancet.* 1983;II:482.

274. Myhre BA. Fatalities from blood transfusion. *JAMA.* 1980; 244:1333.

275. Centers for Disease Control: Report: yersinia enterocolitica bacteremia and endotoxin shock associated with red blood cell transfusions—United States 1991. *JAMA.* 1991;265:2174.

276. Braine HG, Kickler TS, Charache P, et al. Bacterial sepsis secondary to platelet transfusion: an adverse effect on extended storage at room temperature. *Transfusion.* 1986; 26:391.

277. Morrow JF, Braine HG, Kickler TS, et al. Septic reactions to platelet transfusions. *JAMA.* 1991; 266:555.

278. Wood EE. Brucellosis as a hazard of blood transfusion. *Br Med J.* 1955;1:27.

279. Guerrero IC, Weniger BC, Schults MG. Transfusion malaria in the United States: 1972-1981. *Ann Intern Med.* 1983;99:221.

280. Siegel SE, Lunde MN, Yelderman AH, et al. Transfusion of toxoplasmosis by leukocyte transfusions. *Blood.* 1971; 37:388.

281. Smith RP, Evans AT, Popovsky M, et al. Transfusion acquired babesiosis and failure of antibiotic treatment. JAMA 1986; 256:2726.

282. Rosner F, Zarrabi MH, Benach J, et al. Babesiosis in splenectomized adults: review of 22 reported cases. *Am J Med.* 1984;76:696.

283. Jacoby GA, Hunt JV, Kosinski KS, et al. Treatment of transfusion-transmitted babesiosis by exchange transfusion. *N Engl J Med.* 1980;303:1098.

284. Schumunis GA. Chagas' disease and blood transfusion. In: Dodd RY, Barker LF. eds. *Infection, Immunity, and Blood Transfusion.* New York, NY: Alan R. Liss; 1985:127.

285. Peltola H, Rapola J, Jokipii L. Fever, hepatosplenomegaly and hypergammaglobulenemia caused by Kala-azar in a child. *Duodecim.* 1980;96:1145.

286. AABB. *Memorandum 91-14.* American Association of Blood Banks; November 1991.

287. Lee CL, Henry JB. Blood banking and hemotherapy. In: Henry JB, ed. *Todd, Sanford, Davidsohn Clinical Diagnosis and Management by Laboratory Methods.* Philadelphia, Pa: WB Saunders Co; 1984.

288. Simon TL, Marcus CS, Nelson EJ. Effects of AS-3 nutrient-additive solution on 42 and 49 days of storage of red cells. *Transfusion.* 1987;27:178.

289. Luban NLC, Strauss RG, Hume HA. Commentary on the safety of red cells preserved in extended-storage media for neonatal transfusions. *Transfusion.* 1991;31:229.

290. Miller RD: Transfusion therapy. In: Miller RD, ed. *Anesthesia.* 3rd ed. New York, NY: Churchill Livingstone; 1990:1467-1499.

# 2

# COAGULATION AND HEMOSTASIS

*Edward A. Czinn and Juan R. Chediak*

## INTRODUCTION

Nature has designed a unique and complex hemostatic system that normally limits the amount of hemorrhage and blood loss associated with damage to blood vessels. However, excessive hemorrhage may occur when the hemostatic system is overwhelmed by wounds to major blood vessels or when hemostatic mechanisms are impaired by congenital and acquired disorders. Dilution and/or consumption of coagulation factors may also be associated with secondary bleeding and excessive hemorrhage.

The appropriate utilization of blood and blood products requires a fundamental understanding of coagulation and hemostasis. This knowledge is essential in order to both minimize perioperative bleeding in the surgical patient and prevent unnecessary transfusion of blood products. This chapter addresses basic concepts necessary to evaluate normal and abnormal hemostasis including: (1) physiology of normal hemostasis; (2) clinical tests and monitors used to evaluate hemostatic mechanisms; and (3) pathophysiology of common inherited and acquired hemostatic disorders. For those patients in whom a hemostatic abnormality exists, rationale will be provided for selecting among the available forms of treatment.

## NORMAL HEMOSTASIS: AN OVERVIEW

Normal hemostasis is dependent on precisely regulated interactions between endothelial cells of the blood vessel wall, subendothelium, platelets, and plasma coagulation factors. Normal endothelial cells have a thromboresistant surface that allows blood to maintain its fluid nature as it circulates throughout the body. When a blood vessel is injured, circulating blood elements become exposed to the highly thrombogenic subendothelium which initiates a series of events designed to minimize blood loss. Within seconds of the vessel injury, activated platelets aggregate, forming a hemostatic plug in an initial process called primary hemostasis. These series of events are superimposed by secondary hemostasis, a process in which the plasma coagulation system is activated and a definitive fibrin clot is formed. Primary and secondary hemostasis are closely linked, in that activated platelets stimulate the plasma coagulation system, and products of the plasma coagulation system (i.e., thrombin) stimulate platelet aggregation.

## COMPONENTS OF THE COAGULATION SYSTEM

### Endothelium and Subendothelium

In addition to its thromboresistant surface, endothelial cells of vessels possess both antithrombotic and prothrombotic factors (Table 2–1). Normally, these opposing factors are in balance, maintaining the thromboresistant environment; however, even minor distur-bances in the vasculature can activate either one of these factors. Activation of antithrombotic factors may lead to ineffective hemostasis and excessive bleeding, while activation of prothrombotic factors promote clotting and thrombosis.[1]

Endothelial cells have several antithrombotic mechanisms that protect against the unchecked action of thrombin, the terminal enzyme of the plasma coagulation system. Thrombomodulin is a surface protein that downregulates the coagulation system by binding thrombin and activating the natural anticoagulant protein C.[2,3] The endothelium also has heparin-like molecules on its surface that potentiate the effects of antithrombin III, a plasma protein that inactivates thrombin.[4] Thrombin itself induces endothelial cells to synthesize and release prostacyclin ($PGI_2$), a prostaglandin derivative that is a potent inhibitor of platelet aggregation. In addition to these mechanisms, endothelial cells are capable of producing tissue-type plasminogen activator (tPA) which stimulates the fibrinolytic system to dissolve blood clots.

Endothelial cells are able to counterbalance these antithrombotic activities by secreting platelet-activating factor (PAF), a substance that induces platelet aggregation,[5] and synthesizing von Willebrand factor (vWF), a cofactor necessary for platelet adherence to the subendothelium. In addition, the endothelium is able to secrete plasminogen-activator inhibitor (PAI) which inhibits the fibrinolytic system from dissolving clots.[6]

Damage to the endothelial monolayer exposes blood to a highly thrombogenic subendothelial connective tissue which initiates clot formation. This connective tissue consists of

**Table 2–1.   Endothelial antithrombotic and prothrombotic factors**

| Antithrombotic factors | Prothrombotic factors |
| --- | --- |
| Thrombin inhibition<br>  Thrombomodulin conversion of protein C to<br>    activated protein C<br>  Antithrombin III acceleration of surface heparin-like<br>    molecules | Coagulation factors<br>  Tissue factor/thromboplastin |
| Platelet inhibition<br>  Prostacyclin ($PGI_2$) | Platelet aggregation<br>  von Willebrand factor<br>  Platelet activating factor (PAF) |
| Fibrinolysis enhancement<br>  Tissue plasminogen activator (tPA) | Inhibition of fibrinolysis<br>  Tissue plasminogen activator inhibitor (PAI) |

various types of compounds including fibrillar collagen, which is a potent stimulus for platelet adhesion and activation. Simultaneously, subendothelial components convert inactive coagulation factors into powerful enzymes, initiating intrinsic stimulation of the plasma coagulation system.

## Platelets

Platelets are produced by megakaryocytes in bone marrow and play a crucial role in hemostasis. Not only are platelets recruited when vascular integrity is disturbed, but they maintain the integrity of normal endothelium, as evidenced by the tendency of patients with platelet deficiencies to develop purpuric bleeding. With vascular and endothelial injury, the following sequence of platelet-mediated events occur.

### ADHESION

Platelets recognize sites of endothelial injury and become activated, adhering to exposed subendothelial collagen. von Willibrand factor (vWF) is necessary for adhesion, serving as a molecular bridge between platelets and collagen.[7] After being stimulated, platelets change their shape, utilizing their internal actin and myosin microfilaments to spread broadly and become tightly adherent.

### SECRETION

With activation, platelets secrete granules, the two major types being $\alpha$-granules and dense bodies.[8] $\alpha$-granules contain platelet-specific proteins that include fibrinogen, fibronectin, vWF, factor V, platelet-derived growth factor, and an antiheparin known as platelet factor 4. Dense bodies are rich in ionized calcium, adenosine diphosphate (ADP), histamine, epinephrine, and serotonin. Following platelet activation and granule secretion, a phospholipid complex known as platelet factor 3, becomes exposed on the platelet surface. Platelet factor 3 provides a site where several clotting factors (particularly factor X) are able to bind and ultimately form thrombin.

### PLATELET AGGREGATION

Adenosine diphosphate is a potent stimulator of platelet aggregation. Activated platelets synthesize thromboxane $A_2$ (TxA$_2$), a prostaglandin that locally increases ADP release. The aggregation associated ADP release results in an enlarging mass that serves as the primary hemostatic plug. Excessive platelet aggregation is inhibited by prostacyclin (PGI$_2$) via its ability to elevate cyclic AMP in the platelet cytoplasm. Recently, endothelium-derived relaxing factor (EDRF), one form of which is nitric oxide (NO), has similarly been shown to inhibit platelet aggregation by stimulating guanylate cyclase, increasing the level of cyclic GMP in the cytoplasm.[9]

## Plasma Coagulation System

The third component of the hemostatic process involves a series of plasma coagulation proteins which initiate the formation of a stronger hemostatic plug. This system consists of a series of reactions involving the conversion of inactive precursor enzymes (zymogens) to activated proteolytic enzymes (Fig. 2–1; Table 2–2). Traditionally, this system is divided into an extrinsic and intrinsic coagulation pathway, converging to a common pathway at the point where factor X is activated. Both pathways culminate in the formation of thrombin (factor IIa) which converts soluble fibrinogen (factor I) into fibrin clots. These reactions are accelerated by calcium, as well as various plasma cofactors and other cellular components.

Tissue factor, a form of thromboplastin, is released from injured cells and activates the extrinsic pathway of coagulation.[10] Tissue factor and factor VII form a complex which activates factor X to factor Xa. Factor Xa itself is able to activate factor VII, which further accelerates the conversion of factor X to Xa. In addition to activating factor X, factor VII also activates factor IX of the intrinsic pathway, providing an important link between the two pathways.[11]

The intrinsic pathway or contact phase of coagulation is initiated when blood makes contact with a foreign surface or abnormal vascular surface (subendothelium), activating factor XII (Hageman factor). In addition to factor XII, the intrinsic pathway requires the participation of five other clotting factors: plasma prekallikrein (PK), high molecular weight kininogen (HMWK), factor XI, factor IX (Christmas factor), and factor VIII (antihemophilic factor). Initially, factor XII, HMWK,

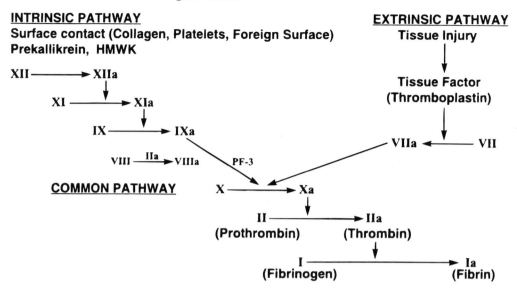

**Fig. 2–1.**   Plasma coagulation system.

and PK are thought to form a complex on subendothelial collagen. Factor XII is slowly converted to an active protease (factor XIIa) which converts PK to kallikrein. Kallikrein accelerates the activation of factor XII which activates factor XI. Factor XIa activates factor IX which joins factor VIII and factor X to form a calcium-dependent complex. Factor X becomes activated with the formation of this complex.[12]

The common pathway is the final step of the plasma coagulation system. Prothrombin (factor II) is converted to thrombin (factor IIa) in the presence of factor V, calcium, and phospholipid. The conversion of prothrombin to thrombin can occur on any phospholipid surface but is accelerated by several thousand fold on platelet surfaces. Thrombin is a powerful platelet agonist which itself induces platelet contraction in association with ADP and TxA$_2$. Thrombin then converts the fibrinogen within the platelet mass to fibrin, further stabilizing the platelet plug. The fibrin monomers produced by thrombin polymerize into an insoluble gel. These monomers join thrombin to activate factor XIII (fibrin stabilizing fac-

**Table 2–2.**   **Nomenclature and synonyms for coagulation factors**

| Roman Numeral | Descriptive name | Synonyms |
|---|---|---|
| I | Fibrinogen | |
| II | Prothrombin | |
| III | Tissue factor | Thromboplastin |
| IV | Calcium ions | |
| V | Proaccelerin | Labile factor, thrombogen, accelerator globulin (AcG) |
| VII | Proconvertin | Stable factor |
| VIII | Antihemophilic factor | Antihemophilic globulin |
| IX | Plasmin thromboplastin component (PTC) | Christmas factor |
| X | Stuart factor | Prower factor |
| XI | Plasma thromboplastin antecedent (PTA) | Antihemophilic factor C |
| XII | Hageman factor | Contact factor |
| XIII | Fibrin stabilizing factor | Laki-Lorand factor (LLF) |
| — | Prekallikrein | Fletcher factor |
| — | HMW kininogen | High molecular weight kininogen, contact activation cofactor |

tor), which stabilizes the fibrin polymer by cross-linking its individual chains. Fibronectin anchors the plug to the site of injury, completing the formation of the definitive secondary hemostatic plug.

## Fibrinolytic System

The fibrinolytic system provides an important mechanism for the dissolution of fibrin clots as vessel repair begins.[6] Fibrin is primarily digested by plasmin, a potent plasma proteolytic enzyme (Fig. 2–2). Plasminogen, a normal plasma protein produced in the liver, is converted to plasmin by the action of specific enzymes, referred to collectively as plasminogen activators. Plasminogen activators can be divided into intrinsic (blood-borne) and extrinsic factors. Intrinsic factors include fragments of factor XII, HMWK, and prekallikrein. Extrinsic factors include tissue-type plasminogen activator (tPA), urokinase, and streptokinase.

Tissue-type plasminogen activator is the primary physiologic activator of plasminogen. It is synthesized by endothelial cells and converts the plasminogen located in the fibrin clot to plasmin. Plasmin then degrades the fibrin polymer into small fragments, referred to as fibrin degradation products (FDP) or fibrin split products (FSP). Fibrin degradation products are potent anticoagulants that are ultimately removed by macrophages.

In addition to degrading fibrin, plasmin also lysis fibrinogen; however, these effects are limited by the presence of $\alpha_2$ plasmin inhibitor which rapidly inactivates free circulating plasmin. The fibrinolytic system is also regulated by plasminogen activator inhibitor (PAI), a substance secreted by endothelial cells to counterbalance the activity of tPA.

## Regulatory Mechanisms of Hemostasis

Normally, only small amounts of inactive precursor enzymes are converted into active forms, resulting in a clot that is localized to the site of injury. This tight regulation of the plasma coagulation system is important because there exists enough potential in even 1mL of blood to clot all the fibrinogen in the human body. Important regulatory mechanisms responsible for maintaining blood fluidity and ensuring tight hemostatic control include blood flow, plasma inhibitors, and hepatic clearance of activated factors.

### BLOOD FLOW

As previously discussed, the surface of normal endothelium is thromboresistant, with both antithrombotic and prothrombotic factors serving to maintain the fluid nature of blood as it circulates through the body. However, even minor disturbances in the endothe-

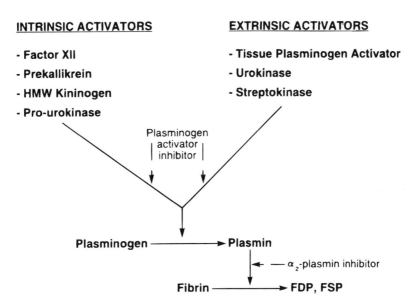

Fig. 2–2. Fibrinolytic pathway.

lium can activate prothrombotic factors, leading to the coagulation of blood. The bulk flow of blood through vessels minimizes the concentration of active coagulants at the site of injury, ensuring localized hemostasis and avoiding excessive coagulation.

## PLASMA INHIBITORS

Antithrombin III (ATIII) is an important plasma protein that inhibits the coagulation process by forming complexes with thrombin, as well as with several other coagulation factors. The rates of formation of these complexes are accelerated by heparin and the heparin-like molecules on the vascular endothelium. The ability of heparin to accelerate the action of ATIII is the basis for its potent anticoagulant activity.

Protein C and protein S (Fig. 2–3) are vitamin K-dependent plasma proteins that limit the formation of thrombin by a series of feedback mechanisms.[13] Thrombin binds to thrombomodulin on the vascular endothelium and activates protein C, which inhibits factors V and VIII, slowing the coagulation process.[14] Activated protein C also promotes fibrinolysis by inactivating a plasminogen activator inhibitor (PAI).[15] Protein S binds to activated protein C on the surface of platelets and endothelium, enhancing the anticoagulant activity of protein C.

Plasma concentrations of these inhibitors are much higher than those of the coagulation factors or plasminogen, comprising nearly 20% of the globulin fraction in human plasma. Reduced concentrations of ATIII, protein C, and protein S may lead to a hypercoagulable state.[16-18]

## HEPATIC CLEARANCE OF ACTIVATED FACTORS

The liver and reticuloendothelial systems appear to play an important role in the removal of fibrin and activated coagulation factors from the circulation. Only activated clotting factors, not precursor factors, are removed by the liver. Similarly, macrophages remove only fibrin, not fibrinogen.

# CLINICAL AND LABORATORY EVALUATION OF HEMOSTASIS

## Medical History

The medical history is universally accepted as being the first and most important aspect of the preoperative evaluation of hemostasis. The history helps localize a hemostatic defect to the platelet or plasma coagulation system. Platelet disorders generally result in bleeding from superficial sites such as skin and mucous membranes, and respond to local measures such as applying pressure to the site of injury. In contrast, disorders in the plasma coagulation system result in deep subcutaneous bleeding and bleeding into muscles, joints, and body cavities. Bleeding from plasma coagulation disorders often manifests days after an

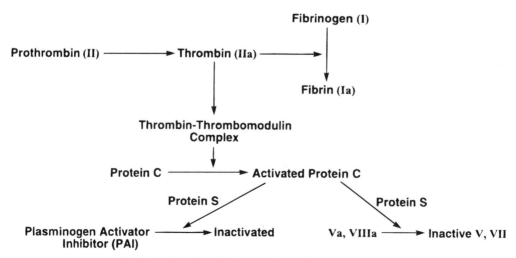

**Fig. 2–3.** Thrombin-thrombomodulin and protein C pathway.

injury and does not generally respond to local measures.

Bleeding problems during infancy and childhood, such as those associated with umbilical cord separation at birth, circumcision, tonsillectomy, and dental extraction are often the result of a congenital deficiency in a clotting factor. Menorrhagia and excessive bleeding during childbirth are common in women with thrombocytopenia and platelet disorders. Bleeding during previous surgery that was severe enough to require a blood transfusion deserves special attention. A detailed account of recently ingested medication (particularly aspirin and nonsteroidal anti-inflammatory drugs), potential exposure to toxins, and an assessment of the patient's general medical health also need to be obtained. Renal disease, hepatic disease, malignancies, and dysproteinemias can alter hemostatic responses. Finally, patients need to be questioned about nonsurgical trauma (i.e., bruising), excessive gingival bleeding, epistaxis, and gastrointestinal bleeding. Any positive findings on history warrant further laboratory investigation.

## Physical Exam

The physical exam complements the medical history in determining the patient's preoperative hemostatic status. The most easily identifiable sign of abnormal bleeding is the presence of purpuric lesions. Petechiae is another sign of abnormal bleeding that consists of pinpoint hemorrhages into the dermis. Petechia are the result of red blood cells leaking through capillaries, and are suggestive of either abnormal platelet function, thrombocytopenia, or defects in the integrity of the vascular endothelium. Larger collections of subcutaneous blood, ecchymoses (bruises), and hematomas (deeper and palpable) may result from platelet abnormalities, but more often occur with defects in the plasma coagulation system. Bleeding into joints, the retroperitoneum, and body cavities almost always occurs with defects in the plasma coagulation system. Hemarthrosis is particularly common with factor VIII and factor IX deficiencies. Bleeding into the retroperitoneum may present with symptoms of lower extremity nerve compression. The most serious complication associated with coagulation factor deficiencies

is intracerebral hemorrhage, the leading cause of death in these patients.

## Laboratory Testing: Preoperative Screening Tests

The routine use of laboratory screening tests to evaluate the hemostatic system is a controversial issue.[19-21] In the absence of positive findings on history and physical, routine preoperative screening tests have a proven low yield for identifying coagulation abnormalities and unnecessarily increase the cost of medical care.[22-25] Despite this, the ability to predict perioperative bleeding based on clinical history and physical alone has been questioned. Inadequate history taking by physicians, incomplete information provided by patients, and the occurrence of perioperative hemorrhage secondary to occult coagulopathies in the presence of "normal" clinical histories, motivate many clinicians to continue ordering screening tests.[26] Personal interest, medicolegal considerations, and academic interest are other factors that motivate physicians to order screening tests.[27]

Currently, the use and indications for preoperative coagulation screening tests vary from institution to institution. When employed, these tests should complement the history and physical and are particularly warranted in the presence of easy bruisability and/or a history of previous bleeding or blood transfusion. The most common preoperative screening tests employed are the platelet count, the bleeding time, the partial thromboplastin time, and the prothrombin time (Table 2–3).

### PLATELET COUNT

With the exception of trauma, thrombocytopenia is the most frequent cause of clinical bleeding. The platelet count is a screening test that estimates the amount of circulating platelets and closely correlates with the tendency for patients to bleed. Although many automated methods have been designed to count platelets, inspection of the blood smear is the most accurate method, and provides additional descriptive information.

A normal platelet count ranges from 150,000 to 300,000/$\mu$L. Providing that platelets are functioning normally, increased

**Table 2–3.  Perioperative screening tests for evaluating coagulation disorders**

| Coagulation disorder | Platelet count<br>nl ≈ 300,000/mm³ | BT<br>nl < 9 min | PT<br>nl ≈ 12 sec | APTT<br>nl ≈ 33–45 sec | TT<br>nl ≈ 12–20 sec |
|---|---|---|---|---|---|
| Thrombocytopenia | ↓ | ↑ | nl | nl | nl |
| Vessel defects | nl | ↑ | nl | nl | nl |
| Qualitative platelet disorders | nl | ↑ | nl | nl | nl |
| Extrinsic coagulation system | | | | | |
|   Factor VII deficiency | nl | nl | ↑ | nl | nl |
|   Factor II, V, or X deficiency | nl | nl | ↑ | ↑ | nl |
| Intrinsic coagulation system | | | | | |
|   Factor VIII & IX deficiency | nl | nl | nl | ↑ | nl |
|   von Willebrand's disease | nl | ↑ | nl | nl→↑ | nl |
| Afibrinogenemia, dysfibrinogenemia | nl | variable | nl | nl | ↑ |
| DIC, severe hepatic disease | ↓ | ↑ | ↑ | ↑ | ↑ |

bleeding does not occur until platelet counts decrease below 100,000/$\mu$L, and is not problematic until they decrease below 50,000/$\mu$L. The risk of spontaneous bleeding is increased at platelet counts below 30,000/$\mu$L. An increased risk for spontaneous intracranial hemorrhage exists with platelet counts less than 10,000/$\mu$L. Accordingly, a minimum platelet count of 50 to 100,000/$\mu$L is recommended before elective surgical procedures.

## BLEEDING TIME

The bleeding time (BT) is the most widely accepted clinical test for evaluating platelet function. It measures the interaction of platelets with blood vessels during the formation of a primary hemostatic plug. The BT assesses both platelet quantity and quality; it is prolonged with thrombocytopenia, as well as with defects in platelet function.

The most common method for performing the BT is one in which the venous pressure is maintained at 40 mm Hg by a sphygmomanometer, while standardized, template incisions of 1 mm depth and 9 mm length are made on the volar surface of the forearm.[28] The timing begins with the incision. Filter paper is used to blot the blood at 30-second intervals until blood no longer appears on the filter paper. The normal BT is 3 to 8 minutes. The BT is technician dependent and can be difficult to reproduce. Ideally, the same technician should be used when doing repeated tests on an individual patient.

The predictive value of the BT as a screening test is currently being reevaluated. A recent exhaustive review of the literature concluded that in individual patients, the bleeding time was: (1) not a specific indicator of in vivo platelet function; (2) not predictively useful in determining an adequate platelet count; and (3) not able to predict the risk of hemorrhage.[29] Other studies have shown that the bleeding time rarely provides information that could not be elicited from the clinical history and physical examination,[30] and that it may be normal in the face of aspirin-induced platelet dysfunction.[31] Nevertheless, the BT is useful in identifying bleeding disorders within large populations (i.e., epidemiologic use) and is likely to remain in use as a diagnostic screen for congenital platelet disorders until a more sensitive, specific, and cost-effective test is designed.

## ACTIVATED PARTIAL THROMBOPLASTIN TIME

The activated partial thromboplastin time (APTT) is a global screening procedure used primarily to evaluate abnormalities of the intrinsic and common pathways of the plasma coagulation system. This test is particularly sensitive to functional deficiencies of factors VIII, IX, XI, XII, prekallikrein, and HMW kininogen, but will also detect severe functional deficiencies (below 25% of normal) in factors I (fibrinogen), II (prothrombin), V, and X. The APTT is prolonged in the presence of heparin, which inhibits enzymatic action of several coagulation factors. In patients taking oral anticoagulants, the circulating levels of factors II, VII, IX, and X are depressed, resulting in a prolonged APTT, as well.

In this test, a partial thromboplastin, such

as purified soy phosphatides or cephalin, is added to citrated plasma at 37° C. Calcium is subsequently added and clot formation is initiated. Since the contact of plasma to a foreign surface can initiate clot formation, kaolin or some other plasma activator is added to citrated plasma to produce maximal "contact activation" prior to adding the partial thromboplastin and calcium.[32] Hence, the term activated partial thromboplastin time. In the past, a timer was started and the test-tube was rolled gently and observed until fibrin strands were formed. Photometric clot detection devices are presently used to determine the coagulation endpoint by measuring change in optical density of the plasma specimen. Alternatively, a mechanical mixing device with a timer known as a fibrometer, is used to assess clot formation. The normal APTT value is usually between 25 and 35 seconds.

## PROTHROMBIN TIME

The prothrombin time (PT) is a screening test for single or combined deficiencies of clotting factors of the extrinsic and common coagulation pathways (factors I, II, V, VII, and X) indicative of hereditary coagulation disorders, liver disease, or vitamin K deficiency. Unlike the APTT, the PT is sensitive to deficiencies in factor VII. Because it bypasses the early intrinsic coagulation pathway, the PT is normal when there are deficiencies in factors VIII, IX, XI, XII, prekallikrein, and HMW kininogen. The PT is also not sensitive for factor I (fibrinogen) deficiencies, unless the concentration of factor I is below 100 mg/dL. The PT is, however, exquisitely sensitive and prolonged in the presence of warfarin (coumarin) which inhibits the activity vitamin K-dependent coagulation factors (See Vitamin K Deficiency).

This test is performed by adding a thromboplastin such as rabbit brain thromboplastin to citrated blood at 37° C. Calcium is added and clot formation is initiated. The methods used to determine the clotting endpoint are similar to those described for the APTT. The normal prothrombin time has been standardized from 11 to 13 seconds.

## OTHER COAGULATION TESTS

### Thrombin Time

The thrombin time (TT) bypasses all but the final stage of the plasma coagulation system, and measures the rate of conversion of fibrinogen to fibrin. The TT is performed by adding thrombin to citrated plasma at 37° C and utilizing the methods previously described to determine the clotting endpoint (when fibrin is formed). The normal TT is 12 to 20 seconds. The thrombin time is prolonged by: (1) a fibrinogen level less than 80 mg/dL; (2) the presence of heparin; (3) the presence of high titers of fibrin degradation products (FDP); and (4) abnormal fibrinogens. Although the TT is not a routine screening test, it is valuable in identifying patients with abnormal fibrinogens in whom the APTT and PT may be only minimally prolonged. Another useful application of the TT is for the detection of heparin in patients bleeding after cardiopulmonary bypass.

### Fibrinogen Concentration

Normal fibrinogen concentrations range from 200 to 400 mg/dL. Low plasma concentrations of fibrinogen may result from consumption secondary to excessive clotting, decreased production (i.e., liver disease), and increased lysis (fibrinogenolysis).

### Fibrin Degradation Products

Fibrin degradation products (FDP) are the breakdown products of fibrinogen and fibrin. Normally, the plasma FDP concentration is less than 4 $\mu$g/mL but is increased in the face of excessive fibrinolysis. High FDP titers lead to the inhibition of fibrin polymerization and excessive bleeding. Primary fibrinolysis is rare, but can occur in association with cardiopulmonary bypass,[33] hepatic disease,[34] and in the presence of various malignancies, including cancer of the prostate and pancreas.[35] Primary fibrinolysis is best treated with an antifibrinolytic agent such as $\epsilon$-aminocaproic acid (EACA). Although $\epsilon$-aminocaproic acid is a potent inhibitor of fibrinolysis, it can cause widespread thrombosis when administered in the wrong setting. If given in excessive doses, EACA can also inhibit platelet aggregation by decreasing fibrinogen binding and lead to bleeding. Fibrin degradation products are also increased from secondary fibrinolysis, accompanying disseminated intravascular coagulation (see Disseminated Intravascular Coagulation).

### Specific Coagulation Factor Assays

Plasma samples, known to be deficient in a specific coagulation factor, are used to identify factor deficiencies in a patient's plasma. For example, if a patient has a prolonged PT, a deficiency in factors I, II, V, VII, or X may exist. The patient's plasma is mixed with plasma known to be deficient in a particular coagulation factor, and the PT is repeated. If the PT is now normal, another plasma sample deficient in a different coagulation factor is used, and the process is repeated until the PT is again prolonged. The factor-deficient plasma sample that maintains a prolonged PT when mixed with the patient's serum, identifies the deficient factor. This same test can be done with the APTT to identify deficiencies in factors VII, IX, XI, XII, prekallikrein, and HMWK.

The only coagulation factor not tested for by the PT and APTT is factor XIII. Factor XIII is activated in the presence of thrombin and causes covalent cross-linking in the fibrin clot. A specific test for factor XIII deficiency does exist; however, it is rarely used because only a small amount of factor XIII is necessary for normal hemostasis.[36]

### SPECIAL TESTS FOR PLATELET FUNCTION

The BT is the only test which directly measures the in vivo role of platelets in hemostasis. A prolonged BT in the presence of a normal platelet count, constitutes a vascular abnormality or a qualitative platelet disorder. In vitro platelet function tests are helpful in diagnosing qualitative platelet diseases.

### Platelet Aggregation

Platelet aggregation refers to the capacity of platelets to clump to one another in the presence of an aggregating agent. In this test, platelet-rich plasma is placed in a cuvette of a spectrophotometer and light transmission is measured. An aggregating agent is then added to the solution. As platelet aggregates are formed, light transmission increases. One way of assessing the sensitivity of platelets is to measure the amount of agent necessary to stimulate aggregation;[37] another way is to measure the velocity of the reaction.

The most common aggregating agents used are adenosine diphosphate (ADP), epi-nephrine, collagen, and arachidonic acid. When these agents are added to a platelet-rich plasma, thromboxane $(TxA_2)$ is formed and ADP is released from the platelets, promoting aggregation. Platelet aggregation tests are essential for diagnosing a variety of qualitative platelet disorders.[38]

### Assay for Ristocetin Cofactor

Ristocetin is an antibiotic that was withdrawn from clinical use because it produced thrombocytopenia. Ristocetin-induced thrombocytopenia occurred secondary to agglutination, an in vivo clumping of platelets. The ristocetin-cofactor refers to the ability of noral plasma to induce agglutination of normal platelets in the presence of ristocetin.[39] Ristocetin-induced platelet agglutination is decreased or absent in von Willebrand's disease and with the Bernard-Soulier syndrome, a disease in which platelets lack receptors for vWF.[40]

## PERIOPERATIVE MONITORS OF COAGULATION

### Activated Clotting Time

The activated clotting time (ACT) is a widely-used test to monitor the effectiveness of heparin therapy, particularly during procedures requiring extracorporeal circulation.[41,42] The ACT is performed by collecting small amounts of blood into a test tube containing celite or kaolin. These substances promote the activation of factor XII and, therefore, measure the intrinsic stimulation of coagulation. The tube is then placed in an automated, temperature-controlled device that measures the time for the blood to clot. Normal ACT values vary by manufacturer of the automated device but are generally between 90 to 120 seconds. Extracorporeal membrane oxygenation (ECMO) or cardiopulmonary bypass (CPB) require the use of heparin, in order to avoid clotting of blood on the foreign surfaces of the extracorporeal circuit. During prolonged use of ECMO, an ACT of 180 to 200 seconds has been shown to be effective in providing an adequate level of anticoagulation.[41] In routine CPB, an automated ACT of above 400 seconds has been recommended to avoid the formation of fibrin monomers.[43] (See Cardiopulmonary Bypass.)

## Whole Blood Viscoelastic Tests

Viscoelastic tests measure the shear elasticity (i.e, strength) of a blood clot. These tests quantitate parameters reflecting the overall coagulation process and not the specific steps involved. The Thromboelastograph (TEG, Haemoscope, Park Ridge, Illinois) and Sonoclot (Sienco, Denver, Colorado) are the viscoelastic tests presently used in clinical practice.

With thromboelastography, whole blood is placed in a metal cuvette that rotates. Mineral oil is spread on the blood surface to prevent evaporation. A pin is suspended in the blood. While the blood remains fluid, the motion of the metal cuvette does not influence the pin. As coagulation begins, fibrin strands form from the walls of the cuvette to the pin, gradually strengthening their hold on the cuvette and pin. The shear elasticity of the blood clot is transferred to the pin, which is recorded by a moving pen on thermal paper (Fig. 2–4).

The thromboelastograph produces a tracing which provides information about the entire clotting process including cellular and humoral interactions between red blood cells, platelets, plasma coagulation factors, and calcium. The reaction time (R) measures the onset of clot formation, and is the time necessary for initial fibrin formation (normal = 7 to 14 minutes). The R is prolonged by anticoagulants and factor deficiencies, and shortened by hypercoagulable conditions. The K time measures the time from R, or the beginning of clot formation, to a fixed level of clot firmness (amplitude of 20 mm). The K time measures the speed of fibrin/platelet interaction, including fibrin cross-linking (normal = 3 to 7 minutes). The K time is shortened by increased platelet function, and is prolonged by anticoagulants that affect platelet function. The maximum amplitude (MA) measures the absolute strength of the clot and is dependent on platelet function and fibrinogen levels. $\alpha$ value is the slope of the divergence or the angle of the tracing from R and also reflects the speed at which the clot is forming (normal = 40 to 60°). $A_{60}$ is the clot strength or MA, 60 minutes after the initial measurement.

The TEG has been found to be useful in guiding replacement of blood products and treatment for fibrinolysis during liver transplantation.[44,45] It has also been shown to be a more effective indicator of postCBP bleeding than the routine coagulation profile or ACT.[46,47]

The Sonoclot provides the same information as the TEG; it differs from the TEG in that it utilizes a vibrating pin in a stationary cuvette. When compared to the TEG, the Sonoclot has been shown to be equally effective in predicting postcardiopulmonary hemorrhage.[48] The Sonoclot is also particularly sensitive to platelet dysfunction, and may provide information faster than the TEG.[49]

# CONGENITAL DISORDERS OF HEMOSTASIS

Congenital disorders of hemostasis are usually due to the absence or decreased presence of a single coagulation factor. Although a congenital deficiency in virtually all clotting factors has been identified, the most common disorders are hemophilia A, hemophilia B, and von Willebrand's disease. The goal during the perioperative period is to maintain adequate levels of the deficient factor to promote adequate hemostasis. Intramuscular injections and medications that inhibit platelets should be avoided in these patients. In addition, the intraoperative use of cautery should be limited, as the cauterized tissue may slough and bleed later.

## Hemophilia A

Hemophilia is an inherited X-chromosome linked coagulation disorder characterized by a decreased activity, or the absence of factor VIII or factor IX. The X-chromosome linkage limits this disorder almost exclusively to males. Hemophilia A, or classic hemophilia, is due to the functional deficiency of factor VIII and

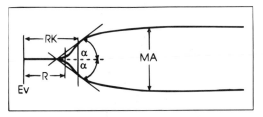

**Fig. 2–4.** Native TEG profile. R = Reactive Time, RK = Clot Time, MA = Maximum Amplitude, $\alpha$ = Angle, Ev = Event Marker. Courtesy of Haemoscope Corporation, Skokie, IL.

accounts for 75% of all patients with hemophilia. Its occurrence in the male population is estimated to be 1 in 100,000 worldwide[50] and affects about 12,000 individuals in the United States.[51]

Factor VIII exists in plasma as a noncovalent complex with vWF. The factor VIII coagulation component (factor VIII:C) is under control of a gene on the X-chromosome and is required for activation of factor X in the intrinsic coagulation system. The deficiency of factor VIII:C is responsible for hemophilia A. vWF is a large protein which exists as a series of multimers of various sizes and accounts for 99% of the factor VIII complex. vWF facilitates the adhesion of platelets to subendothelial collagen and its absence leads to the bleeding associated with von Willebrand's disease (see von Willebrand's disease). von Willebrand factor is produced by endothelial cells and megakaryocytes, while factor VIII:C is synthesized primarily by the liver. These two components of factor VIII complex circulate in the plasma as a unit, promoting both formation of a platelet plug and the coagulation of blood at the site of an injury.

CLINICAL PRESENTATION

The clinical manifestations of classic hemophilia vary in severity among affected individuals. Patients with a mild factor VIII deficiency do not usually suffer from bleeding episodes, except after dental or surgical procedures. Other patients have a virtually total deficiency and exhibit manifestations of the hemorrhagic diathesis from birth, including deep tissue bleeding, hemarthrosis, and hematuria. Central nervous system bleeding is the major cause of death in these patients, and femoral neuropathy is known to occur secondary to hemorrhage into surrounding skeletal muscles.

The diagnosis of classic hemophilia is made by family history and by measuring the plasma concentration of factor VIII and the APTT. The degree of factor VIII deficiency parallels the severity of a patient's symptoms. The APTT is a useful screening test and is prolonged in all patients, except those with very mild disease (factor VIII level between 20 and 30% of normal). The PT is normal because it does not test for the presence of factor VIII.

PERIOPERATIVE CONSIDERATIONS

The perioperative goal is to establish a plasma concentration of factor VIII that will assure hemostasis. A factor VIII concentration of greater than 30% of normal is adequate for hemostasis after major surgery.[52] Ideally, the factor VIII concentration is raised to 100% prior to elective surgery, in order to ensure that the level does not decrease below 30% during surgery. Factor VIII has a half-life of 10 to 12 hours and needs to be given twice a day. Continuous infusions of factor concentrates have also been used safely and efficaciously in hospitalized patients with hemophilia, and offer a convenient alternative therapeutic approach.[53]

Cryoprecipitate is the portion of plasma that remains insoluble after it is thawed and is rich in fibrinogen and factor VIII. Each mL of cryoprecipitate contains 5 to 10 units/mL of factor VIII. The advantages of cryoprecipitate include: (1) simplicity of preparation; (2) ease of administration; and (3) low cost. Disadvantages include: (1) variability of preparation from one unit to another; (2) the presence of trapped red blood cells which may be antigenic; and (3) the risk of hepatitis and human immunodeficiency virus (HIV). Screening tests and careful selection of donors have significantly reduced the risk of hepatitis and HIV infection.

Factor VIII concentrates have been isolated from cryoprecipitate and contain 30 to 40 units/mL of factor VIII. Less volume is infused with factor VIII concentrates, but the risks of HIV and viral hepatitis persist. Recently, factor VIII has been produced by recombinant DNA techniques and appears to behave identically (immunologically and functionally) to plasma-derived factor VIII.[54,55] It has been used successfully in human clinical trials, but issues such as price and availability have limited its therapeutic use.

Desmopressin (DDAVP) is a synthetic analogue of vasopressin and induces the release of vWF from endothelial cells. Because vWF may be decreased in the presence of Factor VIII:C deficiency, desmopressin may be useful in patients with mild hemophilia A, undergoing minor surgery (e.g., dental extraction). When administered, 0.3 to 0.4 $\mu$g/kg of desmopressin should be given intravenously in normal saline 30 minutes prior to surgery.

Approximately 6% of patients with hemophilia develop a specific inhibitor to factor

VIII and must be tested for it prior to elective surgery. It may be difficult to reach an adequate factor VIII level in these patients and surgery is avoided, if at all possible. If surgery is necessary, large amounts of factor VIII are given just prior to surgery, as antibody titers rise quickly. Experimental methods for improving factor VIII levels such as plasmapheresis, inhibition of antibody production, and immunoabsorption are currently under investigation.

## Hemophilia B

Hemophilia B, or Christmas disease, is due to the functional deficiency of factor IX. The inheritance pattern and clinical features of the disease are indistinguishable from classic hemophilia. Its occurrence in the male population is approximately 1 in 100,000.[50] Like classic hemophilia, Christmas disease is associated with a prolonged APTT, and specific assay shows an absence of factor IX activity in the presence of normal factor VIII activity. The severity of the disease generally parallels the degree of factor IX deficiency.

### PERIOPERATIVE CONSIDERATIONS

The therapeutic goal prior to elective surgery, is to raise plasma concentrations of factor IX to levels of at least 30% of normal during the perioperative period to ensure adequate hemostasis. Replacement therapy consists of concentrates of factor IX which are recovered from pooled plasma, although fresh frozen plasma may be adequate in those patients with mild-to-moderate deficiencies.[56] The dosing intervals are based on half-life of about 12-16 hours. Like factor VIII, factor IX has been used effectively as a continuous infusion in hospitalized patients.[52] Inhibitors to factor IX can develop over time, and these patients need to be tested for them prior to surgery.

In addition to the risks of HIV and hepatitis, the infusion of factor IX concentrates is associated with thrombotic complications and disseminated intravascular coagulation.[57] There have also been several reports of acute myocardial infarction associated with factor IX concentrate infusion.[58] The recent development of more pure, less thrombogenic factor IX concentrates, should reduce the incidence of these complications.[59]

## von Willebrand's Disease

von Willebrand's disease is most often inherited as an autosomal dominant trait, although rare autosomal recessive inheritance has been described.[60] von Willebrand's disease is a heterogeneous disorder, and several variants have been identified. All variants involve either a deficiency of vWF in plasma. or the production of a dysfunctional protein. The incidence of von Willebrand's disease is difficult to estimate because the clinical manifestations of the disease are often mild and the condition may pass undetected.

The classic and most common variant of von Willebrand's disease, type I, is characterized by a mild reduction circulating vWF in plasma. Although the synthesis of vWF is not impaired, its release into plasma is inhibited by some unknown mechanism. In type II, a less common variant, the production of vWF is altered, yielding a dysfunctional protein. In type I disease and in some variants of type II, the level of factor VIII:C is decreased, suggesting that vWF plays an additional role in either the release, binding, or molecular stability of factor VIII:C. Therefore, von Willebrand's disease is a disorder that affects both platelet-subendothelium interaction (i.e., decreased adhesiveness) and the coagulation pathway (i.e., factor VIII:C deficiency).

### CLINICAL PRESENTATION

Although the clinical presentation of von Willebrand's disease varies among patients, common characteristics include mucous membrane bleeding, epistaxis, superficial bruising, excessive bleeding from wounds, and menorrhagia. Trauma and surgical procedures performed on previously undiagnosed patients can result in severe bleeding localized to the area of injury. Pregnancy is associated with increased levels of factor VIII:C and vWF, permitting vaginal delivery without excessive hemorrhage in parturients with mild forms of the disease. In severe cases, caesarian section is recommended because levels of these factors in an affected fetus are decreased, despite adequate levels in the parturient.

### DIAGNOSIS

Patients suspected of having von Willebrand's disease should have the following tests performed: bleeding time, platelet count, APTT, factor VIII:C assay, vWF antigen assay with multimeric distribution, ristocetin-induced platelet aggregation, and ristocetin cofactor assay. More than one of these tests are likely to be abnormal in patients who have the disease.

The BT is a useful screening test and is prolonged in the face of a normal platelet count in virtually all variants of the disease. Patients with normal bleeding times tend to have milder clinical disease.

The APTT is usually prolonged, reflecting a decreased level of factor VIII:C. It should be noted that the APTT is not prolonged until factor VIII:C has decreased to 25 to 30% of normal, and may be normal in milder forms of the disease. The majority of patients with type I disease have a normal APTT, while those with type II variants often have prolonged times.

Factor VIII coagulant activity assay is a test used in the initial evaluation of patients with von Willebrand's disease. Nearly all patients with Type I disease have a normal to mildly reduced factor VIII:C, while type II variant patients generally have reduced levels.

Several assays exist for the measurement of vWF-antigen. These assays are sensitive for detecting a deficiency in vWF, as well as detecting molecularly abnormal forms of vWF.

The addition of ristocetin to platelet-rich plasma normally induces clumping; however, this effect is altered in 65 to 75% of patients with von Willebrand's disease.[39] The ristocetin cofactor assay quantitatively measures the ability of plasma vWF to agglutinate platelets in the presence of ristocetin; it is the most sensitive and specific test for detection of von Willebrand's disease.[61]

### PERIOPERATIVE CONSIDERATIONS

With the appropriate perioperative therapy, the surgical risk in patients with von Willebrand's disease is no greater than in unaffected patients.[62] Patients are generally treated before surgery with cryoprecipitate (40 units/kg), or specially derived plasma fractions, which provide both vWF and factor VIII:C. However, because of the viral risks associated with cryoprecipitate and plasma-derived fractions, desmopressin (DDAVP) is being used more frequently. Desmopressin (DDAVP; 1-deamino-8-D-arginine vasopressin) is a synthetic analogue of vasopressin which induces the release of vWF from endothelial cells, and may be adequate therapy in patients with milder forms of the disease, or patients undergoing minor surgical procedures.[63]

# ACQUIRED DISORDERS OF HEMOSTASIS

## Drug-Induced Platelet Abnormalities

### ANTIPLATELET MEDICATION

Antiplatelet medications are often used in the management of patients with arterial lesions and thromboembolic diseases.[64] These medications are associated with mild bleeding disorders, the most common of which result from the ingestion of aspirin and nonsteroidal antiinflammatory drugs (NSAID). These drugs inhibit platelet cyclo-oxygenase, which in turn, inhibits the platelet production of thromboxane $A_2$ ($TxA_2$), an important mediator of platelet aggregation.

Aspirin is the most potent of these agents and the most widely studied. Aspirin irreversibly acetylates cyclo-oxygenase[65] and inhibits thromboxane production with a single dose as low as 160 mg. This inhibition lasts for the normal lifespan of the platelets, which is 8 to 10 days. NSAID are competitive and reversible inhibitors of cyclo-oxygenase, and have more transient effects. Patients with drug-induced cyclo-oxygenase inhibition usually have mildly prolonged bleeding times. At higher chronic doses, aspirin also decreases the production of prothrombin, leading to an increased PT. Patients taking oral warfarin may have increased plasma concentrations of free warfarin, secondary to reduced protein binding in the presence of aspirin.

Patients generally have minimal symptoms, but will occasionally have prolonged oozing after surgery, particularly with procedures involving mucous membranes, such as periodontal and oral surgery. The antiplatelet effect of these drugs may be particularly dramatic in patients with underlying defects like von Willebrand's disease and hemophilia. Evidence is also accumulating that aspirin contributes to excessive perioperative bleeding in patients undergoing CPB surgery.[66] (See Cardiopulmonary Bypass.) Therefore, it is reasonable to defer elective surgical procedures associated with significant blood loss, until the effects of antiplatelet medications have dissipated. Epidural and spinal anesthesia are often avoided, because of the associated prolongation of the bleeding time and potential risk for hematoma formation; however, recent studies suggest that patients receiving usual doses of preoperative antiplatelet medication can safely undergo these anesthetic procedures.[67] Caution is warranted when major regional blocks are performed on patients receiving higher doses of antiplatelet medications.

## ANTIBIOTICS

The administration of high doses of antibiotics, particularly the penicillins, has been shown to produce platelet dysfunction by interfering with ADP receptors on the platelet membrane.[68] An increased bleeding time in patients undergoing antibiotic therapy, is associated with an increased risk of clinical bleeding.[69,70]

## NITRATES

The preservation of platelet function needs to be considered when using nitrates to control arterial blood pressure and vascular resistance. Traditionally, sodium nitroprusside and nitroglycerine have been used for this purpose during cardiac surgery and procedures requiring induced hypotension (e.g., scoliosis, head and neck procedures); however, these two agents significantly alter hemostatic mechanisms and inhibit platelet function, resulting in increased bleeding times at clinically relevant doses.[71-75] Recent studies suggest that this platelet inhibition is related to the generation of nitric oxide (NO), an endothelium-derived relaxing factor.[76-78] Trimethaphan, a ganglionic blocker, is also used to control arterial blood pressure and vascular resistance. Unlike the nitrates, platelet function is preserved in the presence of trimethaphan and is not associated with increased bleeding times.[79] Trimethaphan may be a more appropriate vasodilator during surgical procedures that are associated with abnormalities in hemostasis (e.g., CPB).

There are many other drugs (Table 2–4) that affect platelet function and bleeding

**Table 2–4. Drugs inhibiting platelet function**

Antiinflammatory agents (inhibitors of thromboxane synthesis)
  Aspirin
  Nonsteroidal antiinflammatory agents
  Corticosteroids
  Furosemide
Antibiotics
  Penicillin derivatives
  Nitrofurantoin
Bronchodilators
  Methylxanthines (aminophylline, theophylline)
  β-sympathomimetic agents (isoproterenol)
Psychoactive drugs
  Diazepam
  Phenothiazines
  Tricyclic antidepressants (amitriptyline)
Anesthetic agents
  Halothane, isoflurane
  Nitrous oxide
  Local anesthetics (procaine, lidocaine)
Cardiovascular drugs
  Adenosine
  β-adrenergic blockers (propanolol)
  Calcium channel blockers (verapamil, diltiazem)
  Dipyridamole
  Hydralazine
  Nitroglycerine
  Nitroprusside
  Protamine
Miscellaneous drugs
  Ethanol
  Antihistamines (chlorpromazine)
  Caffeine

times, including bronchodilators, β-adrenergic blockers),[80] calcium-channel blockers,[81] dipyridamole,[82] and inhaled anesthetic agents, including nitrous oxide.[83,84] In addition to affecting platelet function, many drugs including antibiotics, diuretics, and certain cardiovascular drugs can cause thrombocytopenia, resulting in increased bleeding times. (Table 2–5)

## Vitamin K Deficiency

Vitamin K, a fat soluble vitamin, is a cofactor that is essential to the integrity of plasma coagulation system. Vitamin K incorporates γ-carboxylglutamic acid into the polypeptide chains of factors II, VII, IX, and X. γ-carboxylglutamic acid residues are the sites at which calcium binds to these proteins and are required for their biologic function. Vitamin K is supplied in part by the diet; the rest is syn-

**Table 2–5.  Drugs causing thrombocytopenia**

Antibiotics
  Cephalothin
  Gentamicin
  Sulfonamides
Diuretics
  Acetazolamide
  Chlorothiazide
  Ethacrynic acid
  Furosemide
Cardiovascular drugs
  Amrinone
  Heparin
  Protamine
  Quinidine
Miscellaneous drugs
  Acetaminophen

thesized by bacterial flora, resident in the small intestine and colon. Adequate amount of bile salts are necessary to absorb vitamin K from the gastrointestinal tract. Vitamin K is metabolized by microsomal enzymes in the liver to vitamin K epoxide, but is regenerated by a liver membrane reductase.[85] Warfarin, a coumarin derivative, inhibits the activity of the reductase enzyme and blocks the regeneration of vitamin K, limiting its action. Vitamin K is also required for the synthesis of the hemostatic regulatory plasma proteins, protein C and protein S (see Regulatory Mechanisms of Hemostasis).

The major causes of vitamin K deficiency are: (1) inadequate dietary intake; (2) intestinal malabsorption; and/or (3) antibiotic-induced elimination of intestinal bacterial flora. Although a normal liver can store vitamin K for 30 days, acutely ill patients can become deficient in less than 7 days. Patients recovering from biliary tract surgery, without dietary intake of vitamin K and on broad spectrum antibiotics, are particularly prone to deficiencies. Neonatal vitamin K deficiency causes hemorrhagic disease of the newborn; however, routine supplemental administration of vitamin K has virtually eliminated this disease.

Vitamin K deficiency results in a reduction in all vitamin K-dependent coagulation factors. Because factor VII has the shortest half-life, a mild vitamin K deficiency will be readily reflected in the PT, while the APTT is normal. As the deficiency persists, the other factors fall and the APTT will also become prolonged.

The treatment for vitamin K deficiency depends on the urgency of the situation. Parenteral administration of vitamin K restores vitamin K levels in the liver and permits production of these coagulation factors within 6 to 8 hours. In the face of active hemorrhage, FFP immediately corrects the hemostatic defect.[86] Patients with either malabsorption problems, or those receiving total parenteral nutrition, require regular supplementation of vitamin K. Patients on long-term antibiotic therapy should be considered for supplementation, as well.

## Anticoagulant Medications

### HEPARIN

Heparin is a water soluble, organic acid that is present in high concentrations in the liver and in the granules of mast cells and basophils. The anticoagulant effect of heparin stems from its ability to bind with antithrombin III (ATIII), inducing a conformational change that greatly enhances the ability of ATIII to inhibit activated factors XII, XI, IX, X, and II (thrombin).[87] Commercially, heparin is prepared from bovine lung and bovine or porcine gastrointestinal mucosa. It is a heterogeneous biochemical substance, and its anticoagulant activity may vary per unit weight. Therefore, the anticoagulant potency of heparin is measured in standardized units and should always be prescribed in units.

Clinically, heparin is primarily used to produce anticoagulation, although it also induces a release of lipid-hydrolyzing enzymes which reduce plasma triglyceride concentrations. The clinical indications for heparin include anticoagulation during CPB, prophylaxis to reduce the risk of deep vein thrombosis and pulmonary embolism, and as an additive to continuous intravenous infusions used to maintain the patency of intravascular catheters.

The anticoagulant effect of heparin is instantaneous when given intravenously, and occurs within 20 to 30 minutes after subcutaneous injection. It is not effective when given orally. Intramuscular injection is avoided, as there is risk of hematoma formation.

Heparin is metabolized to inactive metabolites in the liver and is excreted by the kidney. It has an elimination half-life of approximately 150 minutes and a duration of action that is generally less than 6 hours. Larger doses are eliminated more slowly, and hypothermia prolongs the anticoagulant effect, as well. The duration of action is also prolonged in patients with hepatic and renal disease.

The heparin effect is monitored by the APTT and/or the ACT. A therapeutic APTT that inhibits thrombus formation is considered to be 1.5 to 2.5 times the patient's pre-drug baseline value. Very prolonged APTT values are readily managed by either omitting a single dose of heparin, or reducing the dose because the half-life is very short. The ACT is widely used to monitor the effectiveness of heparin therapy during CPB and extracorporeal circulation (See Perioperative Monitors of Coagulation; Cardiopulmonary Bypass).

## Adverse Effects of Heparin

*Hemorrhage.* Hemorrhage is the most serious complication associated with the use of heparin; however, close monitoring of laboratory measurements should minimize this risk. Heparin should be used cautiously in patients taking antiplatelet medication, and avoided completely in patients with a history of a bleeding disorder. Patients at risk for subclinical vitamin K deficiency (e.g., antibiotic therapy, malnutrition, hepato-renal disease) may develop severe hemorrhage with even small amounts of heparin[88], and should receive parenteral vitamin K prior to heparin administration. Heparin is best avoided in patients undergoing intraocular or intracranial surgery.

The use of major regional anesthetic techniques is controversial in patients who are receiving, or will subsequently receive heparin. With spinal or epidural anesthesia, the concern is related to the potential for an epidural hematoma to develop if a blood vessel were punctured, and subsequent compression of the spinal cord.[89] Performing a peripheral nerve block might also result in hematoma formation and compression of peripheral nerves in an anticoagulated patient. Although there are studies that demonstrate that major regional techniques can be performed safely in anticoagulated patients,[90] the potential for severe complications associated with these techniques make it prudent to avoid them in patients with a prolonged PT and APTT (more than 20% above normal). This issue is even less clear in patients who receive heparin anticoagulation after administration of a spinal or epidural anesthetic (e.g., major vascular surgery). Although studies utilizing large numbers of patients show no increased incidence of hematoma formation with subsequent heparin administration,[91,92] it seems prudent to postpone surgery if the regional technique is associated with trauma or bleeding. The use of regional techniques is safe in patients receiving subcutaneous heparin injections as prophylaxis for deep vein thrombosis, providing the APTT is confirmed to be normal prior to performing the regional block.

*Allergy.* Allergic reactions are rare, but do occur and are associated with fever and urticaria. Heparin should be given cautiously to patients with a history of allergy to beef or pork products.

*Decreased Antithrombin III (ATIII) Activity.* Patients receiving intermittent or continuous heparin therapy develop a reduction in ATIII activity to approximately 10 to 20% of normal.[93] These patients may require increased dosage requirements for adequate anticoagulation from heparin.[94] This heparin-induced reduction may cause a paradoxical tendency for thrombotic complications in patients with a mild ATIII deficiency. The administration of FFP or ATIII concentrate restores adequate levels of ATIII, and will promote adequate anticoagulation in these patients showing resistance to heparin, secondary to acquired or congenital decreases in ATIII.

*Heparin-Induced Thrombocytopenia.* Heparin-induced thrombocytopenia (HIT) is an uncommon, but well documented complication of heparin therapy. Most studies show a higher incidence of HIT when bovine-lung heparin is used.[95] Two types of HIT exist: one that occurs early and another that is delayed.[96,97] Type I HIT has an early onset, appearing 1 to 5 days after onset of heparin therapy and occurs in approximately 15% of patients. In Type I HIT, platelet counts fall significantly, but are usually greater than $50,000/mm^3$. The platelet count improves during continued therapy and often returns to normal. Type I has few clinical sequelae and is probably due to a direct heparin-induced platelet agglutination and removal of the agglutinates by the reticuloendothelial system.

Type II is more severe and referred to as

heparin-associated thrombosis (HAT). It occurs in approximately 6% of patients and is diagnosed by thrombocytopenia occurring between 5 to 7 days after initiation of heparin therapy. Type II is characterized by a severe reduction in platelets, often to $10,000/mm^3$, and is commonly associated with thromboembolic complications. In general, the lower the platelet count, the higher the incidence of thromboembolic complications. Thrombocytopenia is the result of an immune mediated platelet aggregation caused by IgG and IgM antibodies bound to platelets. Treatment consists of discontinuing heparin and switching to oral anticoagulant therapy. In most instances, platelet counts improve and thromboembolic events resolve 5 to 6 days after discontinuing heparin; however, antibody titers can persist for several weeks. Intravenous immunoglobin has been used to correct particularly severe HAT.[98] Early reexposure to heparin can result in a catastrophic secondary immune response. If patients require reexposure to heparin (e.g., CPB), pretreatment with platelet-inhibiting drugs, such as aspirin and dipyridamole, and strict abstinence from heparin after surgery, can minimize the severity of HIT and associated thromboembolic complications.[97,99-101] Iloprost, a stable $PGI_2$ analogue with a short half-life of 15 to 30 minutes, is a potent antiplatelet drug which has been successful in preventing HAT in patients requiring reexposure to heparin.[102-104]

*Effects on Protein Binding Sites.* Following the acute administration of heparin, the circulatory plasma concentration of drugs like diazepam and propranolol may increase.[105] This is probably due to displacement of these alkaline drugs from their protein binding sites by heparin. These drugs may have increased pharmacologic effects in the presence of acute heparin administration.

## Neutralization of Heparin: Protamine

Protamine is commercially prepared from fish sperm and is the only drug currently available in the United States to neutralize heparin. The high arginine content of protamine makes it strongly cationic, enabling it to form a stable complex with the strongly anionic heparin. The heparin-protamine interaction is based on weight, and, in general, 1.0 mg of protamine is necessary to neutralize 100 units

of circulating heparin. However, as much as 3.0 mg of protamine for every 100 units of heparin may be necessary to effectively neutralize heparin.

## Adverse Effects of Protamine

*Hypotension.* Hypotension is the most common side effect and is usually associated with rapid administration. The hypotension appears to be associated with histamine release[106] and is generally minimized by administering protamine slowly over 5 minutes.[107]

*Allergic Reactions.* A high incidence of anaphylactic and anaphylactoid reactions to protamine have been reported in patients with true fish allergies, diabetic patients receiving NPH (neutral-protamine-Hagedorn) insulin, and prior exposure to protamine.[108,109] True protamine allergies with antiprotamine IgE and IgM exist,[110] but anaphylactoid reactions are more common. These allergic reactions can be life threatening, and treatment includes intravascular fluid administration, supplemental oxygen, epinephrine, antihistamines, and steroids.

Patients who require heparin anticoagulation and are known to be hypersensitive to protamine are a clinical dilemma. Clinical options include (1) avoidance of protamine and allowing heparin to be eliminated by the liver and kidney, (2) pretreatment with $H_1$ and $H_2$ antagonists followed by slow infusion of protamine, and (3) neutralizing heparin with hexadimethrine bromide, an agent not currently available in the United States.[111] Allowing heparin to be metabolized without protamine neutralization may be associated with excessive bleeding requiring blood and FFP. Hexadimethrine bromide may be associated with a greater degree of hypotension than protamine and may have its own inherent anticoagulant effect.[112] At the present time, pretreatment with antihistamines and slow administration of protamine with a test dose prior to initiation of the full neutralizing dose, is probably the best option.

*Pulmonary Hypertension.* Occasionally, the administration of protamine is associated with complement activation and release of platelet thromboxane $A_2$, which presents as severe pulmonary vasoconstriction and bronchoconstriction.[113,114] Pretreatment with cyclo-oxygenase inhibitors such as aspirin or

NSAIDs diminishes these effects.[115] However, these drugs may enhance bleeding secondary to platelet dysfunction.

## COUMARIN DERIVATIVES

The anticoagulant effect of coumarin is related to its ability to interfere with the normal production of biologically active vitamin K-dependent clotting factors, resulting in a reduction of their plasma concentrations. Among the coumarin derivatives, warfarin is the most commonly used and can be administered both orally and intravenously. The anticoagulant effect of warfarin is delayed for 8 to 12 hours following either oral or intravenous administration. It generally takes 3 to 5 days of therapy before vitamin K-dependent factors reach their lowest levels. Warfarin has a long half-life (24 to 36 hours) and is metabolized in the liver to inactive metabolites that are conjugated and excreted in the bile and urine.

Clinically, warfarin is primarily used to reduce the incidence of thromboembolism associated with prosthetic heart valves and atrial fibrillation. Warfarin therapy is generally initiated slowly with 5 to 10 mg daily for the first few days, after which the dose is adjusted according to the PT. The PT is very sensitive to reductions in factors VII and X. Since factor VII has a short half-life of 7 hours, its concentration is reduced the earliest, and reflected in the PT. A therapeutic PT, one that inhibits thrombus formation, generally corresponds to approximately 1.5 times normal. The World Health Organization, along with the International Committee on Thrombosis and Haemostasis have recommended that the reporting of PT results for patients on oral anticoagulant therapy, include the use of International Normalized Ratio (INR) values.[116,117] INR results are independent of reagents and methods used, and are specifically intended to assess patients on long-term warfarin therapy. An INR of 3 to 4 is considered to be therapeutic. Unlike heparin, an excessively prolonged PT is not readily reduced by omitting a dose of warfarin, because of the long elimination half-life. Likewise, an inadequate PT is not increased quickly with one additional dose of warfarin.

In order to avoid risks of excessive hemorrhage, warfarin should be discontinued 2 to 3 days prior to elective surgery, in order to reduce the PT to less than 14 seconds.[118] This approach is reasonable in patients with aortic prosthetic valves because of a low incidence of thromboemboli (1 to 3%). Patients with mitral prosthetic valves have a higher risk for thromboemboli (5%), and may be better managed by reversal of warfarin therapy with vitamin K the day before surgery.[119] In high-risk patients, intravenous heparin should be given while the warfarin is discontinued. On the day of surgery, heparin should be discontinued, as well. Anticoagulation may be restarted 12 hours after surgery with heparin, and replaced with oral anticoagulants on the first postoperative day.[120] In the case of emergency surgery, the anticoagulant effects are readily reversed by administration of FFP and vitamin K.

### Drug Interactions with Coumarin

Many drugs interact with warfarin, enhancing or diminishing its anticoagulant effect (Table 2–6). Cimetidine inhibits warfarin clearance in the liver, and has been reported to be associated with clinical bleeding.[121] The use of aspirin concurrently with warfarin, may result in severe gastrointestinal hemorrhage. Other drugs enhancing the anticoagulant effect of warfarin include cotrimoxazole,[122] metronidazole,[123] disulfiram,[124] allopurinol,[125] quinidine,[126] and amiodarone.[127] Barbiturates increase the activity of hepatic microsomal enzymes, which increase the metabolism of warfarin.[128] Warfarin dosages need to be increased in patients receiving barbiturates, and also need to be reduced when barbiturates are discontinued. Other drugs associated with diminishing the anticoagulant effect of warfarin include rifampin[129] and propranolol.[130] Volatile anesthetic agents may

**Table 2–6.   Drugs that interact with coumarin derivatives**

| Enhance anticoagulant effect | Diminish anticoagulant effect |
| --- | --- |
| Cimetidine | Barbiturates |
| Cotrimoxozole | Rifampin |
| Metronidazole | Propanolol |
| Volatile anesthetics | |
| Allopurinol | |
| Amiodarone | |
| Quinidine | |
| Disulfuram | |

prolong the anticoagulant effect of warfarin by prolonging its elimination half-life.[131] Halothane, in particular, has also been shown to displace warfarin from protein binding sites, resulting in increased plasma concentrations of free warfarin.[132]

### Adverse Effects of Coumarin

*Hemorrhage.* As with heparin, hemorrhage is the most serious side effect of warfarin therapy, and may occur in the face of a desired therapeutic PT value. Gastrointestinal hemorrhage is most frequently encountered, and is usually associated with undetected peptic ulcer disease and neoplasm. Warfarin therapy may also be associated with an increased incidence of intracranial bleeding, following a cerebrovascular accident. Mild hemorrhage may be treated with 5 mg intravenous vitamin K over 5 minutes, which generally returns the prothrombin time to normal within 6 to 24 hours. Immediate reversal of warfarin effects is accomplished by administering FFP. As with heparin, the use of major regional anesthetic techniques is best avoided in the presence of PT values greater than 15 seconds.

*Teratogenicity.* Warfarin crosses the placenta and is associated with serious teratogenic effects when used during the first trimester of pregnancy. Approximately one-third of infants exposed to warfarin are born with serious abnormalities, including blindness and nasal hypoplasia. Heparin does not cross the placenta and may be an alternative in parturients requiring anticoagulant therapy.

## Major Organ System Disease

### HEPATIC DISEASE

Coagulation abnormalities, including a high incidence of major hemorrhagic complications, have been reported in more than 70% of patients with hepatic failure.[133] Hepatic failure adversely affects hemostasis by several mechanisms. First, the synthesis of both coagulation factors and inhibitors of fibrinolysis is depressed. Second, the liver is limited in its ability to clear activated clotting factors, plasma activators of the fibrinolytic system, and fibrin degradation products from the circulation. Third, damaged hepatocytes may

release tissue thromboplastin triggering disseminated intravascular coagulation (DIC). Consequently, the hemorrhagic diathesis of hepatic insufficiency is a multifactorial process with reduced levels of coagulation factors, uncontrolled fibrinolysis, and DIC all playing a role.[134]

In biliary obstruction, only vitamin K-dependent factors are decreased because vitamin K absorption is dependent on the presence of bile salts in the gastrointestinal tract. If biliary obstruction is the *sole* abnormality, parenteral vitamin K will replenish these factors. However, when hepatocellular disease is combined with an acquired vitamin K deficiency (e.g., antibiotic therapy, malnutrition), parenteral administration of vitamin K alone may not be effective (see vitamin K deficiency).

Hepatic failure is also associated with platelet abnormalities, including defective platelet aggregation[135] and thrombocytopenia, secondary to sequestration by an enlarged spleen (hepatosplenomegaly). Patients who are alcoholics often have thrombocytopenia, secondary to folic acid deficiency. Alcohol itself may have toxic effects on megakaryocytes within the bone marrow.[136]

### Preoperative Evaluation

Coagulation abnormalities must be suspected in patients with hepatic insufficiency or jaundice. Preoperative laboratory studies should include a PT, APTT, and platelet count. A bleeding time is also useful if platelet dysfunction is suspected. Normally, only 20 to 30% coagulation factors are necessary to maintain normal hemostasis; however, when hepatic failure is severe, these factors can reduce to critical levels quickly. If the PT is prolonged secondary to a vitamin K deficiency, parenteral vitamin K will partially correct it within 48 hours. Persistent prolongation of the PT suggests severe hepatic failure, and preoperative transfusion of FFP is usually required. If PT and APTT are both elevated, evaluation for fibrinolysis and DIC should be done by measuring FDP and fibrinogen levels. Preoperative platelet transfusions should be administered to patients with hepatic disease who either have platelet counts below 75,000/mm$^3$ and/or increased bleeding times.

## Perioperative Management

Surgery in patients with hepatic disease may be associated with excessive oozing from mucosal surfaces, poor capillary hemostasis, and poor clot formation. Administration of FFP and platelets is ideally guided by intraoperative coagulation tests; however, acute clinical bleeding may warrant empiric administration of blood products as coagulation tests are being performed (PT, APTT, platelet count, fibrinogen level, FDP level). Desmopressin may improve hemostatic function by improving platelet function and raising levels of some circulating cofactors.[137,138] Dilution of platelets and coagulation factors may aggravate the coagulopathy of hepatic failure during the massive transfusion of blood and fluids. Treatment is based on replacing blood products that are diluted, as well as treating preexisting deficits.

Major regional anesthetic techniques (e.g., spinal and epidural) should be performed cautiously in patients with hepatic failure. In the face of abnormal coagulation, major regional techniques are best avoided; however, preoperative normalization of PT, APTT, and bleeding time will minimize the potential of developing peridural hematomas.

## Liver Transplantation

Liver transplantation is associated with major alterations in coagulation and fibrinolytic systems. There is a high risk of hemorrhage during this procedure, as virtually all patients have abnormal coagulation preoperatively.[139] During and after the anhepatic stage of the procedure, the concentration of many coagulation factors, including fibrinogen, decreases. Many of these coagulation factors may have already been decreased preoperatively, secondary to the liver disease. Intraoperative thrombocytopenia and transient increases in fibrinolytic activity are additional factors leading to uncontrolled hemorrhage. The pathogenesis of the increased fibrinolytic activity is complex, involving DIC, the release of tissue plasminogen activator (tPA), and loss of the ability of the liver to clear activated clotting factors.[140-142] Once circulation is established to the transplanted liver, transient excessive fibrinolysis occurs, presumably secondary to tPA released from the vessels of the donor liver. This effect may be diminished by treating these patients with $\epsilon$-aminocaproic acid.[45] Postoperatively, the titers of factors V, VIII, and vitamin K-dependent factors VII, IX, and X fall during the first hours of reperfusion, but rise to normal levels a few days after surgery. Persistent thrombocytopenia during the first few days after transplantation, may be due to platelet sequestration in the transplanted liver.[143] Survival after liver transplantation is adversely affected by excessive blood loss and massive transfusion. Although coagulation defects are of major concern during this procedure, much of the blood loss is likely to be of a mechanical nature, rather than coagulation abnormalities.[144]

## RENAL DISEASE

Patients with renal failure frequently present with symptoms of abnormal hemostasis ranging from ecchymosis, purpura, and epistaxis to severe gastrointestinal hemorrhage.[145] Although a number of factors are associated with this bleeding tendency, acquired platelet functional defects, secondary to uremia, are probably the most important.

Uremic patients have impaired platelet adhesion and aggregation. Although the mechanism for this is unknown, it is probably due to the accumulation of metabolic acids and their interference with vWF, and the subsequent aggregation of platelets. In general, platelet dysfunction correlates with the degree of uremia. The frequency and severity of hemorrhagic symptoms are also related to the degree and duration of the uremic state. The bleeding time is prolonged in the absence of thrombocytopenia, and in vitro platelet function tests that assess adhesion and aggregation are also abnormal. Although there is no recognized threshold blood urea nitrogen and creatinine level at which bleeding occurs, most patients with plasma creatinine less than 6 mg/dL, exhibit normal platelet function. Platelet function returns to normal after hemodialysis or renal transplantation,[146] confirming that these abnormalities are reversible, and the result of the uremic environment. Although hemodialysis corrects platelet abnormalities, systemic heparinization is often required to prevent clotting in the extracorporeal circulation and maintain patency of vascular shunts. The effects of heparin may persist postdialysis, contributing to the tendency for these patients to bleed.

Despite hemodialysis, some patients with renal failure continue to present with symptoms of abnormal hemostasis. There is evidence that anemia contributes to platelet dysfunction, since the bleeding time has been shown to shorten after red blood cell transfusions in uremic patients.[147,148] PT and APTT are normal, since there are no abnormalities in the plasma coagulation system or fibrinolysis; however, vitamin K-dependent coagulation factors tend to be low in end-stage renal disease. Other predisposing factors, including the ingestion of aspirin and antiplatelet medications, are likely to aggravate preexisting hemostatic abnormalities.

Although bleeding is the most common hemostatic defect in renal failure, a thrombotic tendency is also associated with certain renal diseases. Thromboembolic phenomenon and renal vein thrombosis are common complications in patients with nephrotic syndrome.[149] Thrombotic thrombocytopenic purpura (TTP) and hemolytic-uremic syndrome (HUS) are two rare conditions characterized by renal failure, hemolytic anemia, thrombocytopenia, and fever. These two conditions are closely related and often indistinguishable from each other. In both conditions, platelet aggregates occlude small vessels, leading to multiple organ failure, including renal failure. HUS is usually seen in infants, while TTP is often seen in older patients and is associated with neurologic deficits.

## Preoperative Evaluation

Preoperative laboratory tests in patients with renal failure should include hematocrit, PT, APTT, platelet count, and bleeding time. The PT should detect any deficiencies in vitamin K-dependent coagulation factors, while the APTT will detect any residual effect from heparin posthemodialysis. The bleeding time may be prolonged beyond the upper limit of normal. Patients should undergo hemodialysis within 24 hours of elective surgery in order to maximize platelet function. In addition, transfusion of red blood cells to a hematocrit of 30% may also improve platelet function. Platelet transfusion is generally not effective in improving hemostasis, since normal platelets quickly become dysfunctional when transfused to uremic patients.[150]

Cryoprecipitate and desmopressin can temporarily correct the bleeding tendency in patients with uremia. Cryoprecipitate has been shown to shorten the bleeding time for a duration of approximately 6 hours in some patients undergoing major surgical procedures, resulting in significantly reduced blood loss.[151] However, the risk of transmission of bloodborne diseases and heterogeneity of preparations have minimized the use of cryoprecipitate. Desmopressin is a synthetic analogue of antidiuretic hormone that effectively improves platelet function and reduces clinical bleeding in uremic patients without the risk of transfusion therapy.[152] Unlike antidiuretic hormone, DDAVP does not have vasoconstrictor activity and does not raise arterial pressure when administered. It appears to exert its effect by increasing circulating factors of vWF.[153] An intravenous infusion of DDAVP (0.3-0.4 $\mu$g/kg) shortens the bleeding time significantly for at least 4 hours, and can be repeated at 12 hour intervals. However, repeated infusions of DDAVP may lead to a progressively diminished response, hyponatremia, and water retention.[152,154]

The administration of conjugated estrogens has also been shown to effectively shorten prolonged bleeding times and prevent excessive postoperative hemorrhage in uremic patients.[155] When a cumulative dose of 3 mg/kg is infused over 5 days, normalization of bleeding time may last up to 2 weeks without side effects. This long-lasting effect may make conjugated estrogens a useful adjunct to the management of uremic patients undergoing major surgery. The mechanism of the estrogen effect is, in part, related to an increase in circulating vWF and improved platelet adhesiveness.

## Perioperative Management

Before undergoing major surgery, all patients should undergo preoperative hemodialysis. If bleeding times remain prolonged, red blood cells should be transfused. DDAVP (0.3 to 0.4 $\mu$g/kg) should be administered 1 hour before surgery. If unexpected bleeding occurs during or after surgery, DDAVP and/or cryoprecipitate should be administered, depending on the severity of bleeding. Conjugated estrogens may be useful for long-term therapy. As with liver failure, abnormal coagulation needs to be considered when performing regional anesthetic techniques on patients with chronic renal failure.

Patients undergoing renal transplantation may develop quantitative and qualitative changes in platelets after the procedure. Use of immunosuppressive drugs may result in thrombocytopenia, secondary to bone marrow toxicity. Graft rejection is also associated with platelet aggregation and adhesion, leading to thrombus formation. Platelet dysfunction may exist in patients with functioning transplants secondary, in part, to decreased intraplatelet concentrations of serotonin.[156]

## DISSEMINATED INTRAVASCULAR COAGULATION

Disseminated intravascular coagulation is a thrombohemorrhagic disorder that occurs as a complication of a variety of diseases including trauma, sepsis, and malignant neoplasms (Table 2–7). The clinical presentation of DIC is variable, since it exists as both an acute and chronic phenomenon. DIC is characterized by an activation of the plasma coagulation system and formation of microthrombi throughout the microcirculation. The microthrombi lead to vascular occlusion and ischemic damage of vital organs including the kidney, liver, adrenal glands, and central nervous system.[157] Platelets, fibrinogen, and other coagulation factors are rapidly consumed, leading to a worsening bleeding diathesis. The presence of thrombin and formation of fibrin and microthrombi result in a secondary activation of the fibrinolytic system, further aggravating the hemorrhagic diathesis.

### Pathogenesis

The main mechanisms responsible for triggering DIC involve the release of tissue thromboplastin into the circulation, widespread endothelial cell damage, and thrombin formation. Tissue thromboplastins activate the extrinsic pathway of the plasma coagulation, and are released into the circulation following massive tissue destruction, as seen with crush injuries, severe head trauma, significant burn injuries, and a variety of obstetrical complications. Endotoxins released by gram-negative bacteria, release thromboplastins from en-

**Table 2–7. Major disorders associated with disseminated intravascular coagulation**

Obstetric complications
  Amniotic fluid embolism
  Intrauterine retention of a dead fetus
  Abruptio placentae
  Eclampsia
  Septic abortion
Infections
  Bacterial: gram-negative and gram-positive sepsis (staphylococci, streptococci, meningococcemia, pneumonococci, endocarditis, gram-negative bacilli)
  Viral: herpes simplex, varicella, rubella, cytomegalic viremia
  Parasitic: malaria
  Mycotic: candidiasis, histoplasmosis, aspergillosis
  Rickettsial: rocky mountain spotted fever
  Other: hepatitis, miliary tuberculosis
Massive tissue injury
  Traumatic shock
  Head injury
  Burns
  Extensive surgery
Malignancy
  Carcinomas of lung, prostate, and pancreas
  Acute promyelocytic leukemia
Miscellaneous
  Acute hemolytic process
  Hypothermia
  Malignant hyperthermia
  Liver disease
  Hemolytic uremic syndrome
  Aortic aneurysm
  Heat stroke
  Anaphylaxis

dothelial and inflammatory cells, making DIC a frequent complication of sepsis. In addition to activating the extrinsic pathway, widespread endothelial injury results in platelet aggregation, activating the intrinsic pathway of the plasma coagulation system. Endothelial injury can be produced directly by microorganisms (e.g., meningococci, rickettsiae), viruses, and disease-related antigen-antibody complexes (e.g., systemic lupus erythematosus, glomerulonephritis). Endothelial injury can also occur secondary to hypoxia, acidosis, hypothermia, and circulatory shock, which commonly coexist with surgical and obstetric complications.

## Clinical Presentation

The onset of DIC may be acute and severe, as seen with gram-negative septic shock and massive trauma, or it may be chronic and insidious, as seen with malignant neoplasms.[158] In general, a hemorrhagic diathesis dominates the clinical picture of acute DIC, while thrombotic complications are associated with the chronic syndrome.

Disseminated intravascular coagulation is a systemic process, and bleeding can occur anywhere platelets and coagulation factors are consumed, including the respiratory and central nervous systems. In the acute syndrome, patients often present with bleeding from skin and mucous membrane surfaces. Hemorrhage from surgical incision, venipuncture, and catheter sites is also common. Occasionally, pregangrenous changes may be present in digits, genitalia, and the nose, secondary to microthrombi and vasospasm. A hemolytic anemia is a common result of fragmentation of red blood cells as they move through narrowed microvasculature. Ischemic organ damage may ensue, with oliguria and acute renal failure dominating the picture. Patients with chronic DIC, such as that associated with malignancy, may be relatively asymptomatic with only mild laboratory abnormalities confirming the diagnosis. Laboratory evidence of DIC includes thrombocytopenia and the presence of fragmented red blood cells, secondary to damage within the microvasculature. Prothrombin time, APTT, and TT are prolonged, secondary to consumption of coagulation factors. The fibrinogen level is reduced and the FDP level is increased from primary, as well as secondary, fibrinolysis. Of all laboratory measurements, a low plasma fibrinogen level most closely correlates with clinical evidence of bleeding.

## Treatment

The treatment of DIC is directed at (1) attempting to correct the underlying disorder causing DIC and (2) controlling the major symptom of either hemorrhage or thrombosis. Treatment will vary depending on the underlying disorder. Bacterial sepsis and certain obstetric etiologies (e.g., abruptio placentae) may be relatively easy to correct, while chronic DIC associated with a malignancy, may require long-term prophylactic measures to control symptoms. Improvement of DIC is associated with the stabilization of the platelet count and fibrinogen level, with a decreased circulating FDP level.

Patients with bleeding as a major symptom should receive platelet concentrates and FFP, as indicated by measurement of platelet count, PT, and APTT. The use of heparin will prevent thrombin formation and has been recommended, but the dose remains controversial. Although it is a reasonable way to reduce consumption of coagulation factors, heparin itself may induce bleeding when given at usual clinical dosages. Therefore, the use of heparin is generally reserved for patients with evidence of thrombosis, or those who continue to bleed despite vigorous treatment. Antithrombin III concentrate infusions in patients with circulatory shock may be useful in reducing the severity of associated DIC.[159] Use of $\epsilon$-aminocaproic acid and other inhibitors of fibrinolysis should be avoided, since fibrinolysis is a secondary protective mechanism and inhibition might be associated with unopposed thrombosis.

Patients with mild DIC may not be symptomatic until they undergo certain systemic stresses, such as those associated with surgery. Most patients with mild presentations will be adequately controlled with platelet and plasma replacement. Patients with chronic DIC and thrombotic complications may require long-term heparin administration by intermittent subcutaneous injection or continuous infusion with a portable pump.

# Massive Transfusion

The ability to transfuse blood with relatively few immediate and long-term complications, has led to increased survival in patients who require massive amounts of blood. However, the transfusion of blood equal to or greater than a patient's own blood volume (8 to 10 units in an adult), may lead to an acquired coagulopathy. The amount of blood transfused and the duration of hypotension and hypoperfusion, are the factors that most closely correlate with the development of a hemorrhagic diathesis.[160] Large amounts of transfused blood are more likely to dilute platelets and coagulation factors to levels that are inadequate for hemostasis. Prolonged hypoperfusion can lead to regional ischemia and release of tissue thromboplastin, worsening any coexisting coagulopathy by producing DIC. In addition, associated conditions such as hypothermia and acidosis, may alter platelet function and impair coagulation further.[161,162]

## EFFECTS OF MASSIVE TRANSFUSION ON COAGULATION

### Thrombocytopenia

Dilutional thrombocytopenia and altered platelet function, often in conjunction with DIC, is the most likely cause of a hemorrhagic diathesis in patients receiving massive blood transfusion.[163-165] Platelets are poorly preserved in banked blood, and platelet counts of less than $100,000/mm^3$ are common following massive transfusion. Recent studies show that after transfusion of 20 or more units of red blood cell products of any kind (packed RBCs, cell-saver units, or whole blood), 75% of patients will have platelet counts less than $50,000/mm^3$.[166] This reduction in circulating platelets correlates closely with the tendency to bleed, since bleeding is likely when platelet counts drop below $75,000/mm^3$ during surgery.[163] In addition, hypothermia, acidosis, drugs, and trauma can alter the function of existing platelets for days after the initial insult.[167] These factors have motivated clinicians to empirically administer platelets in the absence of laboratory or clinical evidence of bleeding. Controlled clinical trials, however, have demonstrated that the prophylactic administration of platelets does not reduce transfusion requirements or coagulopathy during surgery.[168] It is currently recommended that platelets be administered only when indicated by laboratory evidence of thrombocytopenia or severe generalized coagulopathy. Because intraoperative platelet counts below $75,000/mm^3$ are frequently associated with clinical bleeding, platelet transfusions are indicated at that time.

### Dilution of Coagulation Factors

Most coagulation factors are stable in stored blood with the exception of factors V and VIII. The levels of factor V and factor VIII are reduced below 50% of normal after 48 hours of storage and are even lower after 21 days. Only 5 to 20% of factor V and 30% of factor VIII are necessary for adequate hemostasis; these factors are rarely decreased to these low levels despite massive transfusion. Dilution of coagulation factors is rarely the *sole* cause of bleeding;[169] however, it may intensify bleeding stemming from dilutional thrombocytopenia and consumptive coagulopathy. Recent studies show that following transfusion of 12 or more units of relatively plasma free blood products (packed RBCs and/or cell-saver units), virtually all patients have a prothrombin time (PT) and activated partial thromboplastin time (APTT) prolonged by more than 1.5 times mid-range of normal.[166,170] There is, however, no scientific evidence supporting the routine use of FFP as replacement therapy during massive transfusion.[86,169] It is currently recommended that prior to administering FFP, (1) thrombocytopenia should be ruled out as a cause of bleeding by ensuring that platelets are greater than $70,000/mm^3$ and (2) the activated partial thromboplastin time is at least 1.5 times greater than normal, suggesting low levels of factors V and VIII.

### Fluid Resuscitation

Although intravenous fluid resuscitation is routinely prescribed for hypotensive trauma victims, recent studies suggest that this may be detrimental when administered before bleeding is controlled in the operating room.[171,172] These studies have demonstrated that in uncontrolled hemorrhage, aggressive administration of fluids may disrupt thrombus formation, increase bleeding, and decrease survival. Fluid resuscitation during the period of uncontrolled hemorrhage may also lead to early dilution of platelets and coagulation factors. Aggressive fluid resuscitation may be best delayed until the time of surgical intervention. Further research is necessary to verify these findings, as well as to provide new guidelines for fluid resuscitation in the field, emergency room, and operating room.

## DIAGNOSIS AND TREATMENT

When a massive blood transfusion begins to approach a patient's blood volume, a blood specimen should be obtained and tested for platelet count, APTT, PT, and plasma fibrinogen level. Clinical observation becomes critical at this time, and the patient should be continuously evaluated for: (1) evidence of a generalized bleeding tendency; (2) how much more blood replacement will be necessary; and (3) associated conditions that may contribute to a coagulopathy (i.e., trauma, hypotension, liver failure). If initial coagulation times are greater than 1.5 times normal and platelet count is less than 75,000/mm$^3$, one can assume that associated factors such as hypotension, organ failure, and trauma are contributing to the coagulopathy.[173] Fibrinogen is stable in banked blood, and a plasma level below 150 mg/100 mL strongly suggests DIC. When hypofibrinogenemia is associated with thrombocytopenia, DIC is the probable diagnosis. Coagulation studies should be repeated as justified by the clinical picture. Ultimately, treatment must be guided by the clinical picture, and in the face of severe uncontrollable bleeding, empiric administration of platelets and FFP may be warranted.

## Cardiopulmonary Bypass

Cardiopulmonary bypass (CPB) is associated with multiple complex abnormalities affecting all aspects of the hemostatic mechanism. Platelet abnormalities are the most common cause of bleeding following CPB; however, activation of coagulation, fibrinolysis, and the effects of various cardiovascular drugs also play a role. These abnormalities lead to a bleeding diathesis in an estimated 5 to 20% of patients.[174,175] Approximately 5% of patients who undergo CPB procedures require reoperation for excessive bleeding.[176,177]

Cardiopulmonary bypass adversely affects both platelet count and platelet function. Immediately after initiating CPB, hemodilution reduces the platelet count to about 50% of preoperative levels, but it usually remains above 100,000 $\mu$/L.[178] A decreased platelet count often persists for several days following CPB, and may be related to platelet sequestration in the liver.[179] Of greater significance is the progressive loss of platelet function induced by CPB. The bleeding time is prolonged and platelet aggregation studies are abnormal, shortly after the initiation of CPB. Platelet dysfunction appears to be dependent on exposure of platelets to the extracorporeal circuit and hypothermia, while the degree of platelet dysfunction is directly related to the duration of CPB.[178,180] The mechanism for this abnormality is unclear, but may be related to a decrease in platelet synthesis of Thromboxane A$_2$,[161,181] transient platelet activation with impaired aggregation,[180,182] and depleted stores of ADP.[183] Other coexisting factors having adverse effects on platelet function during CPB include the cardiotomy suction (destruction of platelets); filters; antiplatelet drugs; nitrates; and protamine, which produces a transient reduction in circulating platelets. The ingestion of aspirin by these patients is particularly associated with an increased risk of perioperative bleeding.[66,184] Platelet dysfunction associated with CPB is usually transient and returns to normal within 24 hours of surgery. However, prolonged dysfunction can exist.

Hemodilution associated with the initiation of CPB produces approximately a 40% reduction in most coagulation factors.[185] These reductions persist throughout CPB and usually return to normal levels within 24 to 48 hours after surgery. Although these reduced levels are generally still adequate for hemostasis, excessive hemodilution and preexisting coagulation defects can lead to increased perioperative bleeding.

Primary fibrinolysis occurs when plasminogen is activated to plasmin, inducing lysis of fibrinogen and fibrin. Although heparin provides an anticoagulated state during CPB, it does not inhibit factor XII, an intrinsic activator of fibrinolysis. Primary or intrinsic fibrinolytic activity occurs with the initiation of CPB.[186] In addition, secondary or extrinsic fibrinolysis is activated as CPB progresses.[187] Despite this, fibrinolysis itself is rarely a clinically significant cause of perioperative bleeding.[180,185]

### RESIDUAL HEPARIN EFFECT

Heparin anticoagulation is necessary to avoid clotting that would otherwise occur when blood makes contact with the foreign surfaces of the extracorporeal circuit. Heparin is administered either through a central line, or directly into the right atrium. A dose of 300 to 400 units/kg of heparin is used to initiate anticoagulation.

The ACT is the most widely used test to monitor the effectiveness of heparin (see Perioperative Monitors of Coagulation). In routine CPB, an automated ACT above 400 seconds has been recommended to minimize the formation of fibrin monomers and consumption of coagulation factors.[188] Although recent studies suggest that an ACT below 400 seconds may be clinically safe,[189] the safe lower limit of the ACT remains to be defined.

Heparin is neutralized at the conclusion of CPB by protamine, with the usual dose being approximately 1.0 mg of protamine for every 100 units of heparin used (see Anticoagulant Medications: Neutralization of Heparin). The ACT is again used to monitor heparin neutralization. Heparin rebound refers to the recurrence of anticoagulation accompanied by an elevated ACT, despite previous neutralization with protamine. Heparin rebound generally occurs 4 to 6 hours after protamine neutralization, because the half-life of heparin is longer than that of protamine. This usually responds to an additional dose of protamine. Occasionally, the ACT can not be returned to the baseline value despite adequate protamine, indicating the likelihood of a low plasma fibrinogen level.

## MANAGEMENT AND TREATMENT OF BLEEDING POST CARDIOPULMONARY BYPASS

After heparin has been neutralized by protamine, the surgical field should be meticulously inspected for bleeding, and the appropriate hemostatic maneuvers should be employed by the surgeon. If bleeding is significant and diffuse, a coagulation profile consisting of a PT, APTT, fibrinogen level, TT, and platelet count should be performed. If residual heparin is suspected, the thrombin time will be prolonged. Thrombocytopenia should be treated with platelet transfusions in the face of excessive bleeding. Intrinsic impairment of platelet function should be assumed to be the primary hemostatic abnormality, while abnormalities of the plasma coagulation system are less likely. Use of FFP is rational treatment only after platelet abnormalities or excessive heparin have been corrected or ruled out.

## PROPHYLACTIC THERAPY

### Fresh Frozen Plasma and Platelets

There is no evidence that the prophylactic administration of FFP or platelets have a positive clinical effect.[190,191] Fresh frozen plasma is indicated when the PT or APTT exceed 1.5 times the normal value, or when blood transfusion exceeds the patient's calculated blood volume. Transfusion of platelets is indicated when the platelet count is less than 75,000/mm$^2$, or when blood transfusion has exceeded the patients calculated blood volume. If the patient is anemic, the transfusion of fresh whole blood (which provides red cells, FFP, and platelets) has been shown to provide better hemostasis than when platelets are transfused alone.[192,193] Several studies have suggested that performing acute-platelet rich plasmapheresis before CPB and returning the platelet-rich plasma after CPB, reduces both blood loss and blood transfusion requirements;[194,195] However, other studies have shown this procedure to be of little benefit.[196,197]

### Desmopressin Acetate

The usefulness of desmopressinacetate (DDAVP) to reduce perioperative blood loss is a matter of debate. Desmopressin increases the level of circulating factors VIII:C and vWF and is associated with a shortening of the bleeding time. Although studies have shown that intravenous desmopressin (0.3 $\mu$g/kg) at the conclusion of CPB significantly reduces perioperative blood loss associated with CPB,[177,198] more recent studies have demonstrated no significant difference in blood loss and transfusion requirements in patients receiving DDAVP.[199,201] Because of these contradictory studies, DDAVP should not be given routinely, but rather, reserved for those patients with excessive bleeding following CPB. Although the use of DDAVP is generally well tolerated, it may be associated with hypotension, antidiuresis, and activation of fibrinolysis. Tachyphylaxis to DDAVP has also been reported.

### Natural and Synthetic Fibrinolytics

Although fibrinolysis is rarely a clinically significant cause of CPB-related bleeding, the use of antifibrinolytic agents appear to be effective in both the treatment and prevention of excessive bleeding associated with cardiac surgery.[202,203] The exact mechanism by which natural (e.g., aprotinin) and synthetic antifibrinolytics (e.g., $\epsilon$-aminocaproic acid (EACA) and tranexamic acid) exert their effects have been difficult to define, but may be due to platelet preservation, as well as inhibition of fibrinolysis.[204,205] Although use of antifibrinolytic therapy is theoretically associated with an increased risk of thrombosis, controlled studies employing prophylactic use of these agents have not demonstrated an increased incidence of venous, coronary, or cerebrovascular thrombosis.[202,206]

Both EACA and tranexamic acid (TA) are administered as a bolus dose followed by a continuous infusion. An intravenous bolus of 100 to 150 mg/kg of EACA, followed by an infusion of 10 to 15 mg/kg-hr, provides the desired plasma concentration in adults. Higher doses are avoided because EACA may inhibit fibrinogen binding to platelets, resulting in platelet function abnormalities. Tranexamic acid is approximately 10 times as potent as EACA and a bolus of 10 mg/kg, followed by an infusion of 1 mg/kg-hr is adequate in adults.

Aprotonin (Trasylol) is a nonspecific serine protease inhibitor extracted from bovine lung. High dose aprotonin administration, consisting of a bolus of 2,000,000 KIU followed by an infusion of 500,000 KIU/hr, with an additional 2,000,000 KIU added to the priming solution of the extracorporeal circuit, has been shown to consistently reduce postoperative bleeding in patients undergoing CPB procedures.[204,207] Low-dose aprotonin administration has been shown to be as effective at reducing perioperative blood loss;[208] however, high risk patients are best treated with the high dose regimen.[209,210] The topical application of aprotonin into the pericardial cavity prior to surgical closure of the sternotomy, may also reduce postoperative blood loss and need for transfusion.[211] When aprotonin is used, the ACT should be assayed with kaolin as the surface activator, because the ACT is inappropriately elevated when celite is used as the activator.[212]

## ADJUNCTS TO SURGICAL HEMOSTASIS: TOPICAL HEMOSTATICS

Topical hemostatics may help control mucosal bleeding and capillary oozing associated with a wide variety of surgical procedures. Topical agents can usually be tailored for the particular hemostatic defect and surgical problem. Although these substances are usually harmless, they act as foreign bodies in a wound and may contribute to an increased risk of wound infection.

## Absorbable Gelatin Sponge (Gelfoam)

This is a gelatin-based, extremely porous substance that exerts its hemostatic effect by tamponade of the oozing area. It is particularly useful for highly vascular areas that are difficult to suture. The substance can be left in place after closure of the surgical wound and is completely absorbed 4 to 6 weeks after surgery. Scar formation and local inflammation is minimal.

## Oxidized Cellulose (Oxycell). Oxidized Generated Cellulose (Surgicel)

When exposed to blood, these substances are converted to a gelatinous mass composed of cellulose and acid hematin, producing an artificial clot. Oxidized cellulose has a low pH and acts as a local caustic substance, as well. Fibrosis and stricture of vascular prostheses and arterial anastomosis may occur with the use of these substances.

## Microfibrillar Collagen Hemostat (Avitene)

This is a water-insoluble agent that activates and entraps platelets initiating the formation of a fibrin clot. It may not be effective when the platelet count is low, but is particularly useful for treating capillary bleeding associated with platelet dysfunction. It appears to retain its hemostatic effect in heparinized patients, as well.

## Thrombin

Topical thrombin is derived from bovine prothrombin and is used to directly clot fibrinogen, bypassing the plasma coagulation system. Thrombin is particularly useful when bleeding is secondary to the use of heparin. Adequate levels of fibrinogen must exist (greater than 50 mg/dL) and it may be combined with gelatin sponge.

## Fibrin Glue

Fibrin glue is an exogenous source of human fibrinogen which is used with bovine-derived thrombin for local hemostasis, when fibrinogen is deficient or abnormal. It may be useful in a variety of difficult surgical situations including trauma, burns, and in patients with coagulation disorders.[213] It has also been shown to be effective in reducing postoperative mediastinal bleeding in patients requiring reexploration after cardiac surgery.[214]

### REFERENCES

1. Gimbrone MA Jr. Vascular endothelium: nature's blood containers. In: Gimbrone MA Jr. ed. Vascular Endothelium in Hemostasis and Thrombosis. New York, NY: Churchill Livingstone; 1986.
2. Dittman WA, Majerus PW. Structure and function of thrombomodulin: a natural anticoagulant. Blood. 1990;75:329.
3. Esmon NL. Thrombomodulin. Semin Thromb Hemostasis. 1987; 13:454.
4. Marcum JA, Rosenberg RD. Anticoagulantly active heparin sulfate proteoglycan and vascular endothelium. Semin Thromb Hemostasis. 1987;13:464.
5. Prescott SM, Zimmerman GA, McIntyre TM. Platelet-activating factor. J Biol Chem. 1990;265:173.
6. Hekman C, Loskutoff D. Fibrinolytic pathways and the endothelium. Semin Thrombos Hemostas. 1987;13:514.
7. Kroll MH, Harris TS, Moake JL, et al. Von Willebrand factor binding to platelet GPIb initiates signals for platelet activation. J Clin Invest. 1991;88:1568.
8. Shattil SJ, Bennett JS. Platelets and their membranes in hemostasis: Physiology and pathophysiology. Ann Intern Med. 1980;94:108.
9. Ware JA, Heistad DD. Platelet-endothelium interactions. N Engl J Med. 1993;328:628.
10. Nemerson Y. Tissue factor and hemostasis. Blood. 1988; 71:1.
11. Furie B, Furie BC: The molecular basis of blood coagulation. Cell. 1988;53:505.
12. Mann KG. The biochemistry of coagulation. Clin Lab Med. 1984;4:207.
13. Esmon CT. The regulation of natural anticoagulant pathways. Science 1987;235:1348.
14. Esmon CT. The roles of protein C and thrombomodulin in the regulation of blood coagulation. J Biol Chem. 1989; 264:4743.
15. van Hinsbergh VWM, Bertina RM, van Wijngaarden NH, et al. Activated protein C decreases plasminogen activator-inhibitor activity in endothelial cell conditioned medium. Blood. 1985;65:444.
16. Griffin JH, Evatt B, Zimmerman TS, et al. Deficiency of protein C in congenital thrombotic disease. J Clin Invest. 1981;68: 1370.
17. Seligsohn U, Berger A, Abend M, et al. Homozygous protein C deficiency manifested by massive venous thrombosis in the newborn. N Engl J Med. 1984;310:559.
18. Comp PC, Esmon CT. Recurrent venous thromboembolism in patients with a partial deficiency in protein S. N Engl J Med. 1984;311:1524.

19. Bachmann F. Diagnostic approach to mild bleeding disorders. Semin Hematol. 1980;17:292.
20. Kaplan EB, Sheiner LB, Boeckmann AJ, et al. The usefulness of preoperative laboratory screening. JAMA. 1985;253:3576.
21. Suchman AL, Mushlin AI. How well does the activated partial thromboplastin time predict postoperative hemorrhage? JAMA 1986; 256:750.
22. Rapapport SI. Preoperative hemostatic evaluation: Which test, if any? Blood 1983; 61:229.
23. Rhorer MJ, Michelotti MC, Nahrwold DL. A prospective evaluation of the efficacy of preoperative coagulation testing. Ann Surg. 1988;208:554.
24. Bushick JB, Eisenberg JM, Kinman J, et al. Pursuit of normal coagulation screening tests generates modest hidden preoperative costs. J Gen Intern Med. 1989;4:493.
25. Manning S, Beste D, McBride T, Goldberg A. An assessment of preoperative coagulation screening for tonsillectomy and adenoidectomy. Int J Ped Otorhinolaryngol. 1987;13:237.
26. Bolger WE, Parsons DS, Potempa L. Preoperative hemostatic assessment of the adenotonsillectomy patient. Otol Head Neck Surg. 1990;103:396.
27. Mozes B, Lubin D, Modan B, et al. Evaluation of an intervention aimed at reducing inappropriate use of preoperative blood coagulation tests. Arch Intern Med. 1989; 149:1836.
28. Harker L, Slichter SJ. The bleeding time as a screening test for evaluation of platelet function. N Engl J Med. 1972;287:155.
29. Rodgers RPC, Levin J. A critical reappraisal of the bleeding time. Semin Thromb Hemostasis. 1990; 16:1.
30. Barber A, Green D, Galluzo T, et al. The bleeding time as a preoperative screening test. Am J Med. 1985;78:761.
31. Hindman BJ, Koka BV. Usefulness of the post-aspirin bleeding time. Anesthesiology. 1986;64:368.
32. Proctor RR, Rapapport SI. The partial thromboplastin time with kaolin: A simple screening test for first-stage plasma clotting deficiencies. Am J Clin Pathol. 1961;36:212.
33. Lambert CJ, Marengo-Rowe AJ, Leveson JE, et al. The treatment of post-perfusion bleeding using epsilon-aminocaproic acid, cryoprecipitate, fresh frozen plasma, and protamine sulfate. Ann Thorac Surg. 1979;28:440.
34. Grossi CE, Moreno AH, Rousselot LM. Studies on the spontaneous fibrinolytic activity of patients with cirrhosis of the liver and its inhibition by epsilon aminocaproic acid. Ann Surg. 1961;153:383.
35. Tagnon HJ, Whitmore WF, Shulman NR. Fibrinolysis in metastatic cancer of the prostate. Cancer. 1952;5:9.
36. Lorand L, Urayama T, de Kiewiet JWC, et al. Diagnostic and genetic studies on fibrin-stabilizing factor with a new assay based on amine incorporation. J Clin Invest. 1969; 48:1054.
37. Born GVR. Aggregation of blood platelets by adenosine diphosphate and its reversal. Nature. 1962; 194:927.
38. Weiss HJ. Platelet physiology and abnormalities of platelet function. N Engl J Med. 1975;293:580.
39. Howard MA, Firkin BG. Ristocetin—a new tool in the investigation of platelet aggregation. Thromb Diath Haemorrh. 1971;26:362.
40. Olson JD, Brockway WJ, Fass DN, et al. Evaluation of ristocetin-Willebrand factor assay and ristocetin-

induced platelet aggregation. Am J Clin Pathol. 1975;63:210.

41. Bull BS, Korpman RA, Huse WM, et al. Heparin therapy during extracorporeal circulation I. Problems inherent to existing protocols. J Thorac Cardiovasc Surg. 1975;69:674.

42. Jobes DR, Schwartz AJ, Ellison N, et al. Monitoring heparin anticoagulation and its neutralization. Ann Thorac Surg. 1981;31:161.

43. Young JA, Kisker CT, Dory DB. Adequate anticoagulation during cardiopulmonary bypass determined by activated clotting time and the appearance of fibrin monomer. Ann Thorac Surg. 1978;26: 231.

44. Kang YG, Martin DJ, Marquez J, et al. Intraoperative changes in blood coagulation and thromboelastographic monitoring in liver transplantation. Anesth Analg. 1985; 64:888.

45. Kang YG, Lewis JH, Novalgund A, et al. Epsilon-aminocaproic acid for treatment of fibrinolysis during liver transplantation. Anesthesiology. 1987;66: 766.

46. Spiess BD, Tuman KJ, McCarthy RJ, et al. Thromboelastography as an indicator of post-cardiopulmonary bypass coagulopathies. J Clin Monit. 1987; 3:25.

47. Tuman KJ, McCarthy RJ, Djuric M, et al. Evaluation of coagulation during cardiopulmonary bypass with a heparinase-modified thromboelastographic assay. J Cardiothorac Vasc Anesth. 1994;8:144.

48. Tuman KJ, Spiess BD, McCarthy RJ, and others: Comparison of viscoelastic measures of coagulation after cardiopulmonary bypass. Anesth Analg 1989; 69:69.

49. Chapin JW, Becker GL, Hurlbert MC, et al. Comparison of thromboelastograph and sonoclot coagulation analyzer for assessing coagulation status during orthotopic liver transplantation. Transplant Proc. 1989;21:3539.

50. Lawn RM, Vehar GA. The molecular genetics of hemophilia. Sci Am. 1986;254:48.

51. Roberts HR: Hemophiliacs with inhibitors: Therapeutic options. N Engl J Med 1981; 305:757.

52. Ellison N: Diagnosis and management of bleeding disorders. Anesthesiology 1977; 47:171.

53. Bona RD, Weinstein RA, Weisman SJ, et al. The use of continuous infusion of factor concentrates in the treatment of hemophilia. Am J Hematol. 1989; 32:8.

54. Giles A, Tiulin S, Hoogendoorn H, et al. In vivo characterization of recombinant factor VIII in a canine model of hemophilia A (factor VIII deficiency). Blood. 1988;72:335.

55. White GC, McMillan CW, Kingdon HS, et al. Use of recombinant antihemophilic factor in the treatment of two patients with classic hemophilia. N Engl J Med. 1989; 320:166.

56. Dike GWR, Bidwell E, Rizza CR. The preparation and clinical use of a new concentrate containing factor IX, prothrombin, and factor X, and of a separate concentrate containing factor VII. Br J Haematol. 1972;22:469.

57. Conlan MG, Hoots WK. Disseminated intravascular coagulation and hemorrhage in hemophilia B following elective surgery. Am J Hematol. 1990; 35:203.

58. Lusher JM. Prediction and management of adverse events associated with the use of factor IX complex concentrates. Semin Hematol. 1993;30:36.

59. Goldsmith JC, Kasper CK, Blatt PM, et al. Coagulation factor IX: Successful surgical experience with a purified factor IX concentrate. Am J Hematol. 1992;40:210.

60. Ruggeri ZM, Zimmerman TS. von Willebrand factor and von Willebrand's disease. Blood. 1987;70: 895.

61. Rodeghiero F, Castaman G, Dini E. Epidemiological investigation of the prevalence of von Willebrand's disease. Blood. 1987;69:454.

62. Blombäck M, Johansson G, Johnsson H, et al. Surgery in patients with von Willebrand's disease. Br J Surg. 1989; 76:398.

63. Schulman S, Johnsson H, Egberg N, Blombäck M. DDAVP-induced correction of prolonged bleeding time in patients with congenital platelet function defects. Thromb Res. 1987; 45:165.

64. Webster MWI, Chesebro JH, Fuster V. Platelet inhibitor therapy: Agents and clinical implications. Hematol/Oncol Clin N Am. 1990;4:265.

65. Smith JB, Willis AL. Aspirin selectivity inhibits prostaglandin production in human platelets. Nature. 1971; 231:235.

66. Bashein G, Nessly ML, Rice AL, et al. Preoperative aspirin therapy and reoperation for bleeding after coronary artery bypass surgery. Arch Intern Med. 1991;151:89.

67. Horlocker TT, Wedel DJ, Offord KP. Does preoperative antiplatelet therapy increase the risk of hemorrhagic complications associated with regional anesthesia? Anesth Analg. 1990;70:631.

68. Shattil SJ, Bennett JS, McDonough M, Turnbull J. Carbenicillin and penicillin G inhibit platelet function in vitro by impairing the interaction of agonists with the platelet surface. J Clin Invest. 1980;65: 329.

69. Weitkamp MR, Aber RC. Prolonged bleeding times and bleeding diathesis associated with moxalactam administration. JAMA. 1983;249:69.

70. Fass RJ, Copelan EA, Brandt JT, et al. Platelet-mediated bleeding caused by broad-spectrum penicillins. J Infect Dis. 1987;155:1242.

71. Saxon A, Kattlove HE. Platelet inhibition by sodium nitroprusside, a smooth muscle inhibitor. Blood. 1976; 47:957.

72. Graybar G, Lalor D, Jones J. Comparison of nitroprusside and nitroglycerine in perioperative blood loss with open heart surgery. Crit Care Med. 1980; 1:240.

73. Schror K, Grodzinska L, Darius H. Stimulation of coronary vascular prostacyclin and inhibition of human platelet thromboxane $A_2$ after low-dose nitroglycerin. Thromb Res. 1981:23:59.

74. Lichtenthal PR, Rossi EC, Louis G, et al. Dose-related prolongation of the bleeding time by intravenous nitroglycerin. Anesth Analg. 1985;64:30.

75. Hines R, Barash PG. Infusion of sodium nitroprusside induces platelet dysfunction in vitro. Anesthesiology. 1989;70:611.

76. Schaffer AI, Alexander RW, Hardin RI. Inhibition of platelet function by organic nitrate vasodilators. Blood. 1980;55:649.

77. Furlong B, Henderson AH, Lewis MJ, Smith JS. Endothelium-derived relaxing factor inhibits in vitro platelet aggregation. Br J Pharmacol. 1987; 90:687.

78. Moncada S, Palmer RMJ, Higgs EA. The discovery of nitric oxide as the endogenous nitrovasodilator. Hypertension. 1988;12:365.

79. Hines R. Preservation of platelet function during trimethaphan infusion. Anesthesiology. 1990;72: 834.

80. Mehta J, Mehta P, Ostrowski N. Influence of propranolol and 4-hydroxypropranolol on platelet aggregation and thromboxane A₂ generation. Clin Pharmacol Ther. 1983;34:559.

81. Dale J, Landmark KH, Myhr E. The effects of nifedipine, a calcium antagonist, on platelet function. Am Heart J. 1983; 105:103.

82. Serneri GGN, Masotti G, Poggesi L, Morettini A. Enhanced prostacyclin production by dipyridamole in man. Eur J Clin Pharmacol. 1981;21:9.

83. Dalsgaard-Nielssen J, Risbo A, Simmelkjaer P, Gormsen J. Impaired platelet aggregation and increased bleeding time during general anesthesia with halothane. Br J Anaesth. 1981;53:1039.

84. Fauss BG, Meadows JC, Bruni CY, Qureshi GD. The in vitro and in vivo effects of isoflurane and nitrous oxide in platelet aggregation. Anesth Analg. 1986;65:1170.

85. Suttie JW. Vitamin K dependent carboxylase. Ann Rev Biochem. 1985;54:459.

86. NIH Consensus Conference. Fresh frozen plasma: indications and risks. JAMA. 1985;253:551.

87. Rosenberg RD. Actions and interactions of antithrombin and heparin. N Engl J Med. 1975;292: 146.

88. Shah MC, Schwarz KB. Hazards of small amounts of heparin in a patient with subclinical vitamin K deficiency. J Parenteral Enteral Nutr. 1989;13:324.

89. Owens EL, Kasten GW, Hessel EA. Spinal subarachnoid hematoma after lumbar puncture and heparinization. A case report, review of the literature, and discussion of anesthetic implication. Anesth Analg. 1986;65:1201.

90. Odoom JA, Sih IL. Epidural analgesia and anticoagulant therapy. Experience in one thousand cases of continuous epidurals. Anaesthesia. 1983;38:254.

91. Matthews ET, Abrams LD. Intrathecal morphine in open heart surgery (Letter). Lancet. 1980;2:543.

92. Rao TLK, El-Etr AA. Anticoagulation following placement of epidural and subarachnoid catheters. Anesthesiology. 1981; 55:618.

93. Marciniak E, Gockerman JP. Heparin-induced decrease in circulating anti-thrombin III. Lancet. 1977;2:581.

94. Anderson EF. Heparin resistance prior to cardiopulmonary bypass. Anesthesiology. 1986;64:504.

95. Bell WT, Royall RM. Heparin-associated thrombocytopenia: a comparison of three heparin preparations. N Engl J Med. 1980;303:902.

96. Becker PS, Miller VT. Heparin-induced thrombocytopenia. Stroke. 1989;20:1449.

97. Walls JT, Curtis JJ, Silver D, Boley TM. Heparin-induced thrombocytopenia in patients who undergo open heart surgery. Surgery. 1990;108: 686.

98. Frame JN, Mulvey KP, Phares JC, Anderson MJ. Correction of severe heparin-associated thrombocytopenia with intravenous immunoglobin. Ann Int Med. 1989;111:946.

99. Olinger GN, Hussey CV, Olive JA, Malik MI. Cardiopulmonary bypass for patients with previously documented heparin induced platelet aggregation. J Thorac Cardiovasc Surg. 1984;87:673.

100. Smith JP, Walls JT, Muscato MS, et al. Extracorporeal circulation in a patient with heparin-induced thrombocytopenia. Anesthesiology. 1985;62:363.

101. Vender JS, Matthew EB, Silverman IM, et al. Heparin-induced thrombocytopenia: alternative managements. Anesth Analg. 1986;65:520.

102. Ellison N, Kappa JR, Fisher CA, Addonzio Jr VP. Extracorporeal circulation in a patient with heparin-induced thrombocytopenia (Letter). Anesthesiology. 1985;63:336.

103. Addonzio Jr VP, Fisher CA, Kappa JR, Ellison N. Prevention of heparin-induced thrombocytopenia during open heart surgery with Iloprost (ZK 36374). Surgery. 1987;102:796.

104. Kappa JT, Cottrell ED, Berkowitz HD, et al. Carotid endarterectomy in patients with heparin-induced platelet activation: comparative efficacy of aspirin and iloprost (ZK36374). J Vasc Surg. 1987; 5:693.

105. Wood AJ, Robertson D, Robertson RM, et al. Elevated plasma free drug concentrations of propanolol and diazepam during cardiac catheterizations. Circulation. 1980;62:1119.

106. Casthely PA, Goodman K, Fyman PN, et al. Hemodynamic changes after administration of protamine. Anesth Analg. 1986;65:78.

107. Stoelting RK, Henry DP, Verburg KM, et al. Haemodynamic changes and circulating histamine concentrations following protamine administration to patients and dogs. Can Anaesth Soc J. 1984;31: 534.

108. Stewart WJ, McSweeney SM, Kellett MA, et al. Increased risk of severe protamine reactions in NPH insulin-dependent diabetics undergoing cardiac catheterization. Circulation. 1984;70:788.

109. Horrow JC. Protamine: a review of its toxicity. Anesth Analg. 1985;64:348.

110. Sharath MD, Metzger WJ, Richerson HB, et al. Protamine-induced fatal anaphylaxis: prevalence of antiprotamine immunoglobin E antibody. J Thorac Cardiovasc Surg. 1985; 90:86.

111. Campbell FW, Goldstein MF, Atkins PC. Management of the patient with protamine hypersensitivity for cardiac surgery. Anesthesiology. 1984;61:761.

112. Castaneda AR, Gans H, Weber KC, et al. Heparin neutralization: experimental and clinical studies. Surgery. 1967;62:686.

113. Lowenstein E, Johnston W, Lappas D, et al. Catastrophic pulmonary vasoconstriction associated with protamine reversal of heparin. Anesthesiology. 1983;59:470.

114. Morel DR, Zapol WM, Thomas SJ, et al. C5a and thromboxane generation associated with pulmonary vaso- and bronchoconstriction during protamine reversal of heparin. Anesthesiology. 1987; 66:597.

115. Conzen PF, Habzettl H, Gutmann R, et al. Thromboxane mediation of pulmonary hemodynamic responses after neutralization of heparin by protamine in pigs. Anesth Analg. 1989;68:25.

116. WHO Expert Committee on Biological Standardization. 28th Report: WHO Technical Report Series 610, Geneva, 1977, World Health Organization; 14:45.

117. Loeliger EA. ICSH/ISTH recommendations for reporting prothrombin time in oral anticoagulant control. Thrombos Haemostasis. 1985;53:155.

118. Tinker JH, Tarhan S. Discontinuing anticoagulant therapy in surgical patients with cardiac valve prosthesis. Observations in 180 operations. JAMA. 1978;239:738.

119. Roizen MF. Anesthetic implications of concurrent

diseases. In: Miller RD, ed. Anesthesia. New York, NY: Churchill Livingstone;1990.

120. Katholi RE, Nolan SP, McGuire LB. The management of anticoagulation during noncardiac operations in patients with prosthetic heart valves: a prospective study. Am Heart J. 1978;96:163.

121. Silver BA, Bell WR. Cimetidine potentiation of the hypoprothrombinemic effect of warfarin. Ann Intern Med. 1979;90:348.

122. Hassall C, Feetam CL, Leach RH, et al. Potentiation of warfarin by cotrimoxazole (Letter). Lancet. 1975;2:1155.

123. O'Rielly RA. The stereoselective interaction of metronidazole in man. N Engl J Med. 1976;295:354.

124. O'Rielly RA. Interaction of sodium warfarin and disulfuram (Antabuse) in man. Ann Intern Med. 1973;78:73.

125. Rawlins MD, Smith SE. Influence of allopurinol on drug metabolism in man. Br J Pharmacol. 1973; 48:693.

126. Koch-Weser J. Quinidine-induced hypothrombinemic hemorrhage in patients on chronic warfarin therapy. Ann Intern Med. 1968;68:511.

127. Watt AH, Stephens MR, Buss DC, et al. Amiodarone reduces plasma warfarin clearance in man. Br J Clin Pharmacol. 1986;20:707.

128. Udall JA. Clinical implications of warfarin: interactions with five sedatives. Am J Cardiol. 1975;35: 67.

129. O'Reilly RA. Interaction of sodium warfarin and rifampin: Studies in man. Ann Intern Med. 1974; 81:337.

130. Scott AK, Park BK, Breckenridge AM. Interaction between warfarin and propranolol. Br J Clin Pharmacol. 1984;17:559.

131. Ghoneim MM, Delle M, Wilson WR, Ambre JJ. Alteration of warfarin kinetics in man associated with exposure to an operating-room environment. Anesthesiology. 1975;43:333.

132. Calvo R, Aguilera L, Suarez E, Rodriguez-Sasain JM. Displacement of warfarin from human serum proteins by halothane anesthesia. Acta Anaesthesiol Scand. 1989;33:575.

133. Kelly DA, Tuddenham EGD. Hemostatic problems in liver disease. Gut. 1986;27:339.

134. Straub PW. Diffuse intravascular coagulation in liver disease. Ann Rev Med. 1974;25:447.

135. Owen JS, Hutton RA, Day RC, et al. Platelet lipid composition and platelet aggregation in human liver disease. J Lipid Res. 1981;22:423.

136. Cowan DH. Effect of alcoholism on hemostasis. Semin Hematol. 1980;17:137.

137. Agnelli G, De Cunto M, Berretini M, et al. Desmopressin induced improvements of abnormal coagulation in chronic liver disease (Letter). Lancet. 1983;1:645.

138. Burroughs AK, Matthews K, Qudiri M, et al. Desmopressin and bleeding time in cirrhosis. Br Med J. 1985;291:1377.

139. Botempo FA, Lewis JH, Van Thiel DH, et al. The relation of preoperative coagulation findings to diagnosis, blood usage and survival in adult liver transplantation. Transplantation. 1985;39:532.

140. Owen Jr CA, Rettke SR, Bowie EJW, et al. Hemostatic evaluation of patients undergoing liver transplantation. Mayo Clin Proc. 1987;62:761.

141. Dzik WH, Arkin CF, Jenkins RL, et al. Fibrinolysis during liver transplantation in humans: role of tissue-type plasminogen activator. Blood. 1988;71: 1090.

142. Palareti G, de Rosa V, Fortunato G, et al. Control of hemostasis during orthoptic liver transplantation. Fibrinolysis. 1988;2(suppl 3):61.

143. Plevak DJ, Halma GA, Forstrom LA, et al. Thrombocytopenia after liver transplantation. Transplant Proc. 1988;20(suppl 1):630.

144. Iwatsuki S, Shaw Jr BW, Starzl TE. Current status of hepatic transplantation. Semin Liver Dis. 1983; 3:173.

145. Zuckerman GR, Cornette GL, Clouse RE, et al. Upper gastrointestinal bleeding in patients with chronic renal failure. Ann Int Med. 1985;102:588.

146. Di Minno G, Martinez J, McKean ML, et al. Platelet dysfunction in uremia: multifaceted defect partially corrected by dialysis. Am J Med. 1985;79: 552.

147. Livio M, Gotti E, Marchesi D, et al. Uraemic bleeding: role of anaemia and beneficial effect of red cell transfusions. Lancet. 1982;2:1013.

148. Fernandez F, Goudable C, Sie P, et al. Low hematocrit and prolonged bleeding time in uraemic patients: effect of red cell transfusions. Br J Haematol. 1985;59:139.

149. Llach F. Hypercoagulability, renal vein thrombosis, and other thrombotic complications of nephrotic syndrome. Kidney Int. 1985;28:429.

150. Remuzzi G. Bleeding in renal failure. Lancet. 1988; 1:190.

151. Jansen PA, Jubelirer SJ, Weinstein MJ, et al. Treatment of the bleeding tendency in uremia with cryoprecipitate. N Engl J Med. 1980;303:1318.

152. Mannucci PM, Remuzzi G, Pusineri F, et al. Deamino-8-D-arginine vasopressin shortens the bleeding time in uremia. N Engl J Med. 1983;308:8.

153. Gralnick HR, McKeown LP, Williams SB, et al. Plasma and platelet von Willebrand factor defects in uremia. Am J Med. 1988;85:806.

154. Canavese C, Salomone M, Pacitti S, et al. Reduced response of uraemic bleeding to repeated doses of desmopressin (Letter). Lancet. 1985;1:867.

155. Capitanio A, Mannucci PM, Ponticelli C, et al. Detection of circulating released platelets after renal transplantation. Transplantation. 1982;33:298.

156. Fruchtman S, Aledort LM. Disseminated intravascular coagulation. J Am Coll Cardiol. 1986; 8(Suppl. 6):159B.

157. Baker R. Clinical aspects of disseminated intravascular coagulation. Semin Thromb Hemostasis. 1989;15:1.

158. Vinazzer H. Therapeutic use of antithrombin III in shock and disseminated intravascular coagulation. Semin Thromb Hemostasis. 1989;15:347.

159. Collins JA. Recent developments in the area of massive transfusion. World J Surg. 1987;11:75.

160. Valeri CR, Feingold H, Cassidy G, et al. Hypothermia-induced reversible platelet dysfunction. Ann Surg. 1987; 205:175.

161. Ferrara A, MacArthur JD, Wright HK, et al. Hypothermia and acidosis worsen coagulopathy in the patient requiring massive transfusion. Am J Surg. 1990;160:515.

162. Miller RD, Robbins TO, Tong MJ, et al. Coagulation defects associated with massive blood transfusion. Ann Surg. 1971;174:794.

163. Miller RD. Complications of massive transfusions. Anesthesiology. 1973;39:82.

164. Counts RB, Haiseh C, Simon JL, et al. Hemostasis

in massively transfused trauma patients. Ann Surg. 1979; 190:91.

165. Leslie SD, Toy PT. Laboratory hemostatic abnormalities in massively transfused patients given red blood cells and crystalloid. Am J Clin Pathol. 1991; 96:770.

166. Harrigan C, Lucas DE, Ledgerwood AM, Mammen EF. Primary hemostasis after massive transfusion for injury. Am Surg. 1982;48:393.

167. Reed RL, Ciavarella D, Heimbach DM, Baron L. Prophylactic platelet administration during massive transfusion. A prospective, randomized, double blind clinical study. Ann Surg. 1986;203:40.

168. Martin DI, Lucas CE, Ledgerwood AM, et al. Fresh frozen plasma supplement to massive red blood cell transfusion. Ann Surg. 1985;202:505.

169. Horst HM, Dlugos S, Fath JJ, et al. Coagulopathy and intraoperative blood salvage. J Trauma. 1992; 32:646.

170. Martin RR, Bickell WH, Pepe PE, et al. Prospective evaluation of preoperative fluid resuscitation in hypotensive patients with penetrating truncal injury: a preliminary report. J Trauma. 1992;33:354.

171. Bickell WH, Wall MJ, Pepe PE, et al. Immediate versus delayed fluid resuscitation for hypotensive patients with penetrating torso injuries. N Engl J Med. 1994;331:1105.

172. Hewson JR, Neame PB, Kumar N, et al. Coagulopathy related to dilution and hypotension during massive transfusion. Crit Care Med. 1985;13:387.

173. Bick RL, Arbegast NR, Crawford L, et al. Hemostatic effects induced by cardiopulmonary bypass. Vasc Surg. 1975;9:28.

174. Harker LA. Bleeding after cardiopulmonary bypass. N Engl J Med. 1986;314:1446.

175. Bachmann F, McKenna R, Cole ER, et al. The hemostatic mechanism after open-heart surgery. I. Studies on plasma coagulation factors and fibrinolysis in 512 patients after extracorporeal circulation. J Thorac Cardiovasc Surg. 1975; 70:76.

176. Czer LSC, Bateman TM, Gray RJ, et al. Treatment of severe platelet dysfunction and hemorrhage after cardiopulmonary bypass: reduction in blood product usage with desmopressin. J Am Coll Cardiol. 1987;9:1139.

177. Woodman RC, Harker LA. Bleeding complications associated with cardiopulmonary bypass. Blood. 1990;76:1680.

178. Hope AF, Heyns AD, Lotter MG. Kinetics and sites of sequestration of indium III-labeled human platelets during cardiopulmonary bypass. J Thorac Cardiovasc Surg. 1981; 81:880.

179. Harker LA, Malpass TW, Branson HE, et al. Mechanism of abnormal bleeding in patients undergoing cardiopulmonary bypass: Acquired transient platelet dysfunction associated with selective alpha-granule release. Blood. 1980;56:824.

180. Khabbaz KR, Marquardt CA, Wolfe JA, et al. Reversible platelet dysfunction following cardiopulmonary bypass: a temperature dependent defect in platelet thromboxane $A_2$ synthesis. Surg Forum. 1989;40:201.

181. Rinder CS, Bohnert J, Rinder HM. Platelet activation and aggregation during cardiopulmonary bypass. Anesthesiology. 1991;75:388.

182. Beurling-Harbury C, Galvan CA. Acquired decrease in platelet secretory ADP associated with increased post operative bleeding in post-cardiopul-

monary patients and in patients with severe valvular heart disease. Blood. 1978; 52:13.

183. Ferraris VA, Ferraris SF, Lough FC, et al. Preoperative aspirin ingestion increases operative blood loss after coronary artery bypass grafting. Ann Thorac Surg. 1988; 45:71.

184. Mammen EF, Koets BA, Washington BC, et al. Hemostatic changes during cardiopulmonary bypass surgery. Semin Thromb Hemost. 1985;11:281.

185. Tanaka K, Takao M, Yada I, et al. Alterations in coagulation and fibrinolysis associated with cardiopulmonary bypass during open heart surgery. J Cardiothorac Anesth. 1989;3:181.

186. Lijnen HR, Collen D. Interaction of plasminogen activators and inhibitors with plasminogen and fibrin. Semin Thromb Hemost. 1989;8:2.

187. Bull BS, Huse WM, Brauer FS. et al. Heparin therapy during extracorporeal circulation II. The use of dose-response curve to individualize heparin and protamine dosage. J Thorac Cardiovasc Surg. 1975; 69:685.

188. Metz S, Keats AS. Low activated coagulation time during cardiopulmonary bypass does not increase postoperative bleeding. Ann Thorac Surg. 1990; 49:440.

189. Roy RC, Stafford MA, Hudspeth AS, and others: Failure of prophylaxis with fresh frozen plasma after cardiopulmonary bypass. Anesthesiology 1988; 69: 254.

190. Simon TL, Ali BF, Murphy W. Controlled trial of routine platelet concentrates in cardiopulmonary bypass surgery. Ann Thorac Surg. 1984;37:359.

191. Mohr R, Martinowitz V, Lavee J, et al. The hemostatic effect of fresh whole blood versus platelet concentrates after cardiac operations. J Thorac Cardiovasc Surg. 1988; 96:530.

192. Lavee J, Martinowitz V, Mohr R. The effect of fresh whole blood versus platelet concentrates after cardiac operations: a scanning electron microscopic study of platelet aggregation on extracellular matrix. J Thorac Cardiovasc Surg. 1990;97:204.

193. DelRossi AJ, Cernaianu AC, Vertrees RA, et al. Platelet-rich plasma reduces postoperative blood loss after cardiopulmonary bypass. J Thorac Cardiovasc Surg. 1990; 100:281.

194. Boldt J, Zickmann B, Ballesteros M, et al. Influence of acute preoperative plasmapheresis on platelet function in cardiac surgery. J Cardiothorac Anesth. 1993;7:4.

195. Boey SK, Ong BC, Dhara SS. Preoperative plateletpheresis does not reduce blood loss during cardiac surgery. Can J Anaesth. 1993;40:844.

196. Wong CA, Franklin ML, Wade LD. Coagulation tests, blood loss, and transfusion requirements in platelet-rich plasmapheresed versus nonpheresed cardiac surgery patients. Anesth Analg. 1994;78: 29.

197. Salzman EW, Weinstein MJ, Weintraub RM, et al. Treatment with desmopressin acetate to reduce blood loss after cardiac surgery: a double-blind, randomized trial. N Engl J Med. 1986;314:1402.

198. Rocha E, Llorens R, Paramo JA, et al. Does desmopressin acetate reduce blood loss after surgery in patients on cardiopulmonary bypass? Circulation. 1988; 77:1319.

199. Hackmann T, Gascoyne RD, Naiman SC, et al. A trial of desmopressin (1-desamino-8-d-arginine vasopressin) to reduce blood loss in uncomplicated cardiac surgery. N Engl J Med. 1989;321:1437.

200. Horrow JC, Hlavacek J, Strong MD, et al. Prophylactic tranexamic acid decreases bleeding after cardiac operations. J Thorac Cardiovasc Surg. 1990; 99:70.
201. Horrow JC, van Riper DF, Strong MD, et al. Hemostatic effects of tranexamic acid and desmopressin during cardiac surgery. Circulation. 1991;84: 2063.
202. Hardy JF, Desroches J. Natural and synthetic antifibrinolytics in cardiac surgery. Can J Anaesth. 1992; 39:353.
203. van Oeveren W, Harder MP, Roozendaal KJ, et al. Aprotonin protects platelets against the initial effect of cardiopulmonary bypass. J Thorac Cardiovasc Surg. 1990; 99:788.
204. Harder MP, Eijsman L, Roozendaal KJ, et al. Aprotonin reduces intraoperative and postoperative blood loss in membrane oxygenator cardiopulmonary bypass. Ann Thorac Surg. 1991;51:936.
205. DelRossi AJ, Cernaianu AC, Botros S, et al. Prophylactic treatment of postperfusion bleeding using EACA. Chest. 1989;96:27.
206. Havel M, Teufelsbauer H, Knobl P, et al. Effect of intraoperative aprotonin administration on postoperative bleeding in patients undergoing cardiopulmonary bypass operation. J Thorac Cardiovasc Surg. 1991;101:968.
207. Kawasuji M, Ueyama K, Sakakibara N, et al. Effect of low-dose aprotonin on coagulation and fibrinolysis in cardiopulmonary bypass. Ann Thorac Surg. 1993;55:1205.
208. Hardy JF, Desroches J, Belisle S, et al. Low-dose aprotonin infusion is not clinically useful to reduce bleeding and transfusion of homologous blood products in high-risk cardiac surgical patients. Can J Anaesth. 1993;40:625.
209. Biagini A, Comite C, Russo V, et al. High dose aprotonin to reduce blood loss in patients undergoing redo open heart surgery. Acta Anaesthesiol Belg. 1992;43:181.
210. Tater H, Cicek S, Demirkilic U, et al. Topical use of aprotonin in open heart operations. Ann Thorac Surg. 1993; 55:659.
211. Wang JS, Lin CY, Hung WT, et al. Monitoring of heparin-induced anticoagulation with kaolin-activated clotting time in cardiac surgical patients treated with aprotonin. Anesthesiology. 1992;77: 1080.
212. Kram HB, Nathan RC, Stafford FJ, et al. Fibrin glue achieves hemostasis in patients with coagulation disorders. Arch Surg. 1989;124:385.
213. Rousou J, Levitsky S, Gonzalez-Lavin L, et al. Randomized clinical trial of fibrin sealant in patients undergoing resternotomy or reoperation after cardiac operations: a multicenter study. J Thorac Surg. 1989;97:194.

# 3

# PRINCIPLES OF OXYGEN TRANSPORT

## *George J. Crystal and M. Ramez Salem*

The cardiovascular system acts in concert with the respiratory system in transporting oxygen to tissue mitochondria from its store in environmental air. The oxygen serves as an electron acceptor in oxidative phosphorylation, permitting production of adenosine triphosphate (ATP) along efficient aerobic pathways. The high-energy phosphate bonds of ATP provide energy for functional and biochemical processes within the cell, such as the contraction of muscle proteins and the metabolic activity of enzymes.

Figure 3–1 presents the influence of partial pressure of oxygen ($PO_2$) on oxygen consumption ($\dot{V}O_2$) of isolated mitochondria.[1] It shows that above approximately 0.1 mm Hg, $\dot{V}O_2$ is independent of $PO_2$. Accordingly, the objective of the integrated oxygen delivery system in vivo is to ensure that $PO_2$ is maintained above 0.1 mm Hg in the vicinity of all mitochondria. The only function of a $PO_2$ above 0.1 mm Hg is to provide sufficient driving force for diffusion of oxygen to mitochondria remote from capillaries.

## DETERMINANTS OF CONVECTIVE OXYGEN DELIVERY

The amount of oxygen carried from the lungs to tissues by circulating blood, i.e., the convective systemic oxygen delivery ($DO_2$), is given by the equation:

$$DO_2 = CaO_2 \times CO \qquad (1)$$

Where $CaO_2$ is the arterial oxygen content in vol%, and CO is systemic blood flow or cardiac output in L/min.

### Arterial Oxygen Content

$CaO_2$ content is composed of oxygen bound to hemoglobin (HGB) and oxygen dissolved in plasma:

$$CaO_2 = O_2bound + O_2dissolved \qquad (2)$$

#### OXYGEN BOUND TO HEMOGLOBIN

The structure of a human HGB molecule, which is characteristic for all HGB molecules in vertebrates, is presented in Figure 3–2. The HGB molecule is composed of two basic portions.[2] The protein or globin portion is made up of identical polypeptide chains: two $\alpha$ and two $\beta$ chains. The polypeptide chains are folded and assembled as a tetramer. Each of these chains contains one heme group, which serves as an iron-containing, reversible carrier

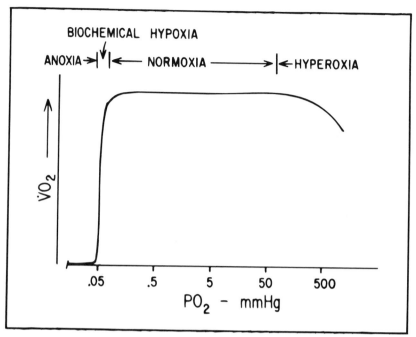

**Fig. 3–1.** Oxygen consumption of isolated mitochondria as a function of $PO_2$. From Honig CR. Modern Cardiovascular Physiology. Boston, 1981, Little, Brown and Company, with permission; 1981.

of one molecule of oxygen. Thus, each molecule of HGB can bind four molecules of oxygen. Oxygen bound is a function of HGB concentration, oxygen-carrying capacity for HGB (1.39 mL $O_2$/g HGB), and oxygen saturation of HGB ($SaO_2$), according to the equation:

$$O_2 bound = (HGB \times SaO_2 \times 1.39) \quad (3)$$

## DISSOCIATION CURVE

$SaO_2$ is a function of $PO_2$ and the oxyhemoglobin dissociation curve, which is a plot of oxyhemoglobin saturation as a function of $PO_2$ (Figure 3–3). The sigmoid shape of the curve reflects the fact that the four binding sites on a given HGB molecule interact with each other.[3] When the first site has bound a molecule of oxygen, the binding of the next site is facilitated, and so forth. The result is a curve that is steep up to $PO_2$ of 60 mm Hg and then becomes more shallow thereafter, approaching 100% saturation asymptotically. At a $PO_2$ of 100 mm Hg, the normal arterial value, 97% of the hemes have bound oxygen; at 40 mm Hg, a typical value for the mixed venous oxygen tension ($P\bar{v}O_2$) in a resting person, the saturation declines to about 75%.

The shape of the oxyhemoglobin dissociation curve has important physiological implications. The flatness of the curve above a $PO_2$ of 80 mm Hg assures a relatively constant oxyhemoglobin saturation for arterial blood, despite wide variations in alveolar oxygen pres-

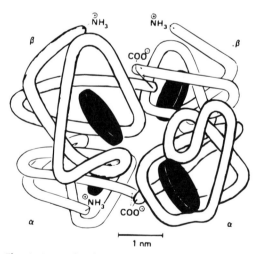

**Fig. 3–2.** Molecular model of human hemoglobin showing its four polypeptides- two $\alpha$ and two $\beta$ chains, each having one heme (indicated by disk) to which oxygen can bind. From Harper HA et al. Physiologische Chemie. Spring-Verlag, with permission; 1975.

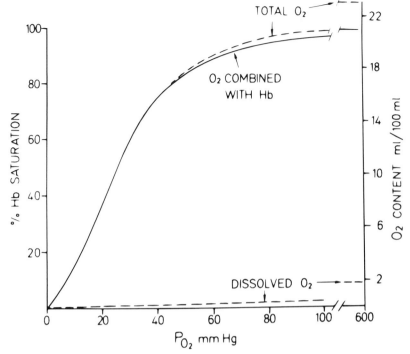

**Fig. 3–3.**  The oxygen content of blood has two components: oxygen binding to hemoglobin follows an S-shaped curve up to full saturation; the amount of oxygen in solution increases linearly with $PO_2$ without limit. From West JB. Best and Taylor's Physiological Basis of Medical Practice. 11th ed. Baltimore, Md: Williams & Wilkins, with permission; 1985.

sure. The steep portion of the curve between 20 and 60 mm Hg, permits unloading of oxygen from HGB at relatively high $PO_2$ values, which favors the delivery of large amounts of oxygen into the tissue by diffusion.

The oxygen binding properties of HGB are influenced by a number of factors, including pH, $PCO_2$, and temperature (Fig. 3–4).

These factors cause shifts of the oxyhemoglobin dissociation curve to the right or left, without changing the slope of the curve. For example, an increase in temperature or a decrease in pH, such as may occur in active tissues, decreases the affinity of HGB for oxygen, and shifts the oxyhemoglobin dissociation curve to the right. Thus, a higher $PO_2$ is required

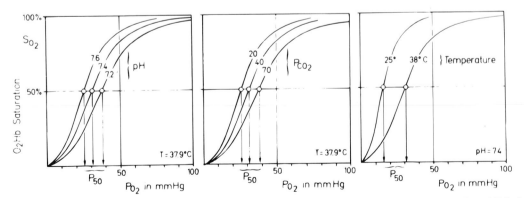

**Fig. 3–4.**  Effects of variations in pH, $PCO_2$, and temperature on oxyhemoglobin dissociation curve. From Weibel ER. The Pathway for Oxygen. Cambridge, MA: Harvard University Press, with permission; 1984.

to achieve a given saturation, which facilitates unloading of oxygen at the tissue. To quantify the extent of a shift in the oxyhemoglobin dissociation curve, the so-called $P_{50}$ is used, i.e., the $PO_2$ required for 50% saturation. The $P_{50}$ of normal adult HGB at 37° C and normal pH and $PCO_2$ is 26 to 27 mm Hg.

## FETAL HEMOGLOBIN

Fetal HGB differs structurally from adult HGB in that two of its polypeptide chains are of the $\gamma$ rather than $\beta$ type.[1] The oxyhemoglobin dissociation curve of the fetus is similar to that of the adult, except that the curve is shifted to the left, resulting in a $P_{50}$ of 20 mm Hg. (See Chapter 5: Perioperative Hemoglobin Requirements.)

## OXYGEN RELEASING FACTOR

The compound 2, 3-diphosphoglycerate (2,3-DPG) is an intermediate in anaerobic glycolysis [the biochemical pathway by which red blood cells (RBCs) produce ATP], which binds to HGB. Increases in intraerythrocytic 2,3-DPG concentration reduce the affinity of HGB for oxygen; they shift the oxyhemoglobin dissociation curve to the right, whereas decreases have opposite effects. Several factors have been found to influence RBC 2,3-DPG concentrations. For example, after storage in a blood bank of only 1 week, 2,3-DPG concentrations are one-third normal, resulting in a shift to the left of the oxyhemoglobin dissociation curve. On the other hand, conditions associated with chronic hypoxia, e.g., chronic anemia or living at high altitude, stimulate production of 2,3-DPG, causing a rightward shift of the oxyhemoglobin dissociation curve.

The amount of oxygen that can be carried per 1 g of HGB is controversial.[4] Originally 1.34 was used, but with the determination of the molecular weight of HGB, the theoretical value of 1.39 became popular. On the basis of extensive human studies, Gregory observed that the appropriate value was 1.306 in human adults.[5] Nevertheless, 1.39 remains in use in most studies.

## DISSOLVED OXYGEN IN PLASMA WATER

Dissolved oxygen is linearly related to $PO_2$ (Figure 3–3). At 37° C, it is defined by the equation:

$$O_2 \text{ dissolved} = 0.003 \text{ vol\%/mm}$$
$$\times \text{ Hg } PO_2 \quad (4)$$

Dissolved oxygen normally accounts for only 1.5% of total oxygen, but this contribution increases when the bound component is reduced during hemodilution. Since HGB is essentially saturated at $PO_2$ of 100 mm Hg, increases in arterial $PO_2$ ($PaO_2$) to levels above 100 mm Hg increase $CaO_2$ by raising the dissolved component.

## CHARACTERISTIC VALUES FOR PARAMETERS OF OXYGEN DELIVERY

For an individual with a HGB concentration of 15 g/100 mL, $PaO_2$ of 100 mm Hg, $P\bar{v}O_2$ of 40 mm Hg , and CO of 5000 mL/min:

$$CaO_2 = (15 \times 0.97 \times 1.39)$$
$$+ (0.003 \times 100) = 20.5 \text{ vol\%;}$$
$$DO_2 = (5000 \times 20.5/100)$$
$$= 1025 \text{ mL/min;}$$
$$C\bar{v}O_2 = (15 \times 0.75 \times 1.39)$$
$$+ (0.003 \times 40) = 15.8 \text{ vol\%;}$$

and the arteriovenous oxygen content difference ($CaO_2 - C\bar{v}O_2$) is:
$$(CaO_2 - C\bar{v}O_2) = 20.5 - 15.8 = 4.7 \text{ vol\%.}$$

# BLOOD FLOW TO PERIPHERAL TISSUES—PRINCIPLES OF BLOOD RHEOLOGY

In addition to $CaO_2$, blood flow (BF) is a primary determinant of tissue oxygen delivery (Eq. 1). BF is a function of the arteriovenous pressure gradient ($Pa - Pv$) and vascular resistance (VR), according to the equation:

$$F \text{ (flow)} = \frac{(Pa - Pv)}{VR} \quad (5)$$

This is analogous to Ohm's law in an electrical circuit. Since arterial and venous blood pressures are normally well maintained within narrow limits, BF usually varies inversely as a function of VR.

## Poiseuille's Law

Poiseuille performed studies that yielded an equation describing the resistance to flow in a straight, rigid tube of length (l) and radius (r):

$$VR \; (resistance) = \frac{\eta 8 l}{r^4} \qquad (6)$$

where $\eta$ is the viscosity. Of note is that blood flow resistance varies inversely with tube radius raised to the fourth power. Thus, small changes in tube radius cause large changes in resistance.

## Geometric Factors

Because the length of blood vessels in situ is fixed, geometric changes in VR occur by variations in vessel radius. These adjustments are the result of contraction or relaxation of the smooth muscle investing the arterioles, which are the principal site of vascular resistance. Chemical factors that are linked to the metabolic activity of the tissue, e.g., adenosine, modulate VR so that BF (and oxygen delivery) are commensurate with the prevailing local oxygen demands.

## Viscosity

Viscosity is the internal friction resulting from the intermolecular forces operating within a flowing liquid.[6] The term "internal friction" emphasizes that as a fluid moves within a tube, laminae in the fluid slip on one another and move at different speeds. The movement produces a velocity gradient in a direction perpendicular to the wall of the tube. This velocity gradient is termed the shear rate. In the circulation, shear rate shows a direct correlation to rate of blood flow. An intuitive understanding of the term "viscosity" can be gained from the experiment shown in Figure 3–5. In this experiment, a homogeneous fluid is confined between two closed-spaced, parallel plates (analogous to playing cards). Assuming the area of each plate is A, the distance between the plates is Y, and the bottom plate is stationary. If a tangential force (a shear stress) is applied to the upper plate, this plate will move with velocity v in the direction of the applied force and a velocity gradient (or shear rate) is developed in the fluid. Viscosity is defined as the factor of proportionality relating shear stress and shear rate for the fluid.

$$Viscosity = \frac{shear \; stress}{shear \; rate} \qquad (7)$$

Newton assumed that viscosity was a constant

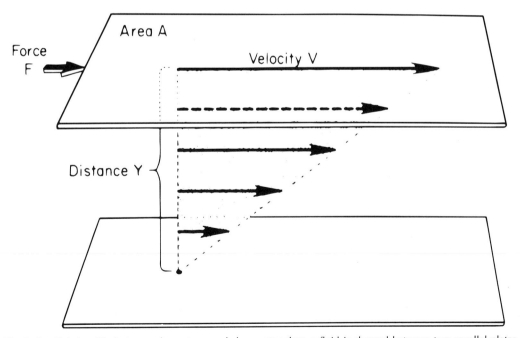

**Fig. 3–5.** Relationship between shear stress and shear rate when a fluid is sheared between two parallel plates. Details included in text. From Fahmy NR. Techniques for deliberate hypotension: Haemodilution and hypotension. In: Enderby GEH, ed. Hypotensive anaesthesia. Edinburgh, Scotland: Churchill-Livingstone, with permission; 1985.

**Table 3–1.   Factors that affect viscosity of whole blood**

HCT
Plasma proteins
RBC deformability
RBC aggregation
Temperature

property of a particular fluid and independent of shear rate. Fluids that demonstrate this behavior are termed "Newtonian." The units of viscosity are dynes per second, per square centimeter or poise.

## Factors Affecting Blood Viscosity

Factors affecting whole blood viscosity are presented on Table 3–1. The viscosity of blood varies as direct function of hematocrit (HCT) (Fig. 3–6), i.e., the greater the HCT,

the more friction there is between successive layers. Plasma is a Newtonian fluid, even at high protein concentrations (Fig. 3–6). However, since blood consists of RBCs suspended in plasma, it does not behave like a homogeneous Newtonian fluid; the viscosity of blood increases sharply with reductions in shear rate (Fig. 3–6). This nonNewtonian behavior of blood has been attributed to changes in the behavior of RBCs at low flow rates. These changes include the following: 1) RBCs lose their axial position in the stream of blood (Fig. 3–7); 2) RBCs lose their ellipsoidal shape; 3) RBCs form aggregates. This tendency toward aggregation appears dependent upon the plasma concentration of large protein molecules, such as fibrinogen, which form cell to cell bridges; and 4) RBCs adhere to the endothelial walls of microvessels. Figure 3–8 demonstrates that nonNewtonian behavior is lo-

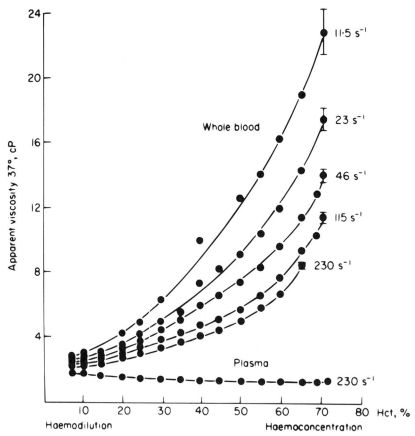

**Fig. 3–6.**   Viscosity of whole blood at various hematocrits as a function of shear rate. Hematocrit was varied by addition of dextran and packed red blood cells. Note that whole blood viscosity increases with hematocrit and that these increases in viscosity are greatest at the lower shear rates. From Messmer K. Hemodilution. Surg Clin N Am. 1975; 55:662, with permission.

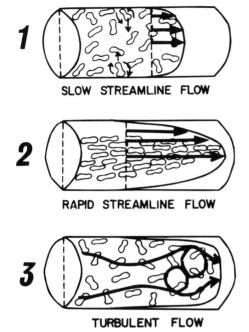

**SLOW STREAMLINE FLOW**

*1*

**RAPID STREAMLINE FLOW**

*2*

**TURBULENT FLOW**

*3*

**Fig. 3–7.** Diagram representing different features of streamline and turbulent flow. From Keele CA, Neil E. Sampson Wright's Applied Physiology, London, England: Oxford University Press, with permission; 1971.

calized in vivo on the venous side of circulation because of its lower shear rates, but that this behavior can be attenuated or abolished by hemodilution.

### Effect of Vessel Size

The tendency for increased HCT to increase blood viscosity is attenuated when blood flows through tubes of capillary diameter (Fig. 3–9). This is because RBCs are normally very deformable, and with a diameter similar to that of the capillary, they can squeeze through the vessel lumen in single file with minimal extra force required. Thus, the rate at which RBCs pass through the capillary has little influence on blood viscosity there; viscosity remains close to that of plasma.

### Effect of Temperature

Blood viscosity varies inversely with temperature. Figure 3–10 shows the decrease in HCT required to maintain a constant viscosity during hypothermia. It indicates that at 20° C, a reduction in HCT from 45 to 25% is required to restore viscosity to the same value evident at 37° C. This is an important consideration during hypothermic cardiopulmonary

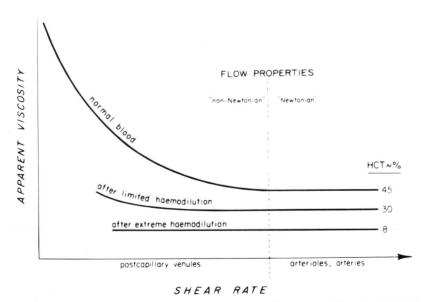

**Fig. 3–8.** Graphic representation of the level of blood viscosity in the different vascular compartments. Under normal condition, (HCT = 45%), viscosity increases in the post-capillary venules because of reduced shear rate. Hemodilution can blunt or even eliminate this regional variation in viscosity. From Messmer K, Sunder-Plassman L. Hemodilution. Prog Surg. 1974;12:208, with permission.

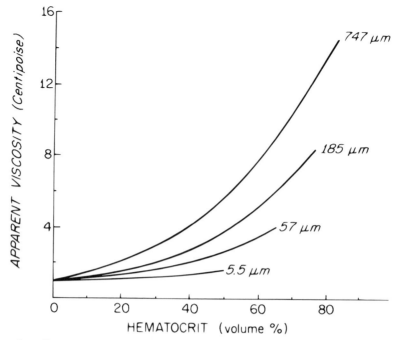

**Fig. 3–9.**  The effect of hematocrit on viscosity of blood in tubes of varying radii. In wide tubes, increasing hematocrit raises viscosity, whereas in narrow tubes it has no effect. From Feigl EO. Physiology and Biophysics II: Circulation, Respiration and Fluid Balance. Philadelphia, Pa: WB Saunders, with permission; 1974.

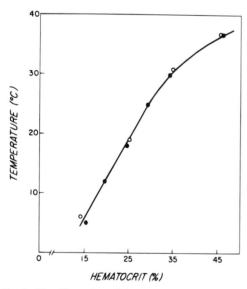

**Fig. 3–10.**  Illustration of decrease in hematocrit that must accompany a reduction in temperature to hold viscosity constant. The measurements were made at low shear rate with an initial hematocrit of 45% at 37° C. Data were obtained with whole blood from two normal adults. From Larson L. Changes in flow properties in human blood. (Master's thesis). Bozeman, Mont: Montana State University; 1973.

bypass. After circulatory arrest, the shear stress required to reinitiate flow and to break up RBC aggregates is likely to be high. Additional rheologic benefit may be gained by a further decrease in HCT.[7]

Turbulent Flow

A principal condition of Poiseuille's law is that flow be laminar. Above a critical flow rate, the laminae break down into eddies that move in all directions. Such flow is said to be turbulent (Fig. 3–7). The tendency for turbulence is given by the Reynolds number (Re):

$$Re = \frac{\rho v r}{\eta} \qquad (8)$$

where ($\rho$) is the fluid density and v is the linear velocity of flow.

In long straight tubes, turbulence occurs when Re exceeds a value of approximately 2000. However, the critical Re in vivo is much less because of pulsatile flow patterns and complicated vessel geometries (8). When flow is turbulent, a greater portion of the total fluid energy is dissipated as heat and vibration; thus,

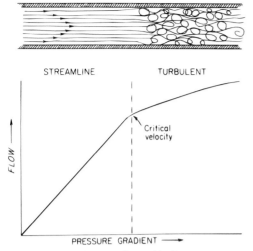

STREAMLINE        TURBULENT

Critical velocity

FLOW

PRESSURE GRADIENT →

**Fig. 3–11.** The linear relationship between pressure gradient and flow is shown. Beyond a critical velocity, turbulence begins and relationship between pressure and flow is no longer linear. From Feigl EO. Physiology and Biophysics II: Circulation, Respiration and Fluid Balance. Philadelphia, Pa: WB Saunders, with permission; 1974.

the pressure drop is greater than that predicted from the Poiseuille equation (Fig. 3–11). The vibrations associated with turbulent flow can often be heard as a murmur during physical examination.

## DIFFUSION OF OXYGEN TO TISSUES

### CAPILLARY TO CELL OXYGEN DELIVERY

The final step in the delivery of oxygen to mitochondria is diffusion from the capillary blood. According to the law of diffusion, this process is determined by the capillary-to-cell $PO_2$ gradient and the diffusion parameters, capillary surface area, and blood-cell diffusion distance. In 1919, Krogh[9] formulated the capillary recruitment model to describe the processes underlying oxygen transport at the tissue level. This basic model was later expanded and refined.[1] Although Krogh's model is limited by multiple simplifying assumptions, it has value as a tool for appreciating the role of vascular control mechanisms in the transport of oxygen to tissue.

### General Features of Krogh Model

The Krogh model consists of a single capillary and the surrounding cylinder of tissue that

it supplies (Fig. 3–12). Two interrelated oxygen gradients are involved: a longitudinal gradient within the capillary (upper panel), and a radial oxygen gradient extending into the tissue (lower panel). Most oxygen in capillary blood is bound to HGB and cannot leave the capillary. This bound oxygen is in equilibrium with the small amount of oxygen dissolved in the plasma. The $VO_2$ creates a transcapillary gradient for oxygen. Diffusion of oxygen into the surrounding tissue shifts the equilibrium between bound and dissolved oxygen, so that more oxygen is released from HGB. By this mechanism, oxygen dissociation from HGB is controlled by $VO_2$.

### LONGITUDINAL OXYGEN GRADIENT

The longitudinal oxygen gradient within the capillary is created by the extraction of oxygen by tissue, as blood passes from the arterial to venous end of the capillary. In accordance with the Fick equation (See Eq. 10 following), the arteriovenous oxygen difference is equivalent to the ratio of $VO_2$ to BF. As shown in Figure 3–12, an increase in $VO_2$, a decrease in BF, or both, will steepen the longitudinal oxygen gradient. Proportional changes in $VO_2$ and blood flow are required for the longitudinal oxygen gradient to remain constant.

A corresponding value for capillary $PO_2$ ($PcO_2$) can be estimated from the value for capillary oxygen content($CcO_2$), taking into account HGB concentration and the oxyhemoglobin dissociation curve. The shape of the longitudinal gradient in $PO_2$ within the capillary is approximately exponential because of the influence of the oxyhemoglobin dissociation curve. The $PcO_2$ is the driving force for diffusion of oxygen into the tissue. Since $PcO_2$ is minimum at the venous end of the capillary, the mitochondria in this region are most vulnerable to oxygen deficits.

### RADIAL OXYGEN GRADIENT (CAPILLARY RECRUITMENT)

The radial $PO_2$ gradient can be described by a value for mean tissue $PO_2$ ($PtO_2$), as calculated according to equation:

$$Mean\ PtO_2 = PcO_2 - A\left(\frac{VO_2 r^2}{4D}\right)$$

(9)

**Fig. 3–12.** Longitudinal and radial oxygen gradients within tissue in accordance with Krogh cylinder model. Details provided in text. Abbreviations: $\dot{V}O_2$, oxygen consumption; Q, blood flow; [$CaO_2$-$CvO_2$], arteriovenous oxygen content difference; $r_c$, capillary radius; R, tissue cylinder radius; A, arterial end of capillary; V, venous end of capillary; x, point within tissue cylinder; $P_{cap}O_2$, oxygen tension of capillary blood; D, diffusion coefficient for oxygen. From Honig CR. Modern Cardiovascular Physiology. Boston, Mass: Little, Brown and Company, with permission; 1981.

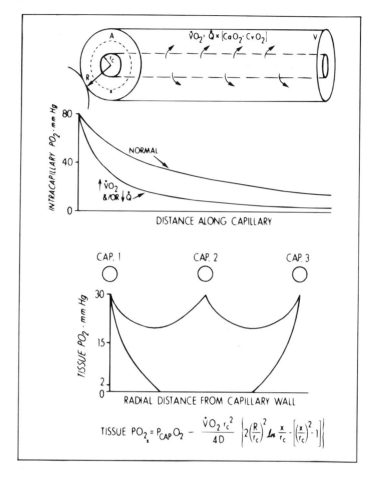

Where $PcO_2$ is blood oxygen tension at a midway point in the capillary, A is a constant related to the relationship between capillary radius and tissue cylinder radius, $\dot{V}O_2$ is oxygen consumption of the tissue cylinder, r is the radius of the tissue cylinder ($\frac{1}{2}$ intercapillary distance), and D is the oxygen diffusion coefficient. r is determined by the number of capillaries perfused with RBCs per volume of tissue and is controlled by the precapillary sphincters. The favorable influence of capillary recruitment on tissue $PO_2$ is evident in Figure 3–12 (lower panel). If only capillaries "1" and "3" are open, diffusion distance is so large that $PO_2$ falls to zero toward the center of the tissue cylinder. The low $PtO_2$ causes relaxation of the precapillary sphincter controlling capillary "2." Perfusion of capillary "2" decreases diffusion distance, and increases $PtO_2$ to an adequate level throughout the tissue.

Mean $PtO_2$ is a reflection of the overall balance between oxygen supply and demand within a particular tissue.[10,11] For example, an increase in BF without a change in oxygen demand, i.e., luxuriant perfusion, raises mean $PtO_2$, whereas a reduction in BF without a change in oxygen demand lowers mean $PtO_2$. If mean $PtO_2$ falls below a critical level, $VO_2$ will become impaired (Figure 3–1). Measurements of mean $PtO_2$ have been obtained in laboratory animals in various tissues, including the myocardium and skeletal muscle, by use of a polarographic technique involving bare-tipped platinum electrodes.[9,10] The invasiveness of the technique has curtailed the use of mean $PtO_2$ measurements in patients. Measurements of local venous $PvO_2$ provide an approximation for average end-capillary $PO_2$, and although they neglect the radial $PO_2$ gradient, they generally show a reasonable correlation to mean $PtO_2$.[12]

# OXYGEN CONSUMPTION AND OTHER MEASURABLE VARIABLES IN VIVO

## Oxygen Consumption

In a clinical setting, there are several methods to measure $\dot{V}O_2$ of the whole body:[13,14] 1) oxygen loss or replacement into a closed breathing system; 2) subtraction of expired from inspired volume of oxygen; and 3) use of the Fick principle.

The first method, oxygen loss or replacement into a closed breathing system, is the most fundamental, is well validated, and has an accuracy well in excess of clinical requirements. However, it is cumbersome and requires meticulous attention to detail if used safely during intensive care. The second method, subtraction of expired from inspired volume of oxygen, is a difficult and potentially inaccurate method to determine systemic $\dot{V}O_2$[14].

Under steady state conditions, the Fick equation can be used to calculate systemic $\dot{V}O_2$:

$$\dot{V}O_2 = CO \times (CaO_2 - C\bar{v}O_2) \quad (10)$$

where $CaO_2$ and $C\bar{v}O_2$ are expressed in vol%, and $(CaO_2 - C\bar{v}O_2)$ is the systemic arteriovenous oxygen content difference. This approach is commonly referred to as the reversed Fick technique. In this technique, CO is usually measured with a thermodilution catheter situated in the pulmonary artery. Samples of blood are collected from an artery and from the pulmonary artery (mixed venous sample), and analyzed for oxygen content. The values for blood oxygen content are used to calculate the systemic arteriovenous oxygen content difference. Using values for CO and $(CaO_2 - C\bar{v}O_2)$ at rest, systemic $VO_2$ can be calculated:

$$\dot{V}O_2 = 5000 \times 4.7/100 = 228 \text{ mL/min}$$

The reverse Fick technique is popular in the intensive care setting since arterial and pulmonary artery catheters are frequently placed in critically ill patients. An important advantage of this method is that it also provides a measurement of $DO_2$ (Eq. 1), which permits analysis of the relationship between systemic $DO_2$ and $\dot{V}O_2$. A drawback of the reverse Fick method is that it excludes $VO_2$ of the lungs. Although this component is negligible in the case of normal lungs, simultaneous measurements of $\dot{V}O_2$ by the Fick and gasometric methods have indicated that it may be significant (as much as 20% of total $\dot{V}O_2$) in critically ill patients.[19] It has been proposed that the increased $\dot{V}O_2$ in the lung is related to the production of the superoxide free radical and, in turn, the hydroxyl free radical, hydrogen peroxide and hypochlorous acid.[16]

## Indices of Mixed Venous Oxygenation

### OXYGEN EXTRACTION RATIO

Oxygen extraction ratio (ER in %) is defined by the equation:

$$ER = \frac{(CaO_2 - CvO_2)}{CaO_2} \quad (11)$$

Combining equations and rearranging terms, it can be demonstrated that ER is also equal to the ratio of systemic $\dot{V}O_2$ to $DO_2$, and, thus, that it reflects the balance between systemic oxygen demand and delivery. Measurements of ER, as well as of $P\bar{v}O_2$, are frequently used clinically to assess the overall adequacy of $DO_2$ (and CO) in critically ill patients.[17-19]

### CRITICAL OXYGEN DELIVERY

At rest, systemic $DO_2$ greatly exceeds $\dot{V}O_2$ (in our example above 1025 versus 228 mL/min) and thus, ER is relatively modest (approximately 25%), resulting in a substantial reserve for oxygen extraction.[20] Figure 3–13A demonstrates that at normal or high levels of $DO_2$, $\dot{V}O_2$ is constant and independent of $DO_2$. As $DO_2$ is gradually reduced, an increased ER maintains $\dot{V}O_2$ (Figure 3–13B). Eventually, a critical point is reached where oxygen extraction cannot increase adequately, and $\dot{V}O_2$ begins to fall. Below this threshold, the so-called "critical $DO_2$,"[21] the level of $\dot{V}O_2$ is limited by the supply of oxygen. In anesthetized dogs, the critical $DO_2$ was found to be approximately 10 mL/min/kg (Figure 3–13A).[21] In some studies, oxygen extraction has been shown to increase further as $DO_2$ is reduced below critical $DO_2$,[22] whereas in

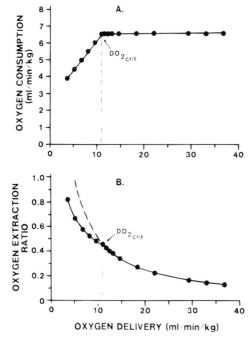

**Fig. 3–13.** Changes in systemic oxygen consumption (A) and oxygen extraction ratio (B) during progressive reduction in oxygen delivery. An increased oxygen extraction ratio maintains oxygen consumption constant until oxygen delivery is lowered to a critical value ($DO_{2crit}$). The dashed line demonstrates the theoretical increase in oxygen extraction required to maintain oxygen consumption for levels of oxygen delivery below $DO_{2crit}$. Modified from Schumaker PT, Cain SM. The concept of critical oxygen delivery. Intensive Care Med. 1987;13: 223, with permission.

others oxygen extraction was maximum at critical $DO_2$ (Figure 3–13B).[23] The normal biphasic $DO_2$—$\dot{V}O_2$ relationship has been demonstrated in patients without respiratory failure undergoing coronary artery surgery,[24] whereas a direct linear relationship between $DO_2$ and $\dot{V}O_2$ has been demonstrated in patients with acute adult respiratory distress syndrome,[25,26] implying a pathological impairment to tissue extraction of oxygen in these patients.[20]

## FACTORS DECREASING OXYGEN DELIVERY

A decrease in systemic $DO_2$ can be produced by a reduction in HCT, $PaO_2$, or cardiac output. Old terminology referred to these conditions as anemic, hypoxic, or stagnant hypoxia. If the reduction in $DO_2$ is severe, it can produce tissue hypoxia, i.e., cause a fall in $PtO_2$ that is sufficient to limit $\dot{V}O_2$ and to stimulate lactate production. Although the value for critical $DO_2$ appears to be similar regardless of the etiology, the corresponding value for critical $P\bar{v}O_2$ differs. The critical $P\bar{v}O_2$ during acute anemia (hemodilution) was 40 mm Hg compared to 17 mm Hg and 31 to 36 mm Hg during hypoxemia and reduced cardiac output, respectively.[21,17,28] A relatively high value for critical $P\bar{v}O_2$ suggests that hemodilution may impair tissue oxygen extraction. This impairment may be attributable to decreased transit time for RBCs through the capillary circulation, thus, limit-

**Table 3–2.** Inter-organ variation in baseline values blood flow, oxygen consumption, and oxygen extraction in average humans

| | Blood flow (mL/min/100 g) | Oxygen consumption (mL/min/100 g) | (a–v) $O_2$ Difference vol% | Oxygen Extraction % |
|---|---|---|---|---|
| Left ventricle | 80 | 8 | 14 | 70 |
| Brain | 55 | 3 | 6 | 30 |
| Liver | 85 } | | | |
| GI tract | 40 } | 2 | 6 | 30 |
| Kidneys | 400 | 5 | 1.3 | 6.5 |
| Muscles | 3 | 0.15 | 5 | 25 |
| Skin | 10 | 0.2 | 2.5 | 12.5 |
| Rest of body | 3 | 0.15 | 4.4 | 22 |

From Folkow B, Neil E: Circulation, New York, 1971; Oxford University Press, with permission.

ing the available time for unloading of oxygen at the tissue, i.e., capillaries within tissues became functional shunts for oxygen.[29] In terms of the Krogh model (Eq. 9), this means that the effective open capillary density was reduced, resulting in a steeper $PO_2$ gradient between the capillary blood and tissue cells. Another potential explanation for the higher values for critical $P\bar{v}O_2$ during hemodilution relates to the possibility that certain regions of the body with high flow rates, such as the kidneys, were overperfused with respect to oxygen demands, which increased values for $P\bar{v}O_2$, while other underperfused regions were producing lactate.

Equations 1, 10, and 11 can be applied to individual tissues by substituting local blood flow for cardiac output and local venous $PO_2$ measurements for $P\bar{v}O_2$ measurements. The individual body tissues vary widely with respect to the relationship between baseline $DO_2$ and $\dot{V}O_2$, and in their baseline ER (Table 3–2). For example, in the left ventricle baseline ER is 70 to 75%, whereas in the kidney it is 5 to 10%. The high baseline ER of the left ventricle renders it extremely dependent on changes in blood flow to maintain adequate oxygen transport.

## REFERENCES

1. Honig CR. Modern Cardiovascular Physiology. Boston, Mass: Little Brown and Company; 1981.
2. Weibel ER. The Pathway for Oxygen. Cambridge, Mass: Harvard Univ Press; 1984.
3. Mines AH. Respiratory Physiology. New York, NY: Raven Press; 1981.
4. Benumof JL. Respiratory physiology and respiratory function during anesthesia. In: Miller RD, ed. Anesthesia. 2nd ed. New York, NY: Churchill Livingstone; 1986.
5. Gregory IC. The oxygen and carbon monoxide capacities of foetal and adult blood. J Physiol (Lond). 1974; 236:625.
6. Fahmy NR. Techniques for deliberate hypotension: Haemodilution and hypotension. In: Enderby GEH, ed. Hypotensive anaesthesia. Edinburgh, Scotland: Churchill-Livingstone; 1985.
7. Laver MB, Buckley MJ, Austen WG. Extreme hemodilution with profound hypothermia and circulatory arrest. Bibliotheca haematologica. 1975;41:225.
8. Hofling B, von Restorff W, Holtz J, Bassenge E. Viscous and inertial fractions of total perfusion energy dissipation in the coronary circulation of the in situ perfused dog heart. Pflugers Arch. 1975;358:1.
9. Krogh A. The number and distribution of capillaries in muscles with calculations of the oxygen pressure

head necessary for supplying the tissue. J Physiol (Lond). 1919; 52:409.
10. Crystal GJ, Weiss HR. $\dot{V}O_2$ of resting muscle during arterial hypoxia: role of reflex vasoconstriction. Microvasc Res. 1980;20:30.
11. Crystal GJ, Downey HF, Bashour FA. Small vessel and total coronary blood volume during intracoronary adenosine infusion. Am J Physiol. 1981;241:H194.
12. Tenny SM. Theoretical analysis of the relationship between venous blood and mean tissue oxygen pressure. Respir Physiol. 1975;20:283.
13. Nunn JF, Makita K, Royston B. Validation of oxygen consumption measurements during artificial ventilation. J Appl Physiol. 1989;67:2129.
14. Makita K, Nunn JF, Royston B. Evaluation of metabolic measuring instruments for use in critically ill patients. Crit Care Med. 1990;10:638.
15. Smithies MN, Makita K, Royston B, et al. A comparison of the measurement of oxygen consumption by indirect calimetry and the reversed Fick method. Crit Care Med. 1991;19:1401.
16. Webster NR, Nunn JF: Molecular structure of free radicals and their importance in biological reactions. Brit J Anaesth. 1988;60:98.
17. Astiz ME, Rackow EC, Kaufman B, et al. Relationship of oxygen delivery and mixed venous oxygenation and to lactate acidosis in patients with sepsis and acute myocardial infarction. Crit Care Med. 1988;16:655.
18. Pinsky MR. Assessment of adequacy of oxygen transport in the critically ill. Appl Cardiopul Pathophysiol. 1990; 3:271.
19. Levy PS, Chavez RP, Crystal GJ, et al. Oxygen extraction ratio: A valid indicator of transfusion need in limited coronary vascular reserve? J Trauma. 1992; 32:769.
20. Schumacker PT, Cain SM. The concept of critical oxygen delivery. Intensive Care Med. 1987;13:223.
21. Cain SM. Oxygen delivery and uptake in dogs during anemic and hypoxic hypoxia. J Appl Physiol. 1977; 42:228.
22. Cain SM. Peripheral oxygen uptake and delivery in health and disease. Clin Chest Med. 1983;4:39.
23. Cain SM, Bradley WE. Critical $O_2$ transport values at lowered body temperatures in rats. J Appl Physiol. 1983; 55:1713.
24. Shibutani K, Komatsu T, Kubal K, et al. Critical level of oxygen delivery in anesthetized man. Crit Care Med. 1983; 11:640.
25. Danek SJ, Lynch JP, Weg JG, Dantzker DR. The dependence of oxygen uptake on oxygen delivery in the adult respiratory syndrome. Ann Rev Resp Dis. 1980;122:387.
26. Mohsenifar Z, Goldbach P, Tachkin DP, Campisi DJ. Relationship between $O_2$ delivery and $O_2$ consumption in the adult respiratory distress syndrome. Chest. 1983;84:267.
27. Cain SM. Appearance of excess lactate in anesthetized dogs during anemic and hypoxic hypoxia. Am J Physiol. 1965; 209:604.
28. Heusser F, Fahey JT, Lister G. Effect of hemoglobin concentration on critical cardiac output and oxygen transport. Am J Physiol. 1989;256:H527.
29. Gutierrez G. The rate of oxygen release and its effect on capillary $O_2$ tension: A mathematical analysis. Respir Physiol. 1986;63:79.

# 4

# BLOOD CONSERVATION TECHNIQUES

## *M. Ramez Salem and Steven Manley*

## INTRODUCTION

Webster's dictionary defines "conservation" as "careful preservation and protection of something; especially: planned management of a natural resource to prevent . . . destruction . . . . " This definition is essential as applied to blood conservation. Efforts to conserve this natural human resource during operative procedures have assumed escalating importance in recent years.[1-6] The increased demands for blood and blood productions for major surgery, the risks and complications of allogeneic blood transfusion (including the transmission of viral infection), the fear of contracting acquired immune deficiency syndrome, and the progress made in studying the physiologic effects of hemodilution have all contributed to the development of blood conservation techniques. The principles of blood conservation have been extended to all surgical subspecialties; therefore, clinicians from various disciplines and practices must become familiar with these principles and practices. The techniques used to conserve blood in surgical operative procedures may be classified as: (1) acceptance of lower perioperative hemoglobin levels; (2) reduction of blood loss; (3) autologous blood transfusion; (4) oxygen therapy; (5) oxygen-carrying blood substitutes; and (6) combination of techniques (Table 4–1).

Specific blood conservation measures are discussed throughout the text. This chapter addresses some general blood conservation measures that are not specifically addressed in other chapters. There has been a tendency in recent years to combine some of these blood conservation measures. When techniques are combined, it is essential for the clinician to understand the physiologic and pharmacologic implications of the "combined maneuvers" and to apply close monitoring of the patient during such "physiologic trespasses" if any real advantages are to accrue to the patients.

## OXYGEN THERAPY

The goal in red blood cell (RBC) transfusion is to increase oxygen delivery to the tissues. Wound healing is a function of arterial oxygen tension ($PaO_2$) in normovolemic patients.[1] Consideration of supplemental oxygen therapy in lieu of transfusion, or combined with transfusion is obviously important[1,7] (see Chapter 3: Principles of Oxygen Transport.) Although hyperbaric oxygen therapy can increase the amount of the dissolved oxygen in the plasma,[7] it is far less popular than it was in the past, and is rarely utilized today for the purpose of increasing oxygen delivery to the tissues.

## SURGICAL TECHNIQUE

Meticulous hemostasis, appropriate operative techniques, and use of certain surgical de-

**Table 4–1.  Blood conservation measures in surgery**

Acceptance of lower perioperative hemoglobin levels
Oxygen therapy
Reduction of blood loss
   Surgical technique
   Anesthetic technique
   Positioning
   Infiltration with vasoconstrictors/topical cocaine
   Tourniquets
   Deliberate hypotension
   Normalizing hemostatic mechanisms/Pharmacologic
     enhancement of hemostatic activity
   Minimizing blood sampling for laboratory testing
Autologous blood transfusion
   Preoperative autologous blood donation
   Acute normovolemic hemodilution
   Blood salvage procedures
Oxygen-carrying blood substitutes
Combination of techniques

tance, airway obstruction, venous obstruction, inadequate muscular relaxation, unintentional positive end-expiratory pressure (PEEP),[9-12] improper positioning, fluid overload, and congestive heart failure can cause a generalized rise in central venous pressure and an increase in venous oozing. Regional obstruction to venous drainage may cause increased venous bleeding during craniotomy or head and neck procedures. Surgery on the head, while the patient is placed in the Trendelenburg position, will be accompanied by venous oozing and therefore, should be avoided.

Partial or complete obstruction to the inferior vena cava during surgery in the prone position, will increase the pressure in the inferior

vices are of paramount importance in decreasing operative blood loss. Prompt surgical intervention may be critical in certain procedures to stop the bleeding. In contrast, staging complex operative procedures, if possible, may be helpful in the Jehovah's Witness patient. The reader is referred to Chapter 11 for further details. (See Chapter 11: Blood Conservation in Jehovah's Witnesses and Chapter 13: Surgical Hemostasis and Blood Conservation.)

## ANESTHETIC TECHNIQUE

Certain factors may increase surgical bleeding in the anesthetized patient including light general anesthesia, intraoperative hypertension, systemic or regional increase in venous pressure, hyperdynamic circulation (increased cardiac output) and hypercapnia. Bleeding may increase during light anesthesia because of selective increases in skin and muscle blood flows and peripheral vasodilation, concomitant with increased cardiac output (CO). The redistribution of CO during light general anesthesia has been known for years, and has been confirmed during isoflurane anesthesia.[8] An intraoperative rise in arterial blood pressure can cause increased bleeding. While no list is all inclusive, excluding measurement errors and limitations, the more common causes of intraoperative arterial hypertension are outlined in Table 4–2.

Coughing, bucking, increased airway resis-

**Table 4–2.  Etiology of intraoperative hypertension**

Inadequate anesthesia & sympathetic stimulation
Hypoxemia
Hypercapnia
Hypothermia
Fluid overload
Pre-existing hypertension
  Essential hypertension
  Secondary hypertension
    Pheochromocytoma
    Hyperthyroidism
    Cushing's syndrome
    Coarctation of the aorta
    Renal parenchymal disease
    Renal artery stenosis
    Pregnancy-induced (i.e., eclampsia or pre-
      eclampsia)
Bladder distention or perforation
Tourniquet pain
Baroreceptor dysfunction
Exogenous induced
  Glucocorticoids
  Mineral corticoids
  Estrogens
  Catecholamines & sympathomimetic drugs
  Ergot derivatives
  Meperidine with monoamine oxidase inhibitors
  Ketamine
Increased intracranial pressure
Autonomic hyperreflexia
Hypermetabolic states
  Burns
  Malignant hyperthermia
  Delirium tremens
Withdrawal or rebound
  Clonidine
  Nitroprusside
  Methyldopa

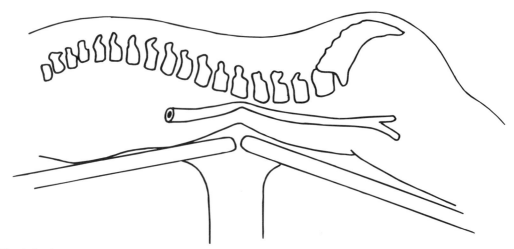

**Fig. 4–1.**   Improper positioning of the patient in the prone position may be accompanied by partial or complete obstruction of the inferior vena cava. The increased pressure distal to the obstruction leads to diversion of blood into the vertebral venous plexus and excessive venous bleeding during spine operations.

vena cava, distal to the obstruction. This obstruction will cause blood to be diverted into the vertebral venous plexuses (Batson's plexus), and lead to increased oozing during surgery on the spine (Fig. 4–1). Any rise in intraabdominal pressure (increased muscle tone, external pressure on the abdomen, gastric inflation, coughing, bucking, airway obstruction, increased airway pressure, and PEEP) will increase inferior vena cava pressure and increase oozing (Table 4–3).[13,14] Com-

**Table 4–3.   Factors affecting blood loss during spinal fusion (prone position)**

| | |
|---|---|
| Surgical factors | |
|   Extent of dissection and number of vertebrae to be fused | |
|   Length of operation | |
|   Site and size of bone graft and phase of operation in which it is obtained | |
|   Previous spinal fusion | |
|   Surgical technique | |
| Anesthetic factors | |
|   Increased arterial pressure | |
|   Increased venous pressure | |
| Postural factors | Increased pressure in inferior vena cava and diversion of blood into vertebral venous plexus |
|   Increased abdominal wall tension | |
|   Increased intraabdominal pressure | |
|   Extrinsic pressure | |
| Respiratory factors | |
|   Intermittent positive-pressure ventilation | |

plete relaxation of the diaphragm and the abdominal musculature decreases intraabdominal pressure, as well as inferior vena cava pressure, and is therefore, desirable to reduce bleeding.[13,14]

## DOES ANESTHETIC CHOICE PLAY A ROLE IN BLOOD LOSS?

It is a common perception among anesthesiologists and surgeons that spinal or epidural anesthesia offers an advantage of decreased blood loss during surgery. Decreased arterial and/or venous pressure, often associated with conduction anesthesia, seems to be the logical explanation. Attempts to validate this common belief remain equivocal at best. A major problem with interpreting the results of some studies is the accuracy of blood loss measurement. Visual assessments have been shown to be unreliable. Some studies have compared postoperative hematocrits (HCT) with preoperative HCT, or have examined the need for transfusion as an endpoint in assessing the degree of blood loss. Clearly, since hydration influences HCT values, the accuracy of blood loss by this method cannot be determined.[15] Certain operative procedures lend themselves to be good sources when comparing regional with general anesthesia, regarding blood loss. Commonly studied procedures are transurethral resection of the prostate, cesarean section, therapeutic abortion, and hip surgery.

Blood loss during transurethral resection of

the prostate has been found to be in the range of 2.6 to 4.6 mL/min.[16,17] It is recognized that factors other than the anesthetic choice influence blood loss, including weight of resected tissue, resection time, and the presence of infection.[16-19] Continuous postoperative bleeding may also be due to release of urokinase from prostatic tissue, which activates plasminogen to plasmin and in turn, causes fibrinolysis.[16,17] Some randomized prospective studies of transurethral resection of the prostate found no significant difference in total perioperative losses or postoperative blood loss between regional and general anesthesia groups.[19,20] Other studies have presented conflicting results, revealing that operative blood losses are substantially greater in patients receiving general, rather than regional anesthesia.[18,21]

In elective cesarean sections examined retrospectively, Gilstrap et al.[22] found increased blood loss during general anesthesia with inhalation drugs, as compared to general anesthesia with nitrous oxide (without inhalation agents) or regional anesthesia. However, the study was not controlled for concentration of inhalation drugs, duration, or timing of exposure to the inhalation drugs. In another retrospective study, there were no differences in blood loss between epidural anesthesia, general anesthesia with "low-dose" halothane-nitrous oxide, or nitrous oxide-opioid anesthesia.[23] Andrews et al.[24] examined blood loss in "uncomplicated" patients undergoing elective repeat cesarean section for singleton cephalic pregnancies. They found that the proportion of patients with a decrease in HCT of 5% or more was greater in patients undergoing general anesthesia supplemented with halogenated agents, than those undergoing regional anesthesia. No patient in either group required transfusion, since blood loss was not clinically significant. In therapeutic abortions, greater blood loss has been observed during the use of potent inhalation anesthetics than with nitrous oxide-opioid anesthesia.[25,26] This phenomenon seems to be related to uterine relaxation. However, low-dose enflurane anesthesia does not increase blood loss, and is therefore, an acceptable technique for use in patients undergoing therapeutic abortion.[27]

Most investigators found no differences in intraoperative blood losses between spinal and general anesthesia during hip fracture surgical procedures.[28-30] However, the decrease in blood pressure that often accompanies subarachnoid block, may contribute to the decrease in blood loss.[31] In total hip arthroplasty, epidural anesthesia is accompanied by reduced blood loss, as compared with general anesthesia.[32,33] Upon further evaluation, investigators found no differences in postoperative HGB or HCT values up to 2 weeks after surgery.[34,35]

It is obvious that studies have not been conclusive as to the role of anesthetic choice in influencing blood loss. Nonetheless, the following conclusions may be drawn: (1) Factors other than anesthetic choice do play a role in influencing blood loss; (2) By causing uterine relaxation, potent inhalation anesthetics increase blood loss during therapeutic abortions and so should be avoided or their concentration limited to "low-dose;" (3) There is no uniform agreement that blood loss increases more during general anesthesia than in regional anesthesia, in transurethral resection of the prostate, cesarean section, or hip surgery; (4) The decreased blood loss sometimes observed during spinal or epidural anesthesia may be attributed to decreased arterial and/or venous pressure that often occurs with these techniques; and (5) Regardless of the choice of anesthetic drug, the anesthetic technique must be well-planned and executed so as to decrease blood loss. For example, increases in arterial or venous pressure may be prevented by adequate preparation, proper intraoperative management, and avoidance of faulty anesthetic technique.

## HYPERCAPNIA DURING ANESTHESIA AND SURGERY

Because prevention of hypercapnia during anesthesia is of utmost importance, a brief discussion of its etiology and detection is warranted. Hypercapnia is simply defined as an arterial carbon dioxide tension ($PaCO_2$) higher than the predicted normal. Hypercapnia may increase bleeding by augmenting CO, raising blood pressure and central venous pressure, and lowering peripheral vascular resistance. To avoid inadvertent hypercapnia, the anesthesiologist must: (1) understand the basic principles of anesthetic equipment and systems, including monitoring devices; (2) be able to detect abnormal $PaCO_2$; (3) recognize the causes of hypercapnia; and (4) be able to correct these problems.[36]

General anesthesia and high spinal and epidural anesthesia may modify the cardiovascular and ventilatory responses to hypercapnia.[37,38] With hypercapnia (up to 60 mm Hg), CO may be slightly increased (predominantly because of increased stroke volume) with most anesthetics, with the notable exception of halothane, which may decrease it. Usually, slight increases in heart rate, blood pressure (except with halothane), right atrial pressure, and pulmonary artery pressure result, while the total peripheral resistance declines slightly. Although cardiac arrhythmias may be seen with high $PaCO_2$ values, they are not reliable indicators of hypercapnia, and may not be present even at very high $PaCO_2$ levels. Similarly, the ventilatory responses commonly seen in awake patients (increased minute ventilation and tachypnea) are usually obtunded during anesthesia, but may not be completely eliminated. Thus, signs of hypercapnia may not be striking during anesthesia and should not be relied upon as diagnostic signs.[37-39] Continuous monitoring of ventilation during anesthesia is, therefore, mandatory. The principle factors that govern $PaCO_2$ during anesthesia include inspired $CO_2$, $CO_2$ output and alveolar ventilation, which is a function of the total ventilation and the physiologic dead space.[39]

## Increased Endogenous Carbon Dioxide Production

During anesthesia, endogenous $CO_2$ production ($\dot{V}CO_2$) is slightly decreased to approximately 80% of the basal state. An increased $\dot{V}CO_2$ may occur in the following situations: fever, sepsis, burns, malignant hyperthermia, shivering, convulsions, excessive production of catecholamines, thyroid storm, airway obstruction, total parenteral hyperalimentation, and following tourniquet deflation. With increased $\dot{V}CO_2$, $PaCO_2$ will rise, unless ventilation is appropriately increased.

In total parenteral nutrition, the respiratory quotient, which is the ratio of $CO_2$ production to oxygen consumption, reflects the composition of the "exogenous fuel." The respiratory quotient is 1.0 for carbohydrates, 0.8 for proteins, and 0.7 for fat. Conversion of carbohydrates to fat (lipogenesis) is associated with a respiratory quotient higher than 1.0, and re-

sults in excessive production of $CO_2$, while with ketogenesis the respiratory quotient is almost zero. Studies have demonstrated that there is an increase in $\dot{V}CO_2$ in patients receiving total parenteral nutrition when high glucose intakes are the primary source of nonprotein calories.[40] The increase in $\dot{V}CO_2$ caused by the administration of a large carbohydrate load could be a critical factor in the awake patient with marginal pulmonary reserve, who is unable to increase minute ventilation. That increase may lead to dyspnea and respiratory distress. Unless ventilatory adjustments are made, patients receiving glucose as the primary source of calories, may exhibit $CO_2$ elevation during anesthesia. Fat emulsions can serve as a source of nonprotein calories and can be associated with lesser degrees of $\dot{V}CO_2$ than is glucose. For this reason, it is advisable to give 50% of the nonprotein calories during total parenteral nutrition as fat emulsions to minimize $\dot{V}CO_2$.[40]

## Exogenous Carbon Dioxide Administration

An increased $PaCO_2$ may be seen when $CO_2$ is injected into a body cavity such as during laparoscopy. Provided that adequate ventilation is maintained, high $PaCO_2$ is not usually seen. A transient increase in $PaCO_2$ occurs following the administration of sodium bicarbonate.[38,39]

## Increased Inspired Carbon Dioxide

This may be encountered when the soda lime absorbing system fails and when a faulty valve allows rebreathing of exhaled gas in a circle system.[41] Significant rebreathing, resulting in increased inspiratory $CO_2$ may also occur when low fresh gas flow is delivered in $CO_2$ washout circuits (such as the Mapleson D system), which is frequently used in pediatric patients.[42]

## Increased Respiratory Dead Space

The respiratory dead space during anesthesia includes several components: apparatus, anatomic, and alveolar dead spaces. The sum of the anatomic and alveolar components is referred to as the physiologic dead space. Anatomic dead space is defined as that part of the inspired tidal volume that is exhaled, unchanged in composition, at the beginning of expiration. The alveolar dead space may be defined as that part of the inspired gas that passes through the anatomic dead space to mix with gas at the alveolar level, but does not take part in gas exchange.[39] Factors influencing the anatomic dead space include patient size, posture, age, position of the neck and jaw, lung volume at the end of inspiration, tracheal intubation and tracheostomy, anesthesia, pneumonectomy, drugs affecting the caliber of bronchi and bronchioles, hypothermia, and hypoventilation.

The alveolar dead space increases when there is lack of effective perfusion of the alveoli to which the inspired gas is distributed. Conditions that reduce pulmonary blood flow or pressure during anesthesia will increase the alveolar component of the dead space. These conditions include hemorrhage, low CO, hypovolemia, deliberate hypotension in adults combined with head-up tilt and/or PEEP, pulmonary embolism, pulmonary atresia or stenosis, tetralogy of Fallot, and kinking or clamping of the pulmonary artery during pulmonary surgery (Table 4–4).[36,39] Factors contributing to increased alveolar dead space during anesthesia include age, tidal volume, use of negative phase during exhalation, short inspiratory phase, and the presence of pulmonary disease (Table 4–4).[39] As a result of the widespread destruction of alveolar septa and capillaries in patients with obstructive pulmonary disease, an increased alveolar dead space ensues. In children with tetralogy of Fallot, subnormal pulmonary blood flow will increase the alveolar dead space. Very high $PaCO_2$ can be found in these patients, despite adequate ventilation during anesthesia.[43] The alveolar

**Table 4–4.  Factors affecting alveolar dead space**

Hydrostatic failure of alveolar perfusion
  Hemorrhage, low cardiac output
  Deliberate hypotension in adults (head-up tilt and/or PEEP)
Obstruction of pulmonary circulation
  Pulmonary embolism
  Pulmonary atresia or stenosis and tetralogy of Fallot
  Surgical interruption of pulmonary artery flow
Anesthesia, PEEP, posture, tidal volume, negative phase, short inspiratory phase
COPD and other lung diseases
  (Destruction of alveoli and capillaries)

**Table 4–5.  Causes of hypoventilation**

Airway obstruction, increased resistance, decreased compliance of lungs and chest wall
Loss of structural integrity of the chest wall and pleural cavity
Impairment of respiratory muscles and diaphragmatic splinting
Anesthetics, narcotics, central depressants
Neuromuscular blocking drugs and neuromuscular diseases
Inadequate tidal volume and/or rate during controlled ventilation
Failure of the respiratory center
Obesity-hypoventilation syndrome
Cervical cordotomy, surgery in the cervical region
Intracranial lesions
Intrathecal and epidural narcotics
High spinal anesthesia and phrenic nerve block
Metabolic alkalosis
High $FiO_2$ in COPD

dead space can be conveniently estimated in patients undergoing surgical procedures by measurement of the arterial to end-tidal $CO_2$ tension difference $[P(a-ET)CO_2]$.[39] Normally, this difference is 2 to 3 mm Hg and is uninfluenced by the actual level of $PaCO_2$. During anesthesia, this difference may increase to 5 mm Hg (range, 0 to 10 mm Hg).

## Decreased Alveolar Ventilation

There are many causes of hypoventilation during anesthesia that lead to hypercapnia.[36,38,39] The etiology of hypoventilation may be simply divided into central and peripheral factors and factors affecting the structural integrity of the respiratory system (Table 4–5).

## Carbon Dioxide Monitoring During Anesthesia

Hypercapnia can be diagnosed by measurement of $PaCO_2$. Measurements of partial pressure of end-tidal $CO_2$ ($PETCO_2$) correlate with $PaCO_2$ values unless there are factors causing an increase in alveolar dead space (Table 4–4). Although anesthesia may be accompanied by a slight increase in alveolar dead space, such an increase is only substantial in patients with pulmonary disease and in elderly patients. Therefore, continuous monitoring of $PETCO_2$ provides a reliable estimate of

$PaCO_2$ in most patients and is useful in the detection of hypercapnia. For appropriate use of $PETCO_2$ monitoring (capnography), it is essential to be able to recognize normal and abnormal waveforms. One must also look for artifacts and trends. Capnography not only measures $PETCO_2$, but also inspiratory $CO_2$. An increase in inspiratory $CO_2$ level (above zero) may indicate rebreathing due to exhausted soda lime or a faulty exhalation valve in a $CO_2$ circle absorber.[41]

## POSITIONING

Much of the physiology of posture can be learned from the giraffe.[45] Because the head of this animal is far from the heart, the task of supplying it with oxygenated blood demands a remarkably high blood pressure. At the heart level, its blood pressure is approximately 260/160 mm Hg. Nevertheless, the pressure that perfuses the brain is the same in giraffes, humans, and most other animals (Fig. 4–2).[45,46]

In the supine position, the arterial and venous pressures are the same in various parts of the body. Moving from the supine to the standing position results in considerable changes in arterial pressures. Parts above the heart are perfused at lower pressures, and parts below the heart are perfused at higher pressures. Similar changes are seen in the veins. In the standing position, the venous pressure is near zero above the heart and is subatmospheric in the cerebral sinuses, where venous collapse is prevented.[47] Below the heart level, the venous pressure progressively increases in the standing position, reaching its highest levels in the feet.

Tilting produces a gradient of about 2 mm Hg for each inch of vertical height, above which the arterial pressure is recorded. It produces increases of the same magnitude below the level of the heart. Thus, in the adult patient of average height (172 cm), the difference between arterial pressure at the head and that at the feet could be 120 mm Hg in the standing position.[47] Because of their small stature, gravitational effects on arterial and ve-

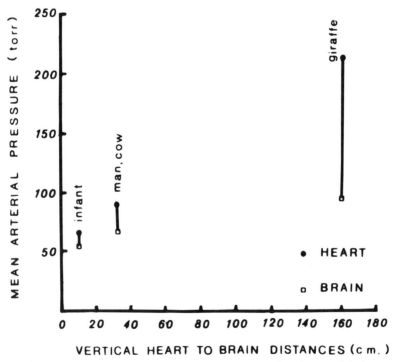

Fig. 4–2.  Mean arterial pressure at the heart and brain levels in various animals and man. While there is an appreciable difference between mean arterial pressure in the giraffe and in man at the heart level, the pressure perfusing the brain is the same in both species. Modified from Warren JV: The physiology of the giraffe. Scientific Am 1974; 231:96, with permission.

nous pressures are less in children (and even much less in infants) than in adults.[46,48]

With vertical tilting, twice as much blood can accumulate in the legs, and even larger volumes can be accommodated in the abdomen. Tilting will also increase the capillary pressure in dependent parts, and, if prolonged, increased filtration results in tissue edema, ultimately reducing blood volume. The converse is seen in elevated parts when tissue fluid is effectively reabsorbed.

In awake individuals, tilting initiates certain cardiovascular reflexes.[47] These reflexes result from baroreceptor activity, which leads to increased production of catecholamines and plasma renin activity, in turn, inducing the formation of the vasoconstrictor angiotensin II with aldosterone release and sodium and water retention. These mechanisms tend to limit the decrease in blood pressure and are evident 15 to 30 minutes after tilting. Increased sympathetic activity results in constriction of the capacitance vessels, thus, maintaining venous return. Constriction of the resistance vessels also minimizes the decrease in arterial pressure. In the normal subject, little change occurs in arterial pressure at the heart level during tilting or standing, although heart rate may increase. Anesthetic drugs, ganglionic, and $\beta$-adrenergic blocking drugs interfere with these compensatory mechanisms. Consequently, head-up (or footdown) tilt in the anesthetized patient will favor the occurrence of arterial hypotension in the upper parts and peripheral venous pooling in the lower parts of the body. These can be facilitated with the use of muscle relaxants, controlled ventilation, myocardial depressant drugs, and peripheral vasodilators.

Positioning the patient so as to place the operative site as the "uppermost" part is a widely practiced maneuver to decrease blood loss. This maneuver has been utilized in a variety of operative procedures, including head, neck, and upper thoracic procedures, as well as in operations on the spine and the hip. Head-up tilt is commonly used; the tilt varies from 10 to 25° in head and neck procedures to 90°, as in sitting-position craniotomy. In operations where head-up tilt is used, pressure gradients must be taken into consideration to assure maintenance of adequate cerebral perfusion. Either an estimate of the pressure gradient is calculated by measuring the vertical distance between the heart and the brain [gradient in mm Hg = distance (inches) × 2], or the pressure transducer (in case of arterial cannulation) is positioned at the brain level.

Although tilting is less effective in infants and children compared with adults, the combination of decreased arterial and venous pressure above the heart, and peripheral venous pooling below the heart, makes tilting useful in reducing bleeding in pediatric head and neck procedures. It can also be used postoperatively to reduce swelling and edema. Added benefit may be derived in reducing postoperative laryngeal and upper airway edema after airway manipulations, instrumentation, and intubation.

If the prone position is used, meticulous attention must be given to positioning. The

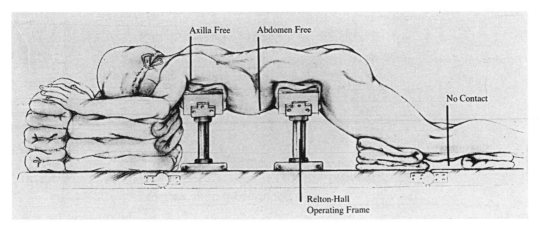

**Fig. 4–3.** Position of patient on Relton-Hall frame. From Schwentker EP: Posterior fusion of the spine for scoliosis. Surg Rounds 1978; 1:12, with permission.

vertebral venous system provides channels into which blood may be diverted from the lower parts of the body, if the inferior vena cava is obstructed. Probably no modification has greater impact on minimizing blood loss during operative correction of scoliosis (spinal fusion and instrumentation), than the use of the Relton-Hall operation frame.[49,50] When the patient is positioned on the frame, the abdomen is free of pressure and thus, pressure on the inferior vena cava is minimized (Fig. 4–3). Also, by avoiding abdominal pressure, the functional residual capacity can be maintained at a near-normal level, helping to prevent atelectasis and hypoxemia.

## INFILTRATION WITH VASOCONSTRICTORS AND TOPICAL COCAINE
### Infiltration with Vasoconstrictors

A commonly used technique for reducing bleeding, involves local infiltration of the skin and subcutaneous tissues with a solution containing a vasoconstrictor drug. Probably, both the local vasoconstrictive effect of the drug, and the hydrostatic pressure exerted by the fluid bulk contribute to the effectiveness of the method. The most common drug used for this purpose is epinephrine. Certain anesthetics, such as halothane, sensitize the myocardium to exogenous catecholamines. The dose of epinephrine needed to produce arrhythmias is, therefore, lower in halothane-anesthetized patients, than in those who are awake. Katz and Bigger[51] suggested that a dosage of 0.15 mg/kg of 1 : 100,000 epinephrine solution per 10-minute period, not to exceed 0.45 mL/kg of the same solution per hour, is safe. Although this claim has not been challenged, a larger dose may be permitted if enflurane or isoflurane is used instead of halothane, since the myocardium is less sensitized by those anesthetic drugs. Johnston et al.[52] determined the median effective dose (ED50) of epinephrine in adult patients; this variable was defined by the appearance of three premature ventricular contractions at any time during, or immediately after, the injection of epinephrine. The ED50 for epinephrine and halothane was 2.1 $\mu$g/kg; and for halothane-lidocaine-epinephrine it was 3.7 $\mu$g/kg. The ED50 for enflurane was 10.9 $\mu$g/kg, while for isoflurane it was 6.7 $\mu$g/kg (Fig. 4–4). Accordingly, for subcutaneous infiltration in adults, the maximum dosages of epinephrine

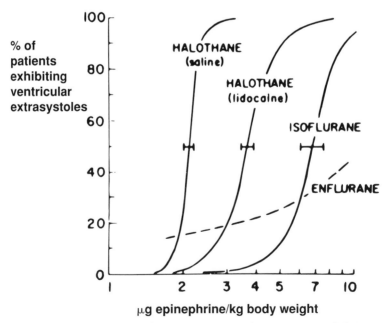

**Fig. 4–4.** Submucosal doses of epinephrine produce PVC's in patients during 1.25 MAC inhalation anesthesia. Notice that the enflurane curve is flat. Modified from Johnston RR, Eger EI, Wilson C: A comparative interaction of epinephrine with enflurane, isoflurane, and halothane in man. Anesth Analg 1976; 55:516, with permission.

recommended as unlikely to produce arrhythmias with halothane, isoflurane, and enflurane are 1, 3.5, and 5.5 $\mu g/kg$, respectively.[52]

Children appear to have a much lower incidence of arrhythmias following epinephrine infiltration. A mean epinephrine dose of 7.8 $\mu g/kg$ given with lidocaine, has been found to be safe during halothane anesthesia for closure of cleft palate.[53] No arrhythmias occurred during various pediatric operations using cutaneous infiltration of 1:100,000 epinephrine (2—15 $\mu g/kg$) with a wide range of halothane concentrations.[54] This may confirm the assumption that children have a higher arrhythmogenic threshold for epinephrine than adults have during halothane anesthesia. Karl and associates[54] concluded that at least 10 $\mu g/kg$ of epinephrine could be used safely with a normal or lower than normal $PaCO_2$. Furthermore, adding lidocaine to the epinephrine solution increases the margin of safety. If a large volume is required, such as in scoliosis correction, a 1:500,000 solution may be used, thus, permitting the injection of as much as 500 mL.[13]

Infiltration with epinephrine solution to reduce bleeding is a technique used in various minor and major surgical procedures, including intranasal and oral procedures, cleft lip repair, cleft palate closure, plastic and reconstructive operations, and correction of scoliosis. One drawback of epinephrine infiltration is that it may produce swelling and distortion of the tissues if an excessive volume is injected. This would interfere with a "precise" repair in certain plastic surgical operations. Electrocardiographic and noninvasive blood pressure monitoring to detect arrhythmias and hemodynamic changes, and pulse oximetry to detect hypoxemia, are essential during and after epinephrine infiltration.

## Topical Cocaine

Topical cocaine combined with local injections of lidocaine and epinephrine is commonly used for anesthesia for intranasal surgery.[55,56] Cocaine is unique among the local anesthetics for its vasoconstrictive properties, secondary to blockade of the uptake of norepinephrine by the postganglionic nerve endings.[57] Its only therapeutic use is topical anesthesia. Pharmaceutical preparations are available in the hydrochloride solutions of 2 to 10% concentrations. The maximum suggested single dose is 150 to 200 mg,[58,59] a dose frequently administered and even exceeded.[60] Peak plasma concentrations are proportional to the dose. However, the time required for peak concentration appears longer with higher doses, suggesting that the absorption is delayed through vasoconstriction.[61] The biologic half-life of cocaine is reported to be 0.5 to 1.5 hours. There appears, however, to be much intersubject variability.[60]

In addition to its local anesthetic effects, cocaine has central nervous system effects. It is a stimulant and causes brief, but intense euphoria and arousal. These effects are felt to be secondary to affected neurotransmitter function, involving norepinephrine, dopamine, serotonin, tryptophan, and acetylcholine. Cocaine may cause sympathetic stimulation due to its blockade of norepinephrine reuptake; however, other mechanisms may play a role. The central and hemodynamic effects decrease more quickly than the plasma levels of cocaine after a dose, suggesting "acute tolerance" at the receptor level or redistribution from the brain to other tissues.[60,62] Cocaine toxicity can lead to death. Reactions have been described as extreme stimulation of the central nervous and cardiovascular systems, followed by collapse. Severe dysrhythmias, seizures, and hyperpyrexia have been reported.[60]

While cocaine's potential for abuse and toxicity is well known, recent reports have further questioned the therapeutic applications of cocaine. Intranasal cocaine has been shown to produce vasoconstriction of the coronary arteries with a decrease in coronary blood flow.[63] Furthermore, nasal administration of 4% lidocaine with 5% phenylephrine solution produced no difference in nasal dilatation than did 5% cocaine solution without cardiovascular side effects.[64]

It is believed by some that epinephrine may decrease the toxicity of cocaine, but this theory remains controversial with limited data to support it.[60] Lidocaine with epinephrine following intranasal cocaine has been shown to cause significant increases in heart rate and arterial pressure. However, esmolol blunts the tachycardia associated with topical cocaine and lidocaine with epinephrine infiltration.[56] The administration of cocaine or cocaine-lidocaine-epinephrine should be carried out judiciously and cautiously with vigilant monitoring. If adverse effects do develop, they should be appropriately managed.

## TOURNIQUETS

Pneumatic tourniquets are often used for surgery on the upper and lower extremities to provide a bloodless operative field and to decrease blood loss. It has been estimated that pneumatic tourniquets are used in about 40% of pediatric orthopedic procedures.[65] Tourniquets may be applied for surgical procedures performed under general, regional (spinal or epidural), and intravenous regional anesthesia. The extremity to be operated upon is raised to a level higher than the rest of the patient's body, and is exsanguinated by an Esmarch bandage. The pneumatic tourniquet is then inflated to a pressure $\geq 75$ mm Hg higher than the patient's systolic pressure. The reader is referred to standard orthopedic, anesthesia, and other texts for details on the use of tourniquets, as well as complications of tourniquet application (e.g., tourniquet pain in the awake patient during regional anesthesia). The following discussion will focus on the hemodynamic and metabolic effects of tourniquet inflation and deflation.

Tourniquet inflation can cause a rise in arterial blood pressure in adult patients.[66,67] Although the usual hemodynamic response to tourniquet deflation is a slight decrease in blood pressure associated with a slight increase in heart rate,[65,68] others reported significant decreases in blood pressure and central venous pressure.[69,70] Data on hemodynamic changes with tourniquet deflation in children are slightly conflicting. Moncorge et al.[71] found that systolic blood pressure fell and heart rate increased by 15 mm Hg and 12 beats/minute, respectively, in 11 children studied; whereas Lynn et al.[65] found a lesser decrease in blood pressure (8 to 10 mm Hg) and no change in heart rate following tourniquet deflation. They concluded that children usually tolerate tourniquet release with fewer hemodynamic changes than adults.

Following tourniquet inflation, progressive decreases in venous pH and $PO_2$ and increases in $PCO_2$ and lactate occur. Wilgis[72] demonstrated that after 1 hour of tourniquet time, venous blood pH reached 7.19, $PO_2$ 20 mm Hg, and $PCO_2$ 62 mm Hg; after 2 hours, pH had decreased to 6.9, $PO_2$ to 4 mm Hg, and

$PCO_2$ to 104 mm Hg. When the tourniquet is deflated, products of anaerobic metabolism enter the circulation, causing a transient state of reactive hyperemia and mixed respiratory and metabolic acidosis. Haljamae and Enger[73] reported a two-to-threefold increase in ischemic muscle lactate content during tourniquet use. Large increases in lactate occur with longer inflation times (more than 75 minutes), or when bilateral tourniquets are used, while the greatest decrease in pH is seen when bilateral tourniquets are deflated simultaneously.[65]

Upon release of the tourniquet, the accumulated acid metabolites are buffered by plasma bicarbonate, resulting in release of $CO_2$ and significant rise in $PaCO_2$ and $PETCO_2$.[73] The respiratory acidosis is quickly compensated, but the metabolic acidosis persists for more than 10 minutes after tourniquet release.[65] Serum potassium levels increase slightly with tourniquet deflation, but the levels remain within the normal range.[65,71] Time for clearance for the increase in $CO_2$, hydrogen ion, and lactic acid from the general circulation after tourniquet deflation varies from patient to patient, and may depend on factors including: duration of inflation; levels of metabolites before deflation; the extremity exsanguinated (upper versus lower, one versus both); efficacy of the buffering capacity; the patient's circulation; ventilation (spontaneous or controlled); and the patient's response to the extra load of metabolites. Reported times of clearance vary from 5 to 15 minutes in some studies[73,74] to 10 to 30 minutes in others.[69,75] With the advent of capnography, anesthesiologists have been able to detect increases in $PETCO_2$ following tourniquet release.[68,76,77] The maximum increase in $PETCO_2$ is about 3 mm Hg (range from 1 to 12 mm Hg) after the release of the upper extremity tourniquet, and about 9 mm Hg (range, 5 to 18 mm Hg) following the release of the lower extremity tourniquet.[77] The increase is approximately threefold higher, following the release of the lower extremity tourniquet, than the upper extremity tourniquet. The time to maximal increase in $PETCO_2$ is 1.5 to 2.5 minutes.

Healthy patients who have adequate spontaneous ventilation respond to the extra $CO_2$ load upon release of tourniquet inflation by increasing their minute ventilation, regardless of the anesthetic given.[68] In these patients, an

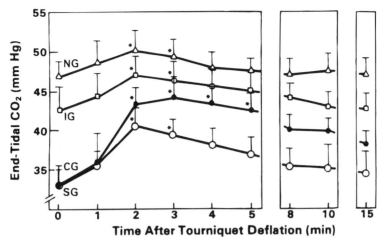

**Fig. 4–5.** Changes in end-tidal $CO_2$ ± SEM after tourniquet deflation for various anesthetic techniques. NG = narcotic group, IG = inhalation group, SG = spinal group, and CG = controlled ventilation group. $n = 10$ for each group. Asterisks indicate values that are significantly different ($P < 0.05$) from values immediately prior to tourniquet deflation. From Bourke DL, Silberman MS, Ortega R, et al: Respiratory responses associated with intraoperative tourniquets. Anesth Analg 1989; 69:541, with permission.

excessive rise in $PETCO_2$ will not occur, and will return to the baseline levels within 3 to 5 minutes. In patients whose ventilation is controlled at a preset level, and who cannot increase their ventilation (because of paralysis, etc), a greater increase in $PETCO_2$ may be seen ($\geq 10$ mm Hg with lower extremity tourniquet deflation), and may take longer than 15 minutes before $PETCO_2$ returns to baseline values[68] (Figs. 4-5 and 4-6).

To minimize the systemic and metabolic effects after tourniquet release, the following recommendations need to be emphasized: (1) Monitoring $PETCO_2$ before and after the release of the tourniquet. $PETCO_2$ provides a reliable estimate of $PaCO_2$ except in patients with increased alveolar dead space (Table 4–4). In those patients, measurement of $PaCO_2$ will be more reliable than $PETCO_2$; (2) Increasing minute ventilation by about 50% just

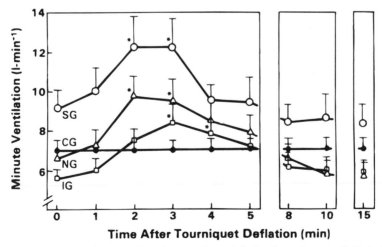

**Fig. 4–6.** Changes in minute ventilation ± SEM after tourniquet deflation for various anesthetic techniques. NG = narcotic group, IG = inhalation group, SG = spinal group, and CG = controlled ventilation group. $n = 10$ for each group. Asterisks indicate values that are significantly different ($P < 0.05$) from values immediately prior to tourniquet deflation. From Bourke DL, Silberman MS, Ortega R, et al: Respiratory responses associated with intraoperative tourniquets. Anesth Analg 1989; 69:541, with permission.

before, and for 5 minutes after, tourniquet deflation;[68,77] This increase should prevent PETCO$_2$ from increasing more than 3 to 5 mm Hg in most patients. These measures may be of utmost importance in patients with head injuries, in whom sudden increase in PaCO$_2$ may result in an undesirable increase in intracranial pressure. Patients with head injuries may undergo surgery on an extremity requiring tourniquet placement.[77]

Because of the greater oxygen consumption and high metabolic rate in infants and children, there has been concern that tourniquet hemostasis may result in greater accumulation of ischemic metabolites, and that physiologic compensation may not be sufficient.[65] Although it has been demonstrated that children do not experience adverse effects from tourniquet release, the recommendations by Lynn et al.[65] should be followed to minimize the systemic and metabolic effects after tourniquet release. These include attempts to limit inflation times to less than 75 minutes and increasing minute ventilation prior to and after tourniquet deflation to prevent the respiratory component of acidosis. It must be emphasized that if the Mapleson D pediatric circuit is being used, controlled ventilation, or simply increasing minute ventilation, may not be adequate in preventing the increase in PaCO$_2$. An increase in fresh gas flow may be necessary to maintain PaCO$_2$ at a near-normal level after tourniquet deflation. Lynn et al.[65] also recommended that blood gas tensions be checked within 5 minutes of tourniquet deflation in children with long tourniquet inflation times (more than 75 minutes), and where bilateral tourniquets are deflated simultaneously or within 30 minutes of each other.

Accurate monitoring of PETCO$_2$ provides a reliable estimate of PaCO$_2$ in children, and therefore, arterial blood sampling may not be necessary following prolonged or bilateral tourniquet deflation. In normal children and in children with acyanotic congenital heart disease, the difference between PaCO$_2$ and PETCO$_2$ is minimal, even during hypotension.[48,78] Provided that the CO$_2$ plateau is observed on capnography and accurate end tidal gas sampling is performed, PETCO$_2$ measurements correlate with PaCO$_2$ values. Exceptions are children with increased alveolar dead space, such as cyanotic congenital heart disease (because of subnormal pulmonary blood flow), and pulmonary disease.[78,79] Accurate sampling of end-tidal gas may be unreliable in infants weighing less than 8 kg when a Mapleson D circuit is used and when PEEP is added.

The use of tourniquets in patients with sickle cell anemia has been discouraged for fear that it may cause circulatory stasis, acidosis, and hypoxemia, the triad known to trigger sickling. Clinical experience suggests that the use of tourniquets in these patients is not associated with harmful effects provided that oxygenation, and mild hyperventilation are maintained, and the usual precautions for tourniquet use are followed.[80] The effect of automatic tourniquets on inducing fractures in children with osteogenesis imperfecta has been recently reported.[81] This disease is a genetic disorder characterized by brittle bones that are easily fractured, or may even fracture simultaneously. Surprisingly, there were no reported fractures associated with the use of tourniquets (or noninvasive automatic blood pressure devices) in 52 patients with osteogenesis imperfecta having 123 operations, confirming that these devices can be safely used in these patients.[81] A progressive increase in temperature (up to 1.6° C) can occur during prolonged leg tourniquet inflation, and a greater increase (up to 2.3° C) occurs with bilateral leg tourniquets.[82,83] This rise in temperature may be related to a reduction in the effective heat loss from the skin and an altered distribution of heat within the body. Thus, close temperature monitoring is suggested during prolonged tourniquet inflation.

## REFERENCES

1. Ellison N. Alternatives to allogeneic (homologous) blood. International Anesthesia Research Society, Review Course Lectures 1993.
2. Walker RH. Is it homologous or is it allogeneic? Transfusion. 1992; 32:397.
3. Stehling LC. Change in transfusion practices. Semin Anesth. 1992; 11:172.
4. Ellison N, Foust RJ. Complications of blood transfusions. In: Benumof JL, Saidman LJ, eds. Anesthesia and Perioperative Complications. Philadelphia, PA: Mosby-Year Book; 1991; 507: chap 21.
5. Sazama K. Report of three hundred fifty-five transfusion-associated deaths: 1976-1985. Transfusion. 1990; 30:583.
6. Curran JW, Lawrence DN, Jaffe H, et al. Acquired immune deficiency syndrome (AIDS) associated with transfusions. N Engl J Med. 1984; 310:69.
7. Grim PS, Gottlieb LJ, Boddie A, et al. Hyperbaric oxygen therapy. JAMA. 1990; 263:2216.
8. Gelman S, Fowler K, Smith L. Regional blood flow

during isoflurane and halothane anesthesia. Anesth Analg. 1984; 65:557.

9. Jardin F, Farcot JC, Boisante L, et al. Influence of positive end-expiratory pressure on left ventricular performance. N Engl J Med. 1981; 304:387.

10. Pick RA, Handler JR, Murata GH, et al. The cardiovascular effects of positive end-expiratory pressure. Chest. 1982; 82:345.

11. Rankin JS, Olsen CO, Arentzen CE, et al. The effects of airway pressure on cardiac function in intact dogs and man. Circulation. 1982; 66:108.

12. Schreuder JJ, Jansen JRC, Bogaard JM, et al. Hemodynamic effects of positive end-expiratory pressure applied as a ramp. J Appl Physiol. 1982; 53:1239.

13. Salem MR, Klowden AJ. Anesthesia for orthopedic surgery. In: Gregory GA, ed. Pediatric Anesthesia. 2nd ed. New York, NY: Churchill Livingstone; 1994: 607.

14. Relton JES. Anesthesia in the original correction of scoliosis. In: Riseborough EJ, Herndon JH, eds. Scoliosis and Other Deformities of the Axial Skeleton. Boston, MA: Little, Brown & Co; 1975.

15. Stehling L, Simon TL. The red blood cell transfusion trigger: physiology and clinical studies. Arch Pathol Lab Med. 1994; 118:429.

16. Hatch PD. Surgical and anaesthetic considerations in transurethral resection of the prostate. Anaesth Inten Care. 1987; 15:203.

17. Agin C. Anesthesia for transurethral prostate surgery. Int Anesthesiol Clin. 1993; 1:31.

18. Abrams PH, Shah PJR, Bryning K, et al. Blood loss during transurethral resection of the prostate. Anaesthesia. 1982; 37:71.

19. McGowan SW, Smith GFN. Anaesthesia for transurethral prostatectomy. Anaesthesia. 1980; 35:847.

20. Nielsen KK, Andersen K, Asbjorn J, et al. Blood loss in transurethral prostatectomy: epidural versus general anaesthesia. Int Urol Nephrol. 1987; 19:287.

21. Mackenzie AR. Influence of anaesthesia on blood loss in transurethral prostatectomy. Scott Med J. 1990; 35:14.

22. Gilstrap LC III, Hauth JC, Hankins GDV, et al. Effect of type of anesthesia on blood loss at cesarean section. Obstet Gynecol. 1987; 69:328.

23. Hood DD, Holubec DM. Elective repeat cesarian section. J Reprod Med. 1990; 35:368.

24. Andrews WW, Ramin SM, Maberry MC, et al. Effect of type of anesthesia on blood loss at elective repeat cesarian section. Am J Perinatol. 1992; 9:197.

25. Cullen BF, Margolis AJ, Eger EI II. The effects of anesthesia and pulmonary ventilation on blood loss during elective therapeutic abortion. Anesthesiology. 1970; 32:108.

26. Dolan WM, Eger EI II, Margolis AJ. Forane increases bleeding in therapeutic suction abortion. Anesthesiology. 1972; 36:96.

27. Sidhu MS, Cullen BF. Low-dose enflurane does not increase blood loss during therapeutic abortion. Anesthesiology. 1982; 57:127.

28. McKenzie PJ, Wishhart HY, Dewar KMS, et al. Comparison of the effects of spinal anaesthesia and general anaesthesia on postoperative oxygenation and perioperative mortality. Br J Anaesth. 1980; 52: 49.

29. McKenzie PJ, Wishart HY, Smith G. Long-term outcome after repair of fractured neck of femur. Br J Anaesth. 1984; 56:581.

30. Sorenson RM, Pace NL. Anesthetic techniques during surgical repair of femoral neck fractures: a meta-analysis. Anesthesiology. 1992; 77:1095.

31. Valentin N, Lomholt B, Jensen JS, et al. Spinal or general anaesthesia for surgery of fractured hip? Br J Anaesth. 1986; 58:284.

32. Keith I. Anaesthesia and blood loss in total hip replacement. Anaesthesia. 1977; 32:444.

33. Modig J, Borg T, Karlström G, et al. Thrombo embolism after total hip replacement: role of epidural and general anesthesia. Anesth Analg. 1983; 62:174.

34. Hole A, Terjesen T, Breivik H. Epidural versus general anesthesia for total hip arthroplasty in elderly patients. Acta Anaesthesiol Scand. 1980; 24:279.

35. Chin SP, Abou-Madi MN, Eurin B, et al. Blood loss in total hip replacement: extradural v. phenoperidine analgesia. Br J Anaesth. 1982; 54:491.

36. Salem MR. Hypercapnia, hypocapnia, and hypoxemia. Semin Anesth. 1987; 6:202.

37. Cullen DJ, Eger EI II. Cardiovascular effects of carbon dioxide in man. Anesthesiology. 1974; 41:345.

38. Don H. Hypoxemia and hypercapnia during and after anesthesia. In: Orkin FK, Cooperman LH, eds. Complications in Anesthesiology. Philadelphia, PA: JB Lippincott Co; 1983: 183-207.

39. Nunn JF. Applied Respiratory Physiology. 4th ed. Boston, MA: Butterworths, 1993.

40. Askanazi J, Weissman C, Rosenbaum SH, et al. Nutrition and the respiratory system. Crit Care Med. 1982; 10:163.

41. Podraza AG, Salem MR, Joseph NJ. Rebreathing resulting from incompetent unidirectional valves in the semi-closed circuit. Anesthesiology 1991; 75:A422. Abstract.

42. Baraka A, Brandstater B, Muallem M, et al. Rebreathing in a double T-piece system. Br J Anaesth. 1969; 41:47.

43. Laver MB, Hallowell P, Goldblatt A. Pulmonary dysfunction secondary to heart disease: aspects relevant to anesthesia and surgery. Anesthesiology. 1970; 33: 161.

44. Salem MR, Paulissian R, Joseph NJ, et al. Effect of deliberate hypotension on arterial to peak expired carbon dioxide tension difference. Anesth Analg. 1988; 67:S194. Abstract.

45. Warren JV. The physiology of the giraffe. Sci Am. 1974; 231:96.

46. Salem MR. Therapeutic uses of ganglionic blocking drugs. Int Anesthesiol Clin. 1978; 16:171.

47. Hainsworth R. Arterial blood pressure. In: Enderby GEH, ed. Hypotensive Anaesthesia. London, England: Churchill Livingstone; 1985:3.

48. Salem MR, Wong AY, Bennett EJ, et al. Deliberate hypotension in infants and children. Anesth Analg. 1974; 53:975.

49. Relton JES, Hall JE. An operation frame for spinal fusion: a new apparatus designed to reduce haemorrhage during operation. J Bone Joint Surg Br. 1967; 49B:327.

50. Schwentker EP. Posterior fusion of the spine for scoliosis. Surg Rounds. 1978; 1:12.

51. Katz RL, Bigger JT. Cardiac arrhythmias during anesthesia and operation. Anesthesiology. 1970; 33: 193.

52. Johnston RR, Eger EI II, Wilson C. A comparative interaction of epinephrine with enflurane, isoflurane, and halothane in man. Anesth Analg. 1976; 55:709.

53. Ueda W, Hirakawa M, Mae O. Appraisal of epinephrine administration under halothane anesthesia for

closure of cleft palate. Anesthesiology. 1983; 58: 574.

54. Karl HW, Swedlow DB, Lee KW, et al. Epinephrine-halothane interactions in children. Anesthesiology. 1983; 58:142.

55. Fairbanks D, Fairbanks G. Cocaine uses and abuses. Ann Plast Surg. 1983; 10:452.

56. Czinn EA, Provenzale D, Friedman M, et al. Esmolol blunts tachycardia associated with topical cocaine and lidocaine with epinephrine infiltration. Anesthesiology. 1991; 75:A37. Abstract.

57. Stoelting RK. Pharmacology and Physiology in Anesthetic Practice. Philadelphia, PA: JB Lippincott Co; 1987: 627.

58. Savarese JJ, Covino BG. Basic and clinical pharmacology of local anesthetic drugs. In Miller EJ, ed. Anesthesia. 3rd ed. New York, NY: Churchill-Livingstone; 1990.

59. Cousins MJ, Bridenbaugh PO. Neural blockade: Pain Management. 2nd ed. Philadelphia, PA: JB Lippincott Co; 1988: 627.

60. Fleming JA, Byck R, Barash PG. Pharmacology and therapeutic applications of cocaine. Anesthesiology. 1990; 73:518.

61. Wilkinson P, VanDyke C, Jatlow P, et al. Intranasal and oral cocaine kinetics. Clin Pharmacol Ther. 1980; 27:386.

62. Fischman MW, Schuster CR, Javaid J, et al. Acute tolerance development to the cardiovascular and subjective effects of cocaine. J Pharmacol Exp Ther. 1985; 235:677.

63. Lange RA, Cigarroa RG, Yancy CW Jr, et al. Cocaine-induced coronary-artery vasoconstriction. N Engl J Med. 1989; 321:1557.

64. Sessler CN, Vitaliti JC, Cooper KR, et al. Comparison of 4% lidocaine/0.5% phenylephrine with 5% cocaine: which dilates the nasal passage better? Anesthesiology. 1986; 64:274.

65. Lynn AM, Fischer T, Brandford HG, et al. Systemic responses to tourniquet release in children. Anesth Analg. 1986; 65:865.

66. Kaufman RD, Walts LF. Tourniquet-induced hypertension. Br J *Anaesth*. 1982; 54:333.

67. Valli H, Rosenberg PH, Kytta J, et al. Arterial hypertension associated with the use of a tourniquet with either general or regional anesthesia. Acta Anaesthesiol Scand. 1987; 31:279.

68. Bourke DL, Silberberg MS, Ortega R, et al. Respiratory responses associated with release of intraoperative tourniquets. Anesth Analg. 1989; 69:541.

69. Modig J, Kolstad K, Wigren A. Systemic reactions to tourniquet ischemia. Acta Anaesthesiol Scand. 1978; 22:609.

70. Valli H, Rosenberg PH. Effects of three anaesthesia methods on haemodynamic responses connected with the use of thigh tourniquet in orthopaedic patients. Acta Anaesthesiol Scand. 1985; 29:142.

71. Moncorge CV, Brzustowicz RM, Kola BV. Systemic and metabolic responses to tourniquet ischemia in children. Anesthesiology. 1982; 57:A420. Abstract.

72. Wilgis EFS. Observations on the effects of tourniquet ischemia. J Bone Joint Surg Am. 1971; 53A:1343.

73. Haljamae H, Enger E. Human skeletal muscle energy metabolism during and after complete tourniquet ischemia. Ann Surg. 1975; 82:9.

74. Benzon HT, Toleikis JR, Meagher LL, et al. Tourniquet pain: changes in SSEP, blood lactate, and venous blood gases Anesth Analg. 1988; 67:S266. Abstract.

75. Fahmy NR, Patel DG. Hemostatic changes and postoperative deep-vein thrombosis associated with use of a pneumatic tourniquet. J Bone Joint Surg Am. 1981; 63A:461.

76. Patel A, Choi C, Giuffrida JG. Changes in end tidal $CO_2$ and arterial blood gas levels after release of tourniquet. South Med J. 1987; 80:213.

77. Dickson M, White H, Kinney W, et al. Effect of extremity tourniquet deflation on end-tidal $pCO_2$ values. Anesth Analg 1989; 68:S71. Abstract.

78. Lindahl SGE, Yates AP, Hatch DJ. Relationship between invasive and noninvasive measurements of gas exchange in anesthetized infants and children. Anesthesiology. 1987; 66:168.

79. Nicodemus HF, Downes JJ. Ventilatory alterations associated with operation for tetralogy of Fallot. Anesthesiology. 1969; 31:265.

80. Adu-Gyamfi Y, Sankarankutty M, Marwa S. Use of a tourniquet in patients with sickle-cell disease. Can J Anaesth. 1993; 40:24.

81. Burnett YL, Brennan MP, Klowden AJ, et al. Effect of automatic tourniquets and automatic noninvasive blood pressure devices on inducing fractures in pediatric patients with osteogenesis imperfect. Anesthesiology. 1994; 81:A507. Abstract.

82. Mostello LA, Casey WF, McGill WA. Does the use of a surgical tourniquet induce fever in infants? Anesth Analg. 1992; 72:S191. Abstract.

83. Bloch EC, Ginsberg B, Binner RA Jr, et al. Limb tourniquets and central temperature in anesthetized children. Anesth Analg. 1992; 74:486.

# 5

# PERIOPERATIVE HEMOGLOBIN REQUIREMENTS

*M. Ramez Salem, Steven Manley,*
*George J. Crystal, and Harold J. Heyman*

## INTRODUCTION

Oxygen is carried in the blood in two forms: the greatest portion is in reversible chemical combination with hemoglobin (HGB), while the smaller part is dissolved in plasma. The ability to carry large amounts of oxygen in HGB is important, since without HGB, the amount carried would be so small that the cardiac output (CO) would need to be increased 20 times to give an adequate oxygen flux.[1] The biological significance of HGB is immense, and it may be compared to chlorophyll in plants, which closely resembles HGB, although containing magnesium in place of iron.

Anemia is generally defined as a reduction in red blood cell (RBC) mass or total body HGB. In clinical practice, HGB concentration is assumed to reflect the circulating RBC mass. These quantitative definitions lack acceptable qualitative correlate based on physiologic or biochemical basis. As a consequence of these arbitrary definitions of anemia, clinicians for years have spent much time arguing as to what HGB level is acceptable for anesthesia and surgery, at what HGB level a patient should be transfused, and whether a certain HGB level is adequate for a patient with chronic lung disease or cyanotic congenital heart disease.[2]

Because HGB levels undergo pronounced changes during the first year of life, the discussion will be separated into: (1) perioperative HGB requirements in infants and children;

and (2) perioperative HGB requirements in adults.

# I. PERIOPERATIVE HEMOGLOBIN REQUIREMENTS IN INFANTS AND CHILDREN

The etiology of anemia is traditionally considered under three general pathophysiologic categories of decreased RBC production, increased RBC destruction, and blood loss (Table 5–1). In infants, this classic approach to anemia is complicated by an HGB concentration that undergoes physiologic changes during the first few months of life.[3] Although anemia in infants is defined as "a reduction in RBC mass or HGB concentration," a more meaningful definition would be "a decrease in the level of HGB content of a unit volume of blood below the level previously established as normal for age and sex."

**Table 5–1.   Pathophysiologic classification of anemia**

Decreased production of red cells
  Congenital
    Red Cell Aplasia
    Infections (Rubella)
    Leukemia
  Acquired
    Nutritional deficiencies: iron, $B_{12}$/folic acid
    Drugs and toxic agents
    Infections and sepsis
    Marrow infiltrates
    Chronic renal failure
Increased destruction of red cells
  "Immune" hemolytic anemia
    Incompatibility
    Autoimmune
    Drug-induced
  Infections
  Vitamin deficiency
  Red cell membrane disorders
    Spherocytosis
    Elliptocytosis
  Red cell enzyme deficiencies
    Glucose 6—phosphodiesterase deficiency
    Pyruvate kinase deficiency
  Hemoglobinopathies
  Thalassemias
Blood loss
  Acute
  Chronic

**Table 5–2.   Normal cord hemoglobin values in premature infants**

| Gestational age (weeks) | Hemoglobin (g/d) | |
|---|---|---|
| | Male | Female |
| 28–29 | 15.00 ± 2.45 | 13.60 ± 2.16 |
| 30–31 | 15.91 ± 1.34 | 14.73 ± 1.07 |
| 32–33 | 16.29 ± 1.89 | 15.21 ± 2.64 |
| 34–35 | 16.29 ± 2.05 | 15.82 ± 2.43 |
| 36–37 | 16.20 ± 2.20 | 15.88 ± 2.45 |
| 38–39 | 16.22 ± 2.24 | 16.68 ± 2.23 |
| 40–41 | | 16.56 ± 1.65 |

Modified from Burman D, Morris AF. Cord hemoglobin in low birth weight infants. *Arch Dis Child* 1974;49:382, with permission.

# NORMAL HEMOGLOBIN LEVELS IN NEWBORN INFANTS

After 28 weeks of gestation, cord HGB levels undergo little changes. The mean HGB concentration in cord blood at birth is 16.8 g/dL, with 95% of all values falling between 13.7 and 20.1 g/dL.[3,4] In male newborns, the HGB levels are maximal at 32 weeks of gestation, whereas female infants have cord HGB levels which increase very gradually from 28 weeks of gestation until term (Table 5–2).[5] Based on this data, cord HGB levels less than 13 g/dL are considered abnormal.[3]

At birth, blood is rapidly transferred from the placenta to the infant, with 25% of the placental transfusion occurring within 15 seconds of birth and 50% by the end of the first minute.[6] The blood volume of an infant can be increased by as much as 40% with delayed cord clamping. Usher and coworkers[7] demonstrated that with immediate cord clamping, the average RBC mass was 31 mL/kg, whereas with delayed cord clamping it was 49 mL/kg.

# PHYSIOLOGIC ANEMIA OF INFANCY

The early anemia of infancy has been termed "physiologic" because of its association with the adaptive factors that preserve the availability of oxygen to tissues.[8–12] After birth there is a transient increase in HGB concentration as plasma moves extravascularly to compensate for the placental transfusion and increase in circulating RBC volume that occurs at the time of delivery.[3,13] Thereafter, the HGB level decreases rapidly as the proportion of hemoglobin F (HGB-F) diminishes, reaching a level between 10.5 and 11.5 g/dL in term infants by age 8 to 12 weeks and 7 to 10 g/dL in premature infants by 6 weeks of age[3,12] (Figs. 5–1, 5–2, 5–3). The rapidity with which the HGB levels decline and the actual nadir in the HGB concentration varies inversely with gestational age.[14]

A regulatory effect of the hormone "erythropoietin" on HGB levels has been demonstrated in full-term infants[15] and premature infants.[16] Erythropoietic hemostasis in the fetus is not dependent on direct maternal control, but is probably endogenously controlled by fetally produced erythropoietin. Erythropoietin levels increase gradually during the latter part of gestation. The rate of increase in HGB levels observed in small-for-gestational age infants is greater than that observed in those with weight appropriate for gestational age.[18] This increase in erythropoietic response may be related to chronic intrauterine fetal hypoxemia, due to placental insufficiency.[8]

The explanation for this characteristic fall in HGB concentration after birth is as follows: the high HGB and reticulocyte values seen in cord blood reflect an erythropoietic response to the hypoxic intrauterine environment (Figs. 5–1, 5–2, 5–3). In response to the in-

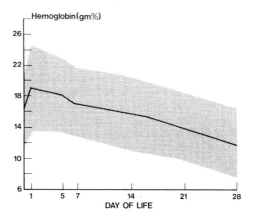

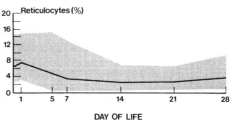

**Fig. 5–2.** These graphs were constructed from studies of 178 normal premature infants (<36 weeks gestation). Measurements were made on Day 0 (cord blood) and Days 1, 5, 7, 14, 21, and 28 (capillary blood). On the graphs the dark solid lines represent means and the shaded areas include 95 percent of the value. From Blanchette VS, Zipursky A. Assessment of anemia in newborn infants. Clin Perinatol. 1984; 11:489, with permission.

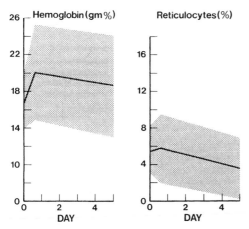

**Fig. 5–1.** These graphs were constructed from studies of 163 normal full-term infants (≥36 weeks gestation). Measurements were made on Day 0 (cord blood) and Days 1, 2, 3, 4, and 5 (capillary blood). On the graphs the dark solid line represents means and the shaded areas include 95% of the value. From Blanchette VS, Zipursky A. Assessment of anemia in newborn infants. Clin Perinatol. 1984; 11:489, with permission.

crease in the arterial oxygen tension ($PaO_2$) after birth, and the increase in arterial oxygen content ($CaO_2$), erythropoietin levels decrease markedly, and there are corresponding falls in reticulocyte levels and marrow erythroid activity.[19-21] Consequently, hematopoiesis virtually ceases after birth. The increase in oxygen delivery following transition from placental to pulmonary oxygenation after birth, with a consequent decrease in erythropoietin production, is the major cause of the physiologic anemia of infancy. Coupled with the shortened RBC survival in term (80 to 100 days) and premature infants (60 to 80 days), progressive fall in HGB concentration occurs during the first 1 to 3 months of life (life-span of normal RBCs is approximately 120 days).[3,22,23] When the HGB concentration falls to a level low enough to affect tissue oxygen delivery, erythropoietin production is stimulated, active marrow erythropoiesis re-

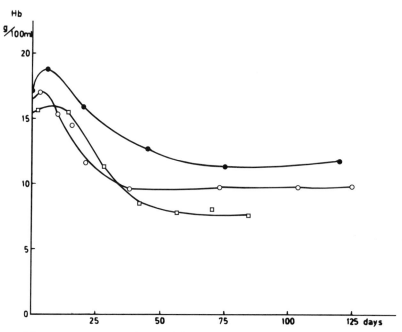

**Fig. 5–3.** Hemoglobin concentration in infants of different degree of maturation at birth. ●, Full term infants; ○, premature infants with birth weights of 1200 to 2350 g; □, premature infants with birth weights less than 1200 g. From Nathan DG, Oski FA. Hematology of infancy and childhood, 3rd ed. Philadelphia, PA: WB Saunders Co; 1987: 29, with permission.

sumes, a reticulocytosis occurs, and the HGB concentration increases.[16] In newborns with congenital cyanotic heart disease, hypoxemia continues to stimulate active erythropoiesis and the postnatal fall in HGB concentration rarely occurs.[3]

## ANEMIA OF PREMATURITY

In preterm infants, the HGB concentration may fall steeply and often reaches 8 g/dL or lower before the peak effect of hematopoiesis is reached. This is referred to as the anemia of prematurity (Figs. 5–2, 5–3). This anemia is attributed mainly to the abrupt increase in oxygen delivery after birth. As anemia develops there is a diminished erythropoietin response to decreased oxygen availability.[24-26] Anemia of prematurity is characterized by reduced erythropoiesis, in association with what appears to be an inappropriately low serum concentration of erythropoietin.[27,28]

Blood loss due to spontaneous prenatal hemorrhage may be an additional cause of anemia, but diagnostic sampling plays a major role in the occurrence of early anemia in sick premature infants in their first weeks of life.

Blanchette and Zipursky[3] found that in the first 6 weeks of life, 90% of sick premature infants received at least one transfusion and nearly 50% received cumulative transfusions in excess of their total circulating RBC mass. During the first 2 weeks of life most transfusions given to preterm infants were for the purpose of replacing blood withdrawn for laboratory tests. After that time, most transfusions were given for an anemia that is not attributable to blood withdrawal.[29] Other factors may contribute to the occurrence of anemia including more rapid destruction of fetal cells, hemodilution due to rapid growth between 30 and 40 weeks gestation,[24, 25] and nutritional deficiencies.

Because of the multifactorial etiology of anemia in premature infants, it has been referred to as "anemias," rather than anemia of prematurity. The view has become obsolete that anemia is "physiologic" in preterm infants.[30] This anemia which may be severe, reduces the amount of available oxygen, and may contribute to apneic spells, mesenteric hypoperfusion, necrotizing enterocolitis, and failure to thrive.[26, 30-32]

## Nutritional Factors in Anemia of Prematurity

The premature infant is unlike a term infant in that rapid growth rates do not usually permit assimilation of certain nutritional substances quickly enough to maintain sufficiency if routine feeds are provided.[11] Three deficiencies have been implicated in the development of anemia of prematurity: iron, vitamin E and folic acid, with iron deficiency being the most important. Iron reserves at birth are quantitatively a direct function of birth weight.[11,33] Consequently, the smaller the preterm infant, the greater the risk of developing iron deficiency anemia. At birth, the majority of body iron is in the HGB fraction, with approximately 15 mg/kg in an actual storage form. During the postnatal period, iron released from the destruction of RBCs is either stored or used for tissue growth, and there is practically no excretion. Because of the diminished iron stores and the need for expansion of the RBC mass with rapid tissue growth, iron deficiency anemia is a common etiology of the late anemia of prematurity. This late anemia occurs at a time when storage iron has been completely utilized in new blood formation and coincides with a doubling of birth weight.[11] Although some investigators have attempted to implicate iron deficiency as a possible factor in the development of the early anemia of prematurity, it is believed that iron deficiency plays no role in the early or physiologic anemia of prematurity.[34,35] Other conditions, including infection, renal disease, malignancy and nutritional deficiencies, may prevent the hematopoietic response to iron and worsen the anemia.

The current opinion is that the addition of iron be deferred in premature infants until supplementation is really necessary.[11] The reasons are twofold. First, the administration of iron can aggravate the anemia of prematurity. Premature infants who receive iron demonstrate lower HGB during the first 1 to 2 months of life, than do infants who do not receive iron.[11,26,37] This has been attributed to iron's acting as a catalyst in the nonenzymatic autoxidation of unsaturated fatty acids and can, in the absence of antioxidant, result in RBC lipase peroxidation.[11] Second, large doses of iron may stimulate the proliferation of microorganisms and affect the host resistance to infection.[38-40]

Obviously, iron supplementation should be provided to preterm infants in order to prevent the "late anemia" of prematurity.[11] A prudent decision would be to delay iron supplementation until the time of doubling of birth weight. It may be given earlier if the infant has been made iron deficient iatrogenically. Supplementation should start no later than 4 months of age in term infants, and no later than 2 months of age in preterm infants. The recommended dose is 1 mg/kg/day for term infants and 2 mg/kg/day for preterm infants. If iron is given, the infant's feedings should be low in content of polyunsaturated acids, in order to prevent RBC lipid peroxidation.

## OXYGEN UNLOADING IN THE NEWBORN, INFANT AND CHILD

The umbilical venous blood in the mother has an oxygen content of approximately 13.5 vol% and oxygen saturation of 65%, but in the fetus, oxygen content is about 17 vol% and more than 80% saturated. The difference is caused by a beneficial leftward shift in the fetal oxyhemoglobin dissociation curve (Fig. 5–4). HGB-F has a relatively low affinity for and a low concentration of 2, 3-diphosphoglycerate (2,3-DPG), compared with adult hemoglobin (HGB-A). Since both oxygen and 2,3-DPG compete for binding to HGB, the reduced availability of 2,3-DPG causes oxygen to bind more tightly to HGB-F than HGB-A. This can be expressed by measuring P50, the $PO_2$ at which HGB is 50% saturated with oxygen.

Before 34 weeks of gestational age, HGB consists of HGB-F 90% and HGB-A 10%. After 34 weeks, a gradual decline in HGB-F and an increase in HGB-A levels occur. The switchover is normally completed by 6 months of age (Fig. 5–5).[41-43] At birth, P50 is only 18 to 20 mm Hg, as compared to 27 mm Hg in the adult. During the first 3 months of life, there is a rapid increase in RBC HGB-A and 2,3-DPG, which results in increases in P50 (shifting of the curve to the right), as well as tissue oxygen unloading (Figs. 5–6, 5–7). At about 10 weeks of age (or 50 weeks postconception), the increase in P50 reaches the adult level of 27 mm Hg. The oxyhemoglobin dissociation curve shifts further to the right of

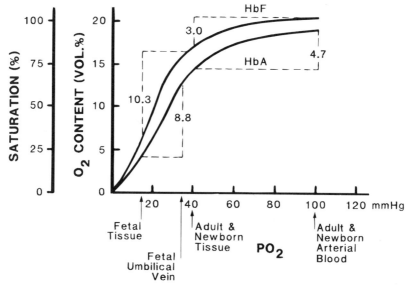

**Fig. 5–4.** Oxygen unloading capacities of fetal and adult HGB before and after birth. In the fetus, fetal hemoglobin (HGB-F) has 15% greater oxygen unloading capacity to the tissues than does adult hemoglobin (HGB-A). In the newborn, HGB-F has 36% less oxygen unloading capacity than HGB-A. Modified from Smith CA, Nelson NM. The Physiology of the Newborn Infant. Springfield, IL: Charles C Thomas; 1976, with permission.

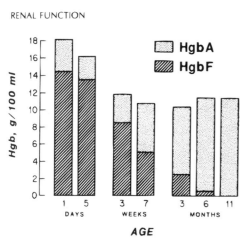

**Fig. 5–5.** The approximate amount of fetal hemoglobin (HGB-F) and adult hemoglobin (HGB-A) present in 100 mL of blood during infancy. Graph constructed from data of Oski FA, Delivoria-Papadopoulos M. The red cell, 2,3-diphosphoglycerate, and tissue oxygen release. J Pediatr. 1970;77:941. Fig. from Goudsouzian N. Anatomy and physiology in relation to pediatric anesthesia. In: Katz J, Steward DJ, eds. Anesthesia and Uncommon Pediatric Diseases. Philadelphia, PA: WB Saunders Co; 1987: 1–11, with permission.

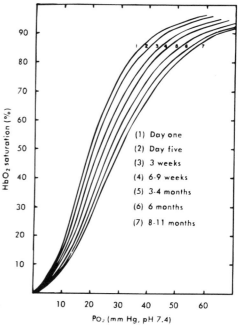

**Fig. 5–6.** Oxyhemoglobin equilibrium curve of blood from normal term infants at different postnatal ages. The P50 on day 1 is 19.4 ± 1.8 mm Hg and has shifted to 30.3 ± 0.7 at age 11 months (normal adults = 27.0 ± 1.1 mm Hg). Modified from Oski FA, Delivoria-Papado-poulos M. The red cell, 2,3-diphosphoglycerate, and tissue oxygen release. J Pediatr. 1970;77:941, with permission.

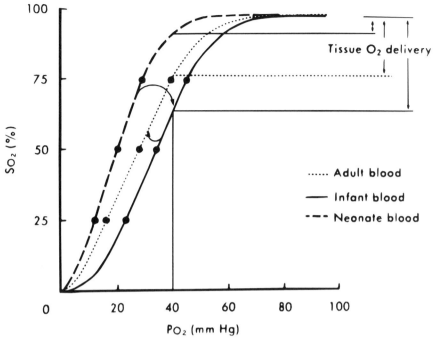

**Fig. 5-7.** Schematic representation of oxyhemoglobin dissociation curves with different oxygen affinities. In infants above 3 months of age with high P50 (30 mm Hg versus 27 in adults), tissue oxygen delivery per gram of HGB is increased. In neonates with a lower P50 (20 mm Hg) and a higher oxygen affinity, tissue oxygen unloading at the same tissue $PO_2$ is reduced. The top arrow indicates the direction of rightward shifting of the oxyhemoglobin dissociation curve (and P50) after birth. By 10 weeks of age, the adult position of the curve is reached. Rightward shifting continues and maximum shifting is observed at 6 to 11 months of age. The lower arrow indicates leftward shifting of the curve (and P50) back to the adult level which is usually completed by approximately 10 years of age. From Motoyama EK. Respiratory physiology in infants and children. In: Motoyama EK, Davis PJ eds. Smith's Anesthesia for Infants and Children. 5th ed. St. Louis, MO: CV Mosby Company; 1990:11–76, with permission.

the adult curve, and a level as high as 30 mm Hg may be reached by 6 to 11 months of age (Figure 7). Thereafter, P50 gradually decreases (shifting of the curve to the left), reaching the adult level of approximately 27 mm Hg during the first decade of life (Figure 7). This is accompanied by a gradual decrease in 2,3-DPG levels toward the adult level by 10 years of age (Fig. 5–8). Even in preterm infants, a decrease in HGB oxygen affinity facilitating release of oxygen to the tissues occurs as a consequence of decline in HGB-F concentrations and improved interactions of HGB with 2,3-DPG during the first few weeks after birth. It must be emphasized that the shift from HGB-F synthesis to HGB-A synthesis appears to be based on postconceptual age and follows a sigmoid curve with a crossover point about 30 to 32 weeks postconception in preterm infants, when HGB-A is produced in significant amounts.[14]

In the fetus, oxygen unloading occurs across the steep portion of the oxyhemoglobin dissociation curve. The leftward shifting of the HGB-F curve makes it steeper than the HGB-A curve, and therefore, HGB-F unloads oxygen to the fetal tissues better than HGB-A would (Figure 4). This is a good example of the efficiency of the fetal circulation in acquiring and distributing adequate nutrients, even though the amount of oxygen supplied to the fetus is reduced because of inefficient gas exchange in the placenta, and because it must be shared with the mother. After birth, HGB-F, despite a high HGB level, puts the newborn at a disadvantage, since its presence reduces the amount of oxygen that would otherwise be unloaded to the tissues.[44] Comparisons of oxygen unloading capacities of HGB-F and HGB-A, before and after birth, are shown in Figure 4. In the fetus, HGB-F can unload 10.3 vol% to the tissues, while HGB-A

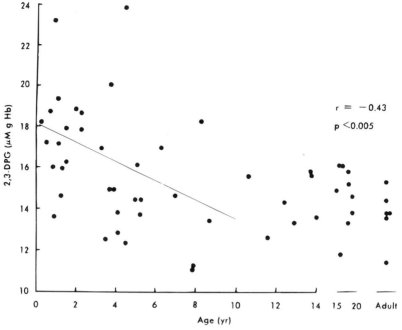

**Fig. 5–8.** Blood 2,3-DPG level versus the age of healthy infants and children. The 2,3-DPG level is high in infants and decreases toward the adult level by age 10. This increase in 2,3-DPG is associated with higher levels of P50. From Motoyama EK, Zigas CJ, Troll G. Functional basis of childhood anemia. Am Soc Anesthesiol. 1974; 283–284, with permission. Abstract.

can unload 8.8 vol%. In contrast, after birth HGB-A has greater unloading capacity than HGB-F.[45]

In terms of oxygen delivery, the newborn is not always at a disadvantage because of the presence of a high affinity HGB-F. During episodes of severe hypoxemia, a leftward shift in the oxyhemoglobin dissociation curve might actually better maintain oxygen delivery.[14] The $PaO_2$ below which shifts to the right in the oxyhemoglobin dissociation curve are no longer of an advantage is known as a "crossover" $PO_2$ (Fig. 5-9).[46] A crossover $PO_2$ is dependent on how low the mixed venous oxygen tension ($P\overline{v}O_2$) falls before oxygen delivery ceases. Wimberley calculated that if $P\overline{v}O_2$ were to fall to 10 mm Hg (a value found in the cerebral venous blood of some sick neonates), the infant would achieve better oxygen delivery with fetal oxyhemoglobin dissociation curve, than with adult curve when $PaO_2$ falls below 50 mm Hg (Fig. 5-9).[47] In contrast, with a higher $PaO_2$, better oxygen delivery would result if the oxyhemoglobin dissociation curve were shifted to the right, such as might be achieved by exchange transfusion.[14] In hypoxemic neonates due to right to left

shunting (cyanotic congenital heart disease and intrapulmonary shunting), rightward shifting of the oxyhemoglobin dissociation curve will tend to lower the venous oxygen saturation at any given $PO_2$, increase arteriovenous oxygen content difference, and improve oxygen delivery.[14,48]

The rapid increase in P50 associated with the decline in HGB levels after birth, seems to be related to the process of general growth and high plasma levels of inorganic phosphate.[49] Normal children have plasma phosphates 50% above the normal adult range "hyperphosphatemia of childhood." Even slight increases in plasma inorganic phosphate concentration produce major alterations in RBC metabolism, and lead to raised levels of RBC adenosine triphosphate (ATP) and 2,3-DPG, with a resultant increase in P50.[49] These observations engendered a hypothesis to explain why HGB levels are lower in children than in adults. Since infants (older than 3 months of age) and children have a lower oxygen affinity for HGB (high P50), oxygen unloading at the tissue level is increased. Thus, a lower level of HGB in these infants and children is just as efficient, in terms of tissue oxy-

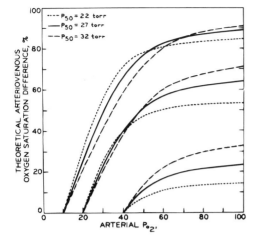

**Fig. 5–9.** The effect of arterial $PO_2$ on theoretical arteriovenous oxygen content difference when venous $PO_2$ is over 40 mm Hg (lower set of curves), 20 mm Hg (middle set of curves), or 10 mm Hg (upper set of curves) at varying P50 values. From Woodson RD. $O_2$ transport. DPG and P50. Basic SRD 1977; 5:1, with permission.

gen delivery, as a higher HGB level in adults (Table 5–3).[2,49-51]

It is evident that the HGB concentration per se, in physiologic, as well as other types of anemia, is neither an adequate descriptor of the severity of anemia, nor is it reflective of the adaptive factors that preserve oxygen delivery to the tissues. This led Oski[2] to introduce the concept of "designation of anemia on a functional basis." Motoyama and associates[50] compared HGB requirements for equivalent tissue oxygen delivery (Table 5–4). Functionally, a 10 g/dL of HGB in an adult, in terms of oxygen unloading capacity, is equivalent to 8.2 g/dL in infants older than 3 months of age, while a 10 g/dL of HGB in preterm infants and in infants under 2 months of age, is only as good as 5 to 7 g/dL of HGB in infants older than 3 months, children, or adults. In contrast, a 9 g/dL of HGB in a 4-month-old infant is equivalent to 11 g/dL in adults.

Although the amount of dissolved oxygen

**Table 5–3. Oxygen unloading changes with age**

| Age | P50 (mm Hg) | $S\bar{v}O_2$ ($P\bar{v}O_2 = 40$ mm Hg) (%) | HGB (gm/dL) | Oxygen unloaded* (mL/dL) |
|---|---|---|---|---|
| 1 d | 19.4 | 87 | 17.2 | 1.84 |
| 3 wk | 22.7 | 80 | 13.0 | 2.61 |
| 6–9 wk | 24.4 | 77 | 11.0 | 2.65 |
| 3–4 mo | 26.5 | 73 | 10.5 | 3.10 |
| 6 mo | 27.8 | 69 | 11.3 | 3.94 |
| 8–11 mo | 30.0 | 65 | 11.8 | 4.74 |
| 5–8 y | 29.0† | 67 | 12.6 | 4.73 |
| 9–12 y | 27.9† | 69 | 13.4 | 4.67 |
| Adult | 27.0 | 71 | 15.0 | 4.92 |

* Assumes arterial oxygen saturation of 95%.
† Derived from data of Card RT, Brain MC: The "anemia" of childhood: evidence for a physiologic response to hyperphosphatemia, N Engl J Med 1973;288:388. The remainder of the P50 data as previously published.
Modified from Oski FA. Designation of anemia on a functional basis. J Pediatr 1973; 83:353, with permission.

**Table 5–4. Hemoglobin requirement for equivalent tissue oxygen delivery***

| | P50 (mm Hg) | Hemoglobin for equivalent oxygen delivery (g/dL) | | | | | | |
|---|---|---|---|---|---|---|---|---|
| Adult | 27 | 7 | 8 | 9 | 10 | 11 | 12 | 13 |
| Infant > 3 mo | 30 | 5.7 | 6.5 | 7.3 | 8.2 | 9.0 | 9.8 | 10.6 |
| Neonate < 2 mo | 24 | 10.3 | 11.7 | 13.2 | 14.7 | 16.1 | 17.6 | 19.1 |

* Data calculated from Motoyama EK, Zigas CJ, Troll G. Functional basis of childhood anemia. Am Soc Anesthesiol 1974;283–284. Abstract. From Motoyama EK. Respiratory physiology in infants and children. In: Motoyama EK, Davis PJ, eds. *Smith's Anesthesia for Infants and Children*, 5th ed. St. Louis, MO: CV Mosby Co; 1990:11–76, with permission.

in plasma is only 2% of the total oxygen-carrying capacity (the rest is reversibly bound to HGB), it is this apparently small portion of the circulating oxygen that provides the gradient that drives oxygen from plasma into tissues. Hence, a high blood oxygen content is of little value if the corresponding oxygen concentration in plasma is too low to sustain adequate tissue oxygenation. A major advantage of an increase in P50 is a higher oxygen tension in plasma for a given level of oxygen saturation.[56] This can produce a substantial increase in the rate of oxygen delivery to tissues, with little change in the degree of saturation of HGB at a high $PaO_2$.

## ACCURACY OF HEMOGLOBIN/ HEMATOCRIT MEASUREMENT

Samples for measurement of HGB and hematocrit (HCT) in infants are usually obtained by heel sticks. There is evidence that HGB levels measured in capillary blood samples (heel sticks) may be significantly higher than values obtained from simultaneously col-

lected venous blood samples. In one study, the mean difference in the HCT level of blood samples obtained by the two collection techniques was 3.7 ± 2.7%, although individual differences as large as 10 percentage points were observed (Fig. 5–10).[3] Prewarming the heel before collection of the capillary samples, reverses circulatory stasis and reduces the average capillary-venous HCT difference from 3.9 to 1.9%.[3,53,54]

## DOES HEMOGLOBIN/ HEMATOCRIT MEASUREMENT REFLECT RED CELL MASS IN INFANTS?

Studies in premature infants failed to show good correlation between capillary HCT and circulating RBC mass.[3,55,56] Wide variations in RBC mass were noted for a given HCT, even if allowances are made for known capillary-venous HCT differences in this age group (Fig. 5–11). Thus, capillary HCT measurement is often a poor reflection of the circulat-

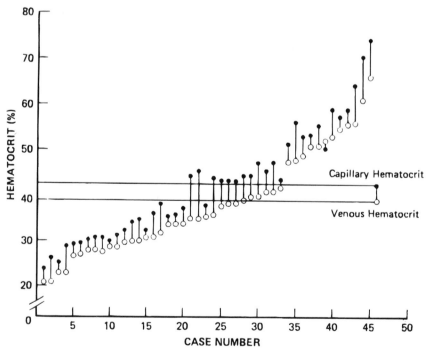

**Fig. 5–10.** Simultaneous capillary (●) versus venous (○) hematocrit levels in 45 premature infants studied during the first six weeks of life. Each vertical line represents values for an individual infant and the horizontal solid lines represent mean capillary and venous HCT levels for the whole group. Data are not shown for five infants in whom capillary and venous HCT levels were identical. From Blanchette VS, Zipursky A. Assessment of anemia in newborn infants. Clin Perinatol. 1984; 11:489, with permission.

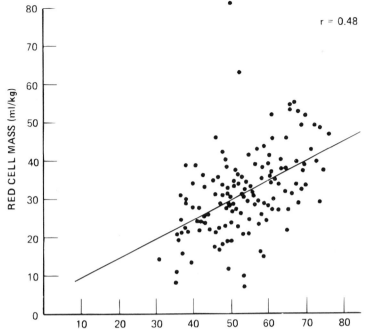

**Fig. 5–11.** Simultaneous capillary HCT and circulating red cell mass levels in 135 premature infants (birth weight <1500 g) studied during the first week of life. r = correlation coefficient. From Blanchette VS, Zipursky A. Assessment of anemia in newborn infants. Clin Perinatol. 1984; 11:489, with permission.

ing RBC mass in newborn infants. This is likely to be noticed in sick infants in whom a poor peripheral circulation may exaggerate capillary-venous HCT difference, and in premature infants during periods of rapid growth, when increases in total circulating blood volume result in hemodilution.[3] These observations in infants are in marked contrast with the excellent relationship that exists between venous HCT and circulating RBC mass in adults.[57] It would be ideal to measure or estimate accurately RBC mass, rather than rely on HGB or HCT measurements in anemic infants. However, methods used for RBC mass estimation have serious drawbacks including inaccuracy (dye-dilution in plasma), infective or radiation hazards (radioisotopes), delay in obtaining results, cost (in vitro neutron activation of $^{50}CO$), and inapplicability (carbon monoxide labeling of HGB).[54,56,58]

## IMPACT OF REPEATED BLOOD SAMPLING ON HEMOGLOBIN LEVEL IN CRITICALLY ILL INFANTS

Repeated blood sampling can have a marked effect on the HGB concentration of

small premature critically ill patients. Blanchette and Zipursky[3] drew attention to the cumulative blood losses through sampling for laboratory monitoring, in spite of using micromethods utilizing small volumes of blood in neonatal units. They observed that

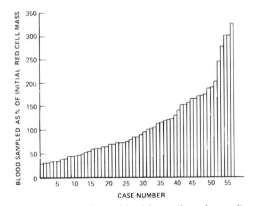

**Fig. 5–12.** Cumulative blood losses through sampling in premature infants expressed as a percentage of their red blood cell mass at birth. Infants were studied during the first six weeks of life, and each vertical bar represents a single infant. From Blanchette VS, Zipursky A. Assessment of anemia in newborn infants. Clin Perinatol. 1984; 11:489, with permission.

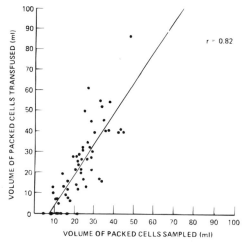

**Fig. 5–13.** Relationship between the cumulative volumes of blood sampled from and transfused into 57 premature infants (birth weight <1500 g) during the first six weeks of life. Volumes represent mL of packed red cells and r = correlation coefficient. From Blanchette VS, Zipursky A. Assessment of anemia in newborn infants. Clin Perinatol 1984; 11:489, with permission.

more than 40% of the infants studied had cumulative losses that exceeded their circulating RBC mass at birth (Fig. 5–12). In a few cases the losses were equivalent to 2 to 3 times the infant's RBC mass at birth. They also made two important observations. First, approximately 10% of all blood loss during sampling for laboratory use is "hidden," and represents blood on swabs, syringes, etc. Second, there was a very close relationship between the volumes of blood sampled and blood transfused (Fig. 5–13), suggesting that much of the transfusion requirements in sick premature infants is a direct consequence of blood loss for laboratory use. Obviously, cumulative blood losses in neonatal units and cardiac catheterization laboratories must be taken into consideration. The removal of 1mL of blood from a 1-kg premature infant, is equivalent to removing 70 mL of blood from an average adult.[3]

## DOES ANEMIA INCREASE ANESTHETIC MORBIDITY AND MORTALITY IN PEDIATRIC PATIENTS?

Infants and children with a HGB level of less than 10 g/dL, have been the subject of controversy as to whether they are acceptable candidates for anesthesia and surgery. Based on the findings that the mean lowest point of HGB level in normal infants is about 11 to 12 g/dL, and the lowest level of the 95% range (two standard deviations below the mean) is 10 g/dL, an arbitrary minimum 10 g/dL for elective surgery has been adopted until recently.[52] One might argue that a minimum value of 10 g/dL will eliminate only the lowest 2.5% of all apparently normal infants. This may seem to be a conservative approach indeed, although it does not take into consideration some important compensatory mechanisms (rightward shifting of the oxyhemoglobin dissociation curve and increased plasma volume).

Even with our modern knowledge of the compensatory mechanisms, some conservative anesthesiologists are reluctant to anesthetize infants and children for elective surgery with HGB levels below 10 g/dL. There seems to be concern that the anemic child, starting with low oxygen stores, (with normal HGB three times as much oxygen is stored in the blood as in the lungs), possibly reduced compensatory mechanisms, and decreased oxygen transport, is at greater risk than the nonanemic child, in the event of critical circulatory or respiratory impairment.[52] The infant is especially susceptible because of his high oxygen requirements, which are almost twice those of the adult.[51]

Earlier studies suggested that preoperative anemia might increase anesthetic morbidity and mortality. Greenberg[59] in 1965 has shown in a series of 20 children who developed cardiac arrest during anesthesia, that 14 had respiratory problems or anemia. Salem and associates[60] (1975) investigated 73 instances in which anesthesia was thought to have been either directly responsible, or had played an important role in the occurrence of cardiac arrest in infants and children. The presence of preoperative anemia, whether unrecognized or underestimated, was considered a contributing factor in the occurrence of cardiac arrest in seven patients; all were successfully resuscitated. All these patients were given halothane, all had HGB levels less than 10 g/dL, in six, controlled ventilation was used, six were between 2 to 4 months old, five were premature infants, and in six, the operation performed was herniorrhaphy. Since cardiac arrest occurred shortly after intubation, while halothane and intermittent positive pressure ventilation were being given, they acknowledged that hypovolemia was probably associated with anemia in these patients.[60]

Several factors might have contributed to the occurrence of greater anesthetic-induced myocardial depression and cardiac arrest in the seven anemic, hypovolemic infants reported by Salem and associates.[60] The institution of controlled ventilation could have enhanced the rate of rise in alveolar halothane concentration, and resulted in rapid deepening of anesthesia by two mechanisms: increased alveolar ventilation and decreased CO.[61] Although higher anesthetic concentrations are required in infants and children than in adults,[62,63] anesthetic requirements of infants younger than 44 weeks gestation are less than that of older children.[64-66] Because a greater portion of the CO in infants and children is directed to their brains and hearts than in adults, the myocardial concentration of an anesthetic might be higher early during induction in infants than in adults.[62,67] This would result in early myocardial depression in the young infant, which is proportional to the depth of anesthesia.[68,69] Based on the observation that inhalational anesthetics depress the force of contraction in isolated neonatal rat atria, far more than in the adult atria, it has been suggested that this may be due to the decreased contractile element in the neonatal myocardium.[70] Systemic blood pressure of infants is decreased more by inhalational anesthetics, than that of adults.[63,71-73] However, protective baroreceptor reflexes, which modulate changes in blood pressure by altering heart rate, may be blunted by anesthetic drugs. In fact, potent anesthetics abolish baroreceptor activity in premature infants.[74,75] Prolonged preoperative fasting, which was designed to reduce the apparent risk of pulmonary aspiration, might have contributed to preoperative dehydration and hypovolemia in the patients reported by Salem and associates.[60] It has been shown that urine specific gravity of more than 1.009 (indicative of dehydration) is associated with hypotension (decrease in blood pressure of more than 30%) in more than 50% of neonates.[76]

It must be emphasized that the studies by Greenberg[59] and Salem et al.[60] were retrospective studies and were published in 1965 and 1975, respectively. Obviously, many pediatric anesthetic advances have taken place since. A more recent prospective survey of anesthesia-related morbidity and mortality in infants and children was carried out in France by Tiret and associates in 1988.[77] The study was conducted on a total of 40,240 anesthetics administered between 1978 and 1982 to patients under 15 years of age. The incidence of major complications related to anesthesia was 0.7 per 1000 anesthetics, while the rate of cardiac arrest was 0.3 per 1000. Although the rate of cardiac arrest was not different from that reported by Salem et al.,[60] preoperative anemia or hypovolemia did not seem to be a major risk factor. Hypovolemia was a factor in only one patient and anemia in another. A recent study of pediatric closed malpractice claims did not show anemia as a factor contributing to damaging events during anesthesia.[78]

In preterm infants, the "physiologic anemia" is usually benign and self-limited, but in some infants it may be associated with apnea[79] and poor weight gain.[14,80] It has been suggested that transfusion with HGB-A blood corrects the anemia, improves oxygen release to the tissues, improves central nervous system oxygenation, and, in some infants, abrogates apneic episodes.[79,81,82] However, these benefits have been refuted by others, or have been attributed to simple correction of hypovolemia, which is often coexistent with anemia.[80,83] Furthermore, blood transfusions are seldom justified to correct anemia for surgery when no blood loss is anticipated.

Recently Welborn and associates[84] examined the association between anemia and postoperative apnea in former preterm infants following general endotracheal inhalational anesthesia supplemented with neuromuscular blockade and controlled ventilation. All infants were less than 60 weeks postconceptual age at the time of operation. They found that anemic infants (HCT < 30%) had an 80% incidence of postoperative apnea, compared to 21% in infants with normal HCT. They also found that infants who developed apnea also had significantly lower HCT, ATP and 2,3-DPG concentrations and had higher levels of HGB-F. Obviously these infants could not increase their ATP and 2,3-DPG in response to anemia. They concluded that anemic preterm infants with HCTs of less than 30% should have elective surgery delayed until such time as their HCT is above 30%. When surgery cannot be deferred, anemic infants must be observed and monitored carefully in the postoperative period.

## MANAGEMENT OF ANEMIA OF PREMATURITY
### Clinical Features

Although infants respond to declines in HGB concentrations approximately by a vigorous erythropoiesis (the sum of RBC production and survival), the response is sometimes insufficient to prevent the occurrence of anemia. Many anemic infants with adequate compensatory mechanisms hardly exhibit any signs or symptoms suggestive of anemia. Some preterm infants become symptomatic with HGB levels of 10.5 g/dL while others remain asymptomatic at significantly lower levels.[85] Early signs of anemia in infants are frequently subtle and may be overlooked until tachycardia and tachypnea are noted at rest. In some preterm infants, signs of anemia could be severe and anemia may worsen the infant's prognosis by interacting with other complications of preterm delivery.[56] As anemia develops, the effects of redistribution of regional flows to favor the heart and the brain become apparent, namely skin pallor and decreased muscular activity (peripheral vasoconstriction). Shunting of blood away from the splanchnic circulation may endanger the integrity of the gastrointestinal tract and the liver.

A clinical suspicion of anemia in an infant is prompted by the presence of pallor, unexplained tachycardia, lethargy, tachycardia, dyspnea exaggerated with feeding, and poor weight gain ($< 25$ g/day). Severe anemia may be associated with apneic attacks in preterm infants (Table 5–5). These clinical signs are manifestations of the high oxygen affinity of fetal HGB. Some of these signs are reversible by correction of the anemia.[31,85]

### Evaluation of Anemia of Prematurity

A consultation with a hematologist knowledgeable of pediatric hematologic disorders may be appropriate in evaluating the etiology of anemia (Table 5-1). The suspicion of anemia should be confirmed by laboratory findings including a HGB or HCT, complete

**Table 5–5. Clinical symptoms and signs of anemia in preterm infants**

| Compensatory (?) | Failure of compensation |
|---|---|
| Tachycardia: raised oxygen consumption | Dyspnea on exertion |
| Tachypnea: even at rest | ? Apneic attacks |
|  | Falls in mixed venous $PO_2$, down to "average critical range" for capillary-tissue oxygen diffusion |
| Blood shunting to heart and brain |  |
| Diminished muscular activity |  |

From Holland BM, Jones JG, Wardrop CAJ. Lessons from the anemia of prematurity. *Hematol/Oncol Clin N Am.* 1987; 1:355, with permission.

blood count including reticulocyte count and a peripheral smear.[8] A HGB measurement will quantitate the decrease in oxygen-carrying capacity, define the degree of anemia and provide a reference value to be followed after therapy is initiated. The reticulocyte count reflects erythroid bone marrow activity. It is elevated in most situations associated with hemolysis and blood loss. The reticulocyte count is decreased when erythroid bone marrow activity is decreased and in most nutritional deficiencies except vitamin E (Table 5–6)[8]. The peripheral blood smear may suggest neutropenia or thrombocytopenia and provide an estimate of bone marrow erythroid activity. It can also reveal morphologic changes in erythrocytes seen in congenial or acquired hemolytic anemias (Table 5–7).[8] Additional tests may be required to aid the diagnosis: bilirubin

**Table 5–6. Reticulocyte count in the laboratory evaluation of the high risk infant with anemia**

| ↓ Decrease reticulocyte count | ↑ Increased reticulocyte count |
|---|---|
| Iron deficiency | Vitamin E deficiency |
| Folic acid deficiency | Blood loss |
| Copper deficiency | Recovery phase of |
| Physiologic anemia | physiologic anemia |
| Congenital or acquired bone marrow (or erythroid) suppression | Congenital or acquired hemolytic anemia |

From Sabio H. Anemia in the high-risk infant. *Clin Perinatol.* 1984; 11:59, with permission.

**Table 5–7.  Laboratory evaluation of anemia in the high-risk infant**

|  | Neutrophils | Platelets | Peroxide hemolysis | Reticulocyte level | Mean red cell volume | Peripheral blood smear |
|---|---|---|---|---|---|---|
| Iron deficiency | N | ↓ or N | N | ↓ | ↓ | Hypochromia; microcytosis |
| Folic acid deficiency | N or ↓ | N or ↓ | N | ↓ | ↑ | Macrocytosis; hypersegmented; neutrophils |
| Copper deficiency | ↓ | N | N | N or ↓ | N | Hypochromia |
| Vitamin E deficiency | N | ↑ | ↑ | ↑ | N or ↑ | Aniso-poikilocytosis; polychromatophilia |
| Physiologic anemia | N | N | N | ↓ | N | — |
| Recovery phase of physiologic anemia | N | N | N | ↑ | N | — |

Modified from Sabio H. Anemia in the high-risk infant. *Clin Perinatol.* 1984; 11:59, with permission.

and direct/indirect Coombs' test (immune hemolytic anemia); mean corpuscular volume (iron deficiency, α-thalassemia syndromes). Quantitative assays for specific enzymes (such as pyruvate kinase and glucose-6-phosphate dehydrogenase) may be indicated particularly in infants with a Coombs'-negative, non-spherocytic hemolytic anemia.[3]

Refractory early anemia of prematurity coincides with the period of maximal brain and neurologic cell differentiation and growth. Prophylaxis, anticipation, diagnosis, and treatment of anemia when appropriate can only benefit long-term neurologic development and intellectual potential especially infants less than 28 weeks gestational age.[56]

## Prophylaxis

The severity of anemia in preterm infants may be limited by 1) optimization of placental transfusion at birth; 2) minimization of blood losses; 3) adequate nutritional intake; 4) clinical and laboratory monitoring for the development of anemia; 5) recombinant human erythropoietin therapy.

In critically ill infants admitted to neonatal units, HGB levels initially determined should be followed closely during the first few weeks of life. Despite the use of micromethods, cumulative blood losses through sampling for laboratory monitoring can have a great impact on HGB levels. Proper charting of iatrogenic blood losses is essential. Iron supplementation should be started at the time doubling of the weight occurs or sooner when anemia is asso-

ciated with iatrogenic blood losses. The infant who does not receive replacement of the iatrogenic blood losses has a decreased available iron pool and could be at increased risk of developing iron deficiency. This may become apparent beyond the period of intensive monitoring.[8] The infant who requires intestinal surgery with resection of the terminal ilium will be at risk of developing vitamin B$_{12}$ deficiency. Parenteral vitamin B$_{12}$ should be administered if deficiency is documented.

## Recombinant Human Erythropoietin Therapy

The successful use of recombinant human erythropoietin to stimulate erythropoiesis in patients with anemia due to renal failure has led neonatologists to investigate its efficacy in reducing the severity of anemias of prematurity.[86-89] Stimulation of the infant's own erythropoiesis could maintain RBC volume and oxygen delivery thus decreasing the need for allogeneic RBC transfusion and minimizing the complications associated with anemia of prematurity.[26,31] Ohls et al.[90] found that the erythroid burst promoting activity of erythropoietin in the serum of patients with anemia of prematurity is similar to that found in adult blood and cord sera. The findings indicate that the anemia of prematurity like the anemia of end-stage renal disease is associated with a specific deficiency of erythropoietin and that erythroid progenitors remain highly sensitive to erythropoietin.[87,89]

Studies demonstrated the safety of recombinant human erythropoietin when given at a subcutaneous dose of 50 U/kg/week to preterm infants.[26] In the doses studied, however erythropoietin therapy failed to demonstrate a hemopoietic response. The lack of a positive response has been attributed to inadequate dosage, suboptimal nutrition including iron deficiency, inflammation, infection, or the requirement for other growth factors. Studies of erythropoietin therapy in preterm infants were carried out utilizing small doses to ascertain its safety whereas much larger doses have been used in adults. Oster and associates[91] administered doses of 300 to 600 U/kg/week to prevent chemotherapy-induced anemia while Goodnough and associates[92] used 1,200 U/kg/week to increase preoperative collection of autologous blood in adult patients.

Preterm infants may require relatively larger doses of erythropoietin to successfully stimulate erythropoiesis than older children and adults. George et al.[93] found that doses of 250 units/kg, given twice weekly produced significant increases in HGB in adults, but no change in newborn animals. Halpérin et al.[94] in a pilot study reported an increase in reticulocytes and stabilization of HCT in preterm infants treated with higher doses (up to 300 units/kg/week) of erythropoietin. Ongoing controlled studies with higher doses of recombinant erythropoietin are expected to demonstrate its efficacy in reducing the severity of anemia of prematurity. It is likely that such efforts will completely reshape the prevention and treatment of the anemia of prematurity.[29]

## Specific Therapy

Specific therapy in the high-risk infant requires identification of the etiologic factors contributing to the development of anemia. When a nutritional deficiency is identified, replacement therapy is indicated within the context of the infant's other medical problems.

Vitamin E deficiency is confirmed when the concentration of serum tocopherol is less than 0.5 mg/dL. The hematologic manifestations can usually be corrected by the oral administration of 50 to 200 units of vitamin E ($\alpha$-tocopherol) daily. Low birth weight infants might require increased doses because of malabsorption.[8]

Iron deficiency anemia is characterized by

a low serum level (< 10 ng/mL) of ferritin, elevated serum transferrin, decreased saturation of transferrin, and decreased RBC volume. Supplemental iron 2 mg/kg/day will prevent the development of iron deficiency anemia in infants weighing less than 2,000 g. However, the infants with established iron deficiency anemia may require up to 6 mg/kg/day. The composition of formulas should be evaluated before initiating iron therapy to ensure an adequate ratio of vitamin E to polyunsaturated fatty acids (< 0.6 mg/g) to prevent oxidative changes in the RBC membrane causing hemolysis.[8,37]

Copper deficiency should be suspected in infants who are requiring parenteral hyperalimentation for long periods and in those with persistent diarrhea or malabsorption syndromes. Therapy consists of 2 to 3 mg daily of 1% copper sulfate solution.[8]

Premature infants have increased folic acid requirements (50 $\mu$g/day) as compared to term infants (10 $\mu$g/day). A decrease in HGB associated with increased mean volume of RBCs suggests folic acid deficiency. Clinically apparent megaloblastic anemia due to folic acid deficiency is unusual, but has occurred in infants who have had diarrheal syndromes associated with malabsorption and in infants who have had infections[8]. Other appropriate therapy for anemia may be indicated. In infants with severe isoimmune hemolytic anemia, early exchange transfusion will remove the antibody and bilirubin, and correct the anemia.[3]

## Blood Transfusion Therapy

A decision to transfuse based on a HGB level alone will be associated with some degree of imprecision. Considerations must be given to the physiologic principles already discussed as well as the clinical status of the infant. Decisions regarding transfusion must be discussed with and explained to the parents or guardians. These considerations are especially important in view of the increasing recognition of the risks encountered with transfusion. Some of the complications of blood transfusion are limited to the nursery setting, including transmission of cytomegalovirus (CMV), human immunodeficiency virus, type 1 (HIV-1) and possibly Epstein-Barr virus.[14,95–97] Yeager and associates found that infants negative for CMV antibody who received CMV-antibody positive donor blood in cumulative amounts greater than 50 mL were at highest risk. Complications included infection (fatal in 20% of affected patients), pneumonia, hepatitis, thrombocytopenia and hemolytic anemia. Awareness of transmission of HIV has resulted in increased concern over allogeneic transfusion. Manifestations of these viral infections can be different in the neonate from similar infections in older children or adults because of the relative immunologic immaturity of the neonate. Other infections such as hepatitis B, non-A, non-B hepatitis, and malaria may be as likely to cause illness in the neonate as at any age.[14]

Non-infectious complications, including sensitization to a variety of blood component antigens, hyperkalemia, hypokalemia (if frozen erythrocytes are used for exchange transfusion) and hypocalcemia, are additional risks.[99] Graft-versus-host disease has been noted in association with intrauterine and postnatal transfusions in infants with erythroblastosis fetalis.[100] Blood donor screening procedures do not include individuals with hemoglobinopathies, and death may follow the use of such blood products in hypoxemic neonates.[14] It has been speculated that transfusions, may potentiate the risk of retrolental fibroplasia because of the replacement of HGB-F with HGB-A and the consequent increase in oxygen delivery.[101] However, it is not clear whether this is related to the transfusion or the high inspired oxygen fraction (FIO$_2$) for long periods of time.[102] Although these risks of transfusion should not be considered contraindications to transfusions when indicated, they do highlight the necessity for making wise decisions based upon sound principles concerning transfusions.

A realistic expression of the physiologic and biochemical efficiency of HGB must be based on both the amount and the properties of circulating HGB. Two expressions have been proposed as a guide to transfuse critically ill anemic infants.[56] Both calculations encompass the steep portion of the oxyhemoglobin dissociation curve which is of paramount physiologic importance.

(A) "Available oxygen," which utilizes the difference in oxygen content between arterial blood based on a measured PaO$_2$ and an assumed PvO$_2$ of 20 mm Hg.[30,56] The expression of available oxygen represents the amount of oxygen available for extraction before the need arises for an increase in CO to cope with extra oxygen demand.[56,103] Available oxygen can be derived from HGB concentration and in vivo P50. It has been suggested that available oxygen should ideally be expressed per kilogram body weight so that the RBC mass would be taken into account. This may be calculated from the following measurements: 1) RBC mass (or HGB) and PaO$_2$ from which arterial blood oxygen content can be derived; 2) P50 adjusted for in vivo pH and PCO$_2$; and 3) body weight in kilograms. If one is unable to measure P50 directly, it may be calculated from the following equation after determination of the functioning 2,3-DPG fraction;[16]

$$P50 = 18.4 + 0.0016 \ [2,3\text{-}DPG] \ functional$$

Investigations demonstrated that the correlation of the clinical signs and symptoms of anemia with HGB concentration was relatively poor compared with a correlation with "available oxygen."[85] Since a linear correlation existed between available oxygen and the age of an infant measured in weeks from the time of conception, this relationship may be expressed by the following formula:

$$Available \ Oxygen = [0.54 + 0.005 \times Age \\ (weeks \ from \ conception)] \times [HGB \ (g/dL)]$$

When the available oxygen is calculated from infants of less than 32 weeks gestational age, an available oxygen of less than 7 mL/dL is often associated clinical signs of anemia some of which respond to transfusion.[14,85]

The calculation of available oxygen may be useful in deciding when to transfuse. However, the "Wardrop" formula would be expected to be applicable only when the HGB-F is predictable based on postconceptual age. Infants who had been exchange transfused or multiply transfused might not have a predictable available oxygen.

In preterm infants, the decrease in HGB reaches a nadir at 6 to 9 weeks of age. Due to the change in P50 that occurs, there is a concomitant increase in the calculated oxygen-releasing capacity but a decline in the oxygen reserve occurs during the same period as reflected in a 38% decrease in the available oxygen (8 mL/dL in babies born at 36 weeks).[56,85] Preterm infants born before 30 weeks' gestational age are still synthesizing predominantly HGB-F at a time when the nadir in HGB level is reached.[56,104] Because of the lack of compensatory changes in oxygen affinity in these infants, the available oxygen at the nadir decreases to about 6.6 mL/dL and may remain decreased for a prolonged time because of persistently high HGB-F levels.[56]

Tiny infants have unexpectedly low RBC mass per kilogram body weight. In predicting RBC mass values optimal for oxygen requirements, it has been suggested that we should take into account the much higher proportion of lean-metabolizing, oxygen-consuming tissue in preterm infants. Perhaps the optimal RBC mass for a 1 kg preterm infant is about 15% higher than in term infants because of the differences in the proportions of adipose tissue.[56] The normal reference values for oxygen transport parameters in preterm infants are those of healthy full-term infants. These values represent minimum desirable levels for optimal oxygen availability in preterm infants. Respiratory distress, fever, infections and other complications demand extra oxygen above basal requirements.

(B) Infant's $P\bar{v}O_2$ (or central venous $PO_2$)

An imbalance between oxygen supply and demand producing clinical signs of anemia would be expected to produce an increase in erythropoietin production. If all the variables involved in oxygen supply and oxygen demand are analyzed, it can be shown that a decline in the infants's $P\bar{v}O_2$ (or central venous $PO_2$) correlates with the stimulus to an increase in erythropoietin production. In a study of 21 preterm infants with birth weights less than 1,500 g, various factors were studied including HGB concentration, RBC oxygen affinity, HGB concentration, plasma erythropoietin, heart rate, stroke volume, $PaO_2$, and $P\bar{v}O_2$.[27] HGB levels ranged from a high 17.7 g/dL to a low of 5.8 g/dL. Of all the variables that were examined, $P\bar{v}O_2$ correlated best with plasma erythropoietin levels (Figure 14). The decline in $P\bar{v}O_2$ thus would seem to be the most sensitive indicator of the presence of anemia as its value represents the integration of all the variables that determine oxygen supply and demand. When $P\bar{v}O_2$ is between 35 and 38 mm Hg (normal being $\geq$ 38 mm Hg),

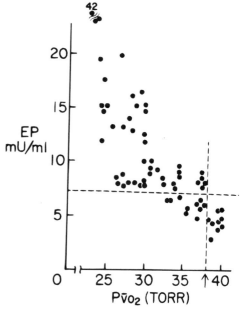

**Fig. 5–14.** Changes in plasma erythropoietin concentrations in response to declines in central venous oxygen tension in preterm neonates. Arrow represents the position of 38 mm Hg which for the purposes of this figure is the lower limit of normal $P\bar{v}O_2$. The horizontal dashed line is the upper limit of normal for erythropoietin, taking $P\bar{v}O_2 \geq 38$ as normal. From Stockman JA III, Graeber JE, Clark DA, et al. Anemia of prematurity: determinants of the erythropoietin response. J Pediatr, 1984;105:786, with permission.

41% of erythropoietin levels are above the normal range; for values between 30 and 35 mm Hg, 79% of erythropoietin levels are increased; at $P\bar{v}O_2$ values less than 30 mm Hg, erythropoietin levels are uniformly above the normal range (Fig. 5–14).

Anemia in preterm infants may be associated with increased or decreased resting oxygen consumption.[105] An increase in oxygen extraction at rest may occur resulting in $P\bar{v}O_2$ values falling to within a critical range of the capillary-tissue oxygen tension gradient, below which oxygen fails to diffuse from blood to tissues.[106] When $P\bar{v}O_2$ is in the 20s, there may be no reserve of oxygen in the blood to meet demands above basal levels.[56] Stockman[11] suggested that the lower oxygen consumption in some premature infants could explain why they are able to tolerate a HGB level 2 to 3 g/dL lower than term infants before the switch to active erythropoiesis occurs.

## Guidelines for Transfusion of Critically Ill Patients

It is apparent that a decision to transfuse based on a HGB level alone will be associated with some degree of imprecision. Most preterm infants have reduced available oxygen during most of the period of the first 3 to 4 months after birth.[56] The HGB levels may be similar over this period to those of more mature infants after the nadir, thus masking the reduction in oxygen availability. The decline in available oxygen (or central venous $PO_2$) is the most sensitive indicator of the presence of anemia and is very useful in deciding when to transfuse. Unfortunately in many nurseries these parameters cannot be determined (central venous $PO_2$ requires central cannulation). Under these circumstances it may be necessary to proceed with transfusion based on the clinical presentation of the infant.

Although precise indications for blood transfusion cannot be given, the following guidelines may be useful.

1. A cumulative record of blood losses should be kept on all critically ill infants admitted to neonatal care units. An infant sufficiently ill to require frequent blood sampling (iatrogenic blood losses) should have such blood losses replaced, especially when 10% of the estimated blood volume has been exceeded. For the infant in respiratory distress or low $PaO_2$, there is a lower threshold for early replacement of blood withdrawn.[8]

2. Infants during the first week of life who weigh less than 1,500 g should have a HGB value greater than 13 g/dL.[3] In the presence of cardiac or pulmonary disease resulting in a lower $PaO_2$, the infant HGB may be maintained in the range of 16 to 17 g/dL.[12]

3. At several weeks of age, when the clinical status of the preterm infant may have been stabilized, transfusion may or may not be needed at the nadir of the anemia. a) Infants without compromised cardiopulmonary function and in whom no unusual metabolic needs exist are unlikely to be aided by transfusions when the HGB level is greater than 10 or 11 g/dL.[14] b) Infants who had been previously transfused are usually able to tolerate lower levels of HGB because of improved tissue oxygen delivery (replacement of HGB-F by HGB-A). c) Premature infants at the nadir of their anemia when HGB levels may be as low as 7 to 8 g/dL should not receive supplemental RBC transfusions unless they manifest clinical signs of tissue hypoxemia.[3] The signs that most commonly result in a need for transfusions are the failure to gain weight appropriately (< 25 g/day) due to easy fatigability during feedings and persistent tachypnea and tachycardia.[8] Some infants with failure to gain weight at several weeks of age may respond to transfusion therapy.[14] Apnea has not unequivocally been shown to improve following transfusion.[14] The simple calculations of available oxygen for central venous $PO_2$ is helpful when it is difficult to ascertain whether clinical signs of anemia exist.

4. Other possible indications for blood transfusion in critically ill infants include improving oxygen delivery in infants with respiratory distress syndrome and stabilizing cardiac dynamics in some forms of acyanotic congenital heart disease.[14] In infants with respiratory distress syndrome, if $PaO_2$ is greater than 50 mm Hg, transfusion of blood containing HGB-A will improve oxygen delivery.[107] Clinical manifestations of large ventricular septal defects are often not apparent until several weeks of age which coincides with the nadir of anemia in infants. It has been postulated that the decrease in HGB reduces the viscosity of blood circulating through the lungs and could contribute to a fall in pulmonary vascular resistance, increased left to right shunting and congestive heart failure.[14,108] Lister et al.[108] found that blood transfusion in anemic infants with large ventricular septal defects results in decreases in pulmonary blood flow and left to right shunting. Thus transfusion may be helpful in stabilizing cardiac dynamics in some forms of acyanotic congenital heart disease.

If blood transfusion is indicated in anemic normovolemic infants, the most common blood component used is packed RBCs which have a HCT value between 70 and 80%. An average of 1 mL/kg packed RBCs will raise the HCT value by 1.5%. Units of packed RBCs are usually supplied in pediatric packs of 50 to 100 mL. The fluid of these stored packed cells is acidic (pH < 7.0), low in ionized calcium and relatively hyperkalemic (15 to 20 mmol/L) while frozen RBCs have a low potassium content. Since transfusion of critically ill infants is carried out slowly and in small quantities, the complications of massive blood transfusion namely hyperkalemia, hypokalemia (if frozen erythrocytes are used), acidemia, volume overload, and pulmonary edema are not usually seen. If large amounts of blood are transfused, electrocardiographic monitoring and measurements of serum potassium and ionized calcium are advisable. Blood must be warmed to near body temperature and air bubbles must be ejected from all the plastic tubing used for infusion. Micropore filters are not routinely used unless massive blood transfusion is given.

The improved tissue oxygenation following transfusion with HGB-A containing erythrocytes leads to a decreased erythropoietic stimulus expressed as a lower reticulocyte count for a given HGB level. Furthermore, because of concomitant plasma volume expansion and resultant hemodilution, the effects of transfusion on HGB level may not be sustained.[56] Although transfused infants will be able to tolerate a lower HGB level better than untransfused anemic infants, HGB measurement must be repeated and followed closely even after these infants are discharged from the neonatal units.

## ANESTHESIA FOR INFANTS AND CHILDREN WITH ANEMIA

From the previous discussion, it is evident that a preoperative HGB value is not an adequate qualitative descriptor of the severity of anemia. The adaptations that accompany changes in HGB concentrations in infants and children have paved the way to better understanding of anemia and consequently a more appropriate management of these patients. It is apparent from Table 4 that if an HGB level of 10 g/dL is acceptable for an adult with a P50 of 27 mm Hg, 8.2 g/dL (HCT = 25%) should theoretically be adequate for an infant older than 3 months of age with a P50 of 30 mm Hg. In contrast, for a 2 month old infant (or younger) with a P50 of 24 mm Hg, a HGB level of 10 g/dL is equivalent to only 6.8 g/dL in adults. This may not be adequate to provide sufficient tissue oxygenation in a 2 month old infant with low CO, decreased PaO$_2$, or increased oxygen consumption.[51]

Recently, the value of routine preoperative HGB determinations in pediatric outpatients has been questioned. In a study from the children's hospital, Vancouver, Canada, several interesting findings have emerged.[109] 1) the prevalence of anemia in their population was remarkably low (0.29%). 2) Anesthesiologists could not reliably predict preoperative anemia in patients presenting for outpatient surgery. 3) In the presence of mild anemia, anesthesia for outpatient pediatric patients can be safely conducted. 4) In view of the costs and patients' discomfort, it was concluded that routine preoperative HGB measurements may not be required in essentially healthy pediatric patients. In centers where patient population has a lower socioeconomic background, the prevalence of anemia might be much higher than that reported among the Canadian population.

The following are general guidelines to the anesthetic management of anemic pediatric patients. 1) In infants older than 3 months of age, HGB levels of 8 g/dL or higher may be acceptable. 2) Infants younger than 2 months of age (or in preterm infants, 50 to 52 weeks postconceptual age), HGB of 9.5 to 10 g/dL is probably the absolute minimum. 3) In infants in their first week of life, infants weighing less than 1,500 g, and infants with cardiac or pulmonary disease, a preoperative HGB of 12 or higher is advisable. 4) If the HGB levels are lower than the above recommended figures and the operation is purely elective, the operation may be postponed for one month or longer (if the risk of postponing surgery is small) especially if the anemia is associated with apneic episodes. The anemia is evaluated and supplemental iron therapy may be given during this time. 5) If surgery cannot be postponed, anesthesia may then be given with extreme care. 6) The decision to transfuse intraoperatively should take into consideration the many factors that comprise clinical judgement. These factors include: blood volume estimates, preoperative HCT, previous blood transfusion (replacement of HGB-F in preterm infants), duration of anemia, general condition of the patient, ability to provide adequate tissue oxygenation (cardiopulmonary function and CO), extent of surgical procedure, probability of massive blood loss and risks versus benefits of transfusion.[51,110]

It is beyond the scope of this chapter to discuss techniques for anesthetizing anemic infants and children. However, the following points need to be emphasized:

1) Avoid excessive preoperative sedation.

2) Shorten the period of preoperative fasting and allow clear fluids up to 2 to 3 hours before the anticipated time of anesthetic induction. For years, strict fasting guidelines were designed to minimize the risk of pulmonary aspiration of gastric contents. Recent studies have questioned the wisdom of these strict fasting guidelines and compared standard fasting (since midnight) with clear liquids 2 to 3 hours before the scheduled induction time.[111-115] Most of these studies showed no difference in gastric residual volume or pH between those patients who fasted for 8 hours or longer versus those who fasted 2 to 3 hours. Allowing clear liquids until 2 to 3 hours before induction would certainly avoid anesthetic induction in a hypovolemic child.

3) Start an intravenous line either prior to or shortly after anesthetic induction.

4) Adequate hydration in essential and therefore fluid deficits must be avoided.

5) Although in experimental animals, it has been demonstrated that anesthetics that depress the myocardium need not be detrimental in all circumstances including chronic anemia,[116,117] these drugs must be used with care since they may cause early and severe myocardial depression in infants and young children. Light anesthesia may be maintained with inhalational anesthetics and/or shorter-acting opioids and relaxants.

6) Airway maintenance is essential and endotracheal intubation is recommended.

7) Unless there is a danger of retinopathy of maturity, an $FIO_2$ greater than 0.4 is desirable.

8) Maintain a near-normal $PaCO_2$ (or end-tidal carbon dioxide) and avoid leftward shift of P50. Hyperventilation, alkalosis and hypothermia should be avoided. The effect of nitrous oxide on P50 is controversial. Contrast media (ionic and non-ionic) cause leftward shift of the oxyhemoglobin dissociation curve and can adversely decrease oxygen unloading

**Table 5–8.   Estimated $PO_2$ at different P50 of hemoglobin***

| | Age | | | | |
|---|---|---|---|---|---|
| | 1 d | 2 wk | 6–9 wk | 6 mo–6 y | Adult |
| P50 (mm Hg)† | 19 | 22 | 24 | 29 | 27 |
| $SO_2$ (%) | Estimated $PO_2$ (mm Hg) at neutral pH (7.40) | | | | |
| 99 | 108 | 130 | 143 | 171 | 156 |
| 98 | 77 | 92 | 101 | 122 | 111 |
| 97 | 64 | 77 | 84 | 101 | 92 |
| 96 | 56 | 68 | 74 | 89 | 82 |
| 95 | 52 | 62 | 68 | 82 | 74 |
| 94 | 48 | 58 | 63 | 76 | 69 |
| 93 | 45 | 55 | 60 | 72 | 66 |
| 92 | 43 | 52 | 57 | 68 | 62 |
| 91 | 41 | 50 | 55 | 66 | 60 |
| 90 | 40 | 48 | 53 | 63 | 58 |
| 88 | 37 | 45 | 49 | 59 | 54 |
| 86 | 35 | 42 | 47 | 56 | 51 |
| 84 | 34 | 40 | 44 | 53 | 49 |
| 82 | 32 | 39 | 42 | 51 | 47 |
| 80 | 31 | 37 | 41 | 49 | 45 |
| 78 | 30 | 36 | 39 | 47 | 43 |
| 76 | 29 | 34 | 38 | 45 | 41 |
| 74 | 28 | 33 | 36 | 44 | 40 |
| 72 | 27 | 32 | 35 | 42 | 39 |
| 70 | 26 | 31 | 34 | 41 | 37 |

* Calculated from Severinghaus's nomogram (1966) assuming that the shift in oxygen dissociation curve of HGB due to changes in its oxygen affinity at neutral pH (7.40) is the same as the shift due to the Bohr effect. † $PO_2$ at which oxygen saturation of hemoglobin ($SO_2$) is 50%. From Motoyama EK. Respiratory physiology in infants and children. In: Motoyama EK, Davis PJ, eds. *Smith's Anesthesia for Infants and Children*, 5th ed. St. Louis, MO: CV Mosby Co; 1990, with permission.

to the tissues.[118] Therefore extreme care is necessary when contrast media are used in anemic infants and children.

9) Close intraoperative and postoperative cardiovascular, respiratory and temperature monitoring are essential. Pulse oximetry is a reliable, accurate, and useful monitor in pediatric patients. Several studies have shown that the margin of error when significant concentrations of HGB-F are present is minimal.[119,120] Estimated $PaO_2$ should be adjusted according to age as shown in Table 8. In the newborn whose P50 is 18 to 20 mm Hg, the range of oxygen saturation to maintain adequate $PaO_2$ (60 to 80 mm Hg) is 97 to 98%, whereas in the adult it is 91 to 96%. In the neonate, a saturation of 91% corresponds to a $PaO_2$ of 41 mm Hg.[121] Motoyama[51] recommends for young infants, maintaining a saturation of 95 to 97% ($PaO_2$ of 50 to 70 mm Hg in newborns and 60 to 80 mm Hg in infants 1 to 2 months old).

10) Extubation is carried out only when these patients are awake and have gained adequate laryngeal reflexes.

11) If surgery cannot be postponed, preterm anemic infants should be monitored closely for apnea during the first 24 hours after surgery.

## II. PERIOPERATIVE HEMOGLOBIN REQUIREMENTS IN ADULTS

### HISTORICAL PERSPECTIVE

Prior to the turn of the century, a HGB level below 30% of normal was considered unsafe because it left no margin for anesthetic errors.[122] It was also erroneously believed that anesthetic drugs destroyed RBCs and this was thought to be most marked in the presence of anemia.[123] Rapid surgery was therefore advocated for anemic patients in order to avoid the "deleterious effects" of prolonged anesthesia on RBCs.[124] Fish in 1899[125] propagated the idea of not subjecting patients to an anesthetic if the HGB level was under 50% of normal.

The theory of RBC destruction by anesthetics was refuted by Da Costa and Kalteyer,[124] but they nevertheless recommended routine preoperative HGB determination. Although figures were not given, they advised employing local anesthesia whenever possible

if there was a low HGB. Potent inhalational anesthetics (chloroform, ether, ethyl chloride) were thought to be contraindicated as the primary anesthetic drugs in anemic patients.[126] Prior to World War II, "anesthetists" held that a minimum HGB level was one that was above the threshold for cyanosis.[122] Predicated on the appearance of cyanosis in the presence of 5 g/dL of reduced HGB, a level of 8 g/dL or higher was considered safe.

In 1941, Adams and Lundy[127] wrote about anemia discovered preoperatively:

"When the concentration of hemoglobin is less than 8 to 10 grams per 100 cubic centimeters of whole blood, it is wise to give a blood transfusion before operation."

This recommendation (later abbreviated to 10 g/dL) was quoted in virtually every anesthesia and surgery textbook, and it became widely practiced until the 1980s.[122] This dictum has been perpetuated by anesthesiologists, surgeons, internists and even hematologists for over half a century.

More than three decades ago, the practice of a minimum HGB requirement for elective surgery was surveyed by mail questionnaires sent to the anesthesia departments of 1,903 United States hospitals, of whom 66% responded.[128] The vast majority (88%) required a HGB of at least 9 g/dL, 44% had a minimum of 10 g/dL and 7.4% had no minimum requirement. This mail survey confirmed the wide acceptance of a HGB value of 10 g/dL as a minimum requirement for elective surgery without any firm clinical or laboratory support.

Experience during the Korean War demonstrated that as long as blood volume was maintained, HGB levels as low as 7 g/dL were tolerated.[129] Shields and Rambach[130] logically suggested balancing the inherent risks of blood transfusion versus the risks of delaying surgery. This was apparently the first plea for evaluation of the patient on an individual basis.[122] With the introduction of cardiopulmonary bypass, it became evident that with crystalloid priming, adequate perfusion can be maintained with lower than normal HCT.[131-134] Surgery on patients of the Jehovah's Witness faith stimulated studies on normovolemic hemodilution. Those studies revealed that normovolemic hemodilution to a hematocrit of 20% is well tolerated.

In 1964, Nunn and Freeman[135] applied the physiological concepts of oxygen delivery and availability to clinical practice. Available oxygen was calculated by multiplying CO by $CaO_2$. $CaO_2$ was equal to the product of HGB concentration and arterial oxygen saturation ($SaO_2$), and the amount of oxygen combined with HGB (the value used was 1.34 mL/g). With HGB = 15 g/dL and $SaO_2$ = 95%:

$$CaO_2 = 15\,g/dL \times 0.95 \times 1.34\,mL/g = 20\,mL/dL \text{ or } 200\,mL/L$$

When multiplied by CO (approximately 5 L/min):

$$Calculated\ available\ oxygen = 200\,mL/L \times 5\,L/min = 1{,}000\,mL/min$$

Approximately one-fourth of the delivered oxygen (250 mL/min) is utilized in normal resting humans (oxygen consumption; $\dot{V}O_2$), corresponding to a systemic arteriovenous oxygen saturation difference of 25% and a mixed venous oxygen saturation ($S\bar{v}O_2$) of 75%. The body tissues show considerable differences in oxygen extraction. For example, the left ventricle normally extracts 70% of available oxygen, whereas the kidney extracts approximately 7%. Since some organs have values for oxygen extraction that are higher than the average, it is imperative that the available oxygen be maintained at a higher level than $\dot{V}O_2$. Nunn and Freeman[135] postulated that 400 mL/min should be the minimum tolerable level of available oxygen during anesthesia. One-third decrease in each of CO, HGB, and $SaO_2$ will result in a substantial decrease in available oxygen, to approximately 300 mL/min, which may not be compatible with survival.

The concept of oxygen availability has made clinicians become aware of the importance of other determinants of oxygen supply (namely, CO and $SaO_2$) when the HGB level is low. However, this approach was an oversimplification since it neither took into account the dissolved oxygen in plasma nor the compensatory mechanisms which come into play in chronic anemia or normovolemic hemodilution; some of which were not truly appreciated at the time the concept of oxygen availability was introduced. The amount of oxygen dissolved in plasma ($0.003 \times$ oxygen tension {$PO_2$}) is ordinarily small during air breathing (0.3 mL/dL), but increases substantially when a high inspired oxygen fraction ($FIO_2$) is given. (See Chapter 3: Principles of Oxygen Transport and Chapter 7: Acute Normovolemic Hemodilution)

The term "available oxygen" was later refined. Of the 1000 mL/min of oxygen normally delivered, 200 mL/min cannot be extracted because of inadequate driving pressure for diffusion of oxygen at low capillary $PO_2$.[136] Thus, the true "available oxygen" should be considered to be 200 mL less than the "oxygen supply."

Under steady state conditions, the utilization of oxygen by the tissues is the product of CO and the difference between $CaO_2$ and mixed venous oxygen content ($C\bar{v}O_2$). It has been shown that changes in $S\bar{v}O_2$ will reflect the relationship between oxygen delivery and oxygen utilization.[137] For example, assuming a constant $\dot{V}O_2$, a decrease in $S\bar{v}O_2$ will be evident when CO is reduced or when a decrease in $CaO_2$ occurs without a sufficient increase in CO. If $\dot{V}O_2$ is constant, monitoring $S\bar{v}O_2$ will quickly reflect changes in oxygen delivery. In the last decade, continuous monitoring of $S\bar{v}O_2$ by oximeters adapted to thermodilution pulmonary artery catheters has been utilized with increasing frequency in critically ill patients.

The oxygen extraction ratio (ER), which is essentially a reflection of $S\bar{v}O_2$, has recently been introduced as an index of myocardial oxygenation in anemia.[138]

$$ER = \frac{CaO_2 - C\bar{v}O_2}{CaO_2}$$

This ratio is normally 25%. In experimental animals, an ER greater than 50% (corresponding to a HCT of 10%) is associated with the onset of myocardial lactate production. Monitoring ER has added a new dimension in assessing the adequacy of oxygen transport and the need for transfusion in critically ill patients.[137,139]

## EFFECTS OF ACUTE ANEMIA

Although both can interfere with oxygen delivery to the tissues, the effects of normovolemic anemia must be separated from those of hypovolemia. A classification of hypovolemia based on blood loss has been established by the American College of Surgeons in 1989.[140] Class I hemorrhage (loss of up to 15% of the total blood volume) usually has little effect other than venous constriction and mild tachycardia. Class II hemorrhage (loss of 15 to 30% of blood volume) usually results in tachycardia and decreased pulse pressure; unanesthetized patients may also exhibit anxiety or restlessness. Class III hemorrhage (loss of 30 to 40%) produces signs of hypovolemia including marked tachycardia, tachypnea and hypotension; unanesthetized patients usually demonstrate altered mental status. In young healthy patients these losses can usually be treated adequately with crystalloid therapy. Class IV hemorrhage, a loss of more than 40% of the blood volume is considered life-threatening and is accompanied by marked tachycardia, very narrow pulse pressure, hypotension, low urine output, and markedly depressed mental status.

In general, the main hemodynamic responses to severe acute normovolemic anemia (HGB < 7 g/dL) are increased CO, left ventricular dP/dtmax, heart rate, coronary blood flow, myocardial $\dot{V}O_2$, along with a significantly reduced systemic vascular resistance (SVR).[117,141-156] CO and coronary blood flow essentially increase in proportion to the decrease in HGB concentration. However, coronary blood flow increases faster than CO during progressive hemodilution; thus a greater portion of the CO is supplied to the myocardium. Blood pressure is usually maintained unless HGB is reduced to extreme levels. Provided that HGB levels are not decreased too rapidly, HGB concentrations above 7 g/dL often result in a few serious hemodynamic alterations.[157,158] In healthy individuals tissue oxygenation is maintained at HGB concentrations as low as 7 g/dL. The myocardium does not begin producing lactic acid until an HCT of 15% is reached,[159] whereas heart failure usually does not occur until the HCT reaches 10%.[139,143]

As HGB levels decrease during acute anemia the arteriovenous oxygen content difference increases. When HGB levels are reduced to levels sufficient to exhaust the oxygen extraction reserve of the tissues, an increased CO becomes the only means of maintaining tissue oxygen uptake. Acute anemia is usually tolerated because of concomitant increases in CO. However, this compensatory mechanism may be limited because of left ventricular dysfunction, pharmacologic intervention, or inadequate intravascular volume. Anesthetic drugs can modulate the hemodynamic responses to acute anemia. By causing myocardial depression, anesthetics may result in decreased oxygen delivery.[160] In contrast, by reducing total body-oxygen consumption, and cerebral and myocardial oxygen demands, lower HGB values can be tolerated during anesthesia and neuromuscular blockade. Thus anesthetized, patients may tolerate lower HGB concentrations during acute anemia than when awake.[161] The magnitude of these effects varies among anesthetics, and as a function of anesthetic concentration.

## EFFECTS OF CHRONIC ANEMIA

The hemodynamic responses to severe chronic anemia differ from those of severe acute anemia in that heart rate is not increased in chronic anemia.[117, 162] However, the CO is usually increased in patients with chronic anemia (HGB < 7 g/dL or less), secondary to larger stroke volume. At extremely low HGB levels (< 3 g/dL), the CO usually does not rise further, but almost always remains above normal. In patients with sickle cell anemia, an elevated resting CO may be found when the HGB level is as high as 9 or 10 g/dL (Fig. 5–15).[143] When HGB levels are chronically reduced to levels sufficient to exhaust the oxygen extraction reserve of the tissues, maintenance of tissue oxygen uptake becomes dependent on an increased CO. At HGB levels below 2 or 3 g/dL, the inability for further increases in CO or oxygen extraction leads to significant tissue hypoxia.[143]

The underlying mechanisms of increased CO and stroke volume during chronic anemia have intrigued investigators. It appears that an increase in ventricular filling pressure, total blood volume, or an intact $\beta$-adrenergic receptor system is not essential for the increase in CO during chronic anemia. A decrease in afterload secondary to decreased SVR and/or decreased blood viscosity probably plays a major role in augmenting the stroke volume in chronic anemia.[143]

The increased oxygen extraction is associ-

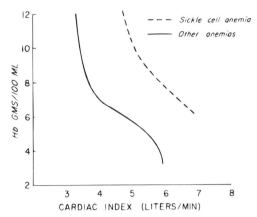

**Fig. 5–15.** Graph illustrating the relation between hemoglobin level and resting cardiac output in several types of anemia. In iron-deficiency anemia and pernicious anemia (solid line), the resting cardiac index is increased with hemoglobin levels below 7 g. In sickle cell anemia (broken line) the cardiac index is elevated at higher hemoglobin levels. From Varat MA, Adolf RJ, Fowler NO. Cardiovascular effects of anemia. Am Heart J. 1972;83:415–426, with permission.

ated with a rightward shift of the oxyhemoglobin dissociation curve, i.e., an increase in P50 from the normal value of 27 mm Hg, because of an increase in intraerythrocytic concentration of 2,3-DPG. As a result of this rightward shift, a 50% decrease in HGB produces only a 27% decrease in oxygen availability.[163] The shift in the oxyhemoglobin dissociation curve is a time-dependent phenomenon and therefore is a feature of chronic but not of acute anemia.[164] Consequently, low HGB levels are better tolerated in chronic anemia than in acute anemia.

The rightward shift in the oxyhemoglobin dissociation curve occurs in all severe chronic anemias, but is more pronounced in patients with sickle cell anemia.[143,165,166] In these patients, P50 can be as high as 42 mm Hg (Fig. 5–16).[167] Although the rightward shift of the curve offers the advantage of facilitating oxygen unloading at the tissues in patients with sickle cell anemia, it also has the disadvantage of requiring a higher level of $PaO_2$ to achieve a given $SaO_2$ at the lungs. Thus a normal $PaO_2$ will produce a lower than normal $SaO_2$. This phenomenon predisposes RBCs to sickling especially in the presence of lower than normal $PaO_2$.[168,169]

Obviously, there is a limit to the body's ability to compensate for chronic anemia.[164]

As the anemia worsens, symptoms become more prominent. With mild anemia (HGB = 9 to 11 g/dL), the only symptoms may be a mild tachycardia or pallor. With a further fall to 7 g/dL, dyspnea on exertion becomes apparent. At a HGB of 6 g/dL, most patients complain of weakness. If HGB falls to 3 g/dL, patients will complain of dyspnea at rest. At a HGB of 2 to 2.5 g/dL, congestive heart failure frequently occurs. In an analysis of anemia in airline flight crews, the critical level of HGB in non-smokers was found to be 7.5 g/dL at rest while 9.5 g/dL was necessary during strenuous exercise. In cigarette smokers, the critical HGB levels were found to be 1.1 g/dL higher. This is due to the significant fraction of HGB bound to carbon monoxide and thus unavailable for oxygen transport.[164,170]

## Chronic Anemia During Pregnancy

Pregnant women usually tolerate chronic anemia without significant adverse maternal or fetal effects. A review of 17 studies of obstetrical patients revealed no effect of HGB concentration on the incidence of stillbirth or intrauterine growth retardation.[171] Murphy et al[172] studied the relation of HGB levels in first and second trimesters to outcome of pregnancy and found increased complications associated with both low (< 10.4 g/dL) and high (> 13.2 g/dL) HGB concentrations. Animal studies of normovolemic anemia suggest normal fetal oxygen extraction until maternal hemoglobin level is reduced by more than 50%.[173] In a study of pregnant sheep with chronic anemia (HCT < 14%), decreased uteroplacental oxygen delivery did not decrease fetal oxygen consumption.[174]

## Chronic Anemia in Renal Failure

Chronic anemia is an almost invariable consequence of progressive renal failure.[175] Although diminished erythropoietin production is the primary cause of anemia, several other factors may also contribute to the development of anemia including: 1) shortening of RBC survival, 2) blood loss associated with platelet dysfunction, 3) depression of erythropoiesis by uremic inhibitors retained in chronic renal failure, and 4) other factors such as residual blood loss in the dialyzer, erythroid suppression from aluminium toxicity, osteitis

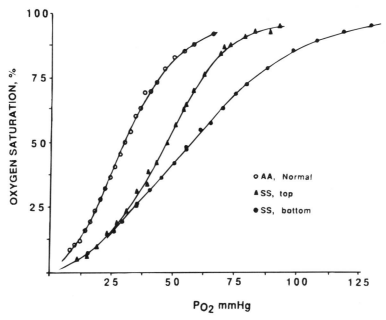

**Fig. 5–16.** Oxyhemoglobin dissociation curves from top and bottom layers of hemoglobin-S red blood cells. Note the heterogeneous nature of the P50 values. From Seakins M, Gibbs WN, Milner PF, Bertles JF. Erythrocyte Hb-S concentration. An important factor in the low oxygen affinity of blood in sickle cell anemia. J Clin Invest. 1973;52: 422–432, with permission.

fibrosa from severe hyperparathyroidism, and, acute or chronic hemolysis. The problem of inadequate erythropoietin production has been resolved by the availability of recombinant DNA technology. At doses of 50 units/kg of recombinant erythropoietin or greater, effective responses were observed. At the highest doses employed (500 units/kg) administered intravenously three times a week after dialysis, increases in HCT by as much as 10% were observed within two to three weeks of therapy in almost all patients.[175] Despite the success of recombinant erythropoietin therapy in increasing HGB concentrations, patients with chronic renal failure may present with HGB levels below 7 g/dL; nonetheless, they are at no greater risk when anesthetized with care.[176-179]

## Anesthetics and Experimentally Induced Anemia

The hemodynamic responses to halothane anesthesia in chronically anemic dogs (mean HGB = 3.4 g/dL) have been studied by Barrera and associates.[117] Control (non-anemic) and anemic animals were exposed to 0.75, 1.5, and 2.25 vol% inspired halothane concen-

trations. Anemic dogs showed progressively decreasing SVR as halothane concentration was increased, whereas nonanemic dogs showed no change in SVR during halothane anesthesia. Cardiac output, coronary blood flow, and myocardial $\dot{V}O_2$, were significantly greater in anemic canines compared with controls at each halothane concentration. The higher coronary blood flow during anemia appears to be an autoregulatory response to a greater myocardial oxygen demand. The lack of myocardial lactate production, and the lack of subendocardial hypoperfusion suggested that myocardial ischemia did not occur. Although these findings should be extrapolated to humans with caution, they suggest that chronic anemia does not necessarily impart a serious hemodynamic handicap in the otherwise healthy patient during anesthesia.[117]

## DOES PERIOPERATIVE ANEMIA INCREASE MORBIDITY AND MORTALITY?

A few retrospective studies suggested that severe perioperative anemia in adult patients increases morbidity and mortality during anesthesia or in the early postoperative period.

In two studies, the low HGB level probably represented the underlying disease.[180,181] In one study of 8 patients who had a mean HGB of 3 g/dL and refused blood transfusion because of religious beliefs, the mortality rate was 87%.[182] Carson and associates[183] found that operative mortality was inversely related to the preoperative HGB level in 125 patients with a mean HGB level of 7.6 g/dL. Although they concluded that the HGB level is an important predictor of postoperative death, they questioned the transfusion threshold of 10 g/dL, since no patient with a HGB level between 8 and 10 g/dL died unless blood loss exceeded 500 mL.[122,183]

A prospective study of 340 patients with HGB levels below 10 g/dL (mean HGB of 8.6 g/dL) who received 473 anesthetics revealed that anemia did not appear to increase morbidity or mortality.[184] To clarify the widespread practice of preoperative transfusion to attain a 10 g/dL of HGB, Spence and coworkers[185] analyzed the relationship among preoperative HGB level, operative blood loss, and mortality in 113 operations in 107 consecutive Jehovah's Witness patients who underwent major elective surgery. Ninety-three patients had HGB values greater than 10 g/dL; 20 had HGB levels between 6 and 10 g/dL. Mortality for preoperative HGB levels greater than 10 g/dL was 3.2% while that for HGB levels between 6 and 10 g/dL was 5%. Mortality was significantly increased with an estimated perioperative blood loss greater than 500 mL, regardless of the HGB level. More importantly, there was no mortality if estimated blood loss was less than 500 mL. They concluded that mortality in elective surgery appears to depend more on estimated blood loss than on preoperative HGB levels and that elective surgery can be done safely in patients with a preoperative HGB level as low as 6 g/dL if estimated blood loss is kept below 500 mL.

Case series reports of Jehovah's Witnesses suggested that some patients tolerate very low HGB concentrations without an increase in mortality in the perioperative period.[185] Kitchens[186] reviewed 16 series published between 1983 and 1990 involving 1,404 operations on Jehovah's Witnesses and found that lack of blood was a primary cause of death in 8 (0.6%) patients and contributed to death in another 12 (0.9%) patients. Viele and Weiskopf[161] identified 23 deaths due to anemia in 4,722 Jehovah's Witnesses. All the deaths except 2 occurred at HGB level < 5 g/dL. In one series of Jehovah's Witnesses,[187] a statistical analysis revealed that HGB alone was not a statistically significant predictor of outcome unless it was <3 g/dL.

The therapeutic goal for HCT value in critically ill postoperative patients was evaluated by Czer and Shoemaker.[188] Mortality was used to define the lower limit for HCT, and improvement in oxygen delivery was used to define the upper limit for postoperative HCT. Both survivors and non-survivors were comparable in terms of age, sex, pretransfusion HCT value and number of transfusions administered. The maximum survival rate was found to occur in the group with pretransfusion HCT values in the 27% to 33% range. In addition, oxygen delivery significantly increased after transfusions when the pretransfusion HCT value was lower than 32%, but not when it was above 33%. The results of the study suggest that when volume therapy is indicated, crystalloids or colloids are adequate when the HCT is greater than 32%, but that blood may be needed in patients with lower HCT values. Other studies of postoperative critically ill or septic patients with HGB levels < 10 g/dL revealed that blood transfusions had little impact on oxygen consumption.[188]

It has been suggested that perioperative anemia may contribute to myocardial ischemia or infarction.[192] A controlled study of 27 high-risk patients undergoing hip arthroplasty showed that the incidence of postoperative myocardial ischemia and other cardiac complications was significantly higher among 14 patients with HCT < 28% as compared to patients with higher HCT.[192] However, the study was not adjusted for confounding variables that increase ischemic risk since the anemic group was significantly older and underwent longer procedures. Furthermore, the study did not examine the impact of RBC transfusion.

## CURRENT STATUS OF PERIOPERATIVE HEMOGLOBIN REQUIREMENTS

It must be emphasized that the importance of HGB has never been questioned. HGB is the primary determinant of the amount of oxygen carried in the blood and without it, the amount of oxygen dissolved in the plasma in a normothermic individual would be so small that the CO would need to be enormously increased (20 fold) to provide adequate oxygen delivery.[1] The fundamental question is what level of HGB is necessary to maintain adequate oxygen delivery to the tissues in the perioperative period.

It is evident that all aspects of oxygen delivery and utilization must be taken into consideration in determining whether perioperative HGB levels are adequate or not.[122] Though the various factors determining oxygen delivery have been known for many years, the emphasis has been on HGB. Obviously, HGB is easy to measure while other determinants of oxygen delivery were, until recently, relatively difficult to obtain and certainly require invasive monitoring.[122] Perioperative HGB determinations also can be misleading. Concomitant administration of colloids and crystalloids can produce artificially low or high HGB values.[193] In critically ill patients who have pulmonary artery (or at least central venous) catheters, it is now possible to determine the adequacy of oxygen delivery and the need for transfusion.[137,139,194,195] These parameters are rather global measures of oxygen utilization and do not reflect specific organ measures of oxygen utilization. Furthermore, decisions regarding the adequacy of oxygen delivery and the need for RBC transfusion are frequently complicated by the abrupt increase in the patient's oxygen requirements due to pain, shivering, fever, sepsis or increased physical activity in the postoperative period.

The 1988 National Institute of Health Consensus Conference[196] on Perioperative Red Cell Transfusion concluded that evidence did not support the use of a single criterion for transfusion, such as a HGB concentration less than 10 g/dL, nor was there evidence that mild to moderate anemia contributed to perioperative mortality. The decision to transfuse a specific patient should take into account the duration of the anemia, the intravascular volume, the extent of the operation, the probability of massive blood loss, and the presence of coexisting factors, such as impaired pulmonary function, increased $\dot{V}O_2$, inadequate CO, myocardial ischemia, or cerebrovascular or peripheral circulatory disease.[196]

No single measure can replace good clinical judgement as the basis for decisions regarding perioperative transfusion. However, current experience would suggest that otherwise healthy patients with HGB values of 10 g/dL or greater rarely require perioperative transfusion, whereas those with acute anemia with resulting HGB values of less than 7 g/dL will frequently require RBC transfusions.[196] It appears that some patients with chronic anemia such as those with chronic renal failure tolerate HGB values of less than 7 g/dL. The decision to transfuse will depend upon clinical assessment aided by laboratory data such as $PaO_2$, $P\bar{v}O_2$, CO, ER, and blood volume, when indicated. It is essential to recognize that the combination of hypovolemia and anemia may lead to severe morbidity and/or mortality and that there is a minimum HGB value for each individual below which severe morbidity and/or mortality due to inadequate oxygen delivery is likely to occur.

In 1992, the American College of Physicians[197] recommended distinguishing between stable and unstable vital signs in determining whether to transfuse anesthetized patients. The College concluded that patients with stable vital signs and no risk of myocardial or cerebral ischemia do not require RBC transfusion, independent of HGB level and recommended transfusing patients with unstable vital signs only if risks of myocardial or cerebral ischemia were present.

In 1994, the American Society of Anesthesiologists Task Force on Blood Component Therapy[198] issued a draft document on perioperative blood component therapy. The Task Force believes that the recommendation of the American College of Physicians to rely solely on vital signs is inappropriate in anesthetized patients. The decision to transfuse is often affected by the dynamic nature of surgical hemorrhage. Changes in vital signs are often masked by anesthetics and other drugs and are frequently a late sign of cardiovascular decompensation.[198] Moreover, silent ischemia of the myocardium and other organs can occur in the presence of stable vital signs. Intraoperative myocardial ischemia, a predictor of cardiac morbidity and mortality is associated with tachycardia in only 26% of patients and with blood pressure changes in less than 10% of patients. The Task Force[198] concluded that (1) transfusion is rarely indicated when the HGB concentration is greater than 10 g/

dL and is almost always indicated when it is less than 6 g/dL; (2) the determination of whether intermediate HGB concentrations (6-10 g/dL) justify or require RBC transfusion should be based on the patient's risk of developing complications of inadequate oxygenation; (3) the use of a single HGB "trigger" for all patients, and other approaches that fail to consider all important physiological and surgical factors affecting oxygenation, are not recommended; (4) where appropriate, preoperative autologous blood donation, acute normovolemic hemodilution, intraoperative and postoperative blood recovery, and measures to decrease blood loss (deliberate hypotension and pharmacologic agents) should be employed; and (5) the indications for transfusion of autologous RBCs may be more liberal than for allogeneic RBCs because of lower risks associated with the former.

## SICKLE CELL DISEASE

Because of sickle cell disease's unique characteristics and perioperative concerns, a more detailed discussion is warranted. Sickle cell disease is manifested by the presence of large quantities of mutant hemoglobins in the blood. The disease is now known to be hereditary and the result of a genetically-determined hemoglobinopathy. The sickle cell gene has worldwide distribution but is most concentrated in West Central Africa. However, the gene is not confined by race or skin color. It is found in Saudi Arabia, India, southern Italy, northern Greece, southern Turkey, and has been reported in Caucasian and other populations.[199] The distribution of sickle cell disease parallels that of malaria. Inheritance of the disease essentially follows the Mendelian principles of autosomal recessive genes. If only one gene determining globin structure is involved the individual is heterozygous (sickle cell trait), having both normal and abnormal globin chains present. The concentration of HGB-S in individuals with sickle cell trait varies between 20 and 40%. If both genes are involved the individual is homozygous (sickle cell anemia) with a predominance of HGB-S. The concentrations of HGB-S in RBCs of these patients is between 80 and 100%. The incidence of sickle cell anemia (SS) in African-Americans in the United States is 1 in 625

births (0.16%), while that of sickle cell trait (AS) is 8 to 9%.[200]

## Pathophysiology

The mutant hemoglobin (HGB-S) results from an altered amino acid sequence in the HGB molecule, whereby valine replaces glutamic acid at position 6 in the $\beta$-globin chain. This mutant chain, although not directly altering oxygen-carrying capacity, causes a conformational change in the HGB molecule which is complementary to the oxygen binding site on the HGB tetramer. Normal RBCs do not sickle because the net energy of interaction, the sum of attractive and repulsive forces between the molecules is negative. In sickle cell disease, the presence of valine at position 6 in the $\beta$-globin chain alters this balance, and a net attractive force develops. As the chains swing outward during deoxygenation, two self-complementary sites fall into alignment. Deoxygenated HGB-S molecules can bind each other, forming long double strands and undergo polymerization (lining up of HGB into strands along the long axis of the RBCs). The molecules stack like building blocks on one another. Within the RBCs, the resulting "rodlets" become packed so tightly that they cannot rotate freely. The higher the concentration of the abnormal HGB, the more the rodlets stack. Dehydration increases the concentration of HGB and enhances the tendency for rodlet formation. As oxygen tension falls, the increase in number of strands results in the formation of complex, multi-stranded fibers sometimes referred to as "tactoids." It is the presence of these tactoids which causes the characteristic sickled shaped-RBCs.

The distortion of sickled RBCs and the loss of the elasticity of their membranes impede the movement of sickled RBCs through the microcirculation and cause an increase in blood viscosity.[200-202] When oxygenated, there is no difference in viscosities of blood containing normal HGB (AA), or blood containing AS or SS HGBs, even at a HCT of 60%. However, deoxygenation of SS or AS HGB results in disproportionate rise in viscosity as a function of HCT, when compared to normal HGB. Deoxygenated SS blood with a HCT of 20% has the same viscosity as that of normal blood at a HCT of 45%, while blood with a HCT of 28%, has the same viscosity as that of normal blood at a HCT of 60%. Sickling of RBCs containing HGB-S at a HCT of 20% leads to a 20% increase in viscosity; at a HCT of 40% viscosity doubles; and a HCT of 60%, it is increased six to eight times.

Increased viscosity in patients with sickle cell disease leads to stasis, sludging, vascular occlusion, tissue ischemia, anoxia and acidosis. This initiates a vicious cycle of sickle cell crisis where ischemia, anoxia, and acidosis precipitate further sickling.[201] Vaso-occlusion can occur at both the arterial and venous ends of the capillary bed, and may result in chronic end-organ damage. Dehydration, diuresis and infection will result in further increase in viscosity and promote sickling.

Although some irreversibly-sickled and fragile RBCs may be seen at high $SO_2$, sickling in SS blood usually begins when $SO_2$ of 85% is reached; at an $SO_2$ of 65%, three-fourths of the RBCs are sickled; and at 50%, all RBCs are sickled.[201,202] Sickling occurs more on the venous rather than the arterial side of the circulation where the low shear rate tends to increase blood viscosity further and is enhanced by factors that decrease $P\bar{v}O_2$ or $S\bar{v}O_2$ such as low CO and increased $\dot{V}O_2$. In patients with sickle cell trait, sickling begins at or below $SO_2$ of 40%. The critical $PO_2$ for sickle cell trait is 20 mm Hg, and 30 mm Hg for patients with sickle cell anemia. The speed of the sickling process is increased by hypoxemia, acidosis, changes in temperature, increase in 2,3 DPG levels, and decreased in the presence of other HGBs such as F and A and to a certain extent C (Table 5–9).[201-203] The presence of these HGBs as well as thalassemia and malaria offer some protection against sickling and may modify the clinical severity of the disease. Newborns who have SS and high concentrations of HGB-F are usually asymptomatic, although extreme conditions may still promote sickling. However, when HGB-F concentrations fall after the neonatal period, the disease becomes manifested.

Although the rightward shift of the oxyhemoglobin dissociation curve promotes increased oxygen delivery to the tissues, it theoretically predisposes to sickling by interfering with oxygen loading at the lungs. In sickle cell anemia, the RBCs are not a homogenous population; but consist of cells of varying HGB concentrations and varying amounts of 2, 3-DPG. The most dense cells (high HGB concentration) are the irreversibly sickled cells. The denser the cells, the greater is the rightward shift in the oxyhemoglobin dissociation curve. This shift, however, does not seem to be attributable to increased 2-3 DPG concentrations. In sickle cell anemia, there is a highly significant correlation between P50 and the mean corpuscular HGB concentration. In RBCs containing HGB-A, the rightward shift in the curve is dependent on the HGB concentration only in the presence of 2,3 DPG levels. In contrast, with HGB-S, the rightward shift in the curve is dependent on HGB concentration irrespective of the 2,3-DPG levels.

The etiology of anemia is primarily related to accelerated destruction of RBCs. The lifespan of sickled RBCs is 10 to 12 days as opposed to 120 days in normal RBCs.[200,203] Other factors contributing to anemia and hemolysis include decreased deformability of sickled cells, adherence of RBCs to vessel wall, formation of dense RBCs and polymerization.[202]

## Clinical Manifestations

The severity of the clinical manifestations is related to the proportion of HGB-S, SS individuals with sickle cell anemia are at particular risk. Sickle cell trait is a relatively benign and asymptomatic condition, frequently discovered incidentally by laboratory testing.[199,204,205] These individuals usually live a normal life and there is no evidence of increased morbidity or mortality. However, vaso-occlusive crises may occur under extreme

**Table 5–9.   Behavior of HGB-S in solution**

| | Resultant effect on | | |
|---|---|---|---|
| Altered critical factor | Minimum gelling concentration | Length of delay | Speed of sickling process |
| ↑ % Deoxyg HGB-S | ↓ | ↓ | ↑ |
| ↑ Temperature | ↓ | ↓ | ↑ |
| ↑ Acidosis | ↓ | ↓ | ↑ |
| ↑ 2,3-DPG levels | ↓ | ↓ | ↑ |
| ↑ Other hemoglobins (F > A > C > D,O) | ↑ | ↑ | ↓ |

From Gibson JR Jr. Anesthesia for the sickle cell diseases and other hemoglobinopathies. *Semin Anesth.* 1987;6:27, with permission.

non-physiologic conditions. Sequestration of blood with splenic infarctions was reported during non-pressurized, high altitude flying.[206] Sickling can also occur in these individuals during extremes of low-flow states and hypoxemia.[202] Conditions reported to predispose to such sickling crises include respiratory depression from drug overdose, severe alcohol intoxication,[208] and high spinal anesthesia resulting in hypotension and splenic pooling.[209]

Sickle cell anemia is a chronic disorder associated with acute crises. Crises are described in four forms: 1) hemolytic crisis, which depletes the circulatory RBC mass, is generally not common unless associated with glucose-6-phosphate dehydrogenase deficiency; 2) aplastic crisis, which is characterized by bone marrow depression associated with an infectious process; 3) sequestration crisis common in children, occurs when RBCs are trapped by the reticuloendothelial system. In this type of crisis, there is pooling of blood in the spleen; and 4) Vaso-occlusive crisis, the most common form, is characterized by pain due to ischemia. Patients with sickle cell anemia are more prone to develop infections as compared to other patients.[210] Environmental factors may have an effect on the severity of the disease. Although in Jamaica up to 9% of the population carry the S gene, the disease is considered relatively more benign as compared to the disease in the United States. It has been suggested that the absence of cold environment in Jamaica might be a contributing factor. If individuals with HGB-S from Jamaica move to a colder climate, the nature of the disease changes, becoming more serious.[200]

## Diagnosis

An accurate diagnosis is important for the patient's long-term prognosis. A reliable history and physical examination are essential. In older children and adults of African ancestry, a sickle preparation test may be performed as a screening test. In this test, a sample of blood is added to a solution of sodium metabisulfite, a reducing agent. A positive test indicates sickling of the RBCs in the blood. Both SS and AS blood will show a positive result. Thus this screening test will not differentiate sickle cell anemia from sickle cell trait. The differentiation can only be made by HGB electrophoresis which is performed on cellulose acetate or

starch and on agar. Electrophoresis on cellulose acetate differentiates most of the abnormal HGBs but not those that migrate toward HGB-S, but agar will recognize these migrating HGBs (Fig. 5–17).[202]

In newborns, history and physical examination may not reveal evidence of the disease. However, early screening in newborns is important since it enables early vaccination and prophylactic antibiotics which reduce infectious processes, a common cause of morbidity and mortality in infants with sickle cell anemia. Folic acid is commonly prescribed to prevent

### A. Cellulose Acetate pH 8.4

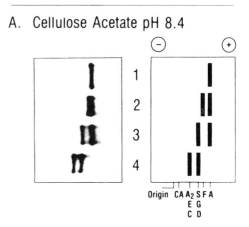

### B. Citrate Agar pH 6.5

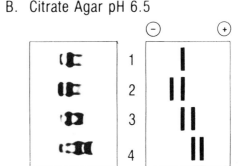

**Fig. 5–17.** Hemoglobin electrophoresis: cellulose acetate and citrate agar—The figures on the left are photographs of the actual laboratory test whereas those on the right are schematic representations of the photos. The numbers 1–4 refer to different patients, each tested by cellulose acetate and citrate agar. Patient 1 shows a normal adult pattern. Patient 2 is a newborn (FA). Patient 3 has sickle cell trait (AS). Patient 4 has sickle cell disease of the SC type (note that there is no HGB-A). From Esseltine DW, Baxter MRN, Bevan JC. Sickle cell states and the anaesthetist. Can J Anaesth. 1988;35:385, with permission.

megaloblastic anemia due to impaired folate turnover.[202] Preventive therapy of vaso-occlusive crises consists of hydration, avoidance of conditions that promote sickling, and prompt and aggressive treatment of infections.

Allogeneic RBC transfusion with HGB-A blood is a mainstay in the treatment of sickle cell anemia. This not only corrects the decreased oxygen-carrying capacity, but also decreases the erythropoiesis associated with the anemia which would produce more HGB-S-laden RBCs. Transfusion is recommended for high morbidity situations, such as severe cerebral ischemic events, acute lung disease with hypoxia, overwhelming infections, high-risk pregnancy and preoperative preparation for major surgery.[202] Patients with sickle cell disease carry considerable risk of transfusion reactions, iron overload, increased blood viscosity and compromised immunocompetency associated with multiple allogeneic blood transfusion. Furthermore, acquired alloimmunizations present crossmatching difficulties and increases the risk of severe delayed hemolytic reactions.[211]

The use of hydroxyurea and bone marrow transplantation have been recommended as therapy for the patient with sickle cell anemia. Hydroxyurea has been demonstrated to increase the circulating levels of HGB-F, with few side-effects.[212] It has been further suggested that adding other agents such as erythropoietin, butyric acid, interleukin 1, and granulocyte macrophage colony stimulating factor may improve the efficiency of hydroxyurea.[213] Bone marrow transplant, which has been shown to cure other hematologic disorders, has been tried in sickle cell anemia. It carries significant risks, with a projected mortality of nearly 10%.[214] With improved immunosuppressive and graft-versus-host disease agents being developed, this mortality rate can be reduced. This treatment modality requires careful consideration of the risk-versus-benefit ratio.

## Perioperative Management

Patients with sickle cell trait require no special perioperative treatment. However, sickle cell crisis, though very rare, can occur in these patients in the presence of severe hypoxemia, acidosis and hypotension. The patient with sickle cell anemia may benefit from a preoperative hematology consultation to assist in preoperative preparation and postoperative optimization. Prime considerations for elective surgery include the extent of the operation, concentration of HGB-S in the patient's blood, anticipated blood loss and problems with oxygenation and whether the patient's condition is stable or in a crisis. Preoperative concern focuses on maintenance of adequate oxygenation, prevention of dehydration, control of infections and/or administration of prophylactic antibiotics, treatment of pre-existing diseases and having an adequate HGB level.

The goals of preoperative preparation are to have HGB level greater than 10 g/dL and HGB-S levels less than 40 to 50%. In certain situations, lower HGB-S levels may be recommended.[215] Three methods of preoperative blood transfusion therapy to increase the levels of HGB-A and reduce the amount of HGB-S have been utilized: 1) A two-volume exchange transfusion which has the advantage of removing most of the abnormal HGB. This technique requires a large catheter in a central vein for blood withdrawal and a second catheter in a peripheral vein for transfusion. In infants it may be necessary to insert a central catheter in the aorta via the femoral artery. This procedure is fraught with dangers including thrombotic complications, vessel injury and septicemia. 2) Serial transfusions commencing one to two weeks prior to surgery eliminate most of the endogenous HGB-S by supplying an excess of HGB-A, which suppresses erythropoietin and allows HGB-S to be cleared from the circulation in about 10 days. This method is costly, cumbersome and cannot be done in emergency situations. 3) Simple preoperative transfusion. It has been suggested by Janik and Seeler[216] that conversion to HGB-A is unnecessary. They proposed a method of preoperative transfusion of 15 to 20 mL/kg of type-specific Sickledex-negative packed RBCs to all children with major hemoglobinopathy (excluding sickle cell trait). This method can be used in elective as well as emergency situations. Pretransfusion HCTs ranged from 10 to 30% and posttransfusion HCTs from 30 to 40%. Post transfusion HGB-S ranged from 20 to 60%. There was no mortality or morbidity related to the hemoglobinopathy, surgery, or anesthesia in any of the 35 children who underwent 46 surgical procedures. The ease of application and absence of morbidity and mortality suggested that this method of preoperative transfusion therapy is more desirable than other methods and that the removal of HGB-S or its complete suppression is not necessary prior to surgery. The addition of HGB-A does not increase the blood viscosity. It must be emphasized that if allogeneic blood is to be ordered, HGB-S-free blood is to be requested from the blood bank. Blood from relatives may not be suitable.

Intraoperatively, attention is directed toward maintenance of adequate tissue oxygenation, CO and hydration and prevention of vasoconstriction, acidosis and hypothermia. Both regional and general anesthetic techniques are acceptable for patients with sickle cell disease.[217-219] If CO decreases, oxygen extraction is increased and $P\bar{v}O_2$ may fall to dangerously low levels despite a normal or high $PaO_2$. If RBCs passing through these hypoxic zones reach the lungs within 15 seconds, sickling may not occur. Hence it is important to maintain hydration and normal CO in these patients. Myocardial depression (deep halothane anesthesia) may not be desirable. During exposure to a cold environment, the temperature in the superficial leg veins may fall to 30° C. Hypothermia not only causes stasis, but may also increase the blood viscosity and tendency to sickling. Acidemia should be prevented and treated promptly. A mild degree of alkalemia maintained by sodium bicarbonate (50 mmol added to each liter of fluids administered) may render HGB-S resistant to sickling. Aseptic techniques must be practiced and antibiotics may be administered as indicated. Proper patient positioning is of prime concern. Although the use of tourniquets in patients with sickle cell anemia is still controversial, their use should be avoided unless absolutely necessary. If used, the extremity should be thoroughly exsanguinated and certain precautions are followed (See Chapter 4: Blood Conservation Techniques). Vasoconstrictors should be used with caution as they may cause undesirable peripheral vasoconstriction.

Adequate monitoring is essential during anesthesia and surgery. For major procedures, monitors should include those for cardiac function (pulse, blood pressure, ECG), hydration (urine output), oxygenation (pulse oximetry, blood gases, pH), capnography, and temperature. It may be helpful to monitor $S\bar{v}O_2$ or $P\bar{v}O_2$ in these patients. Attempts to prevent shivering must be considered during recovery from anesthesia since it may cause marked increase of $\dot{V}O_2$.

Complications including sickle cell crises are most common during the postoperative period, when the potential for hypoxemia is greatest.[202] Close monitoring, adequate hydration, early ambulation and prevention of infection are necessary. Administration of oxygen and the use of other respiratory maneuvers may be necessary.[210] The presence of excessive hemolysis should arouse suspicion as would any rapid deterioration in the patient's condition. Crisis may be manifested as cardiac, pulmonary or central nervous system dysfunction. Management includes maintenance of oxygenation, hydration and blood transfusion. The need for urgency in these circumstances may be sufficient to warrant the transfusion of fresh uncrossmatched O-negative blood.

## Special Concerns

Management of the pregnant patient with sickle cell anemia requires special attention. Although still at an increased risk for spontaneous abortion, intrauterine growth retardation, and possible neonatal death, a decrease in maternal and perinatal morbidity and mortality has been seen over the last few years. This has been attributed to improved perinatal care.[220] All pregnant patients with sickle cell anemia should receive the usual prenatal iron and extra folic acid. Prophylactic transfusions are not recommended. Transfusion should be reserved for complications such as toxemia, septicemia, acute renal failure, severe anemia, hypoxemia, or anticipated surgery. Preoperative transfusion may be indicated to decrease the HGB-S level below 50% if a cesarean section is anticipated.[221] The pregnant patient with sickle cell trait requires no special treatment other than counseling regarding the possibility of having offspring with sickle cell anemia.

Patients with sickle cell anemia who to undergo hypothermic cardiopulmonary bypass (CPB), require special consideration since both hypothermia and stasis promote sickling. Transfusion, either preoperatively or intraoperatively to reduce the quantity of HGB-S to no greater than 50% prior to the initiation of hypothermic CPB is recommended.[222] Other measures may include avoidance of profound hypothermia, use of vasodilators to maintain adequate peripheral perfusion, maintenance of low viscosity and monitoring $S\bar{v}O_2$. CPB has been used successfully without special maneuvers being necessary for the patient with sickle cell trait.

Perioperative complications in patients with sickle cell anemia seem to be decreasing. Although the exact reasons remain unclear, the roles of better preoperative screening, transfusion therapy, and improved anesthetic and monitoring techniques have undoubtedly contributed to improved outcome.[202]

## REFERENCES

1. Nunn JF. Applied Respiratory Physiology. 4th ed. Boston, Mass: Butterworths; 1993.
2. Oski FA. Designation of anemia on a functional basis. J Pediatr. 1973; 83:353.
3. Blanchette VS, Zipursky A. Assessment of anemia in newborn infants. Clin Perinatol. 1984; 11:489.
4. Oski FA, Naiman JL. Hematologic Diseases of the Newborn. 2nd ed. Philadelphia, Pa: WB Saunders; 1982.
5. Burman D, Morris AF. Cord hemoglobin in low birth weight infants. Arch Dis Child. 1974; 49:382.
6. Yao AC, Moinian M, Lind J. Distribution of blood between infant and placenta after birth. Lancet. 1969; II:871.
7. Usher R, Shephard M, Lind J. The blood volume of the newborn infant and placental transfusion. Acta Paediatr Scand. 1963; 52:497.
8. Sabio H. Anemia in the high-risk infant. Clin Perinatol. 1984; 11:59.
9. Schulman I, Smith CH, Stern GS. Studies on the anemia of prematurity. Am J Dis Child. 1954; 88: 567.
10. O'Brien RT, Pearson HA. Physiologic anemia of the newborn infant. J Pediatr. 1971; 79:132.
11. Stockman JA. Anemia of prematurity. Clin Perinatol. 1977; 4:239.
12. Stockman JA, Oski FA. Physiological anaemia of infancy and the anaemia of prematurity. Clin Hematol. 1978; 7:3.
13. Gairdner D, Marks J, Roscoe JD, et al. The fluid shift from the vascular compartment immediately after birth. Arch Dis Child. 1958; 33:489.
14. Stockman JA. Anemia of prematurity. current concepts in the issue of when to transfuse. Pediatr Clin N Am. 1986; 33:111.
15. Finne PH, Halversen S. Regulation of erythropoiesis in the fetus and newborn. Arch Dis Child. 1974; 47:683.
16. Stockman JA, Garcia JF, Oski FA. The anemia of prematurity: factors governing the erythropoietin response. N Engl J Med. 1977; 296:647.
17. Halversen S, Finne PH. Erythropoietin production in the human fetus and newborn. Ann NY Acad Sci. 1968; 149:576.
18. Meberg A. Hemoglobin concentrations and erythropoietin levels in appropriate and small for gestational age infants. Scand J Haematol. 1980; 24: 162.
19. Gairdner D, Marks J, Roscoe JD. Blood formation in infancy Part II: normal erythropoiesis. Arch Dis Child. 1952; 27:214.
20. Seip M. The reticulocyte level, and the erythrocyte production judged from reticulocyte studies, in newborn infants during the first week of life. Acta Paediatr Scand. 1955; 44:355.
21. Garby L, Sjölin S, Vuille J-C. Studies on erythrokinetics in infancy III: disappearance from plasma and red-cell uptake of radioactive iron injected intravenously. Acta Paediatr Scand. 1963; 52:537.
22. Pearson HA. Life-span of the fetal red blood cell. J Pediatr. 1967; 70:166.
23. Bratteby L-E, Garby L, Groth T, et al. Studies on erythro-kinetics in infancy XIII: the mean life span and the life span frequency function of red blood cells formed during foetal life. Acta Paediatr Scand. 1968; 57:311.
24. Dallmann PR. Anemia of prematurity. Annu Rev Med. 1981; 32:143.
25. Brown MS, Garcia JF, Phibbs RH, et al. Decreased response of plasma immunoreactive erythropoietin to "available oxygen" in anemia of prematurity. J Pediatr. 1984; 105:793.
26. Obladen M, Maier R, Segerer H, et al. Efficacy and safety of recombinant human erythropoietin to prevent the anaemias of prematurity: european randomized multicenter trial. Contrib Nephrol. 1991; 88:314.
27. Stockman JA, Graeber JE, Clark DA, et al. Anemia of prematurity: determinants of the erythropoietin response. J Pediatr. 1984; 105:786.
28. Ross MP, Christensen RD, Rothstein G, et al. A randomized trial to develop criteria for administering erythrocyte transfusions to anemic preterm infants 1 to 3 months of age. J Perinatol. 1989; 9: 246.
29. Christensen RD. Recombinant erythropoietic growth factors as an alternative to erythrocyte transfusion for patients with "anemia of prematurity." Pediatrics. 1989; 83:793.
30. Jones JG, Holland BM, Veale KEA, et al. "Available oxygen" a realistic expression of the ability of the blood to supply oxygen to tissues. Scand J Haematol. 1979; 22:77.
31. Stockman JA, Clark DA, Levin EA. Weight gain—a response to transfusion in preterm infants. Pediatr Res. 1980; 14:612.
32. Szabo JS, Stonestreet B, Oh W. Effects of hypoxemia on gastrointestinal blood flow and gastric emptying in the newborn piglet. Pediatr Res. 1985; 19:466.
33. Lanzkowsky P. Iron metabolism in the newborn infant. Clin Endocrinol Metab. 1976; 5:149.
34. Hammond D, Murphy A. The influence of exogenous iron on the formation of hemoglobin in the premature infant. Pediatrics. 1960; 25:362.
35. Brozovic B, Burland WL, Simpson K, et al. Iron status of low birth weight infants and the response to oral iron. Arch Dis Child. 1974; 49:386.
36. Melhorn DK, Gross S. Vitamin E dependent anemia in the preterm infant I: effects of large doses of medicinal iron. J Pediatr. 1971; 79:569.
37. Williams ML, Shott RJ, O'Neal, PL, et al. Role of dietary iron and fat in vitamin E deficiency anemia of infancy. N Engl J Med. 1975; 292:877.

38. Fletcher J. The effect of iron and transferrin on the killing of escherichia coli in fresh serum. Immunology. 1971; 20:493.

39. Gladstone GP, Walton E. The effect of iron and haematin on the killing of staphylococci by rabbit polymorphs. Br J Exp Pathol. 1971; 52:452.

40. Bullen JJ, Rogers HJ, Grittith E. Iron-binding proteins and infections. Br J Haematol. 1972; 23:389.

41. Lister G, Moreau G, Moss M, et al. Effects of alterations of oxygen transport on the neonate. Sem Perinatol. 1984; 8:192.

42. Oski FA, Delivoria-Papadopoulos M. The red cell, 2,3-diphosphoglycerate, and tissue oxygen release. J Pediatr. 1970; 77:941.

43. Goudsouzian N. Anatomy and Physiology in Relation to Pediatric Anesthesia. In: Katz J, Steward DJ, eds. Anesthesia and Uncommon Pediatric Diseases. Philadelphia, PA: WB Saunders Co; 1987:1-11.

44. Shrieber RA. Cardiovascular physiology in infants and children. In: Motoyama EK, Davis PJ, eds. Smith's Anesthesia for Infants and Children. 5th ed. St. Louis, MO: CV Mosby Company; 1990:77-104.

45. Smith CA, Nelson NM. The Physiology of the Newborn Infant. Springfield, Ill: Charles C. Thomas; 1976.

46. Aberman A. Crossover PO₂, a measure of the variable effect of increased P50 on mixed venous PO₂. Am Rev Resp Dis. 1977; 115:173.

47. Wimberley P. Scand J CLin Lab Invest. 1982; 160. (suppl).

48. Rossoff L, Zeldin R, Hew E, et al. Changes in blood P50: effects on oxygen delivery when arterial hypoxemia is due to shunting. Chest. 1980; 77:142.

49. Card RT, Brain MC. The "anemia" of childhood: evidence for a physiologic response to hyperphosphatemia. N Engl J Med. 1973; 288:388.

50. Motoyama EK, Zigas CJ, Troll G. Functional basis of childhood anemia. Am Soc Anesthesiol. 1974; 283. Abstract.

51. Motoyama EK. Respiratory physiology in infants and children. In: Motoyama EK, Davis PJ, eds. Smith's Anesthesia for Infants and Children. 5th ed. St. Louis, MO: CV Mosby Company; 1990:11-76.

52. Rackow H, Salanitre E. Modern concepts in pediatric anesthesia. Anesthesiology. 1969; 30:208.

53. Oh W, Lind J. Venous and capillary hematocrit in newborn infants and placental transfusion. Acta Paedatri Scand. 1966; 55:38.

54. Linderkamp OL, Versmold HT, Strohhacker I, et al. Capillary-venous hematocrit differences in newborn infants. I: relationship to blood volume, peripheral blood flow, and acid-base parameters. Eur J Pediatr. 1977; 127:9.

55. Faxelius G, Raye J, Gutberlet R, et al. Red cell volume measurements and acute blood loss in high-risk newborn infants. J Pediatr. 1977; 90:273.

56. Holland BM, Jones JG, Wardrop CAJ. Lessons from the anemia of prematurity. Hematol/Oncol Clin N Am. 1987; 1:355.

57. Huber H, Lewis SM, Szur L. The influence of anaemia, polycythaemia and splenomegaly on the relationship between venous haematocrit and red-cell volume. Br J Haematol. 1964; 10:567.

58. Phillips H, Holland BM, Jones JG, et al. Determination of red cell mass in assessment and management of anaemia in babies needing blood transfusion. Lancet. 1986; I:882.

59. Greenberg HB. Cardiac arrest in 20 infants and children: causes and results of resuscitation. Dis Chest. 1965; 47:42.

60. Salem MR, Bennett EJ, Schweiss JF, et al. Cardiac arrest related to anesthesia: contributing factors in infants and children. JAMA. 1975; 233:238.

61. Eger EI II. Respiratory and circulatory factors in uptake and distribution of volatile anaesthetic agents. Br J Anaesth. 1964; 36:115.

62. Gregory GA, Eger EI II, Munson ES. The relationship between age and halothane requirement in man. Anesthesiology. 1969; 30:488.

63. Nicodemus HF, Nassiri-Rahimi C, Bachman L, et al. Median effective dose (ED50) of halothane in adults and children. Anesthesiology. 1969; 31:244.

64. Lerman J, Robins S, Willis MM, et al. Anesthetic requirements for halothane in young children 0-1 and 1-6 months of age. Anesthesiology. 1983; 59:421.

65. Cameron CB, Robinson S, Gregory GA. The minimum alveolar concentration of isoflurane in children. Anesth Analg. 1984; 63:418.

66. LeDez KM, Lerman J. The minimum alveolar concentration (MAC) of isoflurane in preterm neonates. Anesthesiology 1987; 67:301.

67. Cook DR, Davis PJ. Pharmacology of pediatric anesthesia. In: Motoyama EK, Davis PJ eds. Smith's Anesthesia for infants and children, 5th ed. St. Louis, Mo: CV Mosby Co; 1990:157.

68. Eger EI II, Smith NY, Cullen DJ, et al. A comparison of cardiovascular effects of halothane, fluorxene, ether and cyclopropane in man: a resume. Anesthesiology. 1971; 34:25.

69. Barash PG, Glanz S, Katz JD, et al. Ventricular function in children during halothane anesthesia: An echocardiographic evaluation. Anesthesiology. 1978; 49:79.

70. Rao CC, Bayer M, Krishna C, et al. Increased sensitivity of the isometric contraction of the neonatal isolated rat atria to halothane, isoflurane, and enflurane. Anesthesiology. 1986; 64:13.

71. Diaz JH, Lockhart CH. Is halothane really safe in infancy? Anesthesiology. 1979; 51:S313. Abstract.

72. Friesen RH, Lichtor JL. Cardiovascular effects of inhalation induction with isoflurane in infants. Anesth Analg. 1983; 62:411.

73. Friesen RH, Henry DB. Cardiovascular changes in preterm neonates receiving isoflurane, halothane, fentanyl, and ketamine. Anesthesiology. 1986; 64:238.

74. Duncan P, Gregory GA, Wade J. The effect of nitrous oxide on the baroreceptor response of newborn and adult rabbits. Can Anaesth Soc J. 1981; 28:339.

75. Gregory GA. The baroresponses of preterm infants during halothane anaesthesia. Can Anaesth Soc J. 1982; 29:105.

76. Robinson S, Gregory GA. Urine specific gravity as a predictor of hypovolemic and hypotensive response to halothane anesthesia in the newborn. Am Soc Anesthesiol. 1978; 37. Abstract.

77. Tiret L, Nivoche Y, Hatton F, et al. Complications related to anaesthesia in infants and children: a prospective survey of 40240 anaesthetics. Br J Anaesth. 1988; 61:263.

78. Morray JP, Geiduschek JM, Caplan RE, et al. A comparison of pediatric and adult anesthesia closed malpractice claims. Anesthesiology. 1993; 78:461.

79. Joshi A, Gerhardt T, Shandloff P, et al. Blood trans-

fusion effect on the respiratory pattern of preterm infants. Pediatrics. 1987; 80:79.

80. Blank JP, Sheagren TG, Vajaria J, et al. The role of RBC transfusion in the premature infant. Am J Dis Child. 1984; 138:831.

81. Kattwinkel J. Neonatal apnea: pathogenesis and therapy. J Pediatr. 1977; 90:342.

82. De Maio JG, Harris MC, Deuber C, et al. Effect of blood transfusion on apnea frequency in growing premature infants. J Pediatr. 1989; 114:1039.

83. Keyes WG, Donohue PK, Spivak JL, et al. Assessing the need for transfusion of premature infants and role of HCT: clinical signs and erythropoietin level. Pediatrics. 1989; 84:412.

84. Welborn LG, Hannallah RS, Luban NLC, et al. Anemia and postoperative apnea in former preterm infants. Anesthesiology. 1991; 74:1003.

85. Wardrop CA, Holland BM, Veale KEA, et al. Non-physiological anemia of prematurity. Arch Dis Child. 1978; 53:855.

86. Winearls CR, Peppard MJ, Downing MR, et al. Effect of human erythropoietin derived from recombinant DNA on the anemia of patients maintained by chronic haemodialysis. Lancet. 1986; II:1175.

87. Shannon KM, Naylor GS, Torkildson JC, et al. Circulating erythroid progenitors in the anemia of prematurity. N Engl J Med. 1987; 317:728.

88. Koch KM, Kühn K, Nonnast-Daniel B, et al. Treatment of renal anaemia with recombinant human erythropoietin. Basel, Switzerland: Karger; 1988.

89. Rhondeau SM, Christensen RD, Ross MP, et al. Responsiveness to recombinant human erythropoietin of marrow erythroid progenitors from infants with "anemia of prematurity." J Pediatr. 1988; 112:935.

90. Ohls R, Liechty KW, Turner MC, et al. Erythroid "burst-promoting" activity in serum of patients with anemia of prematurity. J Pediatr. 1990; 116:786.

91. Oster W, Hermann F, Cicco A, et al. Erythropoietin prevents chemotherapy-induced anaemia. Blut. 1989; 59:341A. Abstract.

92. Goodnough LT, Rudnick S, Price TH, et al. Increased preoperative collection of autologous blood with recombinant human erythropoietin therapy. N Engl J Med. 1989; 321:1163.

93. George JW, Bracco C, Shannin K, et al. Response of rhesus monkeys to recombinant human erythropoietin. Comparison of adults and infants. Pediatr Res. 1989; 25:269A. Abstract.

94. Halpérin DS, Wacker P, Lacourt G, et al. Effects of recombinant human erythropoietin in infants with the anemia of prematurity: a pilot study. J Pediatr. 1990; 116:779.

95. Sandler SG, Grumet FC. Post transfusion cytomegalovirus infections. Pediatrics. 1982; 69:650.

96. Sullivan JL. Epstein-Barr virus and the X-linked lymphoproliferative syndrome. Adv Pediatr. 1983; 30:365.

97. Feorina PM, Jaffee HW, Palmer E, et al. Transfusion-associated acquired immunodeficiency syndrome. Evidence for persistent infection in blood donors. N Engl J Med. 1985; 312:1293.

98. Yeager AS, Grumet FC, Hafleigh EB, et al. Prevention of transfusion-acquired cytomegalovirus infections in newborn infants. J Pediatr. 1981; 98:281.

99. Land DJ, Valeri CR. Hazards of blood transfusion. Adv Pediatr. 1977; 24:311.

100. Parkman R, Mosier D, Umansky J, et al. Graft vs

host disease after intrauterine and exchange transfusions for hemolytic disease of the newborn. N Engl J Med. 1974; 290:359.

101. Aranda JV, Clark TF, Maniello R, et al. Blood transfusions: Possible potentiating risk of retrolental fibroplasia. Pediatr Res. 1975; 9:633.

102. Sacks LM, Schaffer DB, Peckham GJ, et al. Exchange transfusion and retrolental fibroplasia (RLF)—Lack of cause and effect. Pediatr Res. 1978; 12:533.

103. Finch CA, Lenfant C. Oxygen transport in man. N Engl J Med. 1972; 286:407.

104. Brown MS, Phibbs HR, Dallman PR. Postnatal changes in fetal haemoglobin, oxygen affinity and 2,3 DPG in previously transfused preterm infants. Biol Neonate. 1985; 48:70.

105. Stockman JA, Levin EA, Clark DA, et al. Oxygen consumption in premature infants in the first two weeks of life: the response to transfusion. Pediatr Res. 1979; 13:442.

106. Oski FA. Fetal hemoglobin, the neonatal red cell and 2,3 DPG. Pediatr Clin N Am. 1972; 19:907.

107. Gottuso M, Williams M, Oski F. Exchange transfusion in low-birth-weight infants. II. Further observations. J Pediatr. 1976; 89:279.

108. Lister G, Hallenbrand WE, Kleinman CS, et al. Physiologic effects of increasing hemoglobin concentration in left to right shunting in infants with ventricular septal defects. N Engl J Med. 1982; 306:502.

109. Hackmann T, Steward DJ. What is the value of preoperative hemoglobin determinations in pediatric outpatients? Anesthesiology 1989; 71:A1168. Abstract.

110. Bikhazi GB, Cook DR. Perioperative fluid therapy and blood replacement. In: Motoyama EK, Davis PJ, eds. Smith's Anesthesia for infants and children, 5th ed. St Louis, MO: CV Mosby Company; 1990.

111. Miller M, Wishart HY, Nimmo WS. Gastric contents at induction of anaesthesia. is a 4-hour fast necessary? Br J Anaesth. 1983; 55:1185.

112. Maltby JR, Sutherland AD, Sale JP, et al. Preoperative oral fluids: is a five-hour fast justified prior to elective surgery? Anesth Analg. 1986; 65:1112.

113. Sandhar BK, Goresky GV, Maltby JR, et al. Effect of oral liquids and ranitidine on gastric fluid volume and pH in children undergoing outpatient surgery. Anesthesiology. 1989; 71:327.

114. Splinter WM, Stewart JA, Muir JG. The effect of preoperative apple juice on gastric contents, thirst and hunger in children. Can J Anaesth. 1989; 36:55.

115. Schreiner MS, Triebwasser A, Keon TP. Oral fluids compared to preoperative fasting in pediatric outpatients. Anesthesiology. 1990; 72:593.

116. Bland JH, Lowenstein E. Halothane-induced decrease in experimental myocardial ischemia in the non-failing canine heart. Anesthesiology. 1976; 45:287.

117. Barrera M, Miletich DJ, Albrecht RF, et al. Hemodynamic consequences of halothane anesthesia during chronic anemia. Anesthesiology. 1984; 61:36.

118. Kim S-J, Salem MR, Joseph NJ, et al. Contrast media adversely affect oxyhemoglobin dissociation. Anesth Analg. 1990; 71:73.

119. Deckardt R, Steward DJ. Non-invasive arterial hemoglobin oxygen saturation versus transcutaneous oxygen tension monitoring in the preterm infant. Crit Care Med. 1984; 12:935.

120. Solimano AJ, Smyth JA, Mann TK, et al. Pulse oximetry: advantages in infants with bronchopulmonary dysplasia. Pediatrics. 1986; 78:844.

121. Severinghaus JW. Blood gas calculator. J Appl Physiol. 1966; 21:1108.

122. Zauder HL. Preoperative hemoglobin requirements. Anesthesiol Clin N Am. 1990; 8:471.

123. Lyman HM. Artificial Anaesthesia and Anaesthetics. New York: NY: William Wood; 1881.

124. Da Costa JC, Kalteyer FJ. The blood changes induced by the administration of ether as an anesthetic. Ann Surg. 1901; 34:329.

125. Fish H. The importance of blood examinations in reference to general anesthetization and operative procedures. Ann Surg. 1899; 32:269.

126. Gwathmey JT. Anesthesia. 2nd ed. New York, NY: Macmillan; 1924,

127. Adams RC, Lundy JS. Anesthesia in cases of poor surgical risk: some suggestions for decreasing the risk. Surg Gynecol Obstet. 1941; 71:1011.

128. Kowalyshyn TJ, Prager D, Young J. A review of the present status of preoperative hemoglobin requirements. Anesth Analg. 1972; 51:75.

129. Crosby WH. Misuse of blood transfusion. Blood. 1958; 13:1198.

130. Shields TW, Rambach WA. Whole blood transfusion in surgical practice. Surg Clin North Am. 1959; 39:121.

131. Cooley DA, Beal AC, Growdin P. Open heart operations with disposable oxygenators, five percent dextrose prime and normothermia. Surgery. 1962; 53:713.

132. Gollub S, Bailey CP. Management of major surgical blood loss without transfusion. JAMA. 1966; 198:1171.

133. Cosgrove DM, Thurer RL, Lytle BW et al. Blood conservation during myocardial revascularization. Ann Thorac Surg. 1979; 28:184.

134. Aris A, Padro JM, Bonnin JO, et al. Prediction of hematocrit changes in open-heart surgery without blood transfusion. J Cardiovasc Surg. 1984; 25:545.

135. Nunn JF, Freeman J. Problems of oxygenation and oxygen transport during haemorrhage. Anaesthesia. 1964; 19:206.

136. Benumof JL. Respiratory physiology and respiratory function during anesthesia. In: Miller RD, ed. Anesthesia. 2nd ed. New York, NY: Churchill-Livingstone; 1986.

137. Schweiss JF. Continuous Measurement of Blood Oxygen Saturation in the High Risk Patient. vol 1. San Diego, Calif: Beach International; 1883.

138. Wilkerson DK, Rosen AL, Gould SA, et al. Oxygen extraction ratio: a valid indicator of myocardial metabolism in anemia. J Surg Res. 1987; 42:629.

139. Levy PS, Chavez P, Crystal GJ, et al. Oxygen extraction ration: a valid indicator of transfusion need in limited coronary vascular reserve. J Trauma. 1992; 32:769.

140. American College of Surgeons, Committee on Trauma. Advanced Trauma Life Support Course Manual. Chicago, IL: American College of Surgeons; 1989.

141. Michalski AH, Lowenstein E, Austen WG, et al. Patterns of oxygenation and cardiovascular adjustment to acute transient normovolemic anemia. Ann Surg. 1968; 168:946.

142. Vatner SF, Higgins CB, Franklin D. Regional circulatory adjustments to moderate and severe chronic anemia in conscious dogs at rest and during exercise. Circ Res. 1972; 30:731.

143. Varat MA, Adolf RJ, Fowler NO. Cardiovascular effects of anemia. Am Heart J 1972; 83:415.

144. Horstman DH, Gleser M, Wolfe D, et al. Effects of hemoglobin reduction of $\dot{V}O_2$ max and related hemodynamics in exercising dogs. J Appl Physiol. 1974; 37:97.

145. Rodriguez JA, Chamorro G, Rapaport E. Effect of isovolemic anemia on ventricular performance at rest and during exercise. J Appl Physiol. 1974; 36:28.

146. Fowler NO, Holmes JC. Blood viscosity and cardiac output in acute experimental anemia. J Appl Physiol. 1975; 39:453.

147. Biro GP, Beresfor-Kroeger D. Myocardial blood flow and $O_2$-supply following dextran-haemodilution and methaemoglobinaemia. Cardiovasc Res. 1979; 13:459.

148. Loarie DJ, Wilkinson P, Tyberg J, et al. The hemodynamic effects of halothane in anemic dogs. Anesth Analg. 1979; 58:200.

149. Tarnow J, Eberlein HJ, Hess W, et al. Hemodynamic interactions of hemodilution, anesthesia, propranolol pretreatments and hypovolaemia. I. Systemic circulation. Basic Res Cardiol. 1979; 74:109.

150. Tarnow J, Eberlein HJ, Hess W, et al. Hemodynamic interactions of hemodilution, anesthesia, propranolol pretreatments and hypovolaemia. II. Coronary circulation. Basic Res Cardiol. 1979; 74:123.

151. Crystal GF. Coronary hemodynamic responses during local hemodilution in canine hearts. Am J Physiol. 1988; 254:H525

152. Crystal GJ, Rooney MW, Salem MR. Regional hemodynamics and oxygen supply during isovolemic hemodilution alone and in combination with adenosine-induced controlled hypotension. Anesth Analg. 1988; 67:211.

153. Crystal GJ, Rooney MW, Salem MR. Myocardial blood flow and oxygen consumption during isovolemic hemodilution alone and in combination with adenosine-induced controlled hypotension. Anesth Analg. 1988; 67:539.

154. Crystal GJ, Ruiz JR, Rooney MW, et al. Regional hemodynamics and oxygen supply during isovolemic hemodilution in the absence and presence of high-grade beta-adrenergic blockade. J Cardiothorac Anesth. 1988; 2:772.

155. Crystal GJ, Salem MR. Myocardial oxygen consumption and segmental shortening during selective coronary hemodilution in dogs. Anesth Analg. 1988; 67:500.

156. Crystal GJ, Salem MR. Blood volume and hematocrit in regional circulations during isovolemic hemodilution in dogs. Microvasc Res. 1989; 37:237.

157. Pavek K, Carey JS. Hemodynamics and oxygen availability during isovolemic hemodilution. Am J Physiol. 1974; 226:1172.

158. Geha AS. Coronary and cardiovascular dynamics and oxygen availability during acute normovolemic anemia. Surgery. 1976; 80:47.

159. Jan KM, Heldman J, Chien S. Coronary hemodynamics and oxygen utilization after hematocrit variations in hemorrhage. Am J Physiol. 1980–26-32:239.

160. Spahn DR, Leone BJ, Reves JG, et al. Cardiovascular and coronary physiology of acute isovolemic

hemodilution: a review of nonoxygen-carrying solutions. Anesth Analg. 1994; 78:1000.

161. Viele MK, Weiskopf RB. What can we learn about the need for transfusion from patients who refuse blood? the experience with Jehovah's Witnesses. Transfusion. 1994; 34:714.

162. Roy SB, Bhatia ML, Mathur VS, et al. Hemodynamic effects of chronic severe anemia. Circulation. 1963; 28:346.

163. Rosenthal DS, Braunwald E. Hematologic oncology disorders and heart disease. In: Braunwald E, ed. Heart Disease, Philadelphia, PA: WB Saunders Co; 1980.

164. Allen JB, Allen FB. The minimum acceptable level of hemoglobin. Anesthesiol Clin N Am. 1981.

165. Fowler NO, Smith O, Greenfield JC. Arterial blood oxygenation in sickle cell anemia. Am J Med Sci. 1957; 234:449.

166. Rodman T, Close HP, Cathcart R, et al. The oxyhemoglobin dissociation curve in the common hemoglobinopathies. Am J Med. 1959; 27:558.

167. Seakins M, Gibbs WN, Milner PF, et al. Erythrocyte Hb-S concentration: an important factor in the low oxygen affinity of blood in sickle cell anemia. J Clin Invest. 1973; 52:422.

168. Bromberg PA, Jensen WN, McDonough M. Blood oxygen dissociation curves in sickle cell disease. J Lab Clin Med. 1967; 70:480.

169. Milner PF. Oxygen transport in sickle cell anemia. Arch Intern Med. 1974; 133:565.

170. Scott V. Anemia and airline flight duties. Aviat Space Environ Med. 1975; 46:303.

171. Hemminki E, Starfield B. Prevention of low birth weight and pre-term birth: literature review and suggestions. Milbank Mem Fund Q Health Soc. 1978; 56:339.

172. Murphy JF, O'Riordan J, Newcombe RG, et al. Relation of haemoglobin levels in first and second trimesters to outcome of pregnancy. Lancet. 1986; I:992.

173. Paulone ME, Edelstone DI, Shedd A. Effects of maternal anemia on uteroplacental and fetal oxidative metabolism in sheep. Am J Obstet Gynecol. 1987; 165:230.

174. Delpapa EH, Edelstone DH, Milley JR, et al. Effects of chronic maternal anemia on systemic and uteroplacental oxygenation in near-term pregnant sheep. Am J Obstet Gynecol. 1992; 166:1007.

175. Adamson JW, Eschbach JW. Treatment of the anemia of chronic renal failure with recombinant human erythropoietin. Annu Rev Med. 1990; 41:349.

176. Aldrete JA, Daniel W, O'Higgins JW et al. Analysis of anesthetic-related morbidity in human recipients of renal homografts. Anesth Analg. 1971; 50:321.

177. Gopalrao T. Should anemia stop surgery? Int Surg. 1971; 55:250.

178. Slawson KB. Anaesthesia for the patient in renal failure. Br J Anaesth. 1972; 44:277.

179. Stehling LC, Ellison N, Faust RJ, et al. A survey of transfusion practices among anesthesiologists. Vox Sang. 1987; 52:62.

180. Lunn JN, Elwood PC. Anaemia and surgery. Br Med J. 1970; 3:71.

181. Rawstron RE. Anaemia and surgery: a retrospective study. Aust NZ J Surg. 1970; 39:425.

182. Gould SA, Rosen AL, Sehgal LR, et al. Fluosol-DA as a red cell substitute in acute anemia. N Engl J Med. 1986; 314:1653.

183. Carson JL, Spence RK, Poses RM, et al. Severity of anemia and operative mortality and morbidity. Lancet. 1988; 1:727.

184. Stehling L. Perioperative mortality in anemic patients. Transfusion. 1989; 29:37S.

185. Spence RK, Carson JA, Poses R, et al. Elective surgery without transfusion: influence of preoperative hemoglobin level and blood loss on mortality. Am J Surg. 1990; 159:320.

186. Kitchens CS. Are transfusions overrated? Surgical outcome of Jehovah's Witnesses. Am J Med. 1993; 94:117.

187. Spence RK, Costabile JP, Young GS, et al. Is hemoglobin level alone a reliable predictor of outcome in the severely anemic surgical patient? Am Surg. 1992; 58:92.

188. Czer LS, Shoemaker WC. Optimal hematocrit value in critically ill postoperative patients. Surg Gynecol Obstet. 1978; 147:363.

189. Babineau TJ, Dzik WH, Borlase BC, et al. Reevaluation of current transfusion practices in patients in surgical intensive care units. Am J Surg. 1992; 164:22.

190. Lorente JA, Landin L, DePablo R, et al. Effects of blood transfusion on oxygen transport variables in severe sepsis. Crit Care Med. 1993; 21:1312.

191. Marik PE, Sibbald WJ. Effect of stored-blood transfusion on oxygen delivery in patients with sepsis. JAMA. 1993; 269:3024.

192. Nelson CL, Bowen WS. Total hip arthroplasty in Jehovah's Witnesses without blood transfusion. J Bone Joint Surg Am. 1986; 68:350.

193. Stehling L, Simon TL. The red blood cell transfusion trigger: physiology and clinical studies. Arch Pathol Lab Med. 1994; 118:429.

194. Gould SA, Sehgal LR, Sehgal HL, et al. Hypovolemic shock. Crit Care. 1993; 9:239.

195. van Woerkens ECSM, Trouwborst A, van Lanschot JJB. Profound hemodilution: what is the critical level of hemodilution at which oxygen delivery-dependent oxygen consumption starts in an anesthetized human? Anesth Analg. 1992; 75:818.

196. National Institutes of Health Concensus Conference. Perioperative red blood cell transfusion. JAMA. 1988; 260:2700.

197. American College of Physicians. Practice strategies for elective red blood cell transfusion. Ann Intern Med. 1992; 116:403.

198. American Society of Anesthesiologists, Task Force on Blood Component Therapy. Perioperative blood component therapy: Review of the evidence and recommendations, Draft Document 1994.

199. Serjeant GR. Sickle cell anemia: clinical features in adulthood and old age. In: Abramson H, Bertles JF, Nethers DL, eds. Sickle Cell Disease. St. Louis, Mo: CV Mosby Co; 1973.

200. Bennett EJ, Dalal FY. Haemoglobin S and its clinical application. In: Payne JP, Hill DW, eds. Oxygen Measurement in Biology and Medicine. London, Eng: Butterworths; 1975.

201. Gibson Jr. JR. Anesthesia for the sickle cell diseases and other hemoglobinopathies. Semin Anesth. 1987; 4:27.

202. Esseltine, DW, Baxter MRN, Bevan JC. Sickle cell states and the anaesthetist. Can Anaesth Soc J. 1988; 35:385.

203. Aldrete JA, Guerra F. Hematologic diseases. In: Anesthesia and Uncommon Diseases. Katz B, Benu-

mof J, Kadis LB, eds. Philadelphia, PA: WB Saunders; 1981.

204. Hathorn M. Pattern of red cell destruction in sickle cell anemia. Br J Haematol. 1967; 13:746.

205. Diggs WW, Diggs LW. Hospital detection of sickle cell disease. Hosp Pract. 1972; 9:109.

206. Green RL, Huntsman RG, Sergeant GR. The sickle cell and altitude. Br Med J. 1971; 4:593.

207. Bullick FG, Delage C, Frey NS. Sickle cell crisis associated with drugs. Arch Environ Health. 1973; 26:221.

208. Lourie JA, Kontopoulis I. Gin and the sickle cell crisis. Lancet. 1971; 1:1354.

209. Luban N, Epstein B, Watson SP. Sickle cell disease and anesthesia. In: Gallagher TJ, ed. Advances in Anesthesia Vol 1. Chicago, Ill: Year Book Medical Publishers; 1984.

210. Price ME, Kembey TY. Collecting blood for autotransfusion in ectopic pregnancy (written communication). Trop Doct. 1985; 15:67.

211. Castro O. Autotransfusion: a management option for alloimmunized sickle cell patients? Prog Clin Biol Res. 1982; 98:117.

212. Rodgers GP. Recent approaches to the treatment of sickle cell anemia. JAMA. 1991; 265:2097.

213. Vichinsky EP. Comprehensive care in sickle cell disease: its impact on morbidity and mortality. Semin Hematol. 1991; 28:220.

214. Nagel RL. Sickle cell anemia in multigene disease: Sickle painful crises. a case in point. Am J Hematology. 1993; 42:96.

215. Miller DM, Winslow RM, Klein HG, et al. Improved exercise performance after exchange transfusion in subjects with sickle cell anemia. Blood. 1980; 56:1127.

216. Janik J, Seeler RA. Perioperative management of children with sickle cell hemoglobinopathy. J Pediatr Surg. 1980; 15:117.

217. Maduska AL, Guince WS, Henton JA, et al. Sickling dynamics of red blood cells during anesthesia. Anesth Analg. 1975; 54:361.

218. Searle JF. Anesthesia in sickle cell states: a review. Anaesthesia. 1973; 28:48.

219. Atlas SA. The sickle cell trait and surgical complications: A matched pair, patient analysis. JAMA. 1974; 229:1078.

220. Koshy M, Burd L. Management of pregnancy in sickle cell syndromes. Hematol/Oncol Clin North Am. 1991; 5:585.

221. Charache S. Hydroxyurea as treatment for sickle cell anemia. Hematol/Oncol Clin North Am. 1991; 38:571.

222. Chun PKC, Flannery EP, Bowen TE. Open-heart surgery in patients with hematologic disorders. Am Heart J. 1983; 105:835.

# 6

# PREOPERATIVE AUTOLOGOUS BLOOD DONATION

*M. Ramez Salem, Louise Mastrianno, and Ninos J. Joseph*

Preoperative autologous blood donation (PABD) refers to short-term donation of the patient's own blood for storage to provide transfusion back to the patient-donor during or after planned surgical procedures. The objective of PABD is to minimize or even eliminate exposure to allogeneic blood, especially when combined with other blood conservation measures. Of the various autologous blood transfusion options, PABD remains the most feasible and widely practiced.

## HISTORICAL PERSPECTIVES

Probably, the first known preoperative autologous donation of blood was pioneered by Grant in 1921:[1]

### Autotransfusion

"Dr. Francis C. Grant presented a man forty-two years of age, who was admitted to the service of Dr. C. H. Frazier at the University Hospital, presenting a clear-cut picture of cerebellar tumor. A suboccipital exploration was determined upon. It had been their routine practice of late to transfuse postoperatively all cases upon whom a suboccipital exploration has been performed. The procedure is of necessity a prolonged one accompanied by considerable shock to vital centres, and they had found that immediate transfusion insured a prompt reaction and improved the postoperative course. The patient in question had no money to pay for a donor and was of type 3, the least frequent type. They had no donors of this type on their free list. However the patient was large, stout, and plethoric. His B.C.R. totaled, 6,850,000 with 110 per cent. Hgb. confirmed by several counts. Robertson, Rous and Turner, and others. had shown that whole blood could be kept citrated and cold for a considerable time. From observation upon six donors they knew that following the withdrawal of 500 c.c. of blood the cell count and hæmoglobin returned to normal in five to nine days.

The patient was definitely plethoric, his blood pressure was 155 systolic and 110 diastolic. In view of the fact that they could not obtain a suitable donor and that transfusion would be desirable following his operation, it was suggested that they bleed the patient, allow him twenty-four hours to

146

recover from the transfusion, operate upon him, and transfuse him with his own blood. This was accordingly done. The blood was obtained, kept in .2 per cent. sodium citrate solution in a refrigerator and retransfused following operation. Three hours after operation the temperature, pulse, and respiration were 100, 118, and 18, the highest point reached. Clinically no reaction was noted. The postoperative course was favorable. Four days after operation the R.B.C. were 4,919,000, Hgb. 90 per cent and blood pressure 135-100.

In conclusion, they suggest that although the plethora and high blood pressure seemed special indications in this case, autotransfusion might be considered in other conditions. In cases where a donor cannot be obtained for any reason and in which a patient with a high normal blood picture faces an operation known to be attended with shock and hemorrhage, if he be bled sufficiently far enough in advance of his operation to allow his blood picture to return to normal, this blood may be kept with safety and retransfused at a time when such a procedure may be life-saving."

Francis C. Grant, M.D.,1921

When the first blood bank was founded in 1937 in Chicago, Fantus advocated PABD.[2] By the 1960s, PABD was practiced in a few centers.[3-7] In some of these centers, up to 80 to 90% of the blood needed for surgical operations had been met by PABD.[6,7] Despite its success and safety, PABD remained dormant and did not gain wide acceptance until the 1980s.

In 1979, Silvergleid[8] reported his experience at the blood bank of San Bernardino and Riverside Counties in California with the provision of centralized autologous blood services. Despite the obvious success and feasibility of such a program, reservations were initially expressed regarding the ability of a community blood center to provide autologous blood services. However, these reservations were rapidly submerged by tidal waves of enthusiasm, demand, and necessity. Within several years, the issue had shifted from whether to provide such autologous blood services to how to provide them.[9]

The 1980s witnessed dramatic acceptance of PABD. Triggered largely by concerns about blood safety raised by the acquired immune deficiency syndrome scare, interest for PABD grew and became an accepted standard of care. Contributing to the growth in the provision of PABD programs were hospital and physician concerns about litigation, patient fears and concerns, and in some states, hastily conceived legislation. The California Statute CB—37† requires that in addition to the risks and benefits of blood transfusion, alternatives to allogeneic blood be presented to patients. By 1990, as much as 5% of all blood collected for transfusion was intended for use by the patient-donor from whom it was collected.[10] The use of predeposit autologous units, rather than allogeneic stock, helped blood banks maintain availability of blood supplies for patients in whom autologous donation was not possible. After more than 10 years of extensive national and international experience with PABD, controversial issues that surfaced in the 1980s still exist. These issues include indications for donation, extent of testing, disposition of infectious blood, crossover into the homologous blood supply, and indications (or contraindications) for transfusion of autologous blood.[9,11]

## INDICATIONS FOR PREOPERATIVE BLOOD DONATION

Whereas few would disagree that autologous blood is the safest blood, there are definite risks associated with blood donation, and therefore, the risks must be weighed against the potential benefits.[9] Preoperative autologous blood may be donated by patients who are likely to require transfusion during or after surgery. In general, autologous blood is likely to be used for those surgical procedures requiring crossmatch orders for blood. As outlined in the Standards for Blood Banks and Transfusion Services,[12] the ideal patient for PABD is one who: (1) is healthy enough to undergo elective surgery; (2) is likely to need a transfusion during or after surgery; (3) has 2 or more weeks before surgery; and (4) has a hemoglobin > 11 g/dL or hematocrit (HCT) > 33%. Although a hemoglobin > 11 g/dL seems to be a reasonable requirement, some institutions have been accepting slightly lower values, especially when there is strong need for PABD.

Obviously, there are no perfect rules with respect to the indication for PABD. One sug-

---

† The California Statute CB-37, Paul Gann Blood Safety Act, 1990

gested approach would be to base decisions about the need for PABD on the "maximum surgical blood order schedule" (MSBOS) for that procedure in the hospital at which surgery is performed, with consideration given to the patient's medical and emotional condition.[9,13] Patients contemplating an operation prior to which only a type-and-screen procedure is usually performed, might be discouraged from depositing autologous blood, especially if they are less than ideal candidates for phlebotomy. PABD could be provided for MSBOS type-and-screen patients only when they are medically fit, and would be adversely affected psychologically were autologous blood not made available.[9,13]

The fear of transfusion-transmitted diseases from allogeneic blood transfusion has led some panic-stricken patients to offer to participate in an autologous donation program, even for surgical operations that carry little likelihood of requiring transfusion. These patients should be advised against donating their blood for autologous use. This is particularly relevant for those patients whose medical condition increases the potential for an adverse reaction.[9] A typical example is normal obstetric delivery or cesarean section. Data suggests that very few women need transfusion during or after delivery. Furthermore, it is very difficult to accurately predict those likely to require transfusion. Despite the minimal risk to fetus and mother, studies of PABD during pregnancy showed that the donation-to-use ratio in low-risk pregnant women, with neither personal nor family history of blood use at delivery, was approximately 100:1.[14-16] Obviously, PABD in pregnant women seems an unwise and inappropriate utilization of increasingly expensive resources.[14-16] An exception are patients with placenta previa where studies show a high incidence of blood transfusion.[16,17] These patients may be encouraged to donate blood as soon as the diagnosis is made.[16,18]

PABD has been extended to a variety of surgical procedures, including orthopedic, cardiac, vascular, thoracic, abdominal, neurosurgical, maxillofacial, plastic, head and neck, gynecologic, and cancer surgery.[19-27] Patients undergoing total hip or knee replacement and scoliosis correction are ideal candidates.[19,20] PABD in patients undergoing hip and knee joint procedures resulted in a reduction of al-

logeneic blood transfusion from 73 to 18%, and from 71 to 12%, respectively.[28] For cardiovascular-thoracic patients, the benefit must be weighed against the risk of delaying surgery until the appropriate amount of blood is collected. Provided careful monitoring of the cardiovascular function is undertaken, patients with stable coronary artery, stable valvular, and congenital heart diseases, and patients for aortic surgery, can be appropriate candidates for PABD.[29-31] Although worsening angina has been described in a few patients during and after donation, it is unclear whether this was a natural progression of their disease or was actually precipitated by donation.[32] Signs of myocardial ischemia following PABD have been studied. Patients with normal electrocardiographic patterns maintained their normal patterns after phlebotomy. Those with heart disease showed nonspecific ST segment changes. Some patients who had electrocardiographic evidence of ventricular strain before phlebotomy had improved electrocardiograms after phlebotomy, possibly because of the reduced myocardial workload, resulting from decreased blood viscosity.[6] Successful PABD among patients undergoing surgery for cancer has been reported.[22,23,33,34] PABD for cancer patients may be especially beneficial if studies confirm the possible harmful immunosuppressive effects of allogeneic blood transfusion that could lead to metastatic spread of tumor cells.[33-35]

## CONTRAINDICATIONS
### Age

Reservations against PABD in elderly patients probably stem from the assumption that they have limited cardiac reserve and diminished blood volume. Recent data show that the resting cardiac index in fit, active elderly persons is appropriate for their reduced skeletal muscle mass and metabolic rate.[36] Aging, in the absence of disease, produces little effect on circulating red blood cell (RBC) mass, the number or function of platelets, or coagulation.[37] For years, plasma volume has long been assumed to decrease with age in a manner similar to that for intracellular water. It is now realized that plasma volume appears to be well maintained in healthy and physically active men and women.[38] Therefore, age per se is not a contraindication to PABD. In assessing whether an elderly patient may undergo PABD or not, one must separate the effects of aging, per se, from the consequences of age-related diseases. Experience shows that elderly patients can successfully participate in a PABD as long as they are physically active, fit, and free from significant disease. Even those elderly patients who have never donated before, can successfully participate as autologous donors.[39,40] Furthermore, they have lower reaction rates following donation.[41] Needless to say, careful monitoring must be undertaken in these patients during blood donation.

Investigators have shown that autologous transfusion is ideally suited for use in children, adolescents, and young adults, since isoimmunization during youth can complicate future transfusion needs.[3,4] Children and young adults weighing less than 50 kg can safely donate blood, although the volume drawn at each donation is reduced in proportion to body weight.[42] Withdrawal of amounts equal to 10 to 15% of their blood volume is usually well tolerated. PABD has been extended to children as young as 4 years of age.[3] However, technical problems and lack of cooperation often make young children unlikely candidates for PABD. Cowell and Swickard[5] described an autologous transfusion program in 193 children undergoing various orthopedic procedures. These children ranged from 7 to 20 years in age (average age 14), and a total of 1 to 3 units were drawn from each before surgery. The amount of blood withdrawn at each donation was determined by the weight of the child (Table 6–1). The average preoperative decrease of hemoglobin in these children was 2.1 g/dL, resulting in a preoperative level of 11.5 g/dL.

## Bacteriemia

Probably the most important single contraindication to PABD is bacteriemia. Bacteria may proliferate during storage or transport. It is imperative to look for evidence of bacteriemia in the history and physical examination (e.g., osteomyelitis). The presence of bacteriemia should result in routine deferral of autologous donation.

## Decreased Oxygen Delivery

Conditions associated with significant decrease in oxygen delivery probably constitute a relative or absolute contraindication to PABD.[7,43,44] Obviously, medical judgment becomes a valuable tool under these circumstances. In patients with low fixed cardiac output, reduction of hemoglobin concentration may result in significant reduction in oxygen delivery. Similarly, hypoxemic patients (severe respiratory disease) may not be good candidates for PABD. Although most patients who are to undergo heart surgery are reasonable candidates for autologous donations, those with congestive failure, unstable or crescendo angina, critical aortic stenosis, or severe cyanotic congenital heart disease are usually not acceptable donors.

## Chronic Anemias

Chronically anemic patients usually have adequate compensatory mechanisms and adapt to lower hemoglobin levels. In asymptomatic, reasonably active chronically anemic patients, the lower limit of hemoglobin required for donation can be relaxed.[45] Under special circumstances when PABD is essential, and with agreement from the anesthesiologist and surgeon, blood may be drawn from chronically anemic patients whose hemoglobin level is lower than 10 g/dL. Goodnough and coworkers.[21] found that 39% of patients undergoing elective orthopedic procedures who did not donate autologous blood were anemic, suggesting that their physicians might not have considered them suitable candidates for PABD because of anemia. These patients also had a high prevalence of subsequent allogeneic blood exposure (49%). This suggests

**Table 6–1. Preoperative blood donation in children**

| Weight | Blood withdrawn (mL) (each donation) |
|---|---|
| < 30 kg | 100 mL |
| 30–35 kg | 250 mL |
| 36–42 kg | 325 mL |
| 43–48 kg | 400 mL |
| > 48 kg | 450 mL |

Blood collected at 4-day intervals.
Last donation at least 3 days before surgery.
From Cowell HR, Swickward JW: Autotransfusion in children's orthopaedics. *J Bone Joint Surg Br.* 1974; 56B:908, with permission.

that there is a dire need for early identification and treatment of anemia, such as iron therapy for iron-depleted patients to give these patients the same opportunity to participate in PABD as their autologous blood donor counterparts.[21,45]

PABD by patients with sickle cell anemia has been reported. This may be beneficial in patients for whom compatible blood is unavailable because of multiple RBC antibodies.[46-49] However, if sickle cell RBCs are frozen for storage, they become hypertonic with sequential washing solutions, and eventually lyse. This problem can be prevented by screening all African-American donors and using an alternate deglycerolization process if it is necessary to freeze sickle cell RBCs.[50,51]

In summary, absolute contraindications to PABD include bacteriemia, significant decrease in oxygen delivery, and the very young because of technical difficulties. Clinical judgment is vital when there are relative contraindications and when there is any concern that patients may not tolerate phlebotomy because of acute changes in blood volume. In some patients, a separate intravenous line may be established for infusion of isotonic saline or lactated Ringer's solution (1 to 2 times the volume of blood removed). This may help maintain an adequate circulatory volume following phlebotomy. Monitoring the cardiovascular function during and after blood withdrawal may be of utmost importance in critically ill patients.

## DRAWBACKS, CONCERNS AND PROBLEMS
### Reactions

The frequency of reactions during donation of autologous blood is similar to that among allogeneic donors. The reported reaction rate varies between 1.5 and 5.5%.[29,52-54] Most reactions are transient vasovagal attacks that require no treatment other than simple observation. They consist of light-headedness due to transient hypotension and bradycardia. In 10% of these reactions patients lose consciousness. These reactions are more common in women than in men, and occur more frequently among first-time donors. In a series of 187,000 allogeneic and 8900 autologous donors, Stehling[55] reported 2.4% reaction rate for allogeneic and 2.5% for autologous do-

nors. The incidence of reactions among first-time donors was 13% in both groups. In a study conducted by the American Red Cross, serious postdonation complications occurred in fewer than 1% of 5660 PABDs in outpatient, nonhospital settings. Donors who were younger than 17 years of age, weighed less than 45 kg, or had experienced reactions during earlier donations, were most likely to have a reaction. It is interesting that neither donors older than 75 years, nor those with a history of cardiac disease, had a higher reaction rate.[56] Intravenous volume replacement has been shown to decrease or prevent vascular events during PABD, and this should be used in patients scheduled for frequent phlebotomy who are known to have underlying cardiovascular disease.[57,58]

## Delay of Surgical Procedure

The optimal donation period begins 4 to 6 weeks prior to surgery. Some patients may have their surgery scheduled sooner. The benefit of delaying surgery in order to donate blood must be weighed against the risk of deterioration of the patient's condition. This is particularly important in patients with cancer or cardiovascular disease. It is also important to present to the patient alternatives to allogeneic blood transfusion, in addition to the risks and benefits of blood transfusion.

## Need for Allogeneic Blood Transfusion

Although PABD decreases the need for allogeneic blood, it does not completely eliminate the possibility that the patient may need it. The requirement for allogeneic blood depends on many factors, including the number of autologous units donated, type of operative procedure, previous surgery, complications, and whether other methods of blood conservation are utilized or not. In a study of 107 patients who donated between 1 and 6 units of blood (mean 3 units) before cardiac surgery, it was found that only 27% of patients undergoing first-time coronary artery bypass grafting required allogeneic blood. The likelihood of allogeneic transfusion being required was only 10% when 3 or more autologous units were available for transfusion.[31] Data collected from four medical centers revealed that patients undergoing radical prostatectomy lose 44% of their RCM.[22] Toy and associates found that PABD in these patients reduced the rate of transfusion of allogeneic blood from 66 to 20%.[22] Of the patients who donated 1 to 2 units, 32% received allogeneic blood; 14% of those who donated 3 units received allogeneic blood. Donation of 4 units decreased the allogeneic transfusion to 11%. However, only 44% of patients donated 3 units or more. As the number of units donated increased, the number of units not used also increased. Thus, they recommended the donation of 3 units of blood for autologous use for patients who undergo radical prostatectomy.[22] Obviously, the possible need for allogeneic blood, in addition to autologously donated blood, should be explained to and understood by the patient prior to surgery.

## Patient's Inconvenience and Fears

A major impediment to a successful program for PABD is inconvenience for the donor.[59] It has been estimated that a mean of 3.3 visits are required in order to donate 2 units of autologous blood.[60] These extra visits constitute inconvenience to the patient and additional work for the blood bank staff. Despite these inconveniences, concern over blood safety is the most important factor that motivates patients to become donors for autologous transfusion.[59] Deferral, a recognized problem in autologous donation, is mostly due to anemia.[45] Efforts to decrease the patient's inconvenience should be exerted as much as possible. This may be accomplished by having more community hospitals offering this service, or special "bloodmobiles" or donor sites arranged in cooperation with other local community hospitals, at times and places most convenient for the donors.[59]

A critical step in the successful development of an autologous blood transfusion program is physician recruitment and education.[59] As physicians become educated and knowledgeable about the benefits and applicability of autologous blood transfusion, they change their practice habits accordingly. The success of PABD also depends upon patients' cooperation. Patients frequently come up with a list of questions. Some patients are afraid that they may not receive their own blood. The blood bank staff should be prepared to assure these patients, answer their questions, and allay their anxiety.

## Cost

Blood donated for autologous use is slightly more expensive than that from the allogeneic blood supply.[61] Patients are frequently surprised when they discover that donating their own blood costs more than using allogeneic blood. Much of the additional cost can be attributed to the higher procurement cost (approximately $24/unit higher) of autologous blood.[61] Additional costs can also be traced to the collection of blood that is not required and is eventually discarded.[61] Because of concerns about the safety of unused autologous blood units for transfusion to other patients, only 15% of centers currently transfer unused autologous blood to the allogeneic blood supply.[61,62] Even at centers practicing autologous blood crossover, a substantial number of units become outdated before they can be transfused to other patients,[53] the costs of which are incurred by the institution.[61]

Procurement of autologous blood lacks the economies of scale of allogeneic blood collection. Cost effectiveness estimates are high because health benefits of autologous blood donation, the denominator of cost-effectiveness, are low.[61] Birkmeyer et al[61] analyzed the cost-effectiveness of PABD for total hip and knee replacement. Their elegant analysis suggests several ways to reduce the costs associated with PABD: (1) Surgeons can reduce the use of PABD in procedures with low transfusion requirements, by better educating and reassuring their patients about the diminishing risks of allogeneic blood; (2) They can also avoid unnecessary transfusion of autologous blood; and (3) Blood bankers can reassess implications of testing and crossover of autologous blood. It is obvious that the practice of PABD is not likely to be abandoned because of its economic implications and thus, efficient practice of PABD is a necessity. Improving the cost-effectiveness of PABD will become increasingly important as financial pressures on the health care delivery system place greater emphasis on the costs and prioritization of medical interventions.[61]

## CONTROVERSIAL ISSUES
### Testing of Blood Intended for Autologous Use

The 1993 Standards of the American Association of Blood Banks (AABB) specifically require tests on blood intended for autologous use; hepatitis B surface antigen (HbsAg), hepatitis C virus, and antibody to human immunodeficiency virus type 1 (anti-HIV-1) are required on all first autologous units drawn in a 30-day period, unless they remain in the hospital in which they are collected[12] (Table 6–2). In addition, the United States Food and Drug Administration (USFDA) memorandum (February 12, 1990) requires a serologic test for syphilis.[63] The no-test option is available only to hospital-based blood-drawing facilities; for community blood centers, partial testing is a must, and complete testing is often the only practical solution.[9]

Arguments advanced by proponents of minimal or no testing include cost saving, simplified bookkeeping, and avoidance of possible complications where a test is repeatedly reactive. In institutions in which crossover into the allogeneic blood pool is not performed, one might make a strong argument for eliminating testing on units intended for autologous use.[9] In contrast, complete testing renders crossover possible and helps avoid breaks in its standard operating procedures. However, a positive infectious disease test may create a conflict between the patient's right to privacy and the hospital team's right to information that would enable them to take additional precautions.[9]

### Release of Infectious Units

There is a divergence of opinion as to the disposition of units that test positive for an infectious disease. With the absence of firm guidelines, the practice varies considerably from institution to institution. The rationale for a liberal release policy is to protect the patient-donors from the adverse consequences of allogeneic blood exposure, regardless of their own infectious disease status. In contrast, the rationale for not releasing potentially infectious units is to protect health care workers, and to prevent the transmission of an infectious disease to another patient, should the blood be unintentionally transfused to the wrong patient.[9] Availability of more data may help us adopt a better approach in the near future.

### Crossover into the Allogeneic Blood Supply

Depending on patient-donor demographics and other factors, a substantial amount of preoperatively donated autologous blood might be available for allogeneic blood transfusion. Whether unused autologous blood should crossover into the allogeneic supply, remains a highly complex and controversial issue, centered around safety and logistical barriers.[9] Safety of autologous blood is determined by accurate history, frequency of viral markers, and appropriate decisions regarding crossover. Unfortunately, there is no agreement on whether the frequency of viral markers is an adequate measure of safety in a viral marker-negative cohort of donors.[15,56,64]

Silvergleid[9] points out that logistical barriers to widespread crossover are formidable. First, many of the unused units will be with-

**Table 6–2.  Serologic tests after collection of autologous blood**

| Test | AABB standards | IMCC standards |
|---|---|---|
| On unit | | |
| ABO/Rh | Required | Required* |
| Antibody screen | Optional | Required† |
| RPR | Optional | Required† |
| Anti-HIV-1/2 | Required | Required† |
| Anti-HTLV-I | Optional | Required† |
| HbsAG | Required | Required† |
| HBc | Optional | Required† |
| HCV | Required | Required† |
| ALT | Optional | Required† |
| Pretransfusion | | |
| ABO/Rh | Required | Required |
| Antibody screen | Optional | Required |
| Compatibility testing | Optional | Required |

* Each donation
† First donation during a 30 day period
AABB—American Association of Blood Banks; IMMC—Illinois Masonic Medical Center; RPR—rapid plasma reagin; anti-HIV-1/2—combination test for antigen for human immunodeficiency virus types 1 and 2; anti-HTLV-I—antigen for human T-lymphotrophic virus type I; HbsAg—hepatitis B surface antigen; HBc—hepatitis B core; HCV—hepatitis C virus; ALT—alanine aminotransferase. Modified form Kruskall MS: Autologous blood collection and transfusion in a tertiary-care center. In Taswell HF, Pineda AA, eds. Autologous transfusion and hemotherapy. Boston, MA: Blackwell Scientific Publications; 1991:53–77, with permission.

held until nearly outdated to ascertain that they will not be needed by the patient-donor. Second, of the blood donated, 85 to 90% will be used by the patient-donor, leaving the rest available for crossover. From these numbers, it is apparent that less than 10% of autologous units will actually be available for crossover. Given these numbers, and the geometric increase in the complexity of record keeping, documentation, and billing for such a small return, it is no surprise that crossover has become more the exception than the rule in recent years.[9] Recognizing these problems, most centers have abandoned the practice of crossover of preoperatively donated autologous blood into the allogeneic blood supply.

McVay and coworkers[11] provided useful data about the potential recruitment of autologous patient-donors into the allogeneic donor pool. They found that the majority of those recruited for allogeneic blood donation had been such donors, prior to donating for themselves. Since volunteerism is an essential ingredient in the safety of the blood supply, crossover might be restricted to those who had previously participated in the blood program. Other, equally-safe patient-donors whose first contact with the blood program occurs when they donate blood for themselves, might be targeted for special recruitment efforts that are potentially of greater yield than crossover would have been.[11]

## Indications for Transfusion of Autologous Blood

Preoperative autologous blood provides assurance and relative safety for the patient, for whom significant blood loss, during or after surgery, is a real possibility. However, the potential for an adverse outcome to transfusion is not entirely eliminated, merely because the patient will receive his or her own blood.[9] Hemolysis (due to improper handling), infection (bacterial contamination), and transfusion of the wrong unit (misidentification) are rare but recognized complications.

If the anticipated blood loss does not occur, autologous blood may become a risk, rather than a benefit, if transfused. The dangers of hypervolemia and pulmonary edema still exist and make it imperative to transfuse blood only when indicated. It may be reasonable to relax the transfusion "trigger" by transfusing a patient-donor with a hemoglobin $\leq 10$ g/dL rather than $\leq 8$ g/dL with his own autologous blood. However, one should resist the temptation to transfuse autologous blood merely to normalize the hemoglobin, replace lost iron, or promote wound healing, and also resist the temptation to transfuse it just because it is available and may be wasted if not given.[9,65]

## AUGMENTATION OF PREOPERATIVE BLOOD DONATION

Although various techniques for preoperative collection and storage have been described, AABB standards recommend a minimum 4-day interval between phlebotomies and at least 72 hours between the last phlebotomy and surgery. These minimum intervals are required to allow for synthesis and mobilization of proteins, as well as the return of plasma volume to normal. The commonly used schedule for donation is 1 unit a week. For adults, this permits preoperative acquisition of up to 4 units of blood with conventional storage techniques.

Not all donors can donate the number of autologous blood units that their physicians request prior to surgery.[35] As more units are requested, more donors become unable to donate the number of units requested. McVay et al[35] found that 72% of autologous blood donors were able to donate all units if 4 units were requested, whereas only 43% were able to donate all units if 5 units were requested, and 27% were able to donate all units if 6 units were requested. The amount of blood that can be donated preoperatively is limited by the normal 4° C storage period and the erythropoietic regenerative capability of the donor.[35] The shelf-life of RBCs stored in the liquid state can be prolonged to 42 days, when additive solutions (AS-1) are used. (See Chapter 1: Principles of Blood Transfusion) The erythropoietic regenerative capability of the donor and the success of PABD are strongly influenced by the predonation hemoglobin levels. Various methods have been advocated to augment the volume of blood that patients can safely donate preoperatively including: (1) freezing the RBCs to increase the duration of storage; (2) reinfusing citrated blood before it is outdated with simultaneous larger donations (piggyback technique); (3) iron therapy; or (4) recombinant human erythropoietin therapy to increase the rate of endogenous RBC production.

## Cryopreservation (Frozen Storage)

Autologous blood donated preoperatively, can be frozen to $-80°$ C and stored for future use. This is especially applicable if surgery is delayed. More than 80% of the RBCs stored frozen for 10 years can be expected to survive and function normally after transfusion.[47] Advantages of frozen RBCs over blood with added citrate-phosphate-dextrose (CPD) are: longer shelf-life and improved viability of RBCs because of normal levels of 2', 3'—diphosphoglycerate (2,3-DPG) and adenosine triphosphate (ATP); prevention of alloimmunization; a lower incidence of serum hepatitis and human leukocyte antigens (HLA); absence of hyperkalemia with massive transfusion; the possibility of salvaging outdated RBCs by freezing after restoration of 2,3-DPG and ATP; and the use of frozen cells initially intended for autologous use for future allogeneic transfusion.[51,66-74]

In those patients with rare blood types, or patients who have developed alloantibodies from previous transfusions or pregnancies, obtaining compatible blood may become very difficult, and in some cases, next to impossible. Whenever possible, these patients should be encouraged to donate autologous blood at regular intervals so that their blood can be frozen and stored for up to 10 years for future use. When transfusion is required, autologous deglycerolized RBCs can be obtained for these patients in a much more expeditious manner than would occur if the blood bank were faced with the task of screening random donors from the allogeneic donor pool.

Drawbacks of the use of frozen RBCs include: increased costs; unavailability except in large medical centers; 30-minute reconstitution time for each unit; and requirements that once thawed, the previously frozen RBCs must be infused within 24 hours, since longer storage may permit bacterial growth.[74,75] It has been demonstrated that hemolysis is greater after transfusion with frozen RBCs, than after transfusion with fresh blood.[70] Thus, frozen RBCs may not be optimal in patients with renal impairment because of the greater potential for hemolysis. Frozen,

thawed, deglycerolized, washed and resuspended RBCs have decreased levels of intracellular potassium. Intracellular potassium values as low as 4 mMol/$10^{12}$ RBCs can be found.[71] When these RBCs are transfused, potassium ions from the recipient plasma could move into these RBCs, which are low in potassium, thereby, decreasing the serum potassium level of the recipient. Rao and colleagues[76] demonstrated the occurrence of hypokalemia when frozen, thawed RBCs are transfused into patients with normal serum potassium levels. This could be important when frozen RBCs are administered in patients needing massive transfusions, in infants requiring exchange transfusions, and in the presence of other factors associated with low serum potassium levels including alkalemia, hypocapnia, and blood glucose changes.[76] When large amounts of frozen RBCs are administered, it is advisable to monitor serum potassium levels of the recipient, and if hypokalemia occurs, potassium supplementation should be instituted to correct it and prevent occurrence of arrhythmias.

## The Piggyback Technique

The piggyback technique allows collection of 2 to 4 units of fresh blood and up to 6 units of fresh frozen plasma (FFP) before surgery.[43,77] In this technique, blood is stored in CPD solution for 2 weeks, and reinfused as progressively larger volumes of blood are withdrawn. Plasma is separated from the blood after withdrawal and frozen to preserve coagulation factors. A similar "leapfrog" technique, by which 3 or more units of the patient's blood could be obtained before surgery, with none being older than 10 to 14 days, has been described.[43,78] (Fig. 6–1). Although this technique may be valuable in rare patients for whom compatible blood is difficult to obtain, the high cost, availability of newer additive solutions to prolong storage, and the risks involved, including bacteremia, hemolysis, and administration of the wrong unit of blood, made this technique obsolete and of historic interest only.

## Increasing Endogenous Red Cell Production

### IRON THERAPY

In patients with normal hematopoiesis, the bone marrow replenishes lost RBCs after

**CITRATED BLOOD**
**(Piggyback Technique)**
**Storage Duration — 21 days**

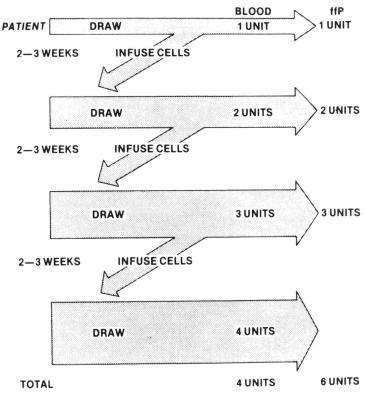

**Fig. 6–1.**  The withdrawal of blood followed by reinfusion and withdrawal of additional units at two- to three-week intervals is useful in collecting fresh blood and fresh-frozen plasma (ffP) in patients with rare blood types or antibodies who require elective operation. Reproduced from Utley JR, Moores WY, Stephens DB: Blood conservation techniques. Ann Thorac Surg. 1981; 31:482, with permission.

blood withdrawal. Marrow reticulocytes appear in the circulation as early as 6 hours after phlebotomy, but a full marrow production (releasing mature RBCs) is not usually reached until 8 to 10 days later.[79,80] Weekly donations (for several weeks) stimulate erythropoiesis by 1.5 times.[81-83] This beneficial effect is lost when a single unit is donated a few days preoperatively. With iron therapy, however, the marrow can double or triple production, and this response can be maintained over several weeks, even with repeated phlebotomies. Studies revealed that preoperative withdrawal of blood is better tolerated if iron supplementation is given.[4] In patients undergoing weekly phlebotomy without added iron, the HCT decreased from 44 to 33% over an 8-week period. In patients who received iron, it decreased from 44 to 38%

during the same period.[84] Oral iron therapy has been shown to be almost as effective as parenteral iron.[82,85,86] In view of the side effects of parenteral iron administration, the oral route is the preferred method.[87,88] The recommended dose is 325 mg, 3 times daily with meals.[89,90] It is preferable to begin iron therapy at least 1 month prior to the first donation, and continue therapy for several months after the last donation.[12]

Because women have less iron reserves than men, fewer women are able to donate as may units as men. McVay et al[35] found that 86% of men were able to donate 4 units with no deferrals for anemia, as compared to 42% of women. In one study,[91] estimates of total iron reserves were 309 mg in premenopausal women and 608 mg in postmenopausal women, whereas men had an average of 776 mg. Since 1-mL RBCs contains an average of 1 mg of iron, the average autologous blood unit donated with an average of 178 mL RBCs contains 178 mg of iron.[35,92] Therefore, without supplemental iron, the premenopausal women have iron reserves sufficient to donate only an average of 1.7 units, whereas a man can donate an average of 4.4 units.[35] Correction of any iron deficiency in women may permit donation of more units. Since elective surgery is sometimes contemplated several months before it is performed, it might be helpful to determine hemoglobin levels and the iron reserves in female patients.[35] If low hemoglobin levels and low iron stores are present, supplemental iron should be administered months before PABD is anticipated.[35]

## RECOMBINANT HUMAN ERYTHROPOIETIN THERAPY

Erythropoietin, a glycoprotein hormone primarily synthesized in the kidney, is the main regulator of RBC production. Erythropoietin levels increase in response to a decrease in oxygen delivery, resulting in increased RBC production, accelerated hemoglobin formation, and premature movement of RBCs into the circulation.[93] The human gene responsible for the production of erythropoietin has recently been cloned, and the recombinant product, epoetin (rHu EPO or EPO), has been made available. The apparent volume of distribution of intravenous EPO approximates the plasma volume. Its efficacy in the treatment of anemia associated with chronic renal dysfunction has been demonstrated. Benefits in these patients include reduced need for blood transfusions, amelioration of symptoms related to anemia, and improved quality of life.[93] Anemias associated with rheumatoid arthritis, sickle cell disease, acquired immune deficiency syndrome, cancer, and prematurity are potential indications. The most frequent adverse effect associated with EPO therapy is hypertension. However, this seems to be limited to patients with chronic renal disease.[94,95] Other less common side effects include thrombocytosis, hyperkalemia, rise in serum urea, iron deficiency, and flu-like symptoms. No drug interactions have been reported.[93,96] The availability of EPO has marked a new era, not only in the therapeutic management of

anemia, but also in enhancing PABD as a blood conservation measure.[89,97,98]

Although PABD provides an inherent and powerful endogenous erythropoietic stimulus to counteract the decrease in hemoglobin levels, the response may not be sufficient to result in maximal marrow erythropoiesis.[83,89] Thus, the success of PABD is limited by the time required for the accumulation of a sufficient amount of blood, and the resultant erythropoietic response. About 40% of patients requested by their physicians to donate blood, could not donate more than 4 units because of ensuing anemia.[99] Furthermore, in patients with coronary artery disease, marked changes in hemoglobin levels may provoke or worsen myocardial ischemia.[100,101] The availability of EPO has prompted a multi-institutional study to investigate its effect in preventing the development of anemia and increasing the procurement of autologous blood in patients before surgery.[89] Its efficacy in increasing the procurement of autologous blood in animals has been reported.[102]

Goodnough and coworkers[89] conducted a randomized control trial of erythropoietin in 47 adults scheduled for elective orthopedic procedures. All patients received iron sulfate 325 mg orally, 3 times daily. Blood was scheduled to be collected from each patient twice a week for 3 weeks, for a maximal collection of 6 units. At each visit for blood collection, the patients received either EPO 600 units/kg or placebo intravenously, whether or not blood was actually collected. Patients were excluded from donation if the HCT was less than 34%. The mean number of units collected per patient was 5.4 for the EPO group and 4.1 for the placebo group. The mean RBC volume donated by the patients who received EPO, was 41% greater than the volume donated by the patients who received placebo (961 versus 683 mL) (Figs. 6–2, 6–3, 6–4). Only 4% of the EPO-treated patients were unable to donate more than 4 units, as compared with 29% of patients receiving placebo. Other clinical trials have shown that the use of EPO can facilitate PABD and reduce allogeneic blood transfusions in autologous blood donors who are anemic at first donation.[103] Some studies demonstrated a dose-response effect of EPO on RBC volume expansion[58,] while others did not find any difference between the effects of 300 units and 600 Units/

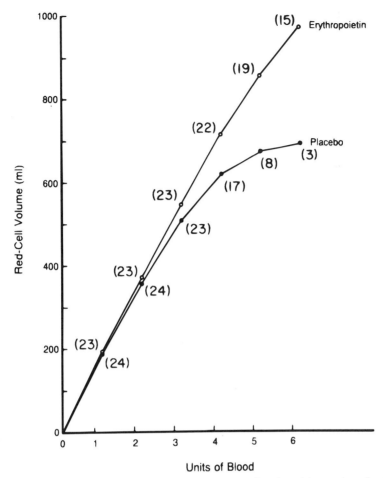

**Fig. 6–2.**  Cumulative red blood cell volume donated per patient as a function of the number of units donated. The numbers in parentheses are the numbers of patients donating blood. The mean cumulative interval between base line and each visit was 3.5 days for visit 1, 7.1 for visit 2, 10.6 for visit 3, 14.2 for visit 4, 17.6 for visit 5, and 20.9 for visit 6. Reproduced from Goodnough LT, Rudnick S, Price TH, et al. Increased preoperative collection of autologous blood with recombinant human erythropoietin therapy. N Engl J Med 1989; 321:1163, with permission.

kg.[103] The ability of EPO to enhance the procurement of autologous blood is now unquestioned.[89,102-105] Its efficacy has led to its wide use as an adjuvant therapy to PABD.[106-110] Without EPO, comparable amounts of autologous blood can be obtained only by prolonging the donation period beyond 3 weeks. By procuring more autologous blood before surgery, there is a greater reduction, or even elimination, of the need for allogeneic blood transfusion.[103] In a recent study of patients undergoing coronary artery surgery, only 1 patient out of 12 receiving EPO required allogeneic blood at surgery, as compared to 8 out of 12 patients who did not receive EPO.[98] It must be emphasized that adequate iron support is a critical factor in the efficacy of treatment. In contrast to anemic patients, no clinical benefit could be demonstrated in autologous donors who were not anemic (HCT > 39%) at first donation.[58] This implies that EPO therapy may not be cost effective in nonanemic patients, even if there is some reduction in the use of allogeneic blood in these patients.

The therapeutic schedules of EPO therapy reported in the literature have short time intervals and high administration frequencies. Some programs required up to nine visits to the hospital or even admission.[110] These requirements had high psychological and physical demands on the patients. Kulier and associates[98] advocated a single weekly dose of EPO (400 units/kg), administered subcutaneously once a week as an outpatient, starting 4 weeks before surgery, combined with 270 mg of iron sulfate and 0.35 of folate by mouth, daily. They found this protocol stimulated erythropoiesis efficiently and compensated for the hemoglobin decrease following donation, which was scheduled once a week. Although peak concentrations of EPO are lower after subcutaneous injection than after intravenous administration, they remain at relatively high levels for up to 24 hours.[96,111] The subcutaneous injection may provide a more constant and more efficient stimulus for erythropoiesis and thus, a smaller dose may be required.[98] In this donation program, patients spent 2 hours at the hospital once a week. This resulted in higher acceptance and motivation. It is possible that subcutaneous administration results in fewer side reactions, as compared to intravenous administration. The authors reported slight pain at the site of injection which was attributed to the volume injected (3 mL per injection).

The efficacy of EPO in increasing PABD is due to increased RBC production through the accelerated conversion of stored iron into circulating iron.[89] Since the initial level of circulating hemoglobin iron is calculated on the basis of blood volume and hemoglobin levels, these two values predict the success of donation in autologous blood donors. Patients who would most benefit from EPO therapy are those with smaller blood volume (such as women), those who are anemic, those with rare blood groups, and those who refuse blood transfusions.[35,89] In these patients, the postoperative administration of EPO may also be useful to accelerate postoperative erythropoiesis.[104] EPO is most useful when relatively large donations are needed, such as in major orthopedic and cardiac surgery, and when maximum collection of blood is needed in a short period (3 weeks).

## PHYSIOLOGICAL EFFECTS OF PREOPERATIVE BLOOD DONATION

In the original technique of PABD, no colloids or crystalloids are infused simultaneously. Consequently, the technique has been described as "hypovolemic hemodilution" to distinguish it from "acute normovolemic hemodilution," a technique that includes phlebotomy immediately after, or sometime after, anesthetic induction and simultaneous hemodilution with a cell-free substitute to maintain a near-normal circulating blood volume.

The major objection to PABD is the "fear" that preoperative phlebotomy will make the patient less fit for the stress of surgery because of the contracted blood volume, and the "presumption" of the patient's inability to compensate fully for the decreased RBC mass. Studies have revealed that the majority of patients can easily tolerate preoperative withdrawal of blood.[4] After the withdrawal of 15% of the blood volume, the plasma volume is replenished more rapidly than the RBC mass. Although no colloids or crystalloids are ordinarily given, full restoration of plasma volume occurs over a period of 12 to 24 hours, as a result of transcapillary refill of the extravascular fluid and protein, immediate increase of albumin production, and a renin-angiotensin response. Therefore, the term hypovolemic hemodilution is not an exact description of the physiologic responses to PABD, and merely indicates that fluids are not simultaneously administered. Erythropoiesis is known to be stimulated by multiple PABD. This beneficial effect often extends well into the postoperative period.

Enhancements in public awareness of the advantages of PABD have resulted in an increased number of highly motivated, but medically high-risk patients, requesting participation.[112] Hemodynamics were studied to assess the relative risk of PABD in 25 high-risk patients with histories of angina, hypertension, myocardial infarction, congestive heart failure, arrhythmias, cerebrovascular disease, or transient ischemia attacks.[57] These patients were on various medications including antihypertensives, nitrates, $\beta$-adrenergic blockers, calcium channel blockers, antiarrhythmics, or digoxin. Decreases in blood pressure were observed during PABD and were most pronounced when patients were asked to sit upright. These changes seemed to be related to a fall in preload. Heart rate remained unaltered throughout the observation period. Contrary to healthy patients who can adequately compensate for donation of 10% of their blood volume by increasing their heart rate, these high-risk patients could not adequately compensate for the fall in pre-load.[57] This is to be expected in patients with angina or myocardial infarction who are receiving β-adrenergic or calcium channel blockers. Despite fluid therapy (500 mL), three patients had their phlebotomy prematurely terminated due to hypotension. One patient with a history of transient ischemic attacks had a near syncopal episode which responded to oxygen and rapid fluid administration.

Because of concern that some patients might not tolerate the acute hypovolemia that initially occurs with PABD, some centers recommend starting a second intravenous line for simultaneous replacement with an equal volume of isotonic saline.[45] Other crystalloids, such as lactated Ringer's solution, may be used instead of isotonic saline. Although an equal volume of a crystalloid is not necessarily adequate to maintain normovolemia, and eventually traverse the vascular endothelium to the extravascular space, it allows better acclimatization to acute blood loss. Intravenous replacement with a crystalloid solution is recommended in patients with cardiovascular disease. Although it has not been recommended for routine PABD, it may become an accepted prophylactic measure in the near future.

# PROCEDURES FOR PREOPERATIVE AUTOLOGOUS BLOOD DONATION
## Donor Recruitment/ Referral/Scheduling

Multicenter studies suggest that PABD for elective surgery is still underutilized.[61,90,113] Successful autologous donor programs depend upon the level of cooperation between the attending physician and the blood bank staff. Selection of candidates for a PABD program begins in the doctor's office. Patients whose anticipated transfusion requirement has been determined as 3 to 4 units will benefit most from the autologous program. With the advent of computerization, many institutions with active PABD programs have developed systems which flag patients who might be potential autologous donors. In many systems, the attending physician is notified that a patient is a potential candidate for PABD when the patient's operative procedure is scheduled.

Anticipated usage should be carefully reviewed prior to sending the patient to the blood bank. Those patients who are not expected to lose blood should not be encouraged to donate autologous units. Drawing such patients places undue concern on the patient and wastes valuable laboratory resources.[60] Patients who are currently bacteriemic or demonstrate symptoms of acute cardiac or cerebrovascular disease, i.e., angina, recent seizures, symptomatic aortic stenosis, or valvular lesions, should be screened carefully before participation in an autologous program.[92] Within the subset of patients in whom transfusion is anticipated, those who are generally in good health, weigh at least 40 kg and have adequate antecubital veins to facilitate multiple venipuncture with 16-gauge needles, should be chosen as candidates for the program. Many pediatric patients are ideal candidates, with the limiting factors being venous access and the ability of the child to cooperate.

Blood may be drawn no more frequently than every 3 days. Blood banks prefer that hemoglobin and HCT levels should be 11 g/ dL or 33%, respectively, at the time of donation. The interval between donations should be a minimum of 72 hours to allow time for the RBC mass to become completely diluted and the HCT to stabilize. The last donation should be completed at least 3 days prior to surgery. Current anticoagulants allow storage for 35 days [citrate-phosphate-dextrose-adenine, formula 1 (CPDA-1)] or 42 days (AS-1). Through careful coordination with surgical staff, many donors can donate 1 unit a week for 4 weeks, and still have 7 days for the patient-donor's hemoglobin level to recover.

## Donor Room Policies & Procedures

When the candidate for PABD presents to the blood bank, it is imperative that the blood bank staff carefully screen the patient. The blood bankers' dictum "first do no harm to the donor," gains new meaning when dealing with patients desiring to predeposit blood for future use. It is crucial that the donor room staff utilize recruitment techniques similar to those used for routine allogeneic blood donors, to give the autologous donors all the

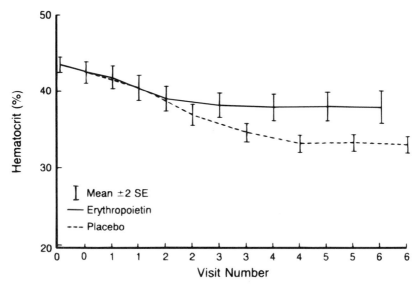

**Fig. 6–3.** Mean hematocrits for each group before the study and at visits 1 through 6. Reproduced from Goodnough LT, Rudnick S, Price TH, and others: Increased preoperative collection of autologous blood with recombinant human erythropoietin therapy. N Engl J Med 1989; 321:1163, with permission.

encouragement necessary to continue in their program. Although preoperative phlebotomy may be performed only at the written request of the patient's physician, it is the responsibility of the drawing facility's medical director to determine, prospectively, the suitability of

each prospective donor prior to each donation.[12]

Each visit to the blood bank begins with a brief interview and obtaining the patient-donor's consent for the phlebotomy, as well as for any disease testing, which will be per-

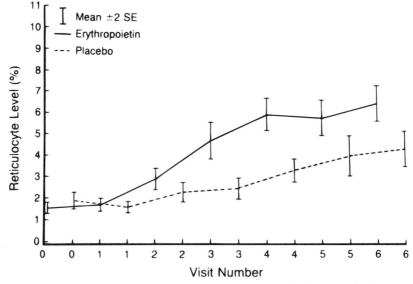

**Fig. 6–4.** Mean reticulocyte counts each group before the study and at visits 1 through 6. The reticulocyte count was corrected for the change in the hematocrit at each visit by the following formula: corrected reticulocyte count = percentage of counted reticulocytes × (measured hematocrit/initial hematocrit). Reproduced from Goodnough LT, Rudnick S, Price TH, and others: Increased preoperative collection of autologous blood with recombinant human erythropoietin therapy. N Engl J Med 1989; 321:1163, with permission.

PATIENT NAME_____ DOB_____
PHYSICIAN_____SSN_____MR_____
PROCEDURE_____DATE OF PROCEDURE_____

The purpose and advantages of autologous transfusion and the risks involved have been explained to me.   Any questions I have regarding autologous transfusion have been answered to my satisfaction.   I understand the following precautions:

1.   I should contact either the Blood Bank or my personal physician should I feel faint, weak, light headed or dizzy after the unit of blood is drawn.
2.   That if the scheduled procedure is delayed for any reason, it will be necessary to discard the unit if more than 35 days have elapsed since the unit was drawn.
3.   I understand that my blood will be tested for the HIV-1&2 viruses (AIDS), HTLV 1 virus, hepatitis C virus, hepatitis B virus and syphilis.   I consent to the notification of my personal physician of the results of these tests, should any of them be positive.

I consent to the withdrawal of blood for autologous transfusion purposes by staff members of the Blood Bank.

| # | SIGNATURE | WITNESS | DATE | UNIT NUMBER | VOL | LOT NUMBER | PHLEB | MD REVIEW |
|---|-----------|---------|------|-------------|-----|------------|-------|-----------|
|   |           |         |      |             |     |            |       |           |
|   |           |         |      |             |     |            |       |           |
|   |           |         |      |             |     |            |       |           |
|   |           |         |      |             |     |            |       |           |

AUTOLOGOUS DONOR PROGRAM
ILLINOIS MASONIC MEDICAL CENTER-DONOR SERVICE, 836 WELLINGTON,CHICAGO, ILLINOIS

| Donation date | Hct (≥33%) | Temp. ≤99.5F | BP 90-180 50-100 | Pulse 50-100 | Weight ≥110 | Tech |
|---------------|------------|--------------|------------------|--------------|-------------|------|
|               |            |              |                  |              |             |      |
|               |            |              |                  |              |             |      |
|               |            |              |                  |              |             |      |
|               |            |              |                  |              |             |      |

| MEDICAL HISTORY | Yes | No |  | Yes | No |  | Yes | No |
|-----------------|-----|----|--|-----|----|--|-----|----|
| Heart disease   |     |    | Hepatitis |     |    | Bleeding tendencies |     |    |
| Lung disease    |     |    | Diabetes |     |    | Dental work (3 days) |     |    |
| Liver Disease   |     |    | Epilepsy or seizures |     |    | Other medical disorders |     |    |
| Blood disorder  |     |    | Skin infections |     |    | Medications (list) |     |    |

| Unit number | Exp. date | Type & Rh | IDAT | DAT | HBSAg | Anti HBc | Anti HCV | STS | alt | HIV 1-2 | HTLV 1 | Tech |
|-------------|-----------|-----------|------|-----|-------|----------|----------|-----|-----|---------|--------|------|
|             |           |           |      |     |       |          |          |     |     |         |        |      |

| Unit Number | Exp. Date | Type | Tech | Unit Number | Exp. Date | Type | Tech | Unit Number | Exp. Date | Type | Tech |
|-------------|-----------|------|------|-------------|-----------|------|------|-------------|-----------|------|------|
|             |           |      |      |             |           |      |      |             |           |      |      |

**Fig. 6–5.**   Illinois Masonic Medical Center Blood Bank Form used to document donor demographic data, history, physical, serology and disease testing at the time of each autologous donation. Based upon FDA guidelines and AABB standards.

**Table 6–3.   Criteria for homologous and autologous blood donation**

| Donor characteristics | Homologous AABB Standards | Autologous AABB Standards | Autologous IMMC Standards |
|---|---|---|---|
| Age (years) | 17–65 | No limit | No limit |
| HGB (gm/dL) | 12.5 | 11.0 | 11.0* |
| HCT (%) | 38.0 | 33.0 | 33.0* |
| Blood pressure (mm Hg) | < 180/100 | Not specified | * |
| Pulse (beats/min) | 50–100 | Not specified | * |
| Donation frequency | 8 weeks | Not specified | As tolerated |
| Bacterial infection | Defer | Defer | Defer |
| Pregnancy | Defer | Not specified | Third trimester |
| Heart disease | Defer | Not specified | Draw† |
| High risk groups (HIV or hepatitis) | Defer | Not specified | Defer |

* Values falling outside AABB Standards must be approved by the Blood Bank Medical Director.
† Exclude only patients with unstable angina or critical aortic stenosis.
AABB—American Association of Blood Banks; IMMC—Illinois Masonic Medical Center; HIV—Human Immunodeficiency Virus.
Modified from Kruskall MS: Autologous blood collection and transfusion in a tertiary-care center. In: Taswell HF, Pineda AA, eds. Autologous transfusion and hemotherapy. Boston, MA: Blackwell Scientific Publications; 1991: 53–77, with permission.

formed during donor processing. A trained staff member, working directly under the guidance and supervision of the facility's medical director, will take a brief medical history, which assures protection of the patient and safety of donation (Fig. 6–5A, B). This history is designed to elicit underlying conditions that are contraindicated in blood donors. Autologous donors need not meet all the criteria established for routine allogeneic donors (Table 6–3). After the interview and history are completed, a brief physical examination is performed. The minimum weight for a standard donation of 450 mL is 50 kg. No more than 12% of the estimated blood volume is usually withdrawn at any one donation. If the donor weighs less than 50 kg, the amount of anticoagulant used should be decreased to accommodate a reduction of the volume of blood drawn. Hemoglobin, pulse, and blood pressure determinations must be performed at the time of the donation. If the hemoglobin falls below 11.0 g/dL (HCT 33%) or if any indications of severe hypertension, hypotension, or arrhythmias are observed, the blood bank medical director should be consulted.

Autologous units are drawn with a standard blood donor collection bag utilizing CPDA-1 or AS-1. Under sterile conditions, the technologist places a 16-gauge needle intravenously (usually the antecubital vein is used). Sterile docking devices now are available which will allow the technologist to replace the standard 16-gauge needle with a smaller needle. If the gauge of the replacement needle is too small, however, the rate of blood collection will be too slow and the blood may clot in the tubing prior to reaching the blood-anticoagulant mixture in the collection bag. In general, the procedure should take only 10 to 15 minutes to perform. After the donation is complete, the patient is given light refreshment and assured of the importance of the donation.

Recently, PABD has been undertaken in high-risk patients with histories of hypertension, coronary artery disease, myocardial infarction, congestive heart failure, and cerebrovascular disease. The risk of hemodynamic compromise and aggravation of preexisting disease states, justify appropriate monitoring of high-risk patients during PABD.[57] With their hemodynamic expertise, anesthesiologists are the most appropriate specialists to monitor and enhance the safety of high-risk patients during blood donation. In these patients, PABD is preferably done in the hospital's postanesthesia care unit where patients can be carefully monitored and observed. Oxygen, fluids, and other measures may need to be given when necessary. Such a service requires coordination and cooperation of the blood bank personnel, anesthesiologists, and recovery room nurses.

## Donor Deferrals

Transfusion medicine specialists have long touted the benefits of autologous donation.

However, in many cases, PABD is not a viable option. Preexisting medical conditions can preclude some patients from participating in such programs; communication between the attending physician and the blood bank medical director is essential to define the risk versus benefit, in an acutely ill patient. Other patients who begin the program may be forced to drop out because of limited venous access, low hemoglobin, or inability of bone marrow to mount an adequate response, even with iron or EPO. Many facilities will not allow participation of those patients whose first donation revealed positive disease testing. In such situations, the risk of exposure to personnel or possible error, and subsequent issue of units testing positive for any of the infectious disease markers to the general inventory, outweigh the potential benefit to the patient. It is essential that these patients be reassured, that even though they could not donate enough blood to satisfy their anticipated transfusion needs, blood from the allogeneic donor pool will be available to them when required.

## Component Preparation

Immediately following donation, FFP can be prepared from autologous whole blood. (See Chapter 1: Principles of Blood Transfusion.) Under certain circumstances, collection of autologous plasma or platelet donations may be indicated. Current apheresis equipment allows efficient collection of single donor platelets and plasma from patients whose condition is stable enough to tolerate these more types of demanding donations. Close communication between the attending physician and the apheresis team is essential if apheresis donation is desired.

## Donor Testing/Labeling/Storage

All autologous units must be tested and labelled in accordance with AABB and USFDA guidelines. (Fig. 6–6). (See Chapter 1: Principles of Blood Transfusion.) In addition, the AABB requires that autologous units be stored under the same conditions mandated for allogeneic blood, but that they be segregated from the allogeneic units to prevent accidental issue to the general inventory. Minimum testing mandated by the USFDA and the AABB includes determination of the ABO and Rh type, hepatitis B surface antigen, hepatitis C virus, anti HIV-1, and syphilis serology (Table 6–2). If crossing the unit over to the allogeneic donor pool is a possibility, all testing must be done, and standard labeling procedures followed.

Collection Date | Unit Number | EXPIRES FORM #AUTO #1

CPDA-1 WHOLE BLOOD

00160

Approx. 450 mL
plus 63 mL CPDA-1.
Store at 1-6° C.

ABO ______
Rh ______

See circular of information for indications, contraindications, cautions and methods of infusion.

AUTOLOGOUS DONOR

This product may transmit infectious agents.
Caution: Federal law prohibits dispensing without a prescription.
PROPERLY IDENTIFY INTENDED RECIPIENT

ILLINOIS MASONIC
MEDICAL CENTER
836 W. Wellington
Chicago, Illinois 60657
#147653

DONOR ______
DONOR SIGNATURE ______
Social Security # ______ Date of Birth ______

**Fig. 6–6.** Illinois Masonic Medical Center Blood Bank autologous donor program unit label.

Prior to transfusion, the same pretransfusion testing protocol used for allogeneic transfusion should be followed. It is imperative that a mechanism be in place which assures that all autologous units be transfused prior to any allogeneic units. Computer-assisted programs in which autologous units are released preferentially are available, and many institutions have developed manual programs which accomplish the same goal. A workable program developed at Illinois Masonic Medical Center prior to computerization consisted of a tie-tag system. At the time of donation, a two-part tag was placed on the unit. The tag was split at the perforation and the donor was given the "Deposit Card" at each donation. The donor was instructed to present all of the cards to the nursing staff on admission. The cards are then sent to the transfusion service when the pretransfusion blood specimen is drawn, alerting the blood bank that this donor has autologous units available.

## Program Development and Implementation

Increased public demand for alternatives to anonymous sources of blood products has facilitated the growth of both hospital-based and blood center-based autologous donor programs. In an effort to promote good community relations, most major blood suppliers have expanded their collection facilities to include autologous donor services, at fixed site locations, as well as at mobile donor sites. Logistically, the actual collection is easily accomplished since facilities, equipment, and personnel required to draw donors are already in place. Each blood center has developed its own unique set of autologous donation policies and procedures based on national guidelines and standard of care within the local health community. The major logistical problems in the blood center setting include making sure that the autologous donations remain separate from routine allogeneic blood donations, and routing the autologous blood products to the appropriate transfusion service in time for the patient's surgical procedure.

One of the major advantages of a hospital-based autologous program is that the units do not have to be shipped to another facility, making it much easier to ensure that the patient's units will be available when needed. In hospitals which do not already have a donor room, establishing an autologous program is a major undertaking. Feasibility studies determining the number of anticipated autologous donation must be done. It may be more feasible to send autologous donors to the local blood center than to develop a new program within the hospital. If the decision is made to initiate an in-house autologous donor program, donor room policies and procedures conforming to AABB and USFDA guidelines must be developed. A location suitable for drawing donors must be identified. This location must afford the donor privacy while being close enough to emergency medical assistance if required. Other location considerations should include easy access for donors confined to wheelchairs, adequate space for screening areas, donor lounge chairs, phlebotomy supplies, and emergency equipment, as well as a cheerful atmosphere which helps maintain the positive attitude of the donor-patient.

Personnel requirements will vary with each program, however, nurses, medical technologists, emergency medical technicians, or paramedics are all good candidates for staffing donor rooms. Donor room phlebotomists must be trained not only in the required phlebotomy procedures, but also must be able to handle emergency situations during phlebotomy and recovery, as well as relate to the emotional requirements of the donor-patient. In smaller programs, the donor room phlebotomist usually becomes a jack-of-all-trades, caring for the patient-donor, scheduling future donations, and being the clerk/receptionist in the donor area.

## REFERENCES

1. Grant FC. Autotransfusion. Ann Surg. 1921; 74: 253.
2. Fantus B. Blood preservation. JAMA. 1937; 109: 128.
3. Cuello L, Vasquez E, Rios R, et al. Autologous blood transfusion in thoracic and cardiovascular surgery. Surgery. 1967; 62:814.
4. Newman MM, Hamstra R, Block M. Use of banked autologous blood in elective surgery. JAMA. 1971; 218:861.
5. Cowell HR, Swickard JW. Autotransfusion in children's orthopaedics. J Bone Joint Surg Am. 1974; 56A:908.
6. Milles G, Langston H, Dalessandro W. Autologous Transfusion. Springfield, IL: Charles C Thomas; 1974.
7. Brzica SM, Pineda AA, Taswell HF. Autologous blood transfusion. Mayo Clin Proc. 1976; 51:723.
8. Silvergleid AJ. Autologous transfusions: experience in a community blood center. JAMA. 1979; 241: 2724.
9. Silvergleid AJ. Preoperative autologous donation: what have we learned? Transfusion. 1991; 31:99.
10. Surgenor DM, Wallace EL, Hao SHS, et al. Collection and transfusion of blood in the United States, 1982—1988. N Engl J Med. 1990; 322:1646.
11. McVay PA, Fung HC, Toy PTCY. Return of autologous blood donors as homologous blood donors. Transfusion. 1991; 31:119.
12. Widman FK. Standards for Blood Banks and Transfusions Services. 14th ed. Arlington, VA: American Association of Blood Banks; 1991.
13. Friedman BA. An analysis of surgical blood use in United States hospital with application to the maximum surgical blood order schedule. Transfusion. 1979; 19:268.
14. Druzin ML, Wolf CFW, Edersheim TG, et al. Donation of blood by the pregnant patient for autologous transfusion. Am J Obstet Gynecol. 1988; 159: 1023.
15. Kruskall MS, Popovsky MA, Pacini DG, et al. Autologous versus homologous donors: evaluation of markers for infectious disease. Transfusion. 1988; 28:286.
16. McVay PA, Hoag RW, Hoag MS, et al. Safety and use of autologous blood donation during the third trimester of pregnancy. Am J Obstet Gynecol. 1989; 160:1479.
17. Andres RL, Piacquadio KM, Resnik R. A reappraisal of the need for autologous blood donation in the obstetric patient. Am J Obstet Gynecol. 1990; 163: 1551.
18. Kruskall MS, Leonard SS, Klapholz N. Autologous blood donation during pregnancy: analysis of safety and blood use. Obstet Gynecol. 1987; 70:938.

19. Thompson JD, Callaghan JJ, Savory CG, et al. Prior deposition of autologous blood in elective orthopaedic surgery. J Bone Joint Surg Br. 1987; 69B: 320.

20. Woolson ST, Marsh JS, Tanner JB. Transfusion of previously deposited autologous blood for patients undergoing hip-replacement surgery. J Bone Joint Surg Am. 1987; 69A:325.

21. Goodnough LT, Vizmeg K, Marcus RE. Blood lost and transfused in patients undergoing elective orthopedic operation. Surg Gyncol Obstet. 1993; 176:235.

22. Toy PTCY, Menozzi D, Strauss RG, et al. Efficacy of preoperative donation of blood for autologous use in radical prostatectomy. Transfusion. 1993; 33:721.

23. Yamada AH, Lieskovsky G, Skinner DG, et al. Impact of autologous transfusions on patients undergoing radical prostatectomy using hypotensive anesthesia. J Urol. 1993; 149:73.

24. Bhasin R, Mahapatra AK, Banerji AK. Autotransfusion in neurosurgical operations. J Indian Med Assoc. 1993; 91:162.

25. Tulloh BR, Brakespear CP, Bates SC, et al. Autologous predonation, haemodilution and intraoperative blood salvage in elective abdominal aortic aneurysm repair. Br J Surg. 1993; 80:313.

26. O'Hara PJ, Hertzer NR, Krajewski LP, et al. Reduction in the homologous blood requirement for abdominal aortic aneurysm repair by the use of preadmission autologous blood donation. Surgery. 1994; 115:69.

27. Yomtovian R, Kruskall MS, Barber JP. Autologous blood transfusion: the reimbursement dilemma. J Bone Joint Surg Am. 1992; 74A:1265.

28. Goodnough LT, Shafron D, Marcus RE. Utilization and effectiveness of autologous blood donation for arthroplastic surgery. J Arthroplasty. 1990; 5:89.

29. Mann M, Sacks HJ, Goldfinger D. Safety of autologous blood donation prior to elective surgery for a variety of potentially "high risk" patients. Transfusion. 1983; 23:229.

30. Love TR, Hendren WG, O'Keife DO, et al. Transfusion of predonated autologous blood in elective cardiac surgery. Ann Thorac Surg. 1987; 43:508.

31. Owings DV, Kruskall MS, Thurer RL, et al. Autologous blood donations prior to elective cardiac surgery: safety and effect of subsequent blood use. JAMA. 1989; 262:1963.

32. Britton LW, Eastland DT, Dziuban SW, et al. Predonated autologous blood use in elective cardiac surgery. Ann Thorac Surg. 1989; 47:529.

33. van Aken WG. Does perioperative blood transfusion promote tumor growth? Transfusion Med Reviews. 1989; III:243.

34. Lichtiger B, Huh YO, Armintor M, et al. Autologous transfusions for cancer patients undergoing elective ablative surgery. J Surg Oncol. 1990; 43: 19.

35. McVay PA, Hoag SH, Lee SJ, Toy PTCY. Factors associated with successful autologous blood donation for elective surgery. Am J Clin Path. 1992; 97: 304.

36. Muravchick S. Anesthesia for the elderly. In Miller RD, ed. Anesthesia. 3rd ed. New York, NY: Churchill Livingstone; 1990:1969-1983.

37. Hussain S. Disorders of hemostasis and thrombosis in the aged. Med Clin N Am. 1976; 60:1273.

38. Fülöp T Jr, Worum I, Csonger J, et al. Body composition in elderly people. I. Determination of body composition by multiisotope method and the elimination kinetics of these isotopes in healthy elderly subjects. Gerontology. 1985; 31:6.

39. Haugen RK, Hill GE. A large-scale autologous blood program in a community hospital: a contribution to the community's blood supply. JAMA. 1987; 257:1211.

40. Pindyck J, Avorn J, Kuriyan M, et al. Blood donation by the elderly: clinical and policy considerations. JAMA. 1987; 257:1186.

41. McVay PM, Andrews A, Kaplan E, et al. Reactions among autologous donors. Transfusion. 1990; 30: 249.

42. Silvergleid AJ. Safety and effectiveness of predeposit autologous transfusions in preteen and adolescent children. JAMA. 187; 257:3403.

43. Utley JR, Moores WY, Stephens DB. Blood conservation techniques. Ann Thorac Surg. 1981; 31:482.

44. Salem MR, Bikhazi GB. Blood conservation. In Motoyama EK, Davis PJ, eds. Smith's Anesthesia for Infants and Children. 4th ed. St. Louis, MO: CV Mosby Co; 1990; 371.

45. Kruskall MS. On measuring the success of an autologous blood donation program. Transfusion. 1991; 31:481.

46. Morrison JC, Whybrew WD, Bucovaz ET. Use of partial exchange transfusion preoperatively in patients with sickle cell hemoglobinopathies. Am J Obstet Gynecol. 1978; 132:59.

47. Chaplin H Jr, Beutler E, Collins JA, et al. Current status of red-cell preservation and availability in relation to the developing national blood policy. N Engl J Med. 1974; 291:68.

48. Castro O, Hardy KP, Winter WP, et al. Freeze preservation of sickle erythrocytes. Am J Hematol. 1981; 10:297.

49. Castro O: Autotransfusion. a management option for alloimmunized sickle cell patients? Prog Clin Biol Res. 2; 98:117.

50. Meryman HT, Hornblower M. Red cell recovery and leukocyte depletion following washing of frozen, thawed red cells. Transfusion. 1973; 13:388.

51. Meryman HT, Hornblower M. Freezing and deglycerolizing sickle-trait red blood cells. Transfusion. 1976; 16:627.

52. Nicholls MD, Janu MR, Davies VJ, et al. Autologous blood transfusion for elective surgery. Med J Aust. 1986; 144:396.

53. Kruskall MS, Glaser EE, Leonard SS, et al. Utilization and effectiveness of a hospital autologous preoperative blood donor program. Transfusion. 1986; 26:335.

54. Rebulla P, Giovanetti AM, Mercuriali F, et al. Autologous predeposit for elective surgery: an Italian experience. World J Surg. 1987; 11:47.

55. Stehling LC. Predeposited autologous blood donation. Acta Anaesthesiol Scand. 1988; 32(suppl):58.

56. AuBuchon JP, Dodd RY. Analysis of the relative safety of autologous blood units available for transfusion to homologous recipients. Transfusion. 1988; 28:403.

57. Speiss BD, Sassetti R, McCarthy RJ, et al. Autologous blood donation: hemodynamics in a high-risk patient population. Transfusion. 1992; 32:17.

58. Goodnough LT, Price TH, Friedman KD, et al. A phase III trial of recombinant human erythropoietin therapy in nonanemic orthopedic patients sub-

jected to aggressive removal of blood for autologous use: dose, response, toxicity, and efficacy. Transfusion. 1994; 33:66.

59. Yomtovian RA, Schrank JY, Betts YM, Kepner JL. Transfusion of previously donated autologous blood in a community hospital. In: Taswell HF, Pineda AA, eds. Autologous Transfusion and Hemotherapy. Boston, Mass: Blackwell Scientific; 1991: 53-77.

60. Kruskall MS. Autologous blood collection and transfusion in a tertiary-care center. In: Taswell HF, Pineda AA, eds. Autologous Transfusion and Hemotherapy. Boston, Mass: Blackwell Scientific; 1991: 53-77.

61. Birkmeyer JD, Goodnough LT, AuBuchon PG, et al. The cost-effectiveness of preoperative autologous blood donation for total hip and knee replacement. Transfusion. 1993; 33:544.

62. Renner SW, Howanitz PH, Bachner P. Preoperative autologous blood donation in 612 hospitals: a College of American Pathologists' Q-Probes study of quality issues in transfusion practice. Arch Pathol Lab Med. 1992; 116:613.

63. Giles KH: Code of federal regulations. Food and drugs, title 21. Washington, DC, 1990, Office of the Federal Register, National Archives and Records Administration.

64. Starkey JM, MacPherson JL, Bolgiano DC, et al. Markers for transfusion-transmitted disease in different groups of blood donors. JAMA. 1989; 262: 3452.

65. Cregan P, Donegan E, Gotelli G. Hemolytic transfusion reaction following autologous frozen and washed red cells. Transfusion. 1991; 31:172.

66. Moss GS, Valeri GR, Brodine CE. Clinical experience with the use of frozen blood in combat casualties. N Engl J Med. 1968; 278:747.

67. Tullis JL, Hinman J, Sproul MT, et al. Incidence of post transfusion hepatitis in previously frozen blood. JAMA. 1970; 214:719.

68. Oski FA, Travis SF, Miller LD, et al. The in vitro restoration of red cell 2,3-diphosphoglycerate level in banked blood. Blood. 1971; 37:52.

69. Blagdon J. The long term storage of blood by freezing. Br J Hosp Med Equip Supplies. 1972:12:23.

70. Valeri CR, Bougas JA, Talarico L, et al. Behavior of previously frozen erythrocytes used during openheart surgery. Transfusion. 1970; 10:238.

71. Valeri CR. Blood Banking and the Use of Frozen Blood Products. Cleveland, Ohio: CRC Press; 1976:177, 192.

72. Valeri CR, Zaroulis CG: Rejuvenation and freezing of outdated stored human red cells. N Engl J Med. 1972; 287:1307.

73. Valeri CR, Szymanski I, Runck AH. Therapeutic effectiveness of homologous erythrocyte transfusion following frozen storage at −80° C for up to seven years. Transfusion. 1970; 10:102.

74. Bryant LR, Wallace ME. Experience with frozen erythrocytes in a private hospital. Transfusion. 1974; 14:481.

75. Kahn RA. Fate of bacteria in frozen red cells. Transfusion. 1975; 15:516.

76. Rao TLK, Mathru M, Salem MR, et al. Serum potassium levels following transfusion of frozen erythrocytes. Anesthesiology. 1980; 52:170.

77. Lubin J, Greenberg JJ, Yahr WZ, et al. The use of autologous blood in open-heart surgery. Transfusion. 1974; 16:602.

78. Ascari WQ, Jolly PC, Thomas PA. Autologous blood transfusion in pulmonary surgery. Transfusion. 1968; 8:111.

79. Hillman RS. Characteristics of marrow production and reticulocyte maturation in normal man in response to anemia. J Clin Invest. 1969; 48:443.

80. Hillman RS. Acute blood loss anemia. In: Williams WJ, Beutler E, Erslev AF, et al, eds. Hematology. New York, NY: McGraw-Hill Book Co; 1972:521.

81. Stehling L. Autologous transfusion. Int Anesthesiol Clin. 1990; 28:190.

82. Coleman DH, Stevens AR, Dodge HT, et al. Rate of blood regeneration after blood loss. Arch Intern Med. 1953; 92:341.

83. Kickler TS, Spivak JL. Effect of repeated whole blood donations on serum immunoreactive erythropoietin levels in autologous blood. JAMA. 1988; 260:65.

84. Finch S, Haskins D, Finch CA. Iron metabolism. Hematopoiesis following phlebotomy: iron as a limiting factor. J Clin Invest. 1950; 29:1078.

85. Cope E, Gillhespy RO, Richardson RW. Treatment of iron-deficiency anaemia: comparison of methods. Br Med J. 1956; 2:633.

86. McCurdy PR. Oral and parenteral iron therapy: a comparison. JAMA. 1965; 191:859.

87. Shafer AW, Marlow AA. Toxic reaction to intramuscular injection of iron. N Engl J Med. 1959; 260:180.

88. Becker CE, MacGregor RR, Walker KS, et al. Fatal anaphylaxis after intramuscular iron-dextran. Ann Intern Med. 1966; 65:745.

89. Goodnough LT, Rudnick S, Price TH, et al. Increased preoperative collection of autologous blood with recombinant human erythropoietin therapy. N Engl J Med. 1989; 321:1163.

90. Goodnough LT, Wasman J, Corlucci K, Chernosky A. Limitations to donating adequate autologous blood prior to elective orthopedic surgery. Arch Surg. 1989; 124:494.

91. Cook JD, Skikne BS, Lynch SR, et al. Estimates of iron insufficiency in the US population. Blood. 1986; 68:726.

92. Walker RH. Technical manual, ed 11. Arlington, VA, 1993, American Association of Blood Banks.

93. Flaharty KK, Grimm AM, Vlasses PH. Epoetin: human recombinant erythropoietin. Clin Pharmacol. 1989; 8:769.

94. Eschbach JW, Egrie JC, Downing MR, et al. Correction of the anemia of end-stage renal disease with recombinant human erythropoietin: results of a combined phase I and II clinical trail. N Engl J Med. 1987; 316:73.

95. Eschbach JW, Kelly MR, Haley NR, et al. Treatment of the anemia of progressive renal failure with recombinant human erythropoietin. N Engl J Med. 1989; 321:158.

96. Zanjani ED, Ascensao JL. Erythropoietin. Transfusion. 1989; 29:46.

97. Goodnough LT, Price TH, Rudnick, S. Preoperative red blood cell production in patients undergoing aggressive autologous blood phlebotomy with and without erythropoietin therapy. Transfusion. 1992; 32:441.

98. Kulier AH, Gombotz H, Fuchs G, et al. Subcutaneous recombinant human erythropoietin and autologous blood donation before coronary artery bypass surgery. Anesth Analg. 1993; 76:102.

99. Goodnough LT. Autologous blood donation. JAMA. 1988; 259:2405.

100. Hagl S, Bornikoel K, Mayr N, et al. Cardiac performance during limited hemodilution. Bibl Haematol. 1975; 41:152.

101. Levy PS, Kim S-J, Eckel PK, et al. Limit of cardiac compensation during acute isovolemic hemodilution: influence of coronary stenosis. Am J Physiol. 1993; 265:H340.

102. Levine EA, Rosen AL, Gould SA, et al. Recombinant human erythropoietin and autologous blood donation. Surgery. 1988; 104:365.

103. Mercuriali F, Zanella A, Barosi G, et al. Use of erythropoietin to increase the volume of autologous blood donated by orthopedic patients. Transfusion. 1993; 33:55.

104. Levine EA, Rosen AL, Sehgal L, et al. Erythropoietin deficiency after coronary artery bypass procedures. Ann Thorac Surg. 1991; 51:764.

105. Levine EA, Rosen AL, Sehgal L, et al. Accelerated erythropoiesis: the hidden benefit of autologous donation. Transfusion. 1990; 30:295.

106. Maeda H, Hitomi Y, Hirata, R. et al. Erythropoietin and autologous blood donation [Letter]. Lancet. 1989; 2:284.

107. Graf H, Watzinger U, Ludvik B, et al. Recombinant human erythropoietin as adjuvant treatment for autologous blood donation. Br Med J. 1990; 300: 1627.

108. Bormann B, Weidler B, Friedrich M, et al. Recombinant human erythropoietin in autologous blood donation. Der Anaesthetist. 1991; 40:396.

109. Gaudiani VA, Mason HD. Preoperative erythropoietin in Jehovah's Witnesses who require cardiac procedures. Ann Thorac Surg. 1991; 51:823.

110. Watanabe Y, Fuse K, Konishi T, et al. Autologous blood transfusion with recombinant human erythropoietin in heart operations. Ann Thorac Surg. 1991; 51:767.

111. Goldberg MA. Biology of erythropoietin. In: Garnick MB, ed. Erythropoietin in Clinical Applications: an international prospective. New York, NY: Marcel Dekker, Inc; 1990:59-104.

112. Sandler SG. Preoperative autologous blood donations by high-risk patients. Transfusion. 1992; 32: 1.

113. Toy PTCY, Strauss RG, Stehling LC, et al. Predeposited autologous blood for elective surgery: a national multicenter study. N Engl J Med. 1987; 316: 517.

# 7

# ACUTE NORMOVOLEMIC HEMODILUTION

## *George J. Crystal and M. Ramez Salem*

## HISTORICAL PERSPECTIVE

Hemodilution was recognized as early as 1882 by Kronecker, who demonstrated that acute dilution of blood to hematocrit (HCT) of 15% was compatible with survival.[1,2] A scientific approach to lowering blood viscosity to improve blood flow in patients was introduced by Muller and Inada in 1904.[3] A few years later, Kottman[4] explained that the beneficial effects of "blood-letting" were the result of "dilution of thick blood." This new concept was based on Poiseuille's law, showing the importance of viscosity on tissue blood flow, especially when the pressure gradient and vessel radius cannot be adjusted further.[3]

Following the introduction of low molecular weight dextran solutions as "flow improvers" by Gelin and Ingelman,[5] hemorrheology

emerged as a scientific field of research and therapy. It shortly became evident that factors other than the viscous nature of red blood cells (RBCs) contributed to the rheology of blood. These factors included the viscosity of plasma and the deformability and aggregation of RBCs.[3] Fahey[6] introduced plasmapheresis to decrease plasma viscosity in paraproteinemias. RBC aggregation and plasma viscosity have been decreased through reduction of plasma fibrinogen concentration.[7] Studies of drug-induced improvement in RBC deformability soon followed.

It was not until the 1960s and 1970s that hemodilution was used clinically as a method to minimize the need for allogeneic blood transfusions.[8-19] Surgery on patients of the Jehovah's Witness faith certainly stimulated studies on hemodilution. In the 1980s therapeutic hemorrheology entered many disciplines, including surgery, anesthesiology, critical care, neonatology, and hematology.[3] Currently, hemodilution alone, or in combination with other measures of blood conservation, e.g., controlled hypotension, has been extended to many types of surgery, including cardiac, orthopedic (especially hip arthroplasty and scoliosis correction), vascular, pediatric, and cancer.[2,13,18-24] In addition, hemodilution is used to prevent the increase in blood viscosity that ordinarily accompanies hypothermic cardiopulmonary bypass (CPB), and to minimize coagulation disorders in cyanotic congenital heart disease when HCT exceeds 65%.[25,26]

## CLASSIFICATION OF HEMODILUTION

Hemodilution refers to decrease in HCT or hemoglobin concentration as a result of dilution of RBCs (dilutional anemia). Several types of hemodilution have been described: (1) hypervolemic hemodilution; (2) hypovolemic hemodilution; and (3) normovolemic (isovolemic) hemodilution.

## Hypervolemic Hemodilution

Hypervolemic hemodilution is the most common type of hemodilution. It can be achieved with infusions of plasma substitutes like dextran, hydroxyethyl starch, or gelatin solutions either acutely, or in a prolonged fashion over days or weeks.[3] A therapeutic decrease in whole blood viscosity occurs (with no change in plasma viscosity) accompanied by an increase in circulating blood volume. RBC deformability is not influenced by hypervolemic hemodilution.[27] RBC aggregation can be reduced with hydroxyethyl starch, whereas low molecular weight dextran has no direct disaggregating effect.[28] Hypervolemic hemodilution has been used with success in stroke patients, and in patients with chronic occlusive arterial diseases.[3,29]

## Hypovolemic Hemodilution

The original technique of preoperative blood donation has been referred to as "hypovolemic hemodilution." Although the descriptor, hypovolemic, is applied to this technique because no colloids or crystalloids are administered simultaneously during preoperative blood donation, it should be kept in mind that normalization of blood volume occurs within 12 to 24 hours via compensatory physiological adjustments. For a more detailed discussion of preoperative blood donation, please refer to Chapter 6. (See Chapter 6: Preoperative Autologous Blood Donation.)

## Acute Normovolemic Hemodilution (ANH)

The technique of acute normovolemic hemodilution (ANH) has been advocated as a method to minimize blood loss during certain major surgical procedures and thus, reduce or even eliminate, the use of allogeneic blood transfusion. ANH entails the intentional decrease of hemoglobin concentration by withdrawal of a calculated volume of the patient's blood, after anesthetic induction or before the critical phases of surgery are started, and si-

multaneous replacement with a cell-free substitute to maintain a near-normal blood volume. The rationale for the use of ANH as a method for blood conservation is that if intraoperative blood loss is relatively constant, the loss of blood constituents, especially RBCs, would be reduced if the blood is diluted by a plasma expander. The patient's own fresh blood is reinfused near the end of the surgical procedure, after major blood loss has ceased. This type of hemodilution has been termed "normovolemic," although there are no simple means of predicting or measuring the accuracy of the normovolemic status. Thus, it is not really possible to exclude slight hypervolemia or hypovolemia when the technique is used experimentally or clinically.

## CARDIOVASCULAR RESPONSES DURING ANH

Before reading the following discussion on the cardiovascular responses during acute normovolemic hemodilution, it is recommended that Chapter 3 be read. (See Chapter 3: Basic Principles of Oxygen Transport.)

Cardiovascular responses during ANH depend on the degree of hemodilution, the circulating blood volume, the nature of the diluent, and the efficacy of compensatory physiologic mechanisms. Although no standard nomenclature for the degree of hemodilution has been established, a decrease in HCT from the normal value of 40% to between 25 and 35%, is referred to as moderate or limited hemodilution, while an HCT below 20% has been referred to as profound or extreme hemodilution.

## Systemic Responses

The decrease in hemoglobin concentration during ANH leads to a proportional decrease in arterial oxygen content ($CaO_2$). Physiological mechanisms available to compensate for this decrease in $CaO_2$ are increased cardiac output (CO) and increased oxygen extraction ratio ($EO_2$).[30]

An increase in CO is the predominant compensatory mechanism operative during moderate ANH.[30] On the basis of in vitro measurements of blood viscosity, Hint[31] predicted

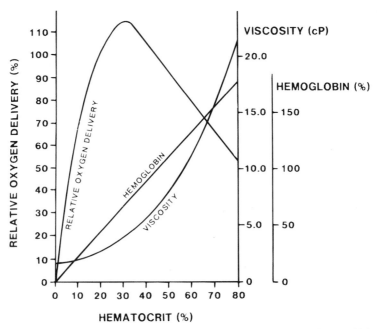

**Fig. 7–1.** Relationship between hematocrit value and theoretical relative oxygen delivery of blood. Values were calculated from the whole blood viscosity assuming that hematocrit value of 45% corresponds with a hemoglobin value of 100%, and that the velocity of flow is inversely proportional to the viscosity of blood. Modified from Hint H. The pharmacology of dextran and clinical background of the clinical use of rheomacrodex. Acta Anaesthesiol Belg. 1968; 19:119, with permission.

that oxygen delivery ($DO_2$) would peak at an HCT of 30%, because the increase in CO would be disproportionate to the decrease in $CaO_2$ (Fig. 7–1). This prediction was corroborated by data obtained in vivo by some investigators,[10,13] but not by others.[32-35] Messmer[30] attributed these conflicting findings simply to differences in the experimental protocols, including the rate of exchange, time of measurements, diluent, and control of blood volume. Von Restorff and associates[34] explained their inability to confirm the theoretical prediction of Hint[31] to problems inherent in estimating the effective viscosity in the circulation from measurements obtained in vitro, because the conditions of Poiseuille's law are not fulfilled in vivo, and they could not explain the opposite findings from other laboratories. Although there remains lack of agreement on the HCT associated with maximal $DO_2$, it is generally accepted that $DO_2$ is reasonably well maintained, as long as HCT is not reduced below 25%.[30]

Most investigators documented increases in CO between 15 and 50% in normal anes-

thetized humans during moderate ANH. The increases in CO during ANH are primarily due to an augmented stroke volume, although an augmented heart rate may assume an important role when basal heart rate is low.[34,36] The increases in stroke volume are attributable to the interaction of several mechanisms: (1) enhanced myocardial contractility via activation of the cardiac sympathetic nerves;[37,38] (2) reduction in impedance to left ventricular ejection, as a result of decreases in blood viscosity and peripheral vascular resistance;[39-41] and (3) increased venous return because of reduced peripheral vascular resistance.[42] An important role for the latter two mechanisms is implied by the significant increases in stroke volume during ANH in animals with denervated hearts, or with hearts having pharmacologically blocked $\beta$-adrenergic receptors.[37,43-46]

It has been suggested that an increase in venomotor tone, via stimulation of $\alpha$-adrenergic receptors by norepinephrine released from sympathetic nerve terminals, increases venous return and stroke volume during ANH.[47] The ability of diluted blood to stimulate aortic body chemoreceptors would provide the sensory limb for this reflex vascular adjustment.[48,49] Such peripheral-to-central translocation of blood by venoconstriction is in apparent conflict with reports of no change in vena caval compliance,[50] and in blood volume within peripheral tissues during ANH in dogs.[51]

When $DO_2$ decreases during extreme ANH, oxygen consumption ($\dot{V}O_2$) can be maintained if mixed venous oxygen content ($C\bar{v}O_2$) falls more than $CaO_2$, i.e., if $EO_2$ increases, resulting in reductions in mixed venous oxygen saturation ($S\bar{v}O_2$) and mixed venous oxygen tension ($P\bar{v}O_2$). Increases in $EO_2$ from the normal value of 25 to 30% to 50% or lower during extreme ANH, have been demonstrated.[34,44,52-54] An increase in $EO_2$ to 50% has been shown to coincide with the onset of lactate production and global dysfunction in normal hearts, and in hearts with a critical coronary stenosis during progressive ANH in animal models.[53,54] On the basis of this finding, it has been proposed that an $EO_2$ of 50% may be used as a trigger for blood transfusion in severely hemodiluted patients.

In chronic anemia, a rightward shift of the oxyhemoglobin dissociation curve may facilitate unloading of oxygen at tissue.[30] This mechanism, which apparently is due to an increased concentration 2,3-DPG within the RBCs, appears to have no important role during ANH.[55]

## Regional Responses

### HEART

The heart, particularly the left ventricular wall, is the principal organ at risk during ANH. This is because of several factors, including: (1) an augmented contractile demand; (2) a low baseline coronary venous $PO_2$, resulting in a small oxygen extraction reserve; and (3) the tendency for subendocardial ischemia, when tachycardia and/or aortic hypotension occur in the presence of a dilated coronary vasculature.

When the coronary arteries are normal, blood flow in both the left and right ventricles increases in proportion to the decreases in HCT during ANH.[34,35,56-60] As long as HCT is not reduced below a critical value (approxi-

mately 10%), the increases in myocardial blood flow are transmurally uniform and sufficient to maintain myocardial oxygen consumption and oxygen delivery. The adequacy of myocardial oxygen delivery is indicated by the unchanged $PO_2$ of coronary venous blood (a reflection of $PO_2$ within the myocardium) and well-preserved myocardial lactate extraction and utilization. It is also indicated by the stability of indices of cardiac performance, including aortic pressure, left atrial pressure, left ventricular $dP/dt_{max}$, CO, and segmental shortening (Fig. 7–2).[59,60]

Inasmuch as aortic pressure (and coronary perfusion pressure) does not increase during ANH, the increases in coronary blood flow reflect reductions in coronary vascular resistance. Although a reduction in blood viscosity has been shown to contribute to the decreased coronary vascular resistance during ANH,[61] significantly diminished reactive hyperemic responses (Fig. 7–3) imply that coronary vasodilation, via metabolic mechanisms (presumably in response to reduced arterial oxygen content), plays a prominent role.[58-61] The dependence on coronary vasodilation during ANH is heightened by an accentuated inertial pressure loss in the coronary circulation.[62] As might be expected, hearts with stenotic coronary arteries (resulting in diminished vasodilator reserve) are less tolerant of ANH, i.e., they exhibit signs of global cardiac dysfunction at a higher HCT.[59,63,64]

A consistent finding associated with the onset of cardiovascular instability during extreme ANH, is a decrease in aortic pressure, which occurs when the heart is incapable of augmenting CO sufficiently to offset the substantially reduced systemic vascular resistance. This decrease in aortic pressure has the effect of decreasing coronary perfusion pressure, while also increasing heart rate via baroreceptor reflex pathways. The combination of decreased perfusion pressure and increased heart rate directs flow away from the subendocardium in the dilated left coronary circulation.[65] The subendocardial hypoperfusion is accompanied by myocardial lactate production and ischemic changes in the electrocardiogram. Subendocardial ischemia leads to global cardiac dysfunction, as manifested by an increase in left ventricular end-diastolic pressure. That pressure is a factor which provides an additional physical impediment to subendocardial

**Fig. 7–2.** Original tracings comparing cardiac effects of selective coronary hemodilution and coronary occlusion in an open-chest, anesthetized dog. The most important point of this figure is that moderate hemodilution at constant perfusion pressure caused an appreciable increase in coronary blood flow accompanied by well maintained regional segmental shortening. In contrast, stoppage of coronary blood flow by arterial occlusion produced regional segmental lengthening, indicative of myocardial ischemia. From Crystal GJ, Salem MR. Myocardial oxygen consumption and segmental shortening during selective coronary hemodilution in dogs. Anesth Analg. 1988; 67:500, with permission.

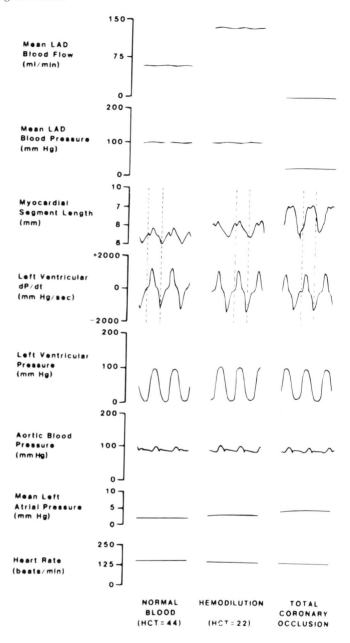

perfusion, causing further limitation to local oxygen supply, and deterioration of global cardiac function. An inadequate CO results in anaerobic metabolism in the body tissues and to lactic acidosis, which may exacerbate the decreases in aortic pressure, subendocardial blood flow, CO, and $DO_2$. The previously mentioned events constitute a vicious cycle, which, if not interrupted by blood transfusion, may lead to irreversible cardiac failure and circulatory collapse.

The improved rheological properties associated with ANH have prompted numerous canine studies to evaluate its effects on ischemic myocardium. In general, these studies have not provided compelling evidence of a benefit. Feola and coworkers[66] reported that ANH with dextran resulted in increased filling pressures and continued progression of ischemic injury, (as assessed from myocardial and epicardial electrograms), in dogs subjected to acute 3-hour occlusion of the

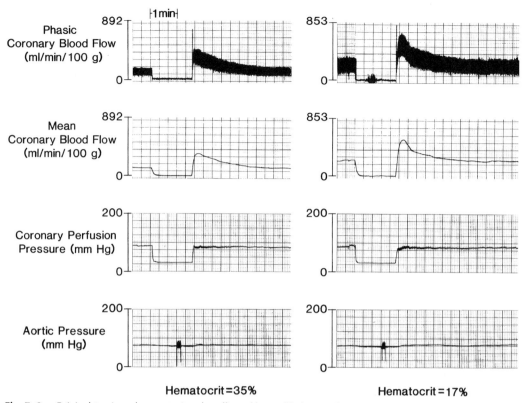

**Fig. 7–3.**  Original tracings demonstrating the effect of hemodilution on the coronary reactive hyperemic response following a 90 sec. occlusion. Note that hemodilution increased the baseline (pre-occlusion) blood flow and peak reactive hyperemic blood flow, and that it also decreased the ratio of peak to pre-occlusion blood flow, implying reduced vasodilator reserve. From Crystal GJ. Coronary hemodynamic responses during local hemodilution in canine hearts. Am J Physiol. 1988; 254:H525, with permission.

left anterior descending coronary artery. Kleinman and associates[67] demonstrated a decrease in oxygen delivery, especially to the subendocardium, via the collateral circulation, following ANH with dextran. Johansson and associates[68] demonstrated a modest increase in coronary collateral flow to acutely (5-minute) ischemic myocardium during ANH with dextran-40. However, these increases were not sufficient to offset the decrease in $CaO_2$, and myocardial oxygen delivery fell.

Cohn and coworkers[69] compared the severity of myocardial ischemia, (as determined by surface electrocardiographic mapping and coronary collateral blood flow), during occlusions of the left anterior descending coronary artery, before and after ANH, with homologous plasma, dextran-70, dextran-40, and lactated Ringer's solution. Although only the dextran solutions improved the surface manifestations of ischemic myocardial injury, they did so without increasing collateral blood flow. The investigators speculated that this benefit of dextran was due to a reduction in myocardial oxygen demand by an uncertain mechanism. In contrast to the above studies, Yoshikawa and colleagues[70] reported that ANH with lactated Ringer's solution reduced ST segment elevation, and increased collateral blood flow in an acutely ischemic region of an isolated heart. The results of clinical investigations have also been inconsistent, with only some studies demonstrating a benefit for ANH in ischemic myocardium.[71] It is evident that the effects of ANH in ischemic myocardium require further elucidation.

In summary, the normal heart appears to tolerate reductions in HCT to as low as 10% during ANH. This is because of transmurally-uniform increases in coronary blood flow, which can compensate fully for the reduction in $CaO_2$. The increases in blood flow during

ANH are secondary to reduced blood viscosity and vasodilation mediated by local metabolic mechanisms. Deterioration of global cardiac function during extreme ANH is largely attributable to the tendency of tachycardia, decreased perfusion pressure, and increased left ventricular end-diastolic pressure to divert blood flow (and oxygen) away from the subendocardium. Factors that diminish coronary reserve, e.g., proximal stenosis, reduce the ability of the heart to tolerate ANH. Whether the improved rheological properties of diluted blood will be beneficial in collateral-dependent regions of myocardium is an open question.

## BRAIN

ANH has been shown to increase blood flow throughout the central nervous system in a variety of species, including humans[57,72-75]. A controversy exists regarding the relative roles of reduced blood viscosity and vasodilation, secondary to reduced $CaO_2$ in the hemodilution-related increases in cerebral blood flow.[76-79] The findings of unimpaired electroencephalographic activity, lack of anaerobic metabolism, and well maintained cerebral $\dot{V}O_2$ in anesthetized dogs and rats,[75, 80,81] suggest that, on a global basis, cerebral oxygenation is adequate during moderate ANH. However, the limitation imposed by venous sampling has made it impossible to rule out the possibility of regional cerebral oxygen deficits. A recent canine study demonstrated that ANH impairs hypocapnia-induced vasoconstrictor responses in the central nervous system.[72] This finding suggests that hyperventilation may have less value as a clinical tool to reduce cerebral vascular volume and intracranial pressure in patients with reduced HCTs.

## OTHER ORGANS

Blood flow in the splanchnic organs and kidney changes minimally during ANH, thus, resulting in decreases in regional oxygen delivery.[73,74] These findings suggest that, in these organs, the favorable influence of reduced viscosity on blood flow is antagonized by vasoconstriction. This selective peripheral vasoconstriction during ANH serves two important functions: (1) It combines with the increased CO to support aortic pressure; and (2) it ensures that the increased CO is preferentially distributed to the vital organs, namely the heart and brain. Although the mechanism(s) responsible for peripheral vasoconstriction during ANH remains to be identified with certainty, a role for the sympathetic nervous system is suggested for two reasons. First, aortic chemoreceptors are stimulated by diluted blood,[48,49] which would provide the obligatory sensory limb for activation of the sympathetic nerves. Second, activation of the sympathetic vasoconstrictor nerves in peripheral beds is an important component of the reflex response to other systemic cardiovascular stresses, including hemorrhagic shock.[82] Simchon and coworkers[83] reported that plasma renin activity declines progressively with ANH to an HCT of 25%, but then increases markedly as HCT is reduced below 20%. Accelerated renin release, and the subsequent increase in angiotensin levels, may also contribute to vasoconstriction in the kidney, as well as to other peripheral tissues, during extreme ANH. The pattern of regional circulatory response during ANH previously described, (preferential perfusion of the heart and brain), remains intact in the presence of high-grade $\beta$-adrenergic blockade.[46]

Although oxygen delivery decreases in the kidney during ANH, renal oxygen consumption is maintained by an increase in local oxygen extraction.[84] An appreciable oxygen extraction reserve is normally evident in the kidney because renal blood flow is very high (owing to its primary function in filtering the blood), and is well in excess of that required to meet the basal oxidative demands of renal tissue.

Sunder-Plassman and colleagues[55] reported that mean tissue $PO_2$, measured with platinum electrodes, remained at control levels in abdominal viscera and skeletal muscle during reductions in HCT to 20% in dogs. The fact that this could occur in the presence of a decreased regional oxygen delivery, may be related to the relative preservation of HCT in the microcirculation during ANH, observed recently by several investigators.[51,85-87] It has been postulated that the maintained microvascular HCT causes a more uniform radial distribution of RBCs in arterioles, resulting in a more uniform supply of RBCs to the capillary network and of oxygen to the surrounding tissue.[85]

## EFFECTS ON COAGULATION

In general, blood coagulation is not impaired, as long as HCT remains above 20%.[88] (See Chapter 2: Coagulation and Hemostasis.) However, ANH may potentially influence coagulation and/or bleeding via three mechanisms: (1) the increase in blood flow associated with ANH can increase oozing from cut surfaces during surgery;[89] (2) the diluent used to maintain normovolemia may adversely influence coagulation, especially if given in excessive amounts; and (3) dilution of fibrinogen, platelets, and other coagulation factors concomitant with ANH, may impair coagulation.[90-92] As the HCT decreases from 39 to 25%, there are proportionate decreases in fibrinogen, platelets, and factors V and VIII.[90,91] The slight prolongation of prothrombin time and partial thromboplastin time observed during ANH, is not associated with any discernible increase in surgical bleeding or blood loss.[90,91] Although Kramer et al.[92] found a 30% decrease in platelets and 50% decrease in fibrinogen levels at an HCT of 25% during ANH for major vascular procedures, the values returned to normal levels by the end of the first postoperative day. Because the patient's own fresh blood is reinfused after most of the surgical bleeding has ceased when ANH is terminated, coagulation may be improved and the need for allogeneic blood and blood products, including plasma and platelets, is reduced. Kaplan et al[93] demonstrated that when autologous blood (whole or in components) collected prior to CBP is reinfused following bypass, clotting is improved and the need for allogeneic blood is reduced in the postbypass period. (See Chapter 12: Blood Conservation in Special Situations—Anesthesiologist's viewpoints: Cardiac Surgery.)

## EFFECTS ON PULMONARY GAS EXCHANGE

The effect of chronic anemia on pulmonary gas exchange has been examined by Barrera et al[94] who found that $PaO_2$ was significantly higher in chronic anemic dogs (hemoglobin = 3-4 g/dL) than nonanemic dogs, suggesting that chronic anemia brings about an improved capacity for oxygenating arterial blood. During ANH, the intrapulmonary shunt ($\dot{Q}s/\dot{Q}t$) may increase or decrease, depending on the ventilation-perfusion ($\dot{V}/\dot{Q}$) relationship.[19] When the $\dot{V}/\dot{Q}$ ratios are low, atelectatic areas may have increased perfusion because of reduced viscosity, despite hypoxic pulmonary vasoconstriction and consequently, a large shunt may be found. When $\dot{V}/\dot{Q}$ ratio is normal, $\dot{Q}s/\dot{Q}t$ may actually decrease during ANH, resulting in well-maintained $PaO_2$.[19] Several studies could not demonstrate any deleterious effects of ANH on pulmonary function.[95-97] In patients undergoing hip arthroplasty, there were no changes in blood gas tensions, or pulmonary function between the patients who had and had not undergone ANH.[95,96] In one study,[96] both groups had changes that were attributed to the lateral decubitus position, but the abnormalities resolved more rapidly in patients who underwent ANH. The authors speculated that the smaller amount of allogeneic blood, or the reduction of the amount of fibrin and platelets trapped in the lung, might have contributed to faster recovery.[96]

## CHARACTERISTICS OF REPLACEMENT FLUIDS

Preoperative ANH can be tolerated only in the presence of an adequate circulating blood volume. Crystalloids, colloids, and combinations of both have been used as diluents during ANH. The most common crystalloid used is lactated Ringer's solution. A number of colloids have been used, including the natural colloid, albumin, and the synthetic colloids, dextran and hydroxyethyl starch. Table 7–1 lists advantages and disadvantages of crystalloids and colloids.[26]

### Crystalloids Versus Colloids

The principal advantages of crystalloid solutions are their lower cost and lack of significant adverse physiological effects. The principal shortcoming of these solutions is their greater tendency to traverse the vascular endothelium and leave the vascular compartment. After infusion, crystalloids rapidly distribute between the intravascular and extravascular compartments, in proportion to the size of these compartments. When crystalloids are given as the sole replacement fluid, they must be administered in a volume 3 times that of the blood withdrawn to maintain normovolemic conditions. Within 2 hours after infu-

**Table 7–1.   Crystalloid versus colloid as the replacement fluid for hemodilution**

|  | Crystalloid | Colloid |
| --- | --- | --- |
| Volume required | 3 times volume of shed blood | 1–2 times volume of shed blood |
| Plasma volume | 80% leaves intravascular compartment in 2 hours | Retained longer in the circulation—a better plasma expander |
| Water balance | Positive water balance, more peripheral edema, responds to diuretics | Less peripheral edema |
| Colloidal osmotic pressure | Reduced, probably not important | Maintained |
| Postoperative HCT | Higher | Lower |
| Coagulation defect | None | May occur with excessive colloid therapy (Dextrans) |
| Cost | Inexpensive | Expensive |

Reprinted with permission from Salem MR, Bikhazi GB: Blood conservation. In: Motoyama EK, Davis PJ, eds. Anesthesia for infants and children. St. Louis, CV Mosby Co, 1990.

sion, 80% of the administered volume of crystalloid moves to the extravascular compartment.[98] In contrast, colloids are retained longer in the circulation, thereby maintaining colloidal osmotic pressure (COP) and plasma volume for several hours. Thus, colloids produce slightly lower HCT, perioperatively, than do crystalloids.[11] Diuresis follows the administration of crystalloids and there is usually a rapid response to furosemide.

Crystalloids have a greater tendency to cause pulmonary edema than colloids. When the lungs are normal, pulmonary edema is usually prevented by intrinsic compensatory factors, including the plasma-interstitial oncotic gradient, the high lymphatic capacity of the lung, the physical-chemical characteristics of the interstitial space, the integrity of the microvascular membrane, and a low vascular hydrostatic driving pressure.[99,100] These factors appear to be less effective in elderly patients and in patients with underlying cardiopulmonary disease, who demonstrate a greater tendency for pulmonary edema when crystalloids are used for volume replacement.

The development of peripheral edema after crystalloid therapy does not necessarily reflect pulmonary edema.[99] It is controversial whether maintenance of normal COP is beneficial in preventing pulmonary edema. In the presence of capillary leakage, the administered albumin crosses the pulmonary capillary endothelium, pulling water with it, thus increasing pulmonary interstitial water. Probably the amount of the fluid administered and the vigilance in monitoring the hemodynamic variables are more important in the development of pulmonary edema than the choice of the fluid.

Extreme positions in the colloid-crystalloid controversy are unwarranted.[98] Although colloid solutions have not been proven to be harmful, and are better plasma volume expanders, most authorities prefer to use lactated Ringer's solution, either as the sole replacement fluid, or in combination with a colloid. Lactated Ringer's solution has been used as the replacement fluid in adults and children belonging to the Jehovah's Witness sect.

While colloids as a group share the ability to expand vascular volume without high risk of tissue edema, they each possess unique physiological properties, some beneficial, and others, deleterious.

## Albumin

Albumin is prepared from pooled human plasma by a process that eliminates the risk of disease transmission associated with blood transfusion. Albumin is usually used in a concentration of 5%, which has a COP of approximately 19 mm Hg. This COP is similar to that of plasma. Albumin is unique because of its monodisperse characteristics with a molecular weight of 69,000 daltons, its multiple negative charges, and the fact that it is not glycosylated.[100] These features favor vascular retention. Beneficial physiological properties attributed to albumin are that it improves immune mechanisms, promotes microvascular integrity, scavenges free radicals, and helps to prevent lipid peroxidation. Deleterious properties attributed to albumin are that it adversely affects blood coagulation, impairs cardiac, renal, and respiratory function, and increases extracellular leakage.[100]

## Dextrans

Dextrans are high-molecular weight polysaccharides produced by specific bacteria grown in a sucrose medium.[101] For intravenous infusion, partial acid hydrolysis is used to produce dextran fractions in specific molecular weight ranges. Two preparations are commonly used: a 10% solution with an average molecular weight of 40,000 daltons (dextran-40 or low molecular weight dextran), and a 6% solution with an average molecular weight of 70,000 daltons (dextran-70). Dextran is primarily excreted unchanged in the urine, the rate of excretion being inversely related to the size of the dextran molecules. The dextran molecules that are not excreted in the urine, slowly diffuse into the spleen, liver, lung, kidney, brain, and muscle, and are broken down completely to carbon dioxide and water at a rate of approximately 70 mg/kg body weight per 24 hours.[102] Dextran solutions have antithrombotic effects, likely mediated by inhibition of platelet aggregation and reduction in clotting factors. Anaphylactic reactions are unusual, occurring in 0.03 to 0.07% of patients, but may be severe and even fatal.[101] Precipitation of acute renal failure by infusion of dextran, especially low molecular weight dextran, has been suggested, but this is controversial.[103,104] A plausible mechanism for this effect is accumulation of dextran molecules in the renal tubules, leading to tubular plugging. Patients with preexisting renal disease or impaired renal perfusion, appear to be more susceptible to renal failure during infusion of dextran. An additional problem reported with dextran infusion is that it causes difficulty in crossmatching blood for a subsequent transfusion.[105] This problem has been attributed to adherence of dextran molecules to antigens on the RBC membrane. Maximum recommended doses for dextran-70 and dextran-40, are 1 and 2 g/kg, respectively.[106]

## Hydroxyethyl Starch Solutions

Amylopectin is an energy storage polysaccharide (glucose polymer) of plants which structurally resembles glycogen. Early studies demonstrated that amylopectin was well tolerated when infused intravascularly into animals, but that it was rapidly hydrolyzed, with a half-life of only about 20 minutes. In the early 1960s, the addition of hydroxyethyl groups to the glucose moieties to create hydroxyethyl starch, made the molecule more stable in plasma.

Commercially available hydroxyethyl starch solutions (Hespan, Hetastarch) are prepared in a 6% solution with an average molecular weight of 69,000 daltons, similar to that of albumin. The range of molecular size is wide, varying from 10,000 to 100,000 daltons. Smaller molecules are excreted unchanged into urine, while larger molecules slowly diffuse into the interstitium where slow enzymatic degradation occurs. In normal subjects, hydroxyethyl starch is nearly completely cleared from the plasma within 2 days (half-life = 17 hours), although approximately 50% of it remains in the body. This hydroxyethyl starch is eliminated slowly over weeks, with some of the larger hydroxyethyl starch molecules accumulating in reticuloendothelial cells.[103]

Hydroxyethyl starch appears to be well tolerated, with adverse effects infrequent and mild. Allergic reactions to hydroxyethyl starch are extremely rare. The only clinically significant adverse effect of hydroxyethyl starch appears to be its ability to cause impairment to coagulation. This effect is dose related. At moderate doses (20 mL/kg), the following effects have been described: (1) platelet counts are normal; (2) platelet function is intact, and bleeding times are normal; (3) prothrombin time and thromboplastin time may be prolonged; and (4) fibrinogen levels may be reduced.[103] Despite these effects, there is no evidence of clinical impairment to clotting with hydroxyethyl starch infusions up to 20 mL/kg.[107] Animal investigations have demonstrated increased incisional bleeding, increased intraoperative blood loss, and spontaneous serosal bleeding in the presence of large volumes of hydroxyethyl starch.[108] In contrast to dextran, hydroxyethyl starch does not interfere with typing or crossmatching of blood, and it has no deleterious effect on renal function.[101] Hydroxyethyl starch reduces blood viscosity less than dextran. This factor, combined with a blunted antithrombotic effect, makes hydroxyethyl starch less useful as therapy for microcirculatory flow disturbances.

## CLINICAL MANAGEMENT OF ANH

The patients or the parents (in the case of children) must be fully informed of the rationale of ANH before surgery. Risks of massive intraoperative blood loss and transfusion of allogeneic blood must be explained. Also, the risks of ANH must be detailed, including ischemia to the vital organs. A realistic assessment of the benefit-to-risk ratio must be presented. For Jehovah's Witness patients who object to withdrawal of their blood and its storage in a reservoir out of contact with their circulation, a special closed-circuit continuous-flow system has been devised.[24,109,110] (See Chapter 11: Blood Conservation in Jehovah's Witnesses.) In such a system, a very slow, continuous circulation of blood from a central (or peripheral) vein into a citrate-phosphate-dextrose reservoir bag, and then back into a peripheral vein, ensures that the blood never loses contact with the patient's body, and that the blood is in constant, although extremely slow, circulation.

Accurate preoperative assessment of the cardiovascular, respiratory, and other systems is essential. A history of drug therapy is important, and steps should be taken to correct any coagulation disorders that may be present. (See Chapter 2: Coagulation and Hemostasis.) Unless they are absolutely necessary, salicylates and other cyclooxygenase inhibitors (aspirin, indomethacin) should be discontinued 1 to 2 weeks before surgery. Since the need for postoperative ventilatory support is a possibility, the patient or the parents should be informed about such a possibility.

The goal of premedication is sedation without an increase in myocardial oxygen consumption. Vagolytic drugs, such as atropine, should be either avoided or their dose decreased. Except in younger children, a peripheral intravenous catheter is inserted before induction of anesthesia. After induction of anesthesia and tracheal intubation, an arterial cannula is inserted and additional large-bore peripheral intravenous cannulas may be placed. A central venous (via external or internal jugular vein) or a pulmonary artery catheter may be placed if indicated. A pulmonary artery catheter allows accurate hemodynamic monitoring and CO determinations. Other monitors should include precordial and/or esophageal stethoscope, electrocardiogram, pulse oximeter, capnograph, skin, and an esophageal temperature probe. An indwelling urinary catheter is placed in the urinary bladder to permit urine volume measurements.

Anesthesia is maintained with an inhalational anesthetic and oxygen. Opioids or combinations of inhalational anesthetics and opioids may also be used. Although nitrous oxide may be given during induction and the early anesthetic phase, it should be discontinued before ANH is started, to permit a maximum increase in the fraction of dissolved oxygen. ANH appears to increase the potencies of both the nondepolarizing and depolarizing muscle relaxants.[111] This has been attributed to an increase in cardiac output, to a decrease in protein binding and, in the case of succinylcholine, to a decrease in plasma cholinesterase activity.[111] Monitoring the neuromuscular function should be performed throughout the operative procedure and after reversal. Ventilation is adjusted to maintain $PaCO_2$ between 30 and 40 mm Hg. End-tidal carbon dioxide monitoring is extremely helpful, and except in infants weighing less than 8 kg and elderly patients, it reflects $PaCO_2$ even during hypotension.[112-114] Arterial and central venous (or pulmonary artery) pH, blood gases, and HCT are measured every 30 minutes, and during the critical stages of surgery and blood loss.

Although ANH can be started in the unanesthetized patient in the "holding area;" it is certainly safer to initiate it in the operating room, under controlled conditions, and after a steady state of anesthesia is achieved. The decrease in total body oxygen consumption during anesthesia, and the availability of continuous monitoring and better care mandate the institution of ANH after anesthetic induction.[89] The amount of blood that can be withdrawn depends on the initial HCT, desired HCT, estimated blood volume, patient's condition, and body weight. A decision should be made regarding the lowest acceptable HCT. Unless hypothermia is planned, the lowest acceptable HCT in normal healthy patients is 20%. A higher HCT may be chosen, depending on the condition of the patient and the anticipated blood loss. The volume of blood to be withdrawn is calculated from formulae that have been devised for estimations of allowable blood loss (Table 7–2).[24,89,115]

A simplified formula that takes into consideration the decrease in HCT that accompanies hemodilution, has been introduced by Gross.[116]

$$V = EBV \times \frac{H_O - H_f}{H_{av}}$$

Where V = the volume of blood to be removed,

EBV = the estimated blood volume (70mL/kg in the adult male and 65mL/kg in the adult female)

$H_O$ = initial HCT,

$H_f$ = the desired HCT,

and $H_{av}$ = the average HCT (average of $H_O$ and $H_f$)

Thus in a 70 kg patient, with an initial HCT of 45% and a desired HCT of 30%, 2,000 mL can be withdrawn,[89] and more volume can be collected if the patient can tolerate a lower HCT.

Using a strictly sterile technique, the predetermined volume of blood is withdrawn in a citrate-phosphate-dextrose (CPD) blood donor bag from either the arterial or central venous lines. Collection of blood from a central venous catheter is facilitated by keeping the bag at a lower level. If a peripheral vein is used, withdrawal of blood can also be enhanced by cycling the cuff of a noninvasive blood pressure monitor at 2- or 3-minute intervals.[117] Employing the system shown in

**Table 7–2. Calculation of volume of blood removed for hemodilution**

| | |
|---|---|
| a. | $ERCV_T = \dfrac{HCT}{100} \times v \times body\ wt\ (kg)$ |
| Where: | $ERCV_T$ = estimated total RBC volume (mL) |
| | V = estimated blood volume/kg |
| | 90 mL/kg (neonates) |
| | 80 mL/kg (infants & children) |
| | 65–75 mL/kg (teenagers) |
| b. | $ERCV_{20} = 0.2 \times V \times body\ wt\ (kg)$ |
| Where: | $ERCV_{20}$ = estimated RBC volume at HCT 20%* |
| c. | $RCW = ERCV_T - ERCV_{20}$ |
| Where: | RCW = RBC volume to be withdrawn |
| d. | $WBW = 3 \times RCW$ |
| Where: | WBW = whole bleed volume to be withdrawn† |

* HCT of 20% is chosen since it is the desired initial level of hemodilution and is commonly employed. A lower HCT may be chosen in Jehovah's Witness patients.
† The average HCT value of the blood withdrawn is assumed to be 33% and thus the total volume withdrawn is 3 times the RBC volume to be withdrawn.
Reprinted with permission from Schaller RT Jr, Schaller J, Morgan A, and others: Hemodilution anesthesia: A valuable aid to major cancer surgery in children. Am J Surg 1983; 146:79.

Fig. 7-4, intraarterial pressure measurements can be intermittently obtained by occluding the withdrawal tube with a clamp.[2] The use of kits that contain two blood bags, a Y-type connector set with a Luer lock adapter, and a blood recipient identification band (Autologous Blood Collection Kit 4R5012, Fenwal Division, Baxter Healthcare, Deerfield, IL) simplifies and facilitates the procedure.[89] The collected blood should be mixed gently with the anticoagulant in the blood bag, and care should be taken to exclude air bubbles which will provide for a gas-blood interface.[2] The volume of collected blood is determined by weighing the bags (1 mL = 1 g) using a scale. In adult patients, each bag should contain no less than 300 mL, and no more than 450 mL to ensure proper blood to anticoagulant ratio.[89] In children, 250 mL blood donor bags may be used.

As blood is being collected, 2 to 3 times this amount of lactated Ringer's solution (or an appropriate amount of other diluents) is infused. The fluids should be warmed before their administration, to prevent a precipitous decrease in the patient's temperature. Central venous and/or pulmonary capillary wedge pressure can serve as a guide to fluid therapy during blood withdrawal. It has been suggested that replacement solutions are infused in quantities sufficient to maintain central venous (and pulmonary capillary wedge) pressure 2 to 4 mm Hg above the prebleeding level.[2] The blood bags are numbered sequentially, labelled, and kept at room temperature for up to 6 hours to preserve platelet function. If it is expected that the blood will not be transfused within this period, the blood bags should be kept in a small cooler containing wet ice or arrangements are made with the blood bank for storage up to 24 hours. Although the surgical procedure may start while blood is being withdrawn, critical phases of surgery during which blood loss may occur, should not be commenced until ANH is completed. This usually requires about 30 minutes. The collection of blood hardly delays the surgery since it is usually performed before or during its initial phase.

During the operative procedure, blood loss is initially replaced with an equal volume of lactated Ringer's solution. Serial HCT measurements during ANH and every 30 minutes thereafter, are essential for determining the

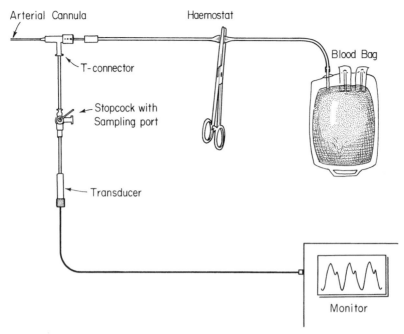

**Fig. 7–4.** Diagrammatic representation of the method of blood withdrawal from the radial artery cannula. Arterial blood pressure is recorded on the monitor by connecting the arterial cannula to a transducer via a T-connector, stopcock, and plastic tubing. Blood is collected into an ACD-containing plastic bag from the arterial cannula. Release of the hemostat causes blood to flow into the bag. Arterial blood pressure is obtained when the hemostat occludes the tubing to the plastic blood bag. From Fahmy NR. Haemodilution and hypotension. In: Enderby GEH, Eckenhoff JE, eds. Hypotensive Anesthesia. London, England: Churchill-Livingstone; 1985, with permission.

need for transfusion. It is important that the HCT measurements are accurate, and it is preferable to do more than one measurement per sample. Conventional laboratory HCT measurements including microcentrifuge technique or the Coulter method, are accurate during ANH. In contrast, HCT values derived by the conductivity of whole blood used in portable compact devices, will report artificially low readings in situations where plasma has been replaced by crystalloid.[118] Additional volumes of lactated Ringer's solution are infused to compensate for third-space losses. If the HCT decreases below the desired level, allogeneic packed RBCs may be infused to maintain the HCT at an acceptable level.

The collected autologous blood is reinfused after most of the blood loss has ceased, or when intraoperative blood loss (in an adult) exceeds 500 mL. Reinfusion is started with the latest collected blood bag. The first obtained blood bag, rich in RBCs, platelets, and coagulation factors, is administered last. The autologous blood collected is given through a 170 $\mu$m filter, rather than through a 40 $\mu$m filter which tends to trap platelets. Fresh autologous blood flows easily through the filter, compared to allogeneic blood, and the filter remains remarkably free from debris. The HCT should be returned to 28 to 30% after surgery. The remaining autologous blood may be refrigerated, and can be used within 24 hours.

Furosemide (0.5 to 1 mg/kg) may be given to promote diuresis and the rapid excretion of excess crystalloids. Large urine volumes with high electrolyte content are expected over the next several hours after ANH is reversed, especially if crystalloids have been given as the sole diluent. Additional doses of furosemide may be needed over the next 2 hours to promote the excretion of excess crystalloids. Blood electrolyte levels may be measured so that hypokalemia resulting from diuresis can be corrected.

## COMBINED ANH AND DELIBERATE HYPOTENSION

The combined use of ANH and deliberate hypotension has been advocated as a logical means of minimizing the need for allogeneic blood and decreasing blood loss.[2,119-121] This technique involves the coexistence of decreased perfusion pressure and reduced oxygen carrying capacity, two factors that may potentially jeopardize tissue oxygen delivery. Thus, its use warrants preoperative evaluation of the patient, extensive monitoring, and experienced and vigilant medical personnel. Patients with clinical evidence of any disease that might compromise blood flow or oxygen delivery to any major organ, are not appropriate candidates for the combined technique. ANH is performed in the immediate preoperative period, after induction of anesthesia. Hypotension is then induced to a mean arterial pressure of approximately 60 to 70 mm Hg. Observations with the combined use of both techniques indicate that CO tends to decrease significantly after hemodilution, when the blood pressure decreases below 60 mm Hg. Therefore, hypotension should be limited and blood pressure monitored accurately. Short-acting hypotensive drugs (trimethaphan, sodium nitroprusside or nitroglycerin) are preferable to long-acting drugs (labetalol), so that blood pressure can be easily restored in case of hemodynamic instability. Since decreases in blood pressure can be achieved easily in hemodiluted patients, the dose of hypotensive drugs should be decreased accordingly to avoid precipitous and uncontrollable hypotension.

Animal studies of the regional hemodynamic responses to the combination of ANH and deliberate hypotension revealed that maintenance of oxygen delivery to selected organs, e.g., the kidney, may be at risk.[56,57,74,122] However, these findings should not detract from the value of the technique. The combination of ANH and deliberate hypotension is designed to aid in minimizing blood loss during major surgery (when severe hemorrhage is likely), and to avoid massive blood transfusion, situations which themselves can jeopardize $DO_2$. The decreases in $DO_2$ with the combined technique are probably far less than those associated with massive blood loss. It is recommended that high $FIO_2$ and continuous monitoring of the arterial, central venous or pulmonary capillary wedge pressures, electrocardiogram, arterial and mixed venous blood gases, blood loss, body temperature, and urine output be employed when the two techniques are combined.

## ANH, DELIBERATE HYPOTENSION AND HYPOTHERMIA

The technique of combined ANH, deliberate hypotension, and hypothermia has been stimulated by the need to carry out major surgical operations, (usually associated with massive blood loss), in patients of the Jehovah's Witness faith who refuse blood or blood products.[14-16,123] This technique requires extensive experience and is undertaken only in specialized medical centers. In this technique, ANH is produced by blood withdrawal and fluid replacement, after induction of anesthesia, but before surgery is commenced. Because the increase in CO may not be sufficient to maintain $DO_2$ during profound ANH, the protective effects of cooling are used, namely, a decreased metabolic oxygen requirement and an increased fraction of dissolved oxygen in the blood. Anesthetics also decrease the metabolic oxygen requirement. Additionally, moderate hypotension decreases both blood loss and myocardial oxygen demand.

During air breathing at normothermia, the dissolved oxygen in the blood represents 0.3 mL/dL (Fig. 7–5). This value increases to 1.3 to 1.5 mL/dL in normal patients with normal hemoglobin at normal temperature when $FIO_2 = 1.0$. This represents 7% of the $CaO_2$ and 30% of the total $EO_2$.[110,123] As temperature decreases during ANH, the fraction of dissolved oxygen increases. During ANH to hemoglobin of 5 g/dL with hypothermia to 30 or 31° C, and an $FIO_2 = 1.0$, the amount of dissolved oxygen increases to 2 mL/dL and represents 30% of the total $CaO_2$ (8.7 mL/dL). This dissolved oxygen accounts for more than half the metabolic requirement. When oxygen consumption decreases by 40%, as a result of anesthesia and cooling to 31° C, $S\bar{v}O_2$ does not change during a reduction in hemoglobin concentration from 15 to 5 g/dL. Therefore, when this technique is used optimally, the combined effects of increased dissolved oxygen in the blood, decreased peripheral resistance, increased CO, and decreased oxygen requirement can balance the induced reduction in $CaO_2$, resulting in an unchanged $EO_2$.

Patients who are to undergo operations

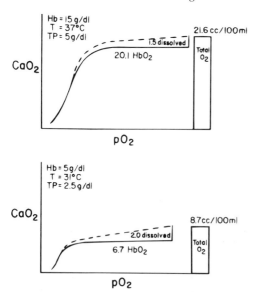

**Fig. 7–5.** Curves plotting total arterial oxygen content (CaO₂) against PO₂ during the awake normal state and during hemodilution. The increase in dissolved oxygen during hemodilution represents approximately 30% of total CaO₂. See text for details. From Singler RC. Special techniques: deliberate hypotension, hypothermia, and acute normovolemic hemodilution. In: Gregory GA, ed. Pediatric Anesthesia. New York, NY: Churchill- Livingstone; 1983, with permission.

where major blood losses are expected, (more than their blood volume), may be considered candidates for ANH combined with mild hypothermia. The use of this technique has been extended to pediatric cardiac surgery, spinal surgery for scoliosis, and operations for malignant disease (Wilms' tumor, neuroblastoma, teratomas, retroperitoneal ganglioneuroma, liver tumors, and pancreatic tumors).[24,124]

Postoperatively, the patient remains in an intensive care environment for 4 to 8 hours while the excess crystalloid is excreted. Furosemide 0.5 to 1 mg/kg may be given to promote diuresis and may be repeated. Any increase in patient's metabolic rate must be prevented by maintaining sedation and muscular paralysis until the temperature returns to normal and the HCT rises to approximately 30%. Shivering may triple the oxygen demand, possibly resulting in a serious decline in SvO₂, even with a normal HCT value. Since third-space losses may continue during the recovery phase, it is essential to continue to infuse crystalloids, colloids, or blood, or a combination of the fluids, as required. Weaning from mechanical ventilation should be commenced

slowly. The trachea is usually extubated within 8 hours after surgery. If there is any doubt about the patient's condition, mechanical ventilation may be continued overnight. Laboratory tests, hemodynamic measurements, chest radiograph, and ventilatory variables are continually checked during the postoperative period, to confirm that the patient's condition remains stable before the arterial and central venous (or pulmonary artery) cannulas are removed.

## EFFICACY OF ANH AS A BLOOD CONSERVATION STRATEGY

ANH alone, or combined with other measures of blood conservation, has been extended to virtually all types of surgical procedures associated with significant blood loss, especially major orthopedic and cardiac operations. The fundamental question that needs to be answered is: Does ANH reduce or eliminate the need for allogeneic blood transfusions? Early investigators addressed this question. Hallowell et al[125] found that the withdrawal of 1250 mL of blood, prior to CPB, decreased the requirement for allogeneic blood by 25%, while Ochsner et al[126] observed a 50% reduction. Others[127,128] found that 60 to 90% of their patients did not require allogeneic blood when they combined ANH with transfusion of shed mediastinal blood. Martin et al[22] reported that the need for allogeneic blood can be decreased by 20 to 90%, depending on the type of surgical procedure. Using extreme ANH in patients undergoing correction of scoliosis with instrumentation, Martin and Ott[129] were able to decrease the transfusion requirement from 4370 mL to 750 mL. In patients undergoing hip arthroplasty, Rosberg and Wulff[96] reported that ANH decreased the transfusion requirement by 1.2 units of blood.

Although the effect of moderate ANH in reducing blood loss is not as great as deliberate hypotension,[130] there is evidence that the combination of both techniques leads to marked reductions in blood loss and in the need for allogeneic blood.[130] In a large series of adult patients, blood replacement was decreased by about 45% when deliberate hypotension was utilized, but was reduced by more than 80% when both techniques were employed.[2] Using the combined technique, Fahmy[2] avoided allogeneic blood in 47 patients undergoing total hip replacement. Significant decreases in the use of allogeneic blood were also noted when ANH was utilized in hepatic resection,[131] major colon surgery,[97] and major vascular procedures.[132]

When clinical trials are conducted to define the efficacy of ANH as a means of blood conservation, the value of the findings is frequently limited by lack of randomization, and by ethical and moral considerations. Since such trials are unblinded, alterations in transfusion practices may become uncredited interventions in both intervention and control groups.[133] Furthermore, criteria for blood transfusion in these trials may account for both the success[134,135] and failure[136,137] of single blood conservation techniques in otherwise well-designed trials.[133] In some of these studies, comparisons of blood or RBCs saved via ANH, were basically made with "historic" control groups.[89] Furthermore, these studies did not examine the relative impact of factors that can affect the total RBCs saved by ANH, and the extent to which the technique may reduce the need for allogeneic blood transfusion,[138] namely: initial HCT; amount of blood removed during ANH; and surgical blood loss.

Two recent studies,[138,139] employed mathematical computer models of ANH to determine the maximum benefit to be expected, and to evaluate how to save RBCs, as much as possible, with the use of ANH. Brecher and Rosenfeld[139] found that because of the decreasing HCT during ANH, and the need to begin transfusion at some minimal HCT, the theoretic savings in RBCs attributable to ANH are less than had previously been appreciated. They also found that additional ANH does not necessarily result in additional patient benefit. Feldman et al[138] data indicated that ANH does indeed save RBCs that would otherwise be lost during surgery; but the savings are not as much as typically reported. They concluded that a degree of ANH more than that which is typically recommended, is necessary to achieve even modest RBC savings.[138]

In an attempt to test the predictions of these mathematical models, Goodnough et al[140] performed a case study analysis of ANH in patients undergoing radical prostatectomy by one surgeon during a 3-year period. They found that the net intraoperative RBC volume saved by this technique was 95 mL, representing only 9.3% of total RBC volume lost during hospitalization. The RBC volume removed by ANH constituted 34% of the total RBC volume transfused.[140] These results essentially confirmed the mathematical model findings.[138,139]

## CURRENT STATUS OF ANH

It is apparent from the aforementioned discussions, that moderate ANH used as the sole method may contribute only modestly to blood conservation.[140] The efficacy of ANH may vary greatly, but is certainly enhanced if a lower posthemodilution HCT level, in the range from 28% to as low as 20%, is targeted.[140,141] This requires an institutional protocol that would allow a lower posthemodilution HCT level at the start of surgery. The effectiveness of moderate ANH can also be enhanced when combined with other blood conservation techniques, including deliberate hypotension and blood salvage procedures, as well as emerging new technologies.[140]

Whether used alone or in combination with other measures, ANH offers certain unique advantages. It can be employed in situations where preoperative blood donation was not planned because of urgency of the operative procedure or scheduling conflicts. It can also be utilized whenever blood salvage could not be performed because of unavailability of technical personnel or lack of equipment. Unlike preoperative blood donation or blood salvage, ANH is performed by the anesthesiologist and, therefore, does not require the presence of blood bank technicians or perfusionists. Furthermore, ANH is the only practical means of providing fresh autologous whole blood for transfusion.

ANH prior to the institution of CPB serves two functions: (1) It provides a source of autologous blood rich in hemoglobin, platelets, and coagulations factors, which is reinfused to the patient after the cessation of CPB; and (2) It prevents the increase in viscosity that accompanies hypothermic CPB (See Chapter 3: Principles of Oxygen Transport.) Although blood can be withdrawn after induction of anesthesia or during the early stage of surgery in patients with normal cardiac function, it is usually done after heparinization and cannulation, immediately before instituting CPB. The blood is withdrawn from the tubing to the oxygenator before the blood passes through the roller pump.[89] Alterations in pump flow can be used to compensate for hemodynamic instabilities associated with blood removal. With the initiation of CPB with a crystalloid (or crystalloid-colloid) prime, a further, and sometimes profound, hemodilution will result, depending on the patient's hemoglobin level prior to bypass. (See Chapter 12: Blood Conservation in Special Situations—Anesthesiologist's Viewpoints: Cardiac Surgery.)

In spite of its simplicity and safety, ANH should not be undertaken in certain situations. Inexperience is the most important absolute contraindication to the use of ANH. The presence of any coexisting disease that may potentially jeopardize tissue oxygen delivery, especially to the heart or brain, constitutes a contraindication to ANH. Since hemoglobin concentration decreases by approximately 1g/dL for each unit of blood withdrawn in adults, ANH should not be performed in anemic patients (hemoglobin < 11%).[89] The technique should not be employed if the anticipated increase in CO, the primary compensatory mechanism in ANH, is neither possible, nor desirable.[89] Although extreme ANH has been used successfully in patients with cardiac disease,[142] its safety in patients with possible myocardial ischemia is still poorly defined.[129,143] The technique is contraindicated in patients with pulmonary disease if they have a significant $\dot{Q}_S/\dot{Q}_T$ interfering with arterial oxygenation. Patients with impaired kidney function may not be suitable candidates for ANH, since they may not be able to excrete large amounts of crystalloids.[89] Age is not an absolute contraindication to ANH. In fact, it has been employed in patients weighing 5 kg, as well as in elderly patients.[24,142]

Finally, the success of the technique is the result of a cooperative effort of the members of the team including surgeons, anesthesiologists, nurses, and laboratory and technical personnel. Communication between the members of the team and cooperation of all individuals involved are essential if any real advantages are to accrue to the patient. Although ANH is a technique performed in the operating room and, thus, is the purview of the anesthesiologist, transfusion medicine specialists must be involved in the approval of protocols, assist in the technical aspects of

blood collection, and in the documentation of quality improvement issues. The protocols also should be approved by the hospital's medical staff committee.

## REFERENCES

1. Kronecker H. Uber die den eweben des korpers gunstigen flussigkeiten. Dtsch Med Wochenscher. 1882; 8:261.
2. Fahmy NR. Techniques for deliberate hypotension: haemodilution and hypotension. In Enderby GEH, ed. Hypotensive Anaesthesia. London, Eng: Churchill-Livingstone; 1985:164.
3. Ehrly AM. Drugs that alter blood viscosity: their role in therapy. Drugs. 1990; 39:155.
4. Kottman K. Über die viskosität des blutes. Correspondence. Schueizer Ärtzte 1907; 5:129.
5. Gelin LE, Ingelman B. Rheomacrodex. A new dextran solution for rheological treatment of impaired capillary flow. Acta Chirurg Scand. 1961; 122:294.
6. Fahey JL. Serum protein disorders causing clinical symptoms in malignant neoplastic disease. J Chronic Diseases. 1963; 16:703.
7. Ehrly AM, Lange B. Reduction in blood viscosity and disaggregation of erythrocyte aggregates by streptokinase. In: Hartert HH, Copley AL, eds. Theoretical and Clinical Hemorrheology. New York, NY: Springer-Verlag; 1971:366.
8. Cooley DA, Bloodwell RD, Beall AC, et al. Open heart surgery in Jehovah's Witnesses. Am J Cardiol. 1962; 13:779.
9. Gollub S, Bailey CP. Management of major surgical blood loss without transfusion. JAMA. 1966; 198: 1171.
10. Sunder-Plassman L, Klovern WP, Holper K, et al. The physiological significance of acutely induced hemodilution. Presented at the Sixth European Conference on Microcirculation; Aalborg, Basel, Switzerland: Karger; 23.
11. Hallowell P, Bland JHL, Dalton BC, et al. The effect of hemodilution with albumen or ringer's lactate on water balance and blood use in open-heart surgery. Ann Thorac Surg. 1978; 25:22.
12. Laver MB, Buckley MJ. Extreme hemodilution in the surgical patient. In: Messmer K, Schmid-Schoembein E, eds. Hemodilution: Theoretical Basis and Clinical Application. Basel, Switzerland: Karger; 1972:215.
13. Laks H, Pilon RN, Klovekorn WP, et al. Acute hemodilution: its effects on hemodynamics and oxygen transport in anesthetized man. Ann Surg. 1974; 180:103.
14. Lawson NW, Ochsner JL, Mills NL, et al. The use of hemodilution and free autologous blood in open heart surgery. Anesth Analg. 1974; 53:672.
15. Laver MB, Buckley MJ, Austen WG. Extreme hemodilution with profound hypothermia and circulatory arrest. Biblioth Haematolog. 1975; 41:225.
16. Lilleaasen P, Frøysaker T, Stokke O. Cardiac surgery in extreme haemodilution without donor blood, blood products or artificial macromolecules. Scand J Thorac Cardiovasc Surg. 1978; 12:248.
17. Cosgrove DM, Thurer RL, Lytle BW, et al. Blood conservation during myocardial revascularization. Ann Thorac Surg. 1979; 28:184.
18. Rosberg B, Wulff K. Hemodynamics following nor-

movolemic hemodilution in elderly patients. Acta Anaesthesiol Scand. 1981; 25:402.

19. Furman EB, Singler RC. Autologous transfusion in pediatric surgery. In: Kasprisin DO, Luban NLC, eds. Pediatric Transfusion Medicine. Boca Raton, Fla: CRC Press; 1987:138.

20. Messmer K. Preoperative hemodilution. In: Rossi EC, Simon TL, Moss GS, eds. Principles of Transfusion Medicine. Baltimore, Md: Williams & Wilkins Co; 1991:405.

21. Kafer ER, Isley MR, Hansen T, et al. Automated acute normovolemic hemodilution reduces homologous blood transfusion requirement for spinal fusion. Anesth Analg. 1986; 65:S76. Abstract.

22. Martin E, Hansen E, Peter K. Acute limited normovolemic hemodilution: a method for avoiding homologous transfusion. World J Surg. 1987; 11:53.

23. Kraft M, Dedrick D, Goudsouzian N. Haemodilution in an eight-month-old infant. Anaesthesia. 1981; 36:402.

24. Schaller RT Jr, Schaller J, Morgan A, et al. Hemodilution anesthesia: a valuable aid to major cancer surgery in children. Am J Surg. 1983; 146:79.

25. Milam JD, Austin SF, Nihill MR, et al. Use of sufficient hemodilution to prevent coagulopathies following surgical correction of cyanotic congenital heart disease. J Thorac Cardiovasc Surg. 1985; 89:623.

26. Salem MR, Bikhazi GB. Blood conservation. In: Motoyama EK, Davis PJ, eds. Anesthesia for Infants and Children. St. Louis, MO: CV Mosby Co; 1990.

27. Landgraf H, Ehrly AM. Hypervolämische hämodilution. Munchener Medizinische Wachenschrift. 1985; 127:117.

28. Landgraf H, Ehrly AM. Effects of an infusion of low molecular weight hydroxyethylstarch (HES) on the rheological properties of blood from healthy volunteers. In: Stoltz F, Drouin P, eds. Hemorrheology and Diseases. Paris, France: Drouin; 1980:665.

29. Gottstein U. Evaluation of isovolemic hemodilution. Clin Hemorheol. 1984; 4:133.

30. Messmer K. Compensatory mechanisms for acute dilutional anemia. Biblthca haemat. 47th ed. Basel, Switzerland: Karger; 1981:31.

31. Hint H. The pharmacology of dextran and clinical background of the clinical use of rheomacrodex. Acta Anesthesiol Belg. 1968; 19:119.

32. Murray JF, Gold P, Johnson BL Jr. Systemic oxygen transport in induced normovolemic anemia and polycythemia. Am J Physiol. 1962; 203:720.

33. Murray JF, Gold P, Johnson BL Jr. The circulatory effects of hematocrit variations in normovolemic and hypervolemic dogs. Am J Physiol. 1963; 42:1150.

34. Von Restorff W, Hofling B, Holtz J, et al. Effect of increased blood fluidity through hemodilution on coronary circulation at rest and during exercise in dogs. Pflugers Arch. 1975; 357:15.

35. Jan K-M, Chien S. Effect of hematocrit variations on coronary hemodynamics and oxygen utilization. Am J Physiol. 1977; 233:36.

36. Glick G, Plath WH, Braunwald E. Role of autonomic nervous system in the circulatory response to acutely induced anemia in anesthetized dogs. J Clin Invest. 1964; 43:2112.

37. Escobar E, Jones E, Rapaport E, et al. Ventricular performance in acute normovolemic anemia and ef-

fects of beta blockade. Am J Physiol. 1966; 211:877.

38. Rodriguez JA, Chamorro GA, Rapaport E. Effect of isovolemic anemia on ventricular performance at rest and during exercise. J Appl Physiol. 1974; 36:28.

39. Murray JF, Escobar E, Rapaport E. Effects of blood viscosity on hemodynamic responses in acute normovolemic anemia. Am J Physiol. 1969; 216:638.

40. Fowler NO, Holmes JC. Blood viscosity and cardiac output in acute experimental anemia. J Appl Physiol. 1975; 39:453.

41. Clarke TNS, Prys-Roberts C, Biro G, et al. Aortic impedance and left ventricular energetics in acute isovolemic anaemia. Cardiovasc Res. 1978; 12:49.

42. Guyton AC, Richardson TQ. Effect of hematocrit on venous return. Circ Res. 1961; 9:157.

43. Chapler CK, Hatcher JD, Jennings DB. Cardiovascular effects of propranolol during acute experimental anemia in dogs. Can J Physiol Pharmacol. 1972; 50:1052.

44. Tarnow J, Eberlein HJ, Hess W, et al. Hemodynamic interactions of hemodilution, anaesthesia, propranolol pretreatment and hypovolaemia.II: systemic circulation. Basic Res Cardiol. 1979; 74:109.

45. Clarke TNS, Foëx P, Roberts JG, et al. Circulatory responses of the dog to acute isovolumic anaemia in the presence of high-grade $\beta$-adrenergic receptor blockade. Br J Anaesth. 1980; 52:337.

46. Crystal GJ, Ruiz JR, Rooney MW, et al. Regional hemodynamics and oxygen supply during isovolemic hemodilution in the absence and presence of high-grade $\beta$-adrenergic blockade. J Cardiothorac Anesth. 1988; 2:772.

47. Chapler CK, Stainsby WN, Lillie MA. Peripheral vascular responses during acute anemia. Can J Physiol Pharmacol. 1981; 59:102.

48. Hatcher JD, Chiu LK, Jennings DB. Anemia as a stimulus to aortic and carotid chemoreceptors in the cat. J Appl Physiol. 1978; 44:696.

49. Szlyk PC, King C, Jennings DB, et al. The role of aortic chemoreceptors during acute anemia. Can J Physiol Pharmacol. 1984; 62:519.

50. Biro GP. Large venous compliance in carboxyhemoglobinemia and hemodilutional anemia. Can J Physiol Pharmacol. 1986; 64:556.

51. Crystal GJ, Salem MR. Blood volume and hematocrit in regional circulations during isovolemic hemodilution in dogs. Microvasc Res. 1989; 20:30.

52. Cain SM, Chapler CK. $O_2$ extraction by hindlimb versus whole dog during anemic hypoxia. J Appl Physiol. 1978; 45:966.

53. Wilkerson DK, Rosen AL, Gould SA, et al. Oxygen extraction ratio: a valid indicator of myocardial metabolism in anemia. J Surg Res. 1987; 42:629.

54. Levy PS, Chavez RP, Crystal GJ, et al. $O_2$ extraction ratio: a valid indicator of transfusion need in limited coronary vascular reserve? Trauma. 1992; 32:769.

55. Sunder-Plassman L, Kessler M, Jesch F, et al. Acute normovolemic hemodilution: changes in tissue oxygen supply and hemoglobin oxygen affinity. Bibl Haematol. 1975; 41:44.

56. Crystal GJ, Rooney MW, Salem MR. Myocardial blood flow and oxygen consumption during isovolemic hemodilution alone and in combination with adenosine-induced controlled hypotension. Anesth Analg. 1988; 67:539.

57. Crystal GJ, Salem MR. Myocardial and systemic he-

modynamics during isovolemic hemodilution alone and combined with nitroprusside-induced controlled hypotension. Anesth Analg. 1991; 72:227.

58. Crystal GJ, Kim S-J, Salem MR. Right and left ventricular $O_2$ uptake during hemodilution and $\beta$-adrenergic stimulation. Am J Physiol. 1993; 265: H1769.

59. Levy PS, Kim S-J, Crystal GJ, et al. Limit to cardiac compensation during acute isovolemic hemodilution: influence of coronary stenosis. Am J Physiol. 1993; 265:H340.

60. Crystal GJ. Myocardial oxygen supply-demand relations during isovolemic hemodilution. In: Bosnjak ZJ, Kampine JP, eds. Advances in Pharmacology: Anesthesia and Cardiovascular Disease. San Diego, CA: Academic Press. 1994; 31:285-312.

61. Crystal GJ. Coronary hemodynamic responses during local hemodilution in canine hearts. Am J Physiol. 1988; 254:H525.

62. Hofling B, von Restorff W, Holtz J, et al. Viscous and inertial fractions of total perfusion energy dissipation in the coronary circulation of the in situ perfused dog heart. Pflugers Arch. 1975; 1:358.

63. Crystal GJ, Salem MR. Myocardial oxygen consumption and segmental shortening during selective coronary hemodilution in dogs. Anesth Analg. 1988; 67:500.

64. Hagl S, Heimisch W, Meisner H, et al. The effect of hemodilution on regional myocardial function in the presence of coronary stenosis. Basic Res Cardiol. 1977; 72:344.

65. Feigl EM. Coronary physiology. Physiol Rev. 1983; 63:1.

66. Feola M, Azar D, Wiener L. Improved oxygenation of ischemic myocardium by hemodilution with stroma-free hemoglobin solution. Chest. 1979; 75: 369.

67. Kleinman LH, Yarbrough JW, Symmonds JB, et al. Pressure-flow characteristics of the coronary collateral circulation during cardiopulmonary bypass: effects of hemodilution. J Thorac Cardiovasc Surg. 1978; 75:17.

68. Johansson B, Linder E, Seeman T. Effects of hematocrit and blood viscosity on myocardial blood flow during temporary coronary occlusions in dogs. Scand J Thorac Cardiovasc Surg. 1967; 1:165.

69. Cohn LH, Lamberti JJ Jr, Florian A, et al. Effects of hemodilution on acute myocardial ischemia. J Surg Res. 1975; 18:523.

70. Yoshikawa H, Powell WJ, Bland JH, et al. Effect of acute anemia on experimental myocardial ischemia. Am J Cardiol. 1973; 32:670.

71. Borchgrevink CF, Enger E. Low molecular weight dextran in acute myocardial infarction. Br Med J. 1966; 11:1235.

72. Czinn EA, Salem MR, Crystal GJ. Hemodilution impairs hypocapnia-induced vasoconstrictor responses in the brain and spinal cord in dogs. Anesth Analg. 1995; 80:492.

73. Fan FC, Chen RY, Schuessler GB, et al. Effects of hematocrit variations on regional hemodynamics and oxygen transport in the dogs. Am J Physiol. 1980; 238:H545.

74. Crystal GJ, Rooney MW, Salem MR. Regional hemodynamics and oxygen supply during isovolemic hemodilution alone and in combination with adenosine-induced controlled hypotension. Anesth Analg. 1988; 67:211.

75. Michenfelder JD, Theye RA. The effects of pro-

76. Todd MM. Cerebral blood flow during isovolemic hemodilution: mechanistic observations. In: Bosnjak ZJ, Kampine JP, eds. Advances in Pharmacology. Vol 31. Anesthesia and Cardiovascular Disease. San Diego, CA: Academic Press; 1994:595-605.

77. von Kummer, Scharf J, Back T, et al. Autoregulatory capacity and the effect of isovolemic hemodilution on local cerebral blood flow. Stroke. 1988; 19: 594.

78. Asplund K. Multicenter trial of hemodilution in acute ischemic stroke. Acta Neurologica Scand. 1986; 73:530. Abstract.

79. Waschke KF, Krieter H, Hagen G, et al. Lack of dependence of cerebral blood flow on blood viscosity after blood exchange with a Newtonian $O_2$ carrier. J Cereb Blood Flow Metab. 1994; 14:871.

80. Borgstrom L, Johansson H, Siesjo BK. The influence of acute normovolemic anemia on cerebral blood flow and oxygen consumption of anesthetized rats. Acta Physiologica Scand. 1975; 93:505.

81. Maruyama M, Shimoj K, Ichikawa T, et al. The effects of extreme hemodilution on the autoregulation of cerebral blood flow, electroencephalogram and cerebral metabolic rate of oxygen in the dog. Stroke. 1984; 16:675.

82. Chien S. Role of sympathetic nervous system in hemorrhage. Physiol Rev. 1967; 47:214.

83. Simchon S, Chen RYZ, Carlin RD, et al. Effects of blood viscosity and plasma renin activity and renal hemodynamics. Am J Physiol. 1986; 250:F40.

84. Wright CJ. The effects of severe progressive hemodilution on regional blood flow and oxygen consumption. Surgery. 1976; 79:299.

85. Lipowsky HH, Firrel JC. Microvascular hemodynamics during systemic hemodilution and hemoconcentration. Am J Physiol. 1986; 250:H908.

86. Kuo L, Pittman RN. Effect of hemodilution on oxygen transport in arteriolar networks of hamster striated muscle. Am J Physiol. 1988; 254:H331.

87. Mirhashemi S, Breit GA, Chavez RH, et al. Effects of hemodilution on skin microcirculation. Am J Physiol. 1988; 254:H411.

88. Messmer K, Sunder-Plassman L. Hemodilution. Prog Surg. 1974; 13:208.

89. Stehling L, Zander HL. Acute normovolemic dilution. Transfusion. 1991; 31:857.

90. Kloevekorn WP, Pichlmaier H, Ott E, et al. Acute preoperative hemodilution—possibility for autologous blood transfusion. Chirurg. 1974; 45:452. Abstract.

91. Rosberg B. Blood coagulation during and after normovolemic hemodilution in elective surgery. Ann Clin Res. 1981; 33:84.

92. Kramer AH, Hertzer NR, Beven EG. Intraoperative hemodilution during elective vascular reconstruction. Surg Gynecol Obstet. 1979; 149:831.

93. Kaplan JA, Cannarella C, Jones EL, et al. Autologous blood transfusion during cardiac surgery. J Thorac Cardiovasc Surg. 1977; 74:4.

94. Barrera M, Miletich DJ, Albrecht RF, et al. Hemodynamic consequences of halothane anesthesia during chronic anemia. Anesthesiology. 1984; 61:36.

95. Fahmy NR, Chandler HP, Patel DG, et al. Hemodynamics and oxygen availability during acute hem-

odilution in conscious man. Anesthesiology. 1980; 53:S84. Abstract.

96. Rosberg B, Wulff K. Regional lung function following hip arthroplasty and preoperative normovolemic hemodilution. Acta Anaesthesiol Scand. 1979; 23:242.

97. Rose D, Coutsoftides T. Intraoperative normovolemic hemodilution. J Surg Res. 1981; 31:375.

98. Gammage G. Crystalloid versus colloid: is colloid worth the cost? Int Anesthesiol Clin. 1987; 25:1.

99. Brinkmeyer S, Safar P, Motoyama EK. Superiority of colloid over electrolyte solution for severe normovolemic hemodilution (NVHD) in concurrent treatment of hemorrhage. Disaster Med. 1983; 1: 171.

100. Carlson RW, Rattan S, Haupt MT. Fluid resuscitation in conditions of increased permeability. Anesthesiol Rev. 1990; 17(suppl 3):14.

101. Tremper KK, Waxman K. Artificial plasma expanders. In: Stoelting RK Barash PG, Gallagher TJ, eds. Advances in Anesthesia, Vol 2. Chicago, IL: Year Book Medical Publishers; 1985.

102. Davies MJ. The role of colloids in blood conservation. Int Anesthesiol Clin. 1990; 28:205.

103. Mailloux L, Schwartz CD, Cappizze R, et al. Acute renal failure after administration of low molecular weight dextran. New Engl J Med. 1967; 277:113.

104. Thoren L. Dextran as a plasma substitute. In: Blood Substitutes and Plasma Volume Expanders. New York, NY: Alan R. Liss, Inc; 1978:265.

105. Murray S, Dewar PJ. Low molecular weight dextran and crossing by enzyme technique. Transfusion. 1971; 11:398.

106. Arfors KE, Bergquist D. Microvascular haemostatic plug formation in the rabbit mesentery. In: Biblioth Haematolog. Basel, Switzerland: Karger; 1975:84.

107. Long IM. Status of plasma expanders in open heart surgery. Chest. 1962; 41:578.

108. Karlson KE, Garson AA, Shafton GW, et al. Increased blood loss associated with administration of certain plasma expanders. Surgery. 1967; 62:670.

109. Laver MB, Bland JHL. Anesthetic management of the pediatric patient during open-heart surgery. Int Anesthesiol Clin. 1975; 13:179.

110. Singler RC. Special techniques: deliberate hypotension, hypothermia, and acute normovolemic hemodilution. In: Gregory GA, ed. Pediatric Anesthesia. New York, NY: Churchill-Livingstone; 1993.

111. Schuh FT. Influence of hemodilution on the potency of neuromuscular blocking drugs. British Journal of Anaesthesia. 1981; 53:263.

112. Salem MR, Paulissian R, Joseph NJ, et al. Effect of deliberate hypotension on arterial to peak-expired carbon dioxide tension difference. Anesth Analg. 1988; 67:S194. Abstract.

113. Badgwell JM, Heavner JE, May WS, et al. End-tidal $PCO_2$ monitoring in infants and children ventilated with either a partial rebreathing or a nonrebreathing circuit. Anesthesiology. 1987; 66:405.

114. Salem MR, Wong AY, Bennett EJ, et al. Deliberate hypotension in infants and children. Anesth Analg. 1974; 53:975.

115. Furman EB, Roman DG, Lemmer LAS, et al. Specific therapy in water, electrolyte and blood-volume replacement during pediatric surgery. Anesthesiology. 1975; 42:187.

116. Gross JB. Estimating allowable blood loss: corrected for dilution. Anesthesiology. 1983; 58:277.

117. Han D, Rosenblatt M. Collecting blood for autologous transfusion. Anesthesiology. 1990; 73:1056

118. McMahon DJ, Carpenter RL. A comparison of conductivity-based hematocrit determinations with conventional laboratory methods in autologous blood salvage. Anesth Analg. 1990; 71:541.

119. Fahmy NR. A comparison of three methods for blood conservation for major orthopedic procedures. Anesthesiology. 1994; 81:A1248.

120. Eerola R, Eerola M, Kaukinen L, et al. Controlled hypotension and moderate hemodilution in major hip surgery. Ann Chir Gynaecol. 1979; 68:109.

121. Wong KC, Webster LR, Coleman SS, et al. Hemodilution and induced hypotension for insertion of a Harrington rod in a Jehovah's Witness patient. Clin Orthop Rel Res. 1980; 152:237.

122. Plewes JL, Farhi LE. Cardiovascular responses to hemodilution and controlled hypotension in the dog. Anesthesiology. 1985; 62:149.

123. Singler RC, Furman EB. Hemodilution: how low a minimum hematocrit? Anesthesiology. 1980; 53: S72. Abstract.

124. Haberkern M, Dangel P. Normovolaemic haemodilution and intraoperative transfusion in children: experience with 30 cases of spinal fusion. Eur J Pediatr Surg. 1991; 1:30.

125. Hallowell P, Bland JHL, Buckley MJ, et al. Transfusion of fresh autologous blood in open-heart surgery. A method for reducing bank blood requirements. J Thorac Cardiovasc Surg. 1972; 64:941.

126. Ochsner JL, Mills NL, Leonard GL, et al. Fresh autologous blood transfusions with extracorporeal circulation. Ann Surg. 1973; 177:811.

127. Weniger J, Shanahan R. Reduction of bank blood requirements in cardiac surgery. Thorac Cardiovasc Surg. 1982; 30:142.

128. Cosgrove DM, Loop FD, Lytle BW. Blood conservation in cardiac surgery. Cardiovasc Clin. 1981; 12:165.

129. Martin E, Ott E. Extreme hemodilution in the Harrington procedure. Bibl Haematol. 1981; 47:322.

130. Barbier-Bohm G, Desmonts JM, Couderc E, et al. Comparative effects of induced hypotension and normovolaemic hemodilution on blood loss in total hip arthroplasty. Br J Anaesth. 1980; 52:1039.

131. Sejourne P, Poirer A, Meakins JL, et al. Effect of haemodilution on transfusion requirements in liver resection. Lancet. 1989; 2:1380.

132. Davies MJ, Cronin KD, Domaingue C. Haemodilution for major vascular surgery—using 3.5% polygeline (haemaccel). Anaesth Intens Care. 1982: 10:265.

133. Goodnough LT. Blood conservation and blood transfusion practices: flipsides of the same coin. Ann Thorac Surg. 1993; 34:176.

134. Ness PM, Bourke DL, Walsh PC. A randomized trial of perioperative hemodilution versus transfusion of preoperatively deposited autologous blood in elective surgery. Transfusion. 1992; 32:226.

135. Eng J, Kay PH, Murray AJ, et al. Post-operative autologous transfusion in cardiac surgery: a randomized, prospective study. Eur J Cardiothorac Surg. 1990; 4:595.

136. Bell K, Scott K, Sinclair J, et al. A controlled trial of intra-operative autologous transfusion in cardiothoracic surgery measuring outcome on transfusion requirements and clinical outcome. Transfus Med. 1992; 2:295.

137. Ward HB, Smith RRA, Landis KP, et al. Prospective randomized trial of auto transfusion after routine cardiac operations. Ann Thorac Surg. 1993; 56: 137.

138. Feldman JM, Roth JV, Bjoraker DG. Maximum blood savings by acute normovolemic hemodilution. Anesth Analg. 1995; 80:108.

139. Brecher ME, Rosenfeld M. Mathematical and computer modeling of acute normovolemic hemodilution. Transfusion. 1994; 34:176.

140. Goodnough LT, Grishaber JE, Monk TG, et al. Acute preoperative hemodilution in patients undergoing radical prostatectomy: a case study analysis of efficacy. Anesth Analg. 1994; 78: 932.

141. Weiskopf RB. Human response to severe hemodilution. In: Proceedings of Autologous Blood Transfusion: Present Status and Controversies. Bethesda, MD: October 21, 1992.

142. Laver MB, Buckley MJ, Austen WG. Extreme hemodilution with profound hypothermia and circulatory arrest. Bibl Haematol. 1975; 41:225.

143. Chapler CK, Cain SM. The physiologic reserve in oxygen-carrying capacity: studies in experimental hemodilution. Can J Physiol Pharmacol. 1986; 64:7.

# 8

# DELIBERATE HYPOTENSION

*Arthur J. Klowden, M. Ramez Salem,*
*Nabil R. Fahmy, and George J. Crystal*

## HISTORICAL BACKGROUND

Poiseuille introduced the mercury manometer in 1828 and Riva-Rocci designed an inflatable cuff for the system; Korotkov described the sounds of systolic and diastolic pressures in 1905. Yet, despite these advances, the routine use and, more importantly, the ability and desire to understand the significance of blood pressure measurement were very slow in their adoption into medical practice. "In principle the surgeon and anesthetist were content with a high or artificially raised head of pressure, but sprang into action to support the circulation of a patient who mysteriously collapsed."[1]

The control of bleeding during surgery constitutes a fundamental tenet of sound surgical practice. Such control is not always easy. Persistent oozing may turn a simple surgical operation into a difficult one. Massive hemorrhage may jeopardize the patient's well-being and affect the outcome of a surgical procedure. Bleeding was undoubtedly a problem from the beginning of modern surgery, but "once the practice of anaesthesia became established, although the surgeon still caused the bleeding, the anaesthetist took the blame. This had some justification,"[2] because, for example, a rapidly performed amputation on a conscious patient possessing intact sympathetic mechanisms would often result in less bleeding than the same procedure using some early anesthetic techniques and volatile anesthetic agents. Anesthesia was done without intubation, without the use of muscle relaxants, and with spontaneous ventilation. Anesthesia was often accompanied by some degree of respiratory obstruction, vasodilation, coughing and straining, and intermittent periods of hypercapnia and hypoxia; these may have contributed to increased bleeding. Furthermore, explosive agents prevented the common usage of electrocautery.

Pitkin in 1912 remarked on the dryness of the operative field when the patient was given a spinal anesthetic.[1,3] It appears to have been Harvey Cushing, in 1917, who first observed the possible benefits of hypotension during surgery.[4] Cushing spoke sadly of the frequent and significant blood loss during neurosurgery but noted that this often led to a drier operative field. Laboratory investigations to demonstrate the interaction and differences between hypotension produced by hemorrhage versus that from neurogenic blockade were conducted by Phemister.[5]

After Kohlstaedt and Page[6] described reversing induced hypotension via the intraarterial reinfusion of removed blood in experimentally hemorrhaged animals, further experiments were initiated. Gardner[7] in 1946 reported on the use of deliberate hypotension to a systolic blood pressure of approximately 80 mm Hg induced via arteriotomy. These patients, for "difficult" neurosurgical procedures, had up to 1600 mL of blood removed via the dorsalis pedis artery; the blood was heparinized, kept in the operating room, and later reinfused. This was a technique fraught with difficulties that produced severe peripheral vasoconstriction, tachycardia, acidosis, and a hemorrhagic shocklike state. It was subsequently realized that vasoconstriction rather than hypotension had yielded the dry operative field. Five years later, Bilsland[8] noted

complications and even fatalities after arteriotomy techniques, and they were quickly abandoned.

Griffiths and Gillies[9] reported that high spinal anesthesia and postural adjustments to produce venous pooling led to a dry surgical wound. They stated that "a low head of arterial pressure associated with vasodilation and normal blood volume carries less potential danger than the illusory higher pressure which accompanies vasoconstriction and a reduced blood volume." Bromage[10] similarly reported on the use of high epidural blocks for a lowering of blood pressure.

Historically, the next step involved neurohumoral blockers. Research in this area had been stimulated by the rediscovery of a 1935 article[11] on the presence of quaternary nitrogen atoms in tubocurarine's structure. The ganglionic blocking agents that followed were linked to research on neuromuscular blocking agents, and the first of them was actually introduced as an antagonist to a neuromuscular blocking drug. In 1946, Acheson and co-workers[12,13] proposed the use of tetraethylammonium to chemically treat hypertension.

In 1948, the tubocurarinelike action of polymethylene bis-quaternary ammonium salts was reported,[14,15] and later Paton and Zaimis[16] wrote specifically on the clinical potentialities of hexamethonium and decamethonium. Hexamethonium was classified as a ganglionic blocking agent "offering possibilities of clinical usefulness in such fields as hypertension and vascular disease," whereas decamethonium was a useful neuromuscular blocking drug not antagonized by prostigmine but by pentamethonium. Combining their work with an anesthetist, these investigators used decamethonium and pentamethonium on themselves and noted postural hypotension and syncope as side effects.[17]

The "side effect" of hypotension was seized upon by investigators who wanted to see whether it could be used during surgery to reduce blood loss. The major advancement with normovolemic hypotension was achieved when ganglionic blockade was combined with foot-down tilt. Enderby actually demonstrated a hypotensive technique in 1950 and published the first definitive article on the subject. His paper, "*Controlled Circulation with Hypotensive Drugs and Posture to Reduce Bleeding in Surgery*,"[18] is perfectly titled and a classic. Enderby initially used pentamethonium, and others also published papers on its use.[19,20] Enderby later switched to hexamethonium and reported easier and more successful control of bleeding;[21] the percentage of successful cases rose from 58 to 85%.[22]

Two other ganglionic blockers were undergoing studies simultaneously: pentolinium and trimethaphan. Pentolinium was chosen by Enderby because of its superior potency and duration when compared with pentamethonium or hexamethonium. He reported on it favorably,[23,24] and it was widely used until its manufacture and distribution in the United States ceased in January 1977.

Trimethaphan (also known as trimetaphan), by contrast, is still in use; its introduction revolutionized the concept of controllability by virtue of its short duration of action and ability to be given by continuous intravenous infusion. The drug was originally studied by Randall and associates[25] and later by McCubbin and Page[26] and Sarnoff and associates.[27] Clinical studies leading to its use soon followed.[28–30]

The obvious advantages of hypotension soon led to considerable demand for its use, but the enthusiastic initial reception was quickly followed by unexplained morbidity and mortality.[31,32] This led some to condemn the technique and totally abandon it, whereas others continued to investigate and refine its possibilities. Those who continued its use were discouraged by the frequent failure of the technique to achieve significant hypotension in healthy young patients.[33] Some surgeons demanded its use in "frankly unsuitable cases and inadvisable circumstances,"[1] and so some authors cautioned a conservative approach.[34,35] Over the years many have attempted to overcome deficiencies in the technique of hypotensive anesthesia by adding on a variety of devices; among the abandoned techniques was Saunders[36] negative pressure device to encase the legs with a suction pressure of 30–40 mm Hg. Another technique attempted was rapid cardiac pacing to produce profound hypotension or circulatory arrest for short periods in selected cases of difficult intracranial aneurysms.[37,38] This method has not gained acceptance because of its inherent dangers and because it requires preoperative insertion of a transvenous pacemaker.

The effects of controlled ventilation and d-tubocurarine on blood pressure had become known by 1952. A more effective control of blood pressure was achieved with the use of positive end-expiratory pressure (PEEP).[39] The introduction of halothane[40,41] was a remarkable breakthrough. It allowed an easier and more gentle induction of hypotension with and without ganglionic blockade.[42] Although the hypotensive effect of sodium nitroprusside was known for many years, it was not introduced into clinical practice until 1962 by Moraca and associates.[43] The action of sodium nitroprusside on vascular smooth muscle produced a dose-dependent hypotension.[44]

With the availability of many drugs, other hypotensive techniques became of merely historic interest. The first scientific report on morbidity and mortality after hypotensive anesthesia in a large series was published in 1961[45] and demonstrated unequivocally that it could be practiced safely. β-Adrenergic blocking drugs were introduced to treat and prevent tachycardia.[46–50] The continued use of β-adrenergic blockers supports the claim that the use of propranolol was another milestone in deliberate hypotension. Advances in knowledge of the physiology of hypotension and the pharmacology of hypotensive agents, along with advances in monitoring methods, have contributed to the evolution and safety of deliberate hypotension. The discovery that labetalol, which has α-adrenergic and β-adrenergic blocking properties, is effective in the treatment of severe hypertension prompted its use to induce deliberate hypotension.[51] Nitroglycerin was introduced as a hypotensive drug by Fahmy in 1978.[52]

Enderby[1] points out that the 40-year history of developing and understanding hypotensive anesthesia has seen a changing attitude toward blood pressure. As noted, all efforts in the past were made to maintain and restore blood pressure to "normal" levels, whereas now it is acceptable for the blood pressure to decrease to a certain extent, and this fall may be beneficial to the patient. Enderby[1] quotes Sir Archibald McIndoe at a 1951 demonstration as saying that, "hypotension was so important that it was up to you anaesthetists to make it safe." Certainly that has been the goal anesthesiologists sought over the years.

## USES OF DELIBERATE HYPOTENSION

The recommended indications in the literature can be found listed in Table 8–1.[53–58] The benefits to be gained by the use of deliberate hypotension depend in part on surgeons and their skills. In this regard, hypotensive anesthesia is not the answer to poor surgical technique, and as Enderby put it, "good surgical technique skillful enough to match the high standards of hypotensive anesthesia is essential if any real advantages are to accrue to the patient."[23]

Hypotensive drugs are used in anesthetic practice to achieve one or more of the following goals:[54,59] (a) reduction of blood loss, (b) facilitation of vessel surgery, and (c) management of threatening hemorrhage.

**Table 8–1.  Indications for the use of deliberate hypotension**

Orthopedic procedures
  Scoliosis
  Total hip arthroplasty
  Miscellaneous, including lumbar spine fusion, disarticulations, bone transplants, etc.
Head and neck surgery
  Orthognathic procedures (maxillo-facial)
  Oncological (radical surgery of head and neck)
  Otolaryngological (middle ear microsurgery)
  Thyroidectomy or parotidectomy
Neurosurgical (including pediatric)
  Aneurysm or arteriovenous malformation
  Vascular tumors
  Craniofacial procedures
Urological surgery
  Radical cystectomy or prostatectomy
Major vascular procedures
  Lieno-renal shunt for portal hypertension
  Coarctation of the aorta and other pediatric vascular anomalies
  Adult vascular procedures
Pelvic surgery
  Abdominoperineal resection
  Radical hysterectomy or pelvic exenteration
Plastic surgery (skin grafts and flaps, etc.)
Chest wall and/or intrathoracic surgery
  Radical mastectomy or thoracoplasty
  Reduction mammoplasty
  Thoraco-abdominal dissection
Transfusion limitations
  Jehovah's witnesses
  Lack of proper blood (e.g., rare agglutinins), etc.

## Reduction of Blood Loss

By producing a relatively dry operative field, deliberate hypotension improves visualization and allows the accurate delineation of lesions. With hypotension, less trauma is inflicted on nerves, vessels, and delicate structures. Hypotension may increase the viability of pedicles and grafts and may diminish the incidence of postoperative hematoma, sepsis, and fibrosis. Accompanying the reduced blood loss is a diminished need for, or avoidance of, massive blood transfusion. In certain operations the need for infiltration with epinephrine-containing solutions may be eliminated with deliberate hypotension, thereby allowing delicate surgery to be performed without distorting the anatomy of the area. Hypotensive anesthesia was shown to reduce the operative time of scoliosis repair by approximately 30 minutes.[60] Reports of blood loss with deliberate hypotension vary widely and may depend on the site of operation, position of the patient, drugs and techniques used, level of blood pressure, heart rate, and the experience of the surgeon and the anesthesiologist.[61]

## Facilitation of Vessel Surgery

Blood pressure control has facilitated surgery on the large vessels.[54,59,61–63] The most common applications include coarctectomy, ligation and division of a large patent ductus arteriosus, surgery on the aorta, clipping of an intracranial aneurysm or arteriovenous malformation, and excision of vascular tumors. By keeping a large vessel soft and preventing excessive stretching and progressive thinning of its wall, blood pressure control makes subsequent suturing or clipping easier. It also reduces the forcefulness of the pulse pounding against a clamped artery, minimizes trauma to a diseased vessel, and helps prevent slippage of the clamp. Control of leakage and prevention of aortic dissection and tearing can also be facilitated. Although no evidence indicates that blood pressure control decreases the incidence of premature intraoperative aneurysm rupture, the reduction in intraaneurysmal pressure decreases the size of the rupture and makes it more mobile, thus facilitating its surgical dissection.

## Management of Threatening Hemorrhage

The rationale for inducing hypotension in the management of threatening hemorrhage is based on the maintenance of capillary blood flow in shock states, the reduction of precapillary sphincteric tone, and the reduction of bleeding from transected vessels, thereby permitting control of the source of hemorrhage and restoration of blood volume.[64–67] Although blood pressure control in the management of hemorrhage has been demonstrated, it has not been widely used for this purpose.

## Mode of Action of Hypotensive Drugs

The cardiovascular effects of hypotensive drugs may be modified by many factors: the anesthetic and other drugs given; position of the patient; degree of hypotension; and relative change from preoperative blood pressure, intrathoracic pressure, acid-base status, circulating blood volume, age of the patient, and mode of action of the hypotensive drug.[54,61]

Normovolemic hypotension can be produced by either a reduction in the cardiac output (CO) or a decrease in the peripheral resistance. Although potent inhalation anesthetics have variable effects on the peripheral circulation, their hypotensive effect is a result of either direct myocardial depression resulting in decreased CO or, in the case of isoflurane, to peripheral vasodilation. Ganglionic blocking drugs and other directly acting vasodilators act primarily on the peripheral circulation. The smaller precapillary arterioles have relatively large amounts of smooth muscle and thus are the major determinants of resistance. Because vascular resistance is inversely related to the fourth power of the radius of the arterioles, relatively small changes in intraluminal diameter have profound effects on peripheral vascular resistance.[68]

## Role of Vascular Endothelium

Up until about 1970 the vascular endothelium was generally regarded as an unstructured cell lining of blood vessels that served passive functions, such as providing a nonthrombogenic barrier for the flowing blood.[69] Investigators paid little attention to the metabolic and functional properties of the vascular endothelium primarily because the relatively small amount of endothelium within the blood vessel made it seem unlikely that these cells could contribute significantly to global organ function and metabolism and suitable procedures to perform such studies of the endothelium had not yet been developed.

The introduction of isolation and cultivation of endothelial cells as a routine technique by Jaffe[70] permitted detailed studies of the specific metabolic and functional properties of the endothelium. The detection of angiotensin-converting enzyme in cultured endothelial cells provided important early evidence that the endothelium can actively alter vascular smooth muscle tone by releasing a vasoactive substance.[70] Subsequent studies provided additional evidence to support this concept. The endothelial cells synthesize many active substances, including large molecules, such as fibronectin and heparin sulfate; interleukin-1; tissue plasminogen activator; various growth-promoting factors; and smaller molecules such as prostacyclin and endothelium-derived relaxing factor (EDRF), which has recently been characterized as nitric oxide.

### PROSTACYCLIN

Prostacyclin was discovered in 1976 and is a major member of the family of prostaglandins produced by endothelial cells. It is a powerful vasodilator and inhibits platelet aggregation via the activation of adenylate cyclase. Prostacyclin is formed from arachidonic acid, which is derived from membrane phospholipids. Its formation is catalyzed by the enzyme cyclooxygenase. Aspirinlike drugs inhibit cyclooxygenase activity and thus prostacyclin production. Once released, prostacyclin is degraded rapidly in plasma to 6-keto-prostaglandin $F_1\alpha$, which is relatively devoid of the biological actions of prostacyclin.[69]

Mechanical or chemical perturbation of cell membranes causes formation and release of prostacyclin, which is not stored by cells. In the endothelial cell, pulsatile pressure, a number of endogenous mediators, and some drugs stimulate prostacyclin production.[69,71,72] The endogenous mediators include substances derived from plasma, such as bradykinin and thrombin, and those liberated from platelets, such as serotonin, platelet-derived growth factor, interleukin-1, and adenine nucleotides. The drugs purported to increase prostacyclin production include calcium antagonists, captopril, dipyridamole, diuretic agents, nitrates, and streptokinase.

From a physiological perspective, prostacyclin is a local hormone rather than a circulating hormone. On the abluminal side of the vessel it causes relaxation of the underlying smooth muscle, and in the lumen it prevents platelets and other cellular elements from adhering to the endothelial surface. The capacity of vascular tissue to produce prostacyclin decreases with age, in diabetes mellitus, and in atherosclerosis.[69]

The instability of prostacyclin restricts its clinical usage. However, when prostacyclin is contained within an alkaline buffer, it has been used to prevent blood coagulation and to preserve platelets in extracorporeal circulations;[73] also, a constant infusion of prostacyclin has been used to treat pulmonary hypertension.[74]

## ENDOTHELIUM-DERIVED RELAXING FACTOR-NITRIC OXIDE

In 1980, Furchgott and Zawadzki[75] discovered a new fundamental mechanism by which the endothelium can modulate vascular smooth muscle tone. They demonstrated that relaxation of isolated arterial strips by acetylcholine is strictly dependent on the presence of intact endothelial cells. They found subsequently that endothelium-dependent relaxation by acetylcholine is initiated by an action of acetylcholine on a muscarinic receptor and that the action of acetylcholine on this receptor stimulates the endothelial cells to release a substance that causes relaxation of vascular smooth muscle. They called this substance endothelium-derived relaxing factor, or EDRF.

It was later demonstrated that EDRF, like the organic nitrates, for example, nitroglycerin, relaxed vascular smooth muscle by stimulating guanylate cyclase to produce cyclic guanosine monophosphate. The fact that the organic nitrates are first metabolized to nitric oxide before producing these effects provided an early clue that EDRF may be nitric oxide. Subsequently, different laboratories provided evidence that EDRF has pharmacological and chemical properties identical to nitric oxide and that a correlation is found between the formation of nitric oxide and the release of EDRF.[76-78] Moreover, it was demonstrated that the amount of nitric oxide released from vascular endothelial cells challenged by bradykinin could account for the actions of EDRF.[79] It is now widely accepted that EDRF is nitric oxide or a very similar compound.

Production of EDRF-nitric oxide is stimulated by arginine[79] and is inhibited by the arginine analog $N^G$-monomethyl-L-arginine.[80] Formation of nitric oxide from arginine appears to be an important component of a widespread intercellular communication system. In addition to the vascular endothelium, nitric oxide is released from a number of other tissues, including neutrophils, brain, renal epithelial cells, adrenal medullary cells, and mast cells.[81-83]

Recent in vivo studies suggested an important role for EDRF-nitric oxide in physiological regulation of the circulation. For example, intravenous injection of the nitric oxide inhibitor $N^G$-monomethyl-L-arginine causes an abrupt and appreciable increase in arterial blood pressure.[84] This suggests that continuous basal release of EDRF may maintain the vasculature in a dilated condition. Animal studies have demonstrated a reduced basal release of EDRF in chronic hypertension, atherosclerosis, and diabetes.[69]

Increments in flow per se caused dilation of epicardial coronary arteries that required intact endothelium.[85] This flow-dependent dilation was not due to endothelial release of prostacyclin, because inhibitors of cyclooxygenase did not blunt the response. The finding that methylene blue (a rather nonspecific inhibitor of soluble guanylate cyclase, nitrovasodilator-induced and EDRF-induced vasodilation) reduced flow-dependent dilation in canine femoral arteries suggests a role for EDRF in the response.[86] It has been speculated that the stimulus for the release of EDRF-nitric oxide in the presence of increased flow is stretching and deformation of endothelial cells because of accentuated luminal shear stresses.[86] In addition to acetylcholine, a number of other compounds are purported to cause vasodilation via the EDRF-nitric oxide mechanism. These include bradykinin, adenosine triphosphate (ATP), arachidonic acid, substance P, and carbon dioxide.[86] Although common hypotensive agents, such as sodium nitroprusside, apparently act independently of both prostacyclin and EDRF-nitric oxide, it seems likely that the activity of these agents will be modified when background vascular tone is altered because of impaired basal release of these endogenous substances from damaged or diseased endothelium.

## Ganglionic Blocking and Direct-Acting Hypotensive Drugs

Ganglionic blocking drugs compete with acetylcholine for the nicotinic receptors on the postjunctional membrane at the autonomic ganglia. There is no change in the membrane potentials of ganglion cells or any alteration in transmission in the preganglionic or postganglionic fibers, and the release of acetylcholine by preganglionic impulses is unaffected. Because most organs are reciprocally innervated by sympathetic and parasympathetic nerves, the overall effect of autonomic blockade depends on the predominance of one or the other system at the end organ. Because the arterioles and venules of the skin and splanchnic viscera have predominantly sympathetic vasoconstrictor innervation, ganglionic blockade usually results in peripheral vasodilation, decreased arteriolar tone, increased venous capacitance, and hypotension. In contrast, the iris, ciliary muscle, gastrointestinal tract, urinary bladder, and sweat glands are all under predominantly parasympathetic control. Thus, ganglionic blockade produces mydriasis, cycloplegia, constipation, urinary retention, and abolition of sweating. Because of these side effects, ganglionic blocking drugs are no longer used for the treatment of hypertension. However, these side effects are of no consequence after intravenous use during anesthesia or in the postoperative period, with the exception of mydriasis and cycloplegia after the use of ganglionic blockade with pentolinium, which may last for several hours. This effect has led to misinterpretation in the neurological assessment of patients after neurosurgical procedures.[59]

Trimethaphan-induced hypotension has been attributed to ganglionic blockade, a direct effect on vascular smooth muscle, $\alpha$-adrenergic blockade, and histamine release.[87] Although histamine release occurs in humans, especially after bolus administration of tri-methaphan, it does not seem to play a predominant role in the production of hypotension.[88]

Both sodium nitroprusside and nitroglycerin produce hypotension by relaxing the vascular smooth muscle. The hypotensive effect of both drugs is independent of either $\alpha$-adrenergic, $\beta$-adrenergic or nicotinic receptors. The site of action is probably within the arteriolar and venular walls. The precise mechanism whereby smooth muscle relaxation is produced is unknown, but molecular mechanisms involving sulfhydryl groups,[89] blocking intracellular calcium activation,[90] or causing reactions with cyclic nucleotides [cyclic AMP or cyclic guanosine 3',5'-monophosphate (GMP)] have been postulated.[91]

Although sodium nitroprusside and nitroglycerin exert profound effects on peripheral vascular resistance, the magnitude of effect on the precapillary resistance vessels and on the capacitance vessels is dissimilar. Sodium nitroprusside exerts its effects mainly on the smaller precapillary resistance vessels. Topically applied sodium nitroprusside (to exclude systemic compensatory hemostatic reflexes) in animal experiments results in potent arteriolar but not venular vasodilation.[92] However, in humans the venous effects are indirectly evidenced by changes in ventricular filling pressure and by changes in oxygenator reservoir volumes during cardiopulmonary bypass.[93,94] Sodium nitroprusside appears to exert its hypotensive action by a combination of decreased systemic vascular (arteriolar) resistance (SVR) and increased capacitance, but the venous effect is minimal and a fall in CO does not occur. In contrast, nitroglycerin has little effect on arteriolar resistance vessels but exhibits relatively pronounced effects on the venous capacitance vessels, resulting in a decreased venous return, decreased ventricular filling pressure, and ultimately reduced CO.[68,95] Because sodium nitroprusside dilates both arterioles and venules, it has proved to be a more potent hypotensive drug than nitroglycerin.[68,95,96]

## EFFECTS OF HYPOTENSIVE DRUGS

### Cardiac Output

High spinal anesthesia decreases the arterial blood pressure primarily by reducing venous return and CO. Deep halothane anesthesia lowers arterial pressure primarily by direct myocardial depression and reduced heart rate. Vasodilator drugs alter the CO through changes in stroke volume and heart rate; they decrease afterload by lowering arterial impedance and reduce preload by increasing venous compliance. Depending on the ventricular function as defined by the Frank-Starling mechanism and the relative effect of the drug on the preload and afterload, stroke volume may rise, remain constant, or even decline.[97] A decrease in afterload shifts the curve to the left. If preload remains constant, stroke volume will increase. If the decrease in afterload is associated with a decrease in preload, then stroke volume will probably remain constant. A decrease in preload without a decrease in afterload will probably result in decreased stroke volume.

Changes in CO during deliberate hypotension are heart rate related.[97,98] Changes in heart rate depend on the predominant autonomic tone existing at the time hypotension is initiated. If sympathetic predominance exists, heart rate decreases; if vagal tone is predominant, heart rate increases. Because children have an increased vagal tone, they respond to hypotensive drugs with tachycardia. Halothane negates the reflex increase in heart rate produced by hypotensive drugs by "resetting the baroreceptors," depressing vasomotor centers, and directly depressing sinoatrial node activity.

In anesthetized humans with normal cardiac function, sodium nitroprusside-induced hypotension is associated with either increased or unchanged CO; hypotension secondary to ganglionic blockade variably affects CO.[88,97–100] In anesthetized dogs, the decrease in CO with trimethaphan was greater than the decrease in blood pressure, resulting in a widening of the arteriovenous oxygen difference. Because of the effect of nitroglycerin on venous capacitance and venous pressure, ventricular filling pressure decreases and ultimately CO is reduced.[52,68,94]

Hypotension associated with "shock states" may be followed by irreversible organ damage. In contrast, well-controlled hypotension is very rarely followed by even minimal organ damage. In the shock state, hypotension is accompanied by severe decreases in organ blood flow, whereas blood flow to vital organs during deliberate hypotension is generally well maintained. In theory, as long as mean arterial blood pressure exceeds the sum of colloid osmotic pressure plus venous pressure, the circulation should be adequate for tissue needs. This calculation suggests that a pressure of 32 mm Hg is satisfactory. However, this value is probably considerably below the safe level for two reasons. First, it ignores specific blood flow requirements; the critical closing pressure (the pressure at which flow ceases despite the existence of a standing head of pressure) varies from organ to organ and from individual to individual. Second, it ignores the limitations set by disease. Therefore, the mean arterial blood pressure should not be allowed to fall below 45–50 mm Hg in any patient unless there is a definite indication or unless additional measures are used to ensure adequate organ protection.

## Cerebral Circulation

As arterial blood pressure decreases, a concomitant parallel decrease in cerebrovascular resistance occurs that serves to maintain a constant cerebral blood flow. The normal cerebral blood flow in the adult is usually maintained at a level of approximately 50 mL/100 g/min within defined limits of blood pressure and cerebral perfusion pressure. The usual limits of such autoregulation are a mean arterial pressure between 50 and 150 mm Hg.[101,102] Below or above these levels flow is pressure dependent. Perfusion pressure is the pressure gradient between arterial-side input and venous-side outflow. Cerebral perfusion pressure is the mean arterial blood pressure minus the mean intracranial pressure; because mean intracranial pressure is normally approximately 10 mm Hg, the cerebral perfusion pressure is mean arterial pressure minus 10 mm Hg.

Patients with chronic hypertension have autoregulation curves that are shifted to the right, and their lower limit for autoregulation is reset at a higher pressure; the cerebral vascular resistance in these patients cannot decrease enough to maintain cerebral blood flow if cerebral perfusion pressure is reduced severely.[103] Hypotension induced in hypertensive patients can decrease cerebral blood flow at higher arterial blood pressures than in normotensive patients and may lead to cerebral hypoxia.[104–107] Because of the fear of a similar event in the anesthetized patient, clinicians have advocated caution with these patients and will not reduce the blood pressure as low as they usually do in a normotensive healthy patient.[108] Effective antihypertensive treatment can move the autoregulatory curve toward normal.[109,110] The cerebral perfusion pressure to cerebral blood flow relationship may be shifted to the left in infants and young children.[61,111,112]

The autoregulatory mechanism may be abolished or attenuated with deep anesthesia, hypoxemia, hypocapnia or hypercapnia, circulatory arrest, and transiently with sudden dramatic changes in systolic arterial blood pressure.[101] Autoregulation may also be absent in abnormal parts of the brain after brain trauma,[113] after subarachnoid hemorrhage,[114] and near brain tumors.[115] In a study of patients with known cerebrovascular disease, small decreases in cerebral perfusion pressure produced marked decreases in cerebral blood flow in certain areas of the brain and produced symptoms of dizziness, neurological deficit, and even stroke.[116] Therefore, if at all possible, hypotension should be avoided in these patients.[117]

If cerebral perfusion pressure falls below a certain critical level, cerebral blood flow decreases. Compensatory mechanisms come into play, including widening of the arteriovenous oxygen content difference; if these are not sufficient, ischemic tissue cell damage will ensue.[118] When cerebral perfusion pressure decreases to 40–50 mm Hg, electroencephalographic (EEG) slowing may be noted. Irreversible damage may occur when the cerebral perfusion pressure falls below 18–20 mm Hg.[119,120] EEG changes have been reported when the cerebral blood flow is reduced 40–50% from control levels, and the EEG may become isoelectric if the cerebral blood flow falls more than 60% below control.[121] Magness and coworkers[122] reported that trimethaphan-induced hypotension sometimes led to an abnormal EEG at or below a mean blood pressure of 50 mm Hg.

Extreme hyperventilation (to $PaCO_2$ 25 mm Hg or less) during deliberate hypotension, particularly when the cerebral perfusion pressure is less than 50 mm Hg, can lead to the depletion of brain energy substances, in-

cluding glucose, glucose-6-phosphate, phosphocreatinine, ATP, and $\alpha$-keto-glutarate;[123] a progressive lactic acidosis in the brain may occur and the susceptibility of the brain to hypoxic damage may increase.[118,124,125] Some investigators found that the cerebral vascular response to carbon dioxide continues during deliberate hypotension.[126,127] Thus, many authors advocate the avoidance of excessive hypocapnia during hypotension.[126–129] Other authors have found that hypocapnia reduces cerebral blood flow only during the phase of moderate hypotension; if $PaCO_2$ loses its influence on cerebral perfusion at extremely low arterial pressures, then hypocapnia may not increase the risk of cerebral ischemia.[130–135] It may be concluded that unless hypocapnia is indicated, it ought to be avoided during deliberate hypotension.

The preservation of cerebral function and metabolism during hypotensive anesthesia, at least in animals, is best obtained by isoflurane, then sodium nitroprusside and nitroglycerin, and then trimethaphan.[136–138] It has been postulated that isoflurane might offer some degree of protection against ischemia or hypoxia, similar to that of thiopental, with a dose-related reduction in cerebral metabolic rate.[139,140]

Sodium nitroprusside can abolish cerebral autoregulation while increasing cerebral blood flow.[141] Sudden increases in arterial pressure will result in sudden increases in cerebral blood flow and intracranial pressure during a sodium nitroprusside infusion. The increases in intracranial pressure vary widely from patient to patient but are seen primarily during the initial phase of sodium nitroprusside administration.[142–144] The rapid rate at which sodium nitroprusside reduces blood pressure may exceed the ability of the cerebral circulation to autoregulate its own blood flow,[145] and intracranial pressure and blood pressure will change simultaneously but in opposite directions.[146] Cottrell and coworkers[144] showed that a 33% reduction in mean arterial pressure produced by sodium nitroprusside led to a 50% reduction in cerebral perfusion pressure but an almost 100% increase in intracranial pressure. Lowering the blood pressure slowly over 5 minutes can overcome much of the intracranial pressure rise (Fig. 8–1).[147] Therefore, sodium nitroprusside should probably not be used in pa-

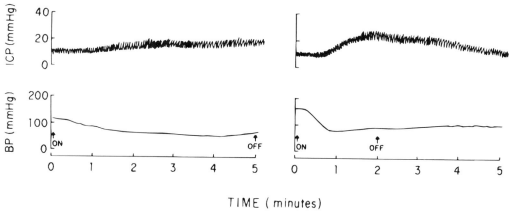

**Fig. 8–1.** Compared with rapid infusion, the slow intravenous administration of sodium nitroprusside does not increase the intracranial pressure. From Marsh ML, Aidinis SJ, Naughton KVH, et al: The technique of nitroprusside administration modifies the intracranial pressure response. Anesthesiology 1979; 51:538, with permission.

tients with low intracranial compliance until the dura has been opened or until drugs (diuretics, barbiturates), hyperventilation, or cerebrospinal fluid drainage have improved intracranial compliance. Similar increases in intracranial pressure are reported during nitroglycerin-induced hypotension.[145] In contrast, trimethaphan does not produce an increased intracranial pressure except during severe intracranial compression.[143]

Knowledge of the patient's preoperative blood pressure may be helpful in deciding on the level of blood pressure during hypotension. In normotensive patients, cerebral ischemia is not expected to occur until the mean cerebral perfusion pressure is decreased by 65% (a 40% reduction during which flow is unchanged because of autoregulation plus a 25% reduction during which cerebral blood flow falls linearly). Using a conservative margin of safety by dividing the calculated allowable reduction in half, the minimum acceptable mean cerebral blood flow would be 67% of the mean normal preoperative cerebral perfusion pressure.[148] Common practice, however, includes a greater reduction in cerebral perfusion pressure by assuming a lower safe blood pressure. In actuality, larger decreases in blood pressure are usually well tolerated. Because infants and children have a normal blood pressure that is lower than that in adults, blood pressure limits established in adult studies may not be appropriate in pediatric patients.[53,54] In general, lower levels of blood pressure must be reached to achieve a comparable dry operative field in pediatric patients.

## The Eye

In the past, many investigators reported that hypotensive anesthesia could decrease intraocular pressure;[149–152] therefore, a reduction in arterial blood pressure was advocated to reduce intraocular pressure and decrease some of the risks of complex intraocular surgery.[153,154]

The effects of general anesthesia and deliberate hypotension on intraocular pressure were studied by Jantzen and associates recently.[155] They compared sodium nitroprusside, adenosine, and isoflurane as hypotensive drugs in pigs. They found that deliberate hypotension does not reduce intraocular pressure and thus is probably of no benefit in surgical ophthalmology. Adenosine, their example of a powerful pure vasodilator, produced an initial increase in intraocular pressure preceding hypotension and produced a further increase in intraocular pressure when arterial pressure recovered rapidly as adenosine was terminated. This intraocular rebound hypertension was not associated with arterial rebound hypertension.

Blurring of vision has been reported with the use of ganglionic blockers after deliberate hypotension. Although blindness was reported as a very rare complication in older studies, it was not proven to be solely due to the hypotension.

## CORONARY CIRCULATION

Oxygen extraction in the left ventricle is nearly maximal under baseline conditions (approximately 70–75%) and remains essentially constant in the face of wide variations in myocardial oxygen consumption.[156] Thus, changes in myocardial oxygen consumption are met by proportional changes in coronary blood flow, secondary to adjustments in coronary vascular resistance. These adjustments in coronary vascular resistance are mediated by vasoactive metabolites, for example, adenosine, released from the myocardium. Such metabolic mechanisms predominate in the physiological regulation of coronary blood flow.

The major determining factor affecting coronary perfusion is the aortic diastolic pressure. Thus, during deliberate hypotension a decrease in arterial pressure may be accompanied by a decrease in coronary perfusion. Two additional factors affect coronary blood flow during deliberate hypotension: metabolic vascular control mechanisms and the direct coronary vascular effects, if any, of the hypotensive agent used. During deliberate hypotension a reduction in left ventricular wall tension reduces cardiac work load and myocardial oxygen demand, as long as reflex tachycardia is avoided. If the hypotensive drug is free of a direct coronary vasodilating action, metabolic factors mediate the changes in coronary vascular tone required to lower coronary blood flow to a level commensurate with this reduced myocardial oxygen demand. However, if the hypotensive drug has a direct vasodilating action in the coronary circulation, for example, exogenous adenosine, the metabolic vascular control mechanisms are overridden and the level of coronary blood flow is excessive or luxuriant.

Because patients with severe ischemic heart disease have limited coronary reserve, coronary blood flow is essentially pressure dependent. Thus, in these patients, deliberate hypotension will cause a decrease in coronary blood flow because of reduced coronary perfusion pressure. Whether this decrease in blood flow leads to myocardial ischemia depends on the extent to which myocardial oxygen demand is also decreased. If blood flow and oxygen demand decrease proportionally, myocardial ischemia will be avoided. If blood flow decreases more than oxygen demand, myocardial ischemia will be evident. The risk of myocardial ischemia is heightened in patients with ischemic heart disease by reflex tachycardia via two mechanisms: the tendency for tachycardia to increase myocardial oxygen demands and a reduction in the duration of diastole, which is the phase of the cardiac cycle in which most of the perfusion of the subendocardium occurs.

During deliberate hypotension, a progressive decrease in the heart rate-systolic pressure product (an index of myocardial oxygen demand) has been observed in adults[97] and children.[98] This may explain the lack of electrocardiographic (ECG) evidence of myocardial ischemia during hypotension.[52,53] However, by increasing the myocardial oxygen demand, tachycardia may increase the potential for myocardial ischemia.

ECG changes suggestive of ischemia were noted in 38–45% of patients during sodium nitroprusside-induced hypotension.[52,157] These changes were attributed to reflex tachycardia, because the incidence of ST-T wave changes was far less during nitroglycerin-induced hypotension that is not associated with increased heart rate.[52] Although nonspecific ECG changes were reported in over 50% of patients during isoflurane-induced hypotension to a mean blood pressure of 50 mm Hg, none of the 33 patients developed enzyme elevation or other evidence of myocardial infarction.[158] Rollason and Hough[159] noted that a 50% decrease in systolic blood pressure could consistently produce transient ECG evidence of ischemia in elderly patients and in patients with preexisting hypertension. They also noted[160] that significant ST-segment or T-wave changes occurred when the decrease in blood pressure was too rapid.

## Renal Circulation

The normal kidneys, although receiving approximately 25% of CO, use only 7% of the total body oxygen consumption; they are thus considered "luxury perfused" and protected from damage even during hypotension. Normally, renal blood flow is autoregulated over a wide range of changes in mean blood pressure from approximately 80–180 mm Hg. There is a system of intrinsic autoregulation as well as the potential for a multiplicity of extrinsic influences via aldosterone and antidiuretic hormone and the autonomic nervous system.[120] This autoregulation is abolished by vasodilators and anesthetics,[56,101,161] making renal blood flow pressure dependent; thus, decreases in renal blood flow can occur with moderate decreases in arterial pressure. Urine formation decreases sharply when renal artery perfusion pressure falls below the level required for glomerular filtration with any hypotensive drug; urine flow may cease when mean arterial pressure falls below 60 mm Hg. Although this level of perfusion pressure may be inadequate to sustain glomerular filtration, it may be adequate for metabolic needs and thus oliguria during hypotension does not, by itself, lead to serious renal damage.[162-165]

Although hypotensive drugs such as sodium nitroprusside decrease the renal vascular resistance in the isolated kidney preparation, the effects of these drugs in the intact kidney are variable and rather complex. This is because of the multiplicity of factors affecting renal blood flow, including the sympathetic nervous system, exogenous or endogenous catecholamines, the renin-angiotensin system, antidiuretic hormone levels, and hypercapnia.

In a rat preparation, deliberate hypotension with nitroglycerin, sodium nitroprusside, or deep enflurane anesthesia did not lead to any significant changes in renal blood flow or kidney function.[109] In the dog, studies have shown that a decrease of 15–50% in systolic blood pressure was associated with normal renal blood flow.[166,167] Even severe hypotension in dogs, to a mean arterial pressure as low as 12–25 mm Hg, was not followed by increases in either serum creatinine or blood urea nitrogen.[168]

In humans, decreases in glomerular filtration rate and effective renal plasma flow may occur during normotensive anesthesia.[169] Similar decreases in glomerular filtration rate and effective renal plasma flow have been noted during hypotensive anesthesia with isoflurane to a mean arterial pressure of 55–65 mm Hg.[170] The lack of further reduction in renal function during deliberate hypotension suggests that renal compensatory mechanisms are preserved during hypotension.[171-173] Thompson and associates[174] found no significant changes in urinary or serum electrolytes, blood urea nitrogen, or creatinine in 30 patients who had deliberate hypotension for total hip arthroplasty. Renal medullary tissue

oxygenation, an index of tissue viability, has been found to be adequate during deliberate hypotension;[164,165] furthermore, various kidney functions, including glomerular filtration rate, effective renal plasma flow, and urine output, all return quickly to normal after blood pressure returns to preoperative levels, even after prolonged hypotension.[170,175,176]

It may be concluded that unless deliberate hypotension reduces renal blood flow below the critical level for the kidney, it is very unlikely that serious renal sequelae will ensue.[61] Monitoring the urine output may be useful, particularly during prolonged periods of hypotension. The presence of known renal artery stenosis may constitute a contraindication to deliberate hypotension, because it may result in a substantial reduction in renal blood flow.

## The Liver and Splanchnic Circulation

The liver has a unique vascular supply from two sources: the hepatic artery supplies 25–30% of the total blood flow to the liver, and the portal vein supplies the remaining 70–75%. The total hepatic blood flow is approximately 100 mL/min/100 g or approximately 25% of the CO.[177] The hepatic oxygen supply is, however, almost equally split with 45–50% from the hepatic artery and 50–55% from the portal vein. Hepatic arterial autoregulation occurs but is rather limited, whereas portal venous autoregulation is virtually nonexistent.[178] Thus, severe hypotension could lead to a decrease in hepatic blood flow that could result in hepatic damage. Dogs subjected to profound arterial hypotension to mean pressures of 12–25 mm Hg showed not only severe enzymatic alterations but also definite pathological changes, including pericentral lobular hepatic necrosis and hepatocyte degeneration.[168] At moderate levels of hypotension, hepatic hypoxia does not occur. In dogs, a 40% decrease in arterial pressure by sodium nitroprusside resulted in a 25% decrease in portal blood flow and a 44% decrease in portal pressure, along with a 13% increase in hepatic arterial blood flow.[179] Sodium nitroprusside decreases portal sinusoidal resistance, allows the liver to increase its arterial flow (in conditions of insufficient portal circulation), and thus does not lead to hepatic hypoxia.[179] Studies in humans subjected to hypotensive anesthesia for hip arthroplasty showed that postoperative liver function tests were essentially unchanged.[174]

It should be noted that anesthetic and surgical factors themselves may have effects on the splanchnic circulation and liver function. Isoflurane, for example, produced a dose-dependent decrease in portal and hepatic blood flows, whereas oxygen consumption in the splanchnic area was unchanged, and consequently the surface oxygen tension was decreased.[180,181] Because the splanchnic circulation has sympathetic nervous system innervation, sympathetic stimulation or catecholamine release could decrease the hepatic blood flow. This effect has been reported with hypoxemia,[182] hypercapnia and acidosis,[101,183] and during mechanical ventilation.[184] These studies lead us to believe that deliberate hypotension per se does not have an adverse effect on the splanchnic circulation or liver function.

## TACHYCARDIA AND TACHYPHYLAXIS

In most patients, the administration of a hypotensive drug results in a decrease in blood pressure and a slight increase in heart rate. After hypotensive anesthesia was introduced into clinical practice, the problem of "failure to maintain hypotension" became apparent (tachyphylaxis). This phenomenon is best described as a diminished response, despite repeated administration of the drug. Resistance to hypotensive drugs is almost always associated with tachycardia. This is more frequently seen in children than in adults and is very rare in the elderly.[53,185] Resistance to hypotension is not a unique feature of one particular drug or technique and has been reported with all ganglionic blockade drugs, $\alpha$-adrenergic blocking drugs, and other direct-acting drugs, including sodium nitroprusside, nitroglycerin, and phentolamine.[46,52,96,99,186-189]

Various mechanisms have been postulated to explain tachycardia or tachyphylaxis during deliberate hypotension (Table 8–2).[190] The relative importance of these mechanisms may differ depending on the hypotensive drug given. Sodium nitroprusside-induced hypotension is associated with increases in heart rate and CO, activation of the renin-angiotensin system, and release of catecholamines.[191-195] In contrast, ganglionic blockade results in less of an increase in circulating catecholamines and no activation of the renin-angiotensin axis.[195,196] The increase in heart rate with the use of ganglionic blocking drugs is probably the result of parasympathetic blockade. This may be more prominent in children because of their increased vagal tone.[53,96,98,195]

Reflex tachycardia, mediated through the baroreceptors, occurs with almost all hypotensive drugs (Fig. 8–2).[54,59,197,198] The increased heart rate results in an increased CO and counteracts the decrease in blood pressure. Both tachyphylaxis and tachycardia are predominantly due to activation of the renin-angiotensin system after the release of catecholamines in response to hypotension. As a result of sympathetic activation, renin is released from the juxtaglomerular apparatus in the kidney. This acts on an $\alpha_2$-globulin from the liver to produce the decapeptide angiotensin I, which is converted in the lungs to the octapeptide angiotensin II, a potent vasoconstrictor. Stimulation of the sympathetic and the renin-angiotensin systems may adversely affect the operative course of patients undergoing deliberate hypotension. A higher concentration of the inhalational anesthetic or

**Table 8–2. Theories postulated to explain tachycardia or resistant hypotension (tachyphylaxis) or both during deliberate hypotension**

1. Parasympathetic blockade causing tachycardia (ganglionic blockade)
2. Reflex tachycardia mediated through the baroreceptors in response to the initial fall in pressure (probably all hypotensive drugs)
3. Stimulation of the sympathetic and renin-angiotensin systems leading to increased plasma renin activity and angiotensin II and catecholamine levels (direct-acting drugs, especially sodium nitroprusside)
4. Constrictive effect of sympathetic blockade on the $\beta$-adrenoceptive blood vessels leading to rise in blood pressure
5. Inappropriate (excessive) fluid therapy before and during hypotension (causing expansion of blood volume and difficulty in controlling pressure.
6. Antagonism of the vasodilator action of sodium nitroprusside by the increased tissue cyanide concentration (disproved)

From Salem MR, Bikhazi GB. Hypotensive anesthesia. In: Motoyama EA, Davis PJ, eds, Smith's Anesthesia for Infants & Children, 5 ed. St. Louis, 1990, C. V. Mosby, p. 356, with permission.

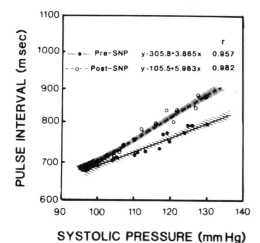

**Fig. 8–2.** Baroreceptor sensitivity increases after nitroprusside-induced hypotension (post-SNP) compared with pre-SNP. From Chen RYZ, Matteo RS, Fan F-C, et al: Resetting the baroreceptor sensitivity after induced hypotension. Anesthesiology 1982; 56:29, with permission.

larger doses of the hypotensive drug may be required to maintain hypotension. With sodium nitroprusside, cyanide toxicity may result if the maximum permissible dose is exceeded. Even when hypotension is achieved, the CO may remain elevated secondary to tachycardia and may result in excessive bleeding.

Tachycardia, even with hypotension, may cause increased oozing because of repetitive spike-filling of the vessels. Tachycardia tends to increase the myocardial oxygen demand and may increase the potential for myocardial ischemia. Rebound hypertension may occur after abrupt termination of the sodium nitroprusside infusion.[191,192,194] This is related to the increase in SVR due to the unopposed persistent stimulation produced by the sympathetic and renin-angiotensin systems. The consequences of rebound hypertension include hematoma formation, wound bleeding, cerebral edema, cerebrovascular accidents, disrupted cerebral autoregulation, and pulmonary edema.[199] The varying sensitivities of vessels to sodium nitroprusside in different organs may cause major changes in the distribution of blood flow among the various organs, as well as a redistribution of blood flow within organs. Considerable evidence suggests that very high circulating catecholamine and angiotensin II levels have deleterious effects on

myocardial and renal tubular cells and may adversely affect arterial and capillary function.[200–202]

The following drugs or techniques have been advocated to prevent tachyphylaxis:

1. Halothane (inactivates the baroreceptor response)
2. Avoiding fluid overload
3. Omitting belladonna drugs
4. Preoperative sedation and the use of intravenous opioids
5. Use of a β-adrenergic blocking drug
6. Pretreatment with angiotensin II competitive antagonist
7. Pretreatment with angiotensin-converting enzyme inhibitor
8. Combining hypotensive drugs
9. Premedication with clonidine

The key to preventing tachyphylaxis is the control of the heart rate. The anesthetic technique must be flawless during hypotension, including all aspects of airway patency, adequate oxygenation, normocapnia, and adequate anesthetic depth. Atropine and similar drugs may be omitted or their dosage decreased. Fluid overload must be avoided when hypotension is induced.

Prevention of tachycardia may be achieved by blocking the β-adrenergic receptors. Propranolol given slowly in small increments up to $60 \mu g/kg$ before or after the administration of a hypotensive drug is effective in preventing the rise in heart rate and in facilitating the control of blood pressure, without the need for high anesthetic concentrations.[53] It is preferable to give propranolol before the onset of tachycardia, because after tachycardia a much larger dose may be required. In this dose range, the action of propranolol is almost exclusively ascribed to blockade of the β-adrenergic receptors. Being a nonselective β-adrenergic blocker, propranolol blocks both $\beta_1$ (predominantly the heart) and $\beta_2$ (predominantly blood vessels and bronchial smooth muscles) receptors. Increased airway resistance in normal subjects and the occurrence of bronchospasm in asthmatics after the use of propranolol led to the development of more selective $\beta_1$-adrenergic blockers.[203] Table 8–3 lists the currently available β-adrenergic blocking drugs that can be used as adjuvants to hypotensive anesthesia and gives information regarding cardioselectivity and elimina-

**Table 8–3.   Dose, cardioselectivity, and elimination half-life of currently available B-adrenergic blocking drugs**

| Drug | Dose | Cardioselectivity ($\beta_1$) | Elimination half-life |
|---|---|---|---|
| Propranolol | 0.06 mg/kg | 0 | 4 hr |
| Practolol | 0.15 mg/kg | + | 10 hr |
| Metoprolol | 0.15 mg/kg | + | 3–4 hr |
| Esmolol | Loading dose 0.5 mg/kg/min followed by 300 μg/kg/min constant infusion | + | 10 min |
| Labetalol | 0.1–0.4 mg/kg depending upon background anesthetic; additional increments until desired effect is achieved | 0 (has $\alpha_1$-$\beta_1$ and $\beta_2$ adrenergic blocking properties) | 3.5–4.5 hr |

Modified from Salem MR, Bikhazi G. Hypotensive Anesthesia. In: Motoyama EA, David RJ, eds. Smith's Anesthesia for Infants and Children, 5 ed. St. Louis, CV Mosby, 1990; 357.

tion half-life. The advantages of the $\beta$-adrenergic blocker esmolol appear to be its rapid onset, titratable action, short duration, and cardioselectivity.[204-206] The drug may be given in a loading dose of 500 μg/kg/min for 2–4 minutes and continued by constant infusion at a rate of 300 μg/kg/min.

Treatment with propranolol or other $\beta$-adrenergic blocking drugs prevents increased heart rate, CO, plasma renin activity, and catecholamine levels (Fig. 8–3).[53,98,191,194,196] $\beta$-Adrenergic blockade also prevents rebound hypertension after cessation of sodium nitroprusside infusion (Fig. 8–4).[191,194] Furthermore, the dose requirements of sodium nitroprusside are decreased by approximately 40% in patients pretreated with propranolol. Because the combination of inhalational anesthetics and $\beta$-adrenergic blockers produces an additive hemodynamic depression, careful monitoring of patients given the combination of these drugs is essential.[207]

Attempts to prevent increased concentrations of vasoactive substances during deliber-

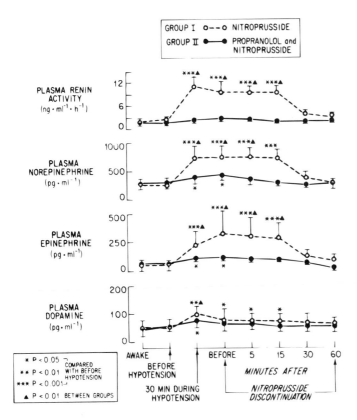

**Fig. 8–3.**  Values (mean ± SD) of plasma renin activity and plasma norepinephrine, epinephrine, and dopamine levels in the awake state, before and during sodium nitroprusside, and after abrupt discontinuation of sodium nitroprusside in two groups of patients: one group received sodium nitroprusside alone and the other group was pretreated with intravenous propranolol before infusion of sodium nitroprusside. From Fahmy NR, Mihelakos PT, Battit GE, et al: Propranolol prevents hemodynamic and humoral events after abrupt withdrawal of nitroprusside. Clin Pharmacol Ther 1984; 36:470, with permission.

**Fig. 8–4.** Hemodynamic events (mean ± SD) in the awake state, before and during sodium nitroprusside infusion, and after abrupt discontinuation of sodium nitroprusside in two groups of patients: one group received sodium nitroprusside alone and the other group was pretreated with intravenous propranolol before infusion of sodium nitroprusside. From Fahny NR, Mihelakos PT, Battit GE, et al: Propranolol prevents hemodynamic and humoral events after abrupt withdrawal of nitroprusside. Clin Pharmacol Ther 1984; 36:470, with permission.

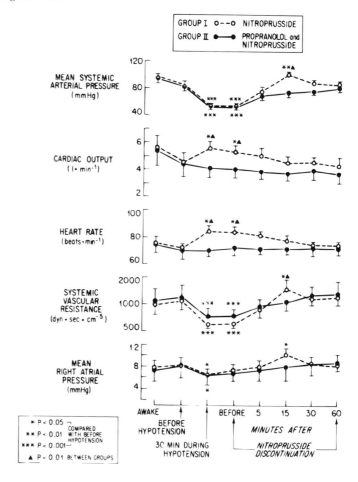

ate hypotension have included pretreatment with saralasin,[208] an angiotensin II competitive antagonist, and captopril,[209] an oral angiotensin-converting enzyme inhibitor. Pretreatment with captopril results in lower dosage requirements and also prevents rebound hypertension.

Resistance to sodium nitroprusside might, at least in part, involve a diminished release of nitric oxide because of the depletion of tissue thiols. Administration of an intravenous thiol, cystine, has been reported to reverse the resistance.[210]

Recently there has been renewed interest in combining hypotensive drugs. A 10 : 1 mixture of trimethaphan (250 mg) and sodium nitroprusside (25 mg) in a solution of 5% dextrose in water has been recommended. The mixture produces controllable hypotension with smaller doses of sodium nitroprusside and trimethaphan than when either drug is used separately. When the mixture is used, the dose of sodium nitroprusside is approximately one-third to one-fifth the amount required when sodium nitroprusside is used alone. The combination has a synergistic rather than an additive effect because the proportional reduction in dose of each drug is greater than half. The use of the mixture has the following advantages (Fig. 8– 5): a drier surgical field, absence of tachyphylaxis, a quiet circulation (less or no increase in CO and heart rate), lower dose requirement for sodium nitroprusside and thus lower cyanide and thiocyanate levels, gradual return of blood pressure without rebound hypertension after termination of the infusion, and absence of the prolonged hypotension sometimes associated with large doses of trimethaphan when used alone.[211–213] In the most recent study,[214] the authors concluded that a 5 : 1 ratio of trimethaphan to sodium nitroprusside was the optimal balance between the tachycardic and excessive sympathetic response induced by the

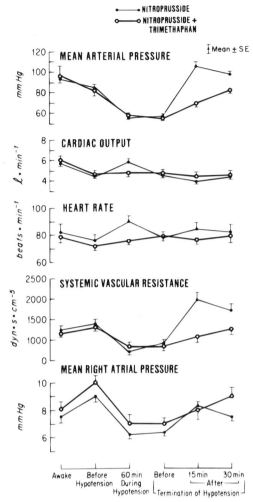

**Fig. 8–5.** Comparison of the hemodynamic effects of sodium nitroprusside and a sodium nitroprusside-tri-methaphan mixture. From Fahmy NR, Almaz MG: Vaso-dilator drugs. In Stoelting RG, Barash PG, Gallagher TJ, eds, Advances in Anesthesia. Chicago, 1989, Year Book Medical Publishers Inc, vol. 6, p. 139, with permission.

sodium nitroprusside and the depressed sympathetic activity induced by trimethaphan.

## TECHNIQUES FOR INDUCING HYPOTENSION

Many varied techniques have been described for the induction of deliberate hypotension during anesthesia (Table 8–4).[54,59,190,215] Preganglionic sympathetic blockade produced by spinal or epidural anes-

thesia has a limited application as a technique for inducing hypotension. If used for this purpose, spinal or epidural anesthesia should be combined with general anesthesia and tracheal intubation. Spinal or epidural catheters are needed to extend the duration of the block. One of the main advantages of spinal or epidural blockade for the induction of deliberate hypotension has been the absence of tachycardia. However, tachycardia associated with the use of intravenous hypotensive drugs can be effectively prevented and treated by the judicious use of a $\beta$-adrenergic blocking drug. Two basic induction techniques are currently in use: the conventional technique and deep anesthesia with or without head-up tilt and PEEP.

## Conventional Technique

Hypotension is to be induced only when the following conditions are satisfied: the patient is in a relatively stable clinical state, the intravenous lines are secured, reliable and adequate monitoring devices are in place and functioning, the airway is secured with an endotracheal tube, controlled ventilation is begun, and a steady state of light anesthesia

**Table 8–4.   Techniques of inducing hypotension**

Requirements before inducing hypotension
   Stable clinical state
   Secure airway (endotracheal intubation)
   Reliable intravenous catheter, basic monitoring
   Means of accurate blood pressure measurements
   Light anesthesia: inhalation anesthetic with relaxants,
     or nitrous oxide, narcotic, relaxant
   Controlled ventilation
Conventional technique
   Steps of inducing gradual hypotension:
     1. Intravenous administration of a vasodilator or a
       ganglionic blocker; a $\beta$-adrenergic blocker may
       be given before the hypotensive drug
     2. Tilting (if feasible)
     3. Gradual increase of inhalation anesthetic
     4. PEEP (very rarely needed)
Alternative technique
   Deep anesthesia (halothane, enflurane, or isoflurane)
     with tilting and/or PEEP

From Salem MR, Bikhazi GB: Hypotensive anesthesia. In: Motoyama EA, Davis PJ, eds, Smith's Anesthesia for Infants & Children, 5 ed. St. Louis, 1990, C. V. Mosby, with permission.

is ensured. This steady state can be achieved with either an opioid and nitrous oxide technique, usually supplemented with a nondepolarizing muscle relaxant, with a low concentration of a volatile anesthetic (halothane, enflurane, or isoflurane), or with a combination of narcotic and of an inhalational agent. All opioid drugs can be given by bolus and/or infusion techniques. If somatosensory-evoked potentials are to be monitored, the inhalational agent must be used in a low concentration to avoid loss of the waveform.

With the patient in the horizontal position, hypotension is induced gradually with the aid of a ganglionic blocking drug or a direct-acting vasodilator (a comparison of five hypotensive drugs is shown in Table 8–5). The drug is administered shortly after intubation and at least 10 minutes before the incision is made. If surgery is to be performed in the prone position (e.g., for scoliosis correction), hypotension is induced only after the patient is carefully positioned and proper placement of the tracheal tube is reconfirmed. It is preferable to give a β-adrenergic blocker before the hypotensive drug is administered, because the tachycardia is better and more easily prevented than treated.[50,53] The time to onset of hypotension depends on the drug given (Table 8–5).

After the effect of the hypotensive drug is assessed, the patient may then be tilted head-up and/or foot-down slowly, if this position is acceptable for the planned surgery. In some patients, hypotension does not occur until this addition of peripheral pooling augments the pharmacological drug effect. The patient should be tilted slowly because cerebral autoregulation requires several minutes.[216] Head-up tilt is not feasible in some operations (hip and back surgery); however, some degree of peripheral pooling may be obtained by lowering the feet alone while maintaining the operative part horizontally, as in scoliosis surgery. A further decrease in arterial pressure can be obtained by a gradual increase in the concentration of the volatile anesthetic. This is particularly useful when tilting is not possible.

Although d-tubocurarine has been used to enhance hypotension, it does not seem to have any real advantages in reducing blood loss.[60] Both atracurium and vecuronium have become popular as relaxants of choice for these procedures, and the two newer longer-acting

agents, pipecuronium and doxacurium, may also be acceptable when titrated for the appropriate duration.

## Deep Anesthesia With or Without Posture and PEEP

Some anesthesiologists prefer to initiate hypotension and maintain the hypotensive state by deepening the anesthetic level or relying on posture, PEEP, or both without intravenous hypotensive drugs.[59,174,217] The dose-related depression of cardiovascular function produced by halothane, enflurane, and isoflurane has been documented in both human and animal experiments.[218–221] However, some qualitative as well as quantitative differences exist among these anesthetics.[222] Halothane and enflurane produce dose-related decreases in arterial pressure and CO, whereas SVR is not significantly affected. Halothane has little effect on heart rate, whereas enflurane produces a significant dose-related increase in heart rate.[222] Isoflurane also produces an increase in heart rate, although the increase is not usually dose related. CO is better preserved with isoflurane, even at twice the minimum alveolar concentration (MAC), because of a decrease in afterload. Thus, in healthy humans both halothane and enflurane have minimal effects on SVR, and the reduction in systemic pressure is secondary to a dose-dependent decrease in left ventricular function, whereas the hypotensive effects of isoflurane are probably related more to its effect on peripheral vasodilation.[221,222]

Because contractile function of the myocardium is impaired with increasing halothane concentration, the use of deep halothane anesthesia as the sole means of inducing hypotension is not recommended.[223] Some patients may exhibit remarkable cardiovascular stability even with deep anesthesia[224]; however, blood pressure control may be difficult with deep anesthesia alone. Furthermore, sluggish return of blood pressure to normal levels may be encountered at the termination of the hypotensive state when the anesthetic is discontinued.

Isoflurane has been used with increasing frequency for the induction of hypotension in the last decade. Lam and Gelb[225] found a rapid (6-minute) onset of hypotension with effective lowering of the arterial blood pres-

**Table 8–5.   Comparisons of five hypotensive drugs**

| Characteristic | Pentolinium tartrate (unavailable in U.S.) | Trimethaphan camphorsulfonate | Sodium nitroprusside | Nitroglycerin | Labetalol |
|---|---|---|---|---|---|
| Onset of action | Gradual onset, slow recovery | Rapid onset, usually rapid recovery | Rapid onset, very rapid recovery | Rapid, but gradual onset, moderately slower recovery | Gradual onset, moderately slow recovery |
| Duration | Long acting | Short acting; but may be prolonged with halothane, propranolol, or in presence of atypical cholinesterase | Evanescent action; may be prolonged if cyanide toxicity develops | Short acting | Long acting |
| Preferred method of administration | IV single injection | IV drip (0.1% to 0.2% in 5% D/W) | IV drip (0.01% solution) | IV drip (0.01% in either 5% D/W or 0.9% NaCl) | IV injection, repeated increments |
| Mode of action | Ganglionic blockade | Ganglionic blockade, direct effect, $\alpha$-adrenergic blockade, histamine release | Direct effect (resistance and capacitance vessels) | Direct effect (capacitance vessels predominantly) | $\alpha$- and $\beta$-adreno-ceptor antagonist |
| Tachycardia | Occurs in children, less likely in adults | Tends to occur in children less likely in adults | Very common | May occur in lightly anesthetized children, unlikely in adults | None, usually slight bradycardia |
| Cardiac output | May remain unchanged, increase, or decrease, depending on posture (venous pooling), changes in heart rate, preload and afterload, anesthetics, other myocardial depressant drugs, ventilation, intravascular volume status. | | | | Slight decrease or no change |
| Blood-brain barrier | Minimal or no derangement | Minimal or no derangement | Pronounced dysfunction | Probably same as sodium nitroprusside | Maintained |
| Metabolism | Excreted unchanged | Unclear; inhibits plasma cholinesterase but not metabolized by it (not an ester), 30% recovered in urine unchanged and active | Metabolized to cyanide and thiocyanate | Degraded rapidly in the liver | Degraded in the liver |
| Stability | Stable | Unstable; kept refrigerated | Available as powder, unstable when reconstituted, protect from light, use within 12 h | Stable; colorless, absorbed by plastics, use high-density polyethylene drip set | Stable |
| Dose | 0.2 mg/kg | Not limited by toxicity; total IV dose should not exceed 10 mg/kg | Initial dose 0.5–1.5 $\mu$g/kg/min. Careful titration, dose usually < 8 $\mu$g/kg/min; total projected dose not to exceed 1.5 mg/kg in 4 h | Recommended dose 10–20 $\mu$g/kg/min. | Recommended dose 0.2–0.4 mg/kg, followed by increments of 0.1–0.2 mg/kg (usually 10–20 mg bolus, then increments of 5–20 mg) |
| Histamine release | None | Histamine release related to administration rate; does not contribute to the hypotensive effect. | Unknown | Unknown | Unknown, probably none |
| Iris and ciliary muscle | Mydriasis and cycloplegia last several hours | Mydriasis and cycloplegia of short duration | Unaffected | Unaffected | Unaffected |
| Neuromuscular function | Probably no effect | A weak nondepolarizing effect in large doses | Probably no effect | A weak nondepolarizing effect | Probably no effect |
| Rebound hypertension | Does not occur | Does not occur | Occurs in absence of $\beta$ blockade | Does not occur | Does not occur |
| Intracranial pressure | Unknown | Variable, but may decrease | Increases in early stages of hypotension, less with hypocapnia | Increases, greater than with trimethaphan | No change |

Modified from Salem MR. Therapeutic Use of Ganglionic Blocking Drugs. Int Anesthesiol Clin 1978; 16:171–200.

sure to a mean of 40 mm Hg. The recovery from hypotension was fairly rapid and the CO was not changed significantly. Maktabi and associates,[226] also taking the mean pressure to 40 mm Hg, found a small yet significant decrease in cardiac index. The intravascular volume status of the patient may be a contributing factor to the possible decrease in CO with isoflurane. In young healthy patients, 2 or 3 vol% isoflurane seems solely to decrease SVR, and this in turn decreases the blood pressure. In contrast, older patients, particularly those who are hypertensive, may show a decrease in CO; in these patients, even isoflurane cannot be recommended as the sole agent for the induction and maintenance of hypotension.[227]

An increase in mean airway pressure has been used to fine-tune hypotension to the desired level.[54,59,215] For example, a decrease of systolic pressure from 80 to 70 mm Hg can be accomplished swiftly by adding PEEP (10 cm $H_2O$) and can be reversed quickly by discontinuing PEEP. However, PEEP may have some undesirable effects when used as the vernier adjustment to deliberate hypotension. PEEP exerts its hypotensive effect by restricting venous return (preload) and thereby reducing CO. Normally, this is opposed by peripheral vasoconstriction. With hypotensive drugs, this potential compensatory mechanism is lost and the circulatory effects of PEEP become apparent.[128]

PEEP may have additional deleterious effects during deliberate hypotension. It tends to increase the intracranial[228,229] and intraocular pressures[230] and tends to raise the cerebral venous pressure, thus reducing perfusion pressure to the brain. From data obtained on patients rendered hypotensive by the application of PEEP, it was observed that some patients developed a critically low jugular bulb oxygen tension, indicating a substantial decrease in cerebral blood flow.[231] Maintenance of high alveolar pressure in normal lungs causes increased physiological dead space and may result in unnecessary distension of the alveoli.[126] Excessive PEEP may result in diminution in urine flow.[232] The use of PEEP in spinal surgery may increase inferior vena cava pressure, with diversion of blood into the vertebral venous plexuses, and lead to increased oozing.[233]

## ANESTHETIC REQUIREMENTS AND DELIBERATE HYPOTENSION

Practitioners of the technique of deliberate hypotension have long been aware of the fact that anesthetic requirements seem to be decreased when deliberate hypotension is used. Rao and colleagues[234] tested this seeming association and demonstrated that the MAC of halothane was decreased by approximately 30% during deliberate hypotension in dogs, independent of the specific drug used for the hypotension. When the blood pressure was allowed to return to normal, the MAC also returned to baseline if the dogs had received either trimethaphan or pentolinium. If the dogs had been given sodium nitroprusside instead, the MAC appeared to remain decreased. In their studies, changes in MAC during deliberate hypotension did not correlate with CO or cerebral blood flow. Although the exact mechanism for these changes has not as yet been elucidated, these findings have potentially important clinical implications. Concentrations of inhalational anesthetic agents must be decreased during deliberate hypotension to avoid a delayed awakening. Similarly, these agents must be terminated sooner if an intraoperative wake-up test is planned during corrective surgery for scoliosis.[235]

## THE DRY OPERATIVE FIELD

A relatively dry operative field and improved operating conditions are the main goals of deliberate hypotension. It is a misconception that these goals are automatically accomplished at a predetermined level of blood pressure. Troublesome bleeding may still continue despite hypotension. The astute anesthesiologist should ascertain that deliberate hypotension did in fact improve the surgical field. A lower level of blood pressure or other hemodynamic adjustments (positioning, control of heart rate) may be needed to improve the success of hypotension.

Controversy surrounds the relative importance of blood pressure and CO (or blood flow at the operative site) in producing a drier operative field. Furthermore, the advantages claimed for a particular technique or drug are erroneously based on the findings that the CO and oxygen delivery are either well maintained or increased during hypotension. Some authors believe that a reduction in CO is essential to reduce bleeding and that even when blood pressure is low, bleeding is not necessarily reduced unless there is a concomitant fall in CO.[98,126,196,236,237] Bennett and associates[60] reported a greater reduction in blood loss with pentolinium than with sodium nitroprusside, which tends to increase the CO. Knight and coworkers[196] found a positive correlation between blood loss and left ventricular stroke work index during hypotensive anesthesia for surgical correction of scoliosis. Other investigators found that blood pressure was the main factor determining blood loss.[100,238] Amaranath and colleagues[239] found a correlation between systolic blood pressure and blood loss. Sivarajan and associates[238] concluded that operative blood loss during deliberate hypotension is determined by mean arterial pressure and not CO. Their study, however, was conducted on patients undergoing mandibular osteotomies placed in a head-up tilt. It is possible that this position resulted in pooling of blood in the dependent areas so that blood flow at the operative site was decreased.

The requirement of a relatively bloodless field may depend on decreased CO and blood flow at the operative site or both. In contrast, when hypotension is used to facilitate vessel surgery (intracranial aneurysms, A-V malformations, or aortic surgery), reduced tension in a large vessel makes suturing, clamping, and the creation of an anastomosis easier, thereby avoiding stretching and tearing of a diseased vessel wall. In these situations, it is the reduction in vessel tension and not the decrease in blood flow that is required;[98] therefore, a hypotensive technique that does not necessarily decrease CO is indicated.

It has been found that in operations where the bleeding is mostly of venous origin, such as orthopedic procedures, blood loss was decreased more with nitroglycerin than with sodium nitroprusside at comparable levels of hypotension.[52] Without hypotension the average blood loss during a total hip arthroplasty is approximately 1475 mL.[240] Fahmy[52] found a mean intraoperative blood loss of 762 ± 93 mL with sodium nitroprusside and only 578 ± 82 mL with nitroglycerin. The decreased blood loss with nitroglycerin despite similar systolic blood pressures was attributed to decreased venous bleeding from the superior venodilation achieved with nitroglycerin. The central venous pressure was significantly lower with nitroglycerin than with sodium nitroprusside,[52] and this lower venous pressure may be partly responsible for the decreased blood loss. Other investigators found that nitroglycerin is less predictable, less potent, and therefore less reliable than sodium nitroprusside. In approximately one-third of patients, blood pressure could not be decreased to a satisfactory level.[241-243] A great variation in effective infusion rates, ranging from 6.6 to 91 $\mu$g/kg/min, has been reported.[241] Yaster and colleagues[96] studied 14 children undergoing scoliosis surgery and found that even at infusion rates up to 40 $\mu$g/kg/min, nitroglycerin could not lower the mean arterial pressure below 60 mm Hg in a high percentage of patients. They concluded that rapid, predictable, and sustained hypotension in children could not be guaranteed with nitroglycerin, whereas sodium nitroprusside was effective in achieving reliable hypotension. All of these studies have also noted a slower return to normotension upon discontinuance of nitroglycerin than after sodium nitroprusside.

Sodium nitroprusside is known to produce an inhibition of platelet aggregation as well as platelet disintegration, in vitro.[244,245] One suggested mechanism is blockade of adenosine diphosphate and serotonin release.[246] A significant reduction in platelet count, 1–3 hours after sodium nitroprusside infusion, has been reported in patients with congestive heart failure; the platelet count returned to normal by 24 hours. A more recent in vivo study[247] supported the earlier in vitro observations demonstrating a detrimental effect of sodium nitroprusside on platelet function in a dose-related manner (Fig. 8–6). When the infusion rate of sodium nitroprusside exceeded 3 $\mu$g/kg/min, there was a dose-related decrease in platelet aggregation. Platelet aggregation was also significantly reduced at a total dose exceeding 16 mg. This was also associated with a concomitant increase in bleeding time from 5.8 to 9.3 minutes.

Nitroglycerin has also been demonstrated to prolong the bleeding time in humans.[248,249] Nitroglycerin has been shown to stimulate prostacyclin (prostaglandin I$_2$) synthesis by both bovine coronary arteries[250] and endothelial cells.[251] Prostacyclin is known to inhibit platelet function.[252,253] Lichtenthal

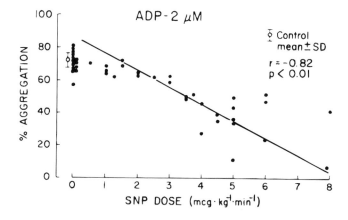

**Fig. 8–6.** Platelet aggregation (%) at varying intravenous infusion rates of sodium nitroprusside. From Hines R, Barash PG: Infusion of sodium nitroprusside induces platelet dysfunction *in vitro*. Anesthesiology 1989; 70:611, with permission.

and coworkers[248] studied intravenous nitroglycerin in patients undergoing coronary artery surgery. Although the platelet count remained unchanged and platelet aggregation was unaltered, a dose-related prolongation of the bleeding time was observed to occur, paralleling the decrease in systolic blood pressure (Fig. 8–7). They postulated that this phenomenon may be due to vasodilation and increased venous capacitance rather than inhibition of platelet aggregation.[248] Trimethaphan seems to be devoid of any effects on platelet aggregation.[254]

## SAFETY FACTORS IN DELIBERATE HYPOTENSION
### Rate of Onset of Hypotension

The induction of hypotension should proceed slowly. At least 10–15 minutes seem to be needed for the vessels of vital organs to dilate maximally, to maintain adequate perfusion in the presence of a lowered head of pres-

sure.[59,128,216] If the blood pressure is allowed to decrease too suddenly, a marked decrease in mixed venous oxygen content ($C\bar{v}O_2$) can occur, reflecting inadequate tissue oxygenation (Fig. 8–8).[255] Complications, including cardiac arrest, during the induction phase of hypotension have been reported and are usually related to the excessive rapidity with which the blood pressure declined;[256] thus, an argument could be made for the use of drugs with a slower onset of action, like trimethaphan and nitroglycerin.[61] There is also some evidence that ischemic ECG changes may occur if the rate of fall of blood pressure is too steep.[160]

The rate of induction of hypotension also has a potential effect on the EEG, biochemical changes in the brain, and the onset of brain ischemia. Autoregulation requires time to be effective; sudden changes in blood pressure may cause rapid changes in flow.[135] If the lower limit of autoregulation is exceeded, the rate at which pressure falls can affect perfu-

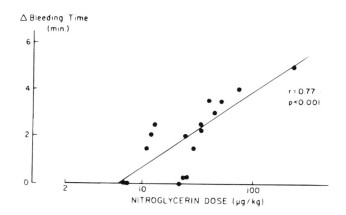

**Fig. 8–7.** Correlation between change in bleeding time and nitroglycerin dose. From Lichtenthal PR, Rossi EC, Louis G, et al: Dose-related prolongation of the bleeding time by intravenous nitroglycerin. Anesth Analg 1985; 64:30, with permission.

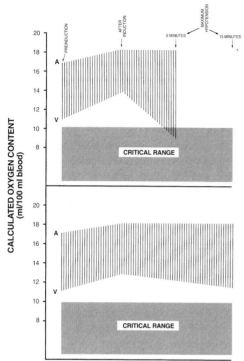

**EFFECT OF SPEED OF ONSET OF HYPOTENSION ON CENTRAL VENOUS OXYGEN CONTENT**

**Fig. 8–8.** *Upper diagram:* Changes in arterial and venous oxygen content (reflecting mixed venous oxygen content) when maximum hypotension was achieved in 5 minutes in six patients. The venous oxygen content fell within the critical range, indicating a state of circulatory inadequacy. *Lower diagram:* In six other patients, hypotension was induced slowly (15 minutes). There was no remarkable increase in a-v oxygen content difference and venous oxygen content was above the critical range. Reproduced from Salem MR: Deliberate hypotension is a safe and accepted anesthetic technique. In: Eckenhoff JE, ed, Controversy in Anesthesiology. Philadelphia, 1979, W.B. Saunders, with permission.

sion; decreases faster than 10 mm Hg/min lead to greater falls in cerebral blood flow than occur when the decreases in pressure are slower.[257,258]

## Safe Level of Hypotension

No one particular blood pressure should be considered safe for all patients. The desired level of blood pressure certainly depends on the age, preoperative blood pressure and condition, position during surgery, and the surgical requirement. Thus, blood pressure should not be decreased to a predetermined level. In young children, a systolic pressure of 55–60 mm Hg in the supine position may be necessary to achieve the desired relatively bloodless field, whereas a higher pressure may be sufficient in adults. As stated earlier, in elderly patients and in patients with chronic untreated hypertension, cerebral blood flow may fall at pressures higher than that in normotensive individuals. In these patients, a higher blood pressure may be sufficient to yield satisfactory operative conditions.

It is the anesthesiologist's duty to look for warning signs concomitant with unwanted severe hypotension, including a very dry operative field, dark venous blood, and the appearance of apneustic gasps. These signs strongly suggest the need to raise the blood pressure. Mixed venous (or central venous) oxygen tension below 30 mm Hg indicates tissue hypoxia; the blood pressure should be increased to improve CO and organ flow.

Tilting produces a gradient of approximately 2 mm Hg for each inch of vertical height above which the blood pressure is recorded. When head-up tilt is used, pressure gradients must be taken into consideration. Either an estimate of this gradient is calculated at the brain level or, in case of arterial cannulation, the transducer is positioned parallel to the site where the perfusion pressure is measured.

If the blood pressure drifts to a level considered too low, attempts should be made to raise the blood pressure by altering the degree of tilt, altering the administration of intravenous fluids, discontinuing the infusion of the hypotensive drug, or lightening the level of anesthesia. Vasopressors are best avoided unless uncontrollable hypotension has occurred.

## Oxygenation

During deliberate hypotension, an increase in the difference between alveolar to arterial oxygen tensions may occur.[259,260] Two possible mechanisms have been proposed to explain this phenomenon: increased intrapulmonary shunt $(\dot{Q}s/\dot{Q}t)$ and decreased CO.

### INCREASED INTRAPULMONARY SHUNT

Changes in functional residual capacity and closing volume during anesthesia and surgery contribute to airway closure and alveolar collapse.[261] This local alveolar hypoxia is normally offset, to a certain degree, by reflex hypoxic pulmonary vasoconstriction (HPV), which directs blood from hypoxic areas of the lung to adequately ventilated alveoli. Blunting or inhibition of this reflex has been noted with pulmonary hypertension, inhalational anesthetics, and vasodilators and leads to increased $\dot{Q}s/\dot{Q}t$.[262,263] Although inhibition of HPV occurs with all vasodilators, it is greater with sodium nitroprusside than with nitroglycerin.[260]

## DECREASED CARDIAC OUTPUT

Decreased CO is accompanied by increased extraction of oxygen, thus resulting in decreased $C\bar{v}O_2$.[264-266] Any portion of blood with decreased $C\bar{v}O_2$ that passes through hypoventilated or nonventilated areas ($\dot{Q}s/\dot{Q}t$) will contribute to a greater decrease in $PaO_2$. A significant reduction in CO during deliberate hypotension will decrease $PaO_2$, although this is significant only in the presence of regional atelectasis.[267]

A high inspired oxygen fraction ($FIO_2$) (above 0.9) during deliberate hypotension has been recommended[53,127] and tends to compensate for ventilation-perfusion imbalance. The lactate:pyruvate ratio does not increase during profound hypotension when the $PaO_2$ is kept above 300 mm Hg.[268] Furthermore, the jugular bulb oxygen tension rises significantly when $FIO_2$ is altered from 0.4 to 1.0

during hypotensive anesthesia in the head-up tilt position, although the oxygen delivery would have increased only slightly with an $FIO_2$ of 1.0.[127] These findings stress the importance of using high $FIO_2$, monitoring oxygenation, and avoiding profound decreases in CO during deliberate hypotension.

## Maintenance of A Near-Normal $PaCO_2$ and Acid-Base Balance

The combination of deliberate hypotension and hypocapnia is undesirable.[127-129,269] Hypocapnia decreases the CO, decreases the coronary, cerebral and spinal cord blood flows, may alter drug action (by altering blood pH), decreases both ionized calcium and serum potassium concentrations, shifts the oxyhemoglobin dissociation curve to the left, may increase the oxygen consumption, and may inhibit HPV. Furthermore, depletion of brain energy supply and the development of brain lactic acidosis can occur when $PaCO_2$ decreases below 25 mm Hg.[118,259] Therefore, unless hypocapnia is needed for certain therapeutic effects, $PaCO_2$ should be kept at a near-normal level during deliberate hypotension.

As a result of redistribution of pulmonary blood during induced hypotension, alveolar ventilation and perfusion may be altered. Eckenhoff and associates[231] demonstrated that the alveolar dead space can increase to as much as 80% of the tidal volume in the hypotensive adult patient who is tilted in the head-up posi-

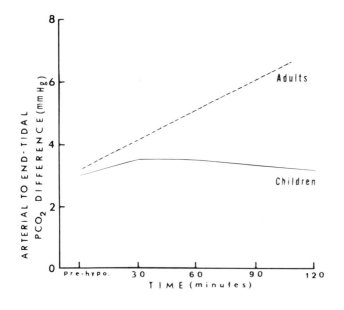

**Fig. 8-9.** Arterial to end-tidal $PCO_2$ difference during deliberate hypotension in adults (Askrog et al, 1964) and in children (Salem et al, 1974). From Salem MR: Therapeutic uses of ganglionic blocking drugs. Int Anesthesiol Clin 1978; 16:171, with permission.

tion and whose airway pressure is increased. Further studies in adult patients showed that the increase in alveolar dead space is less than previously reported.[270] Data from infants and children suggest that the alveolar dead space does not increase during controlled hypotension even with the head-up tilt (Fig. 8–9).[53] Furthermore, Khambatta and colleagues[271] found that deliberate hypotension with sodium nitroprusside did not cause any change in physiological dead space in adequately hydrated adult patients who underwent operations in the prone position.

Many factors tend to influence the alveolar dead space, including degree of hypotension, posture, hemodynamic alterations, filling pressures, CO, pulmonary disease, and age. More recently, the effect of deliberate hypotension on the alveolar dead space has been reevaluated by Salem and associates.[272] The arterial to peak expired carbon dioxide tension difference was used to assess the magnitude of change in alveolar dead space. The increase in arterial to peak expired carbon dioxide tension difference was noted only in older patients and was attributed to changes in pulmonary function due to age or pulmonary disease. Probably the increase in alveolar dead space during deliberate hypotension has been overemphasized and may be seen only in elderly patients or when both PEEP and head-up tilt are used in adult patients. Provided that adequate oxygenation and a near-normal $PaCO_2$ are maintained, metabolic acidosis is not a feature of well-managed deliberate hypotension.[128,268]

## PHARMACOLOGY OF HYPOTENSIVE DRUGS
### Sodium Nitroprusside

Sodium nitroprusside has an unusual structural formula $[Na_2Fe^{++}(CN)_5NO \cdot 2H_2O]$ with five cyanide groups in each molecule. Disodium pentacyanonitrosylferrate dihydrate is the chemical name for this inorganic hypotensive agent that acts as a rapid onset ultrashort duration vasodilator active on both veins and arteries. Known since 1849[273] and used for industrial purposes as a reagent, it was reviewed by Taylor and associates in 1970[274] as a hypotensive agent during anesthesia. Because of its evanescent nature and its freedom from significant actions on systems other than

cardiovascular, it soon became widely accepted in clinical practice.

Although the exact mechanism of action is not proven, recent theory postulates the same activity for sodium nitroprusside as for nitrates. That is, sodium nitroprusside acts as an intracellular nitrate[275] that, after interacting with sulfhydryl groups, decomposes to nitric oxide. Nitric oxide in turn activates the enzyme guanylate cyclase, which increases the concentration of cyclic GMP in vascular smooth muscle.[276] Cyclic GMP appears to inhibit or block calcium activation and/or alter the phosphorylation of protein; the result is vascular smooth muscle relaxation.

Sodium nitroprusside is a direct-acting vasodilator that can produce potent relaxation of both arteriole (resistance) and venous (capacitance) smooth muscle without significant action on nonvascular smooth muscle, autonomic ganglia, or the myocardium.[162] Dilatation of the venous system promotes peripheral pooling of blood, and the result is a decrease in venous return of blood to the heart; left ventricular end diastolic pressure and pulmonary capillary wedge pressures tend to be reduced (i.e., preload). The primary hypotensive action appears to be relaxation of the arterioles, producing a reduction in SVR; mean and systolic arterial blood pressures (i.e., afterload) are reduced. Dilatation of the coronary arteries and a reduction in myocardial oxygen consumption may also occur. It has been suggested that sodium nitroprusside may produce an intracoronary "steal" of blood flow away from already ischemic areas by arteriolar vasodilation of the relatively unaffected vessels;[277] this may lead to an increased area of damage associated with a myocardial infarction.[278]

Sodium nitroprusside-induced reduction in blood pressure tends to produce a reflex response mediated by the baroreceptors, which manifests itself as tachycardia and increased myocardial contractility.[100,146,187,197,279] Such reflex-mediated responses can have a deleterious effect, because they partially counteract the hypotensive action of sodium nitroprusside. CO often tends to increase but may also decrease or remain relatively unchanged depending on a multiplicity of factors, including the rate at which the blood pressure is reduced, the pre-sodium nitroprusside heart rate, the volume status of the patient, the inhalational agents used, the relaxant used, and so on. An improvement in cardiac function has been reported in patients with ischemic cardiac disease and congestive heart failure.[280] CO tends to change with deliberate hypotension on a rate-related basis, particularly in children.[97,98] Such changes in heart rate often depend on the predominant tone of the autonomic nervous system just before the initiation of hypotension; that is, heart rate may increase if vagal tone was predominant, but heart rate could decrease if the dominant tone was sympathetic. Because children tend to have increased vagal tone, they will usually respond with tachycardia when hypotension is induced. "Halothane negates the reflex increase in heart rate produced by hypotensive drugs by 'resetting the baroreceptors,' by depressing vasomotor centers and directly depressing sinoatrial node activity."[61]

Sodium nitroprusside is supplied commercially in 5-mL amber glass vials containing 50 mg of the dihydrate for reconstitution. The vials are to be stored at 15–30° C. The manufacturer recommends dissolving the powder in a minimum of 2–3 mL dextrose in water solution and states that "no other diluent should be used." The reconstituted product must then be further diluted in 250–1000 mL sterile 5% dextrose injection and then protected from light by prompt wrapping with the supplied aluminum foil. If properly reconstituted and wrapped, the solution is stable for 24 hours. Because nitroprusside can be inactivated by trace contaminants, discolored solutions should be discarded. The normal solution is either clear or very faintly brownish.

## CYANIDE TOXICITY

Cyanide release is "part-and-parcel" of the use of sodium nitroprusside; that is, its presence and availability increase pari passu with the use of sodium nitroprusside. The first preliminary evidence suggesting that cyanide poisoning could occur from the use of sodium nitroprusside was reported in 1886.[281] Four dissertations or articles strongly suggesting cyanide poisoning from sodium nitroprusside were published in 1886, 1887, 1897, and 1903. It was also noted that cyanide is excreted by animals as thiocyanate.[282]

Johnson,[283] in a study on humans in 1929,

acknowledged previous cyanide reports, noted that the pharmacological action of sodium nitroprusside was associated with the presence of a nitroso group (NO), and reported that sodium nitroprusside was a vasolytic agent producing cyanide in significant amounts only with excessive dosage. Three reported cases of suicide with oral sodium nitroprusside were acknowledged in two articles.[284,285] In all three cases the presence of free cyanide was noted in the examination of the stomach contents.

Clinical interest in sodium nitroprusside was generated in the early 1950s,[286] as research on oral antihypertensives blossomed. Although the oral preparation was subsequently noted to be disappointingly ineffective,[285] an intravenous preparation was soon available and clinical trials were begun. Initially described as "potent, inexpensive, quick in action, short in duration and non-toxic in clinical dosage,"[43] many investigators thought they had found an almost ideal agent.[287,288] Its wide clinical acceptance was slowed somewhat by the difficulty in its preparation; it required exacting individual daily preparation by each hospital pharmacy.[289] Clinical reports on its use appeared in the 1960s from a variety of sources,[290–292] and the first comprehensive study on the use of sodium nitroprusside to induce hypotension during major surgery appeared in 1970 by Taylor and associates.[274] Nipride (Roche) was finally marketed in 1977. Its ready availability enhanced its use dramatically. In the interim between 1970 and 1977, however, the first documented reports appeared of morbidity and mortality due to cyanide poisoning.

Early studies of sodium nitroprusside toxicity were concerned with documenting and detecting the catabolic product thiocyanate. Prolonged use of sodium nitroprusside was shown to produce elevated thiocyanate levels that were detectable for a prolonged period of time, in part secondary to its tubular reabsorption and low renal clearance.[285,288,293] Because of the belief that the cyanide released from sodium nitroprusside was readily converted to thiocyanate and was not toxic, little attention had been paid to its existence.[283,294]

In 1974 a series of reports began to appear concerning the toxicity of sodium nitroprusside. Few prior reactions to the drug had been recognized. Skin sensitivity had been reported in patients with oral intake of sodium nitroprusside.[285] One patient developed some symptoms of hypothyroidism and elevated thiocyanate levels after a continuous sodium nitroprusside infusion lasting 24 days.[295] Several published reports actually commented on the apparent safety of sodium nitroprusside;[274,296] one article warned about cyanide being a hazard, but only under the very specific circumstances of vitamin $B_{12}$ deficiency, severe hepatic dysfunction, malnourishment, or Leber's optic atrophy.[297]

Davies and coworkers[298] in 1975 stated that past publications had pointed to the potency, efficacious action, and safety of sodium nitroprusside but had failed to properly balance their discussion with adequate mention of the toxic properties inherent in this drug. The dosage of sodium nitroprusside used had been selected empirically to produce the level of hypotension desired. It was believed that young healthy male patients were more resistant or subject to tachyphylaxis, whereas hypertensive patients were more sensitive. The authors went on to state that "there have been no reports of cyanide toxicity during infusion of sodium nitroprusside. In theory such an occurrence is unlikely because of the ease with which tissue rhodanese handles relatively large amounts of cyanide, providing there are adequate amounts of endogenous thiosulphate available."

In fact, the first death believed related to the use of sodium nitroprusside had already been reported in 1974. It occurred 32 hours after the discontinuation of sodium nitroprusside[188] and was suggested but never confirmed as being from cyanide. Also in 1974, the potential for cyanide toxicity was established by Smith and Kruszyna;[299] additional reports[298,300,301] also seemed to point to cyanide as a cause of death from sodium nitroprusside. One article[302] was a clinical report of a patient death. Although the operative procedure and time were not delineated, the author notes that the patients resistance to sodium nitroprusside was "extraordinary" and that a total dose of 750 mg (15 ampules) of sodium nitroprusside was administered. The patient had spontaneous respirations continuously, until a respiratory arrest occurred 50 minutes postoperatively. The patients's initial cyanosis disappeared when the airway was reestablished but was still hypotensive (40/20 mm Hg), and arterial blood gases revealed a pH of 7.12 and a base excess of $-22$ mmol/L with a $PaCO_2$ of 24 mm Hg and a $PaO_2$ of 97 mm Hg. The patient soon died.

The same year an important baboon study was published[189] looking at hemorrhage, halothane, and sodium nitroprusside for hypotension; the blood pressure was lowered to 40 mm Hg and held there for 2 hours using any dose necessary. Two different response levels were found. In one group the dose of sodium nitroprusside was low, and the blood pressure returned to control levels immediately after the drug was discontinued; this group was termed normal. The other group needed much larger doses, did not regain normal pressures when the drug was discontinued, had significantly elevated jugular venous oxygen saturations (i.e., depressed cerebral oxygen consumption) and severe metabolic acidosis, and subsequently died; this group was termed "resistant." The lowest amount required to produce the desired hypotensive effect in the latter group was three times larger than the highest amount in the normal group (4.9 versus 1.6 mg/kg/h). The smallest toxic dose was extrapolated to be equivalent to 320 mg/h in a human, which was a huge amount. The authors recommended selecting a safe maximum possible infusion rate and then supplementing the sodium nitroprusside if adequate hypotension was not achieved at that dose. Another author noted that "there is a paucity of information concerning the total dose of sodium nitroprusside which may be safely administered for deliberate hypotension during anaesthesia in humans."[190]

Davies and coworkers[298] noted that a lethal dose of sodium nitroprusside is 1 g in an adult,[303] and the lethal dose of potassium cyanide is approximately 200 mg; 1 g sodium nitroprusside would release more than twice the lethal cyanide dose. The lethal dose of cyanide is thus approximately 3 mg/kg, which is approximately equivalent to 7 mg/kg of sodium nitroprusside. They went on to state that they recommended "unequivocally that the use of sodium nitroprusside as a hypotensive agent should not be on an empirical basis only related to the blood pressure desired but also with a projected total dose assessed from the initial response which achieves the blood pressure required. If this projected dose exceeds 3.5 mg/kg (half the probable lethal dose) for the anticipated duration of hypotension, it might indicate that the patient is cyanide intolerant."

Vesey and colleagues[297,304] determined that exposure to sodium nitroprusside would produce increases in both red blood cell and plasma cyanide concentrations; they also demonstrated that the cyanide in sodium nitroprusside seemed to be released in a short time period[305] and that the correlation between erythrocyte and plasma cyanide levels and total dosage was linear.[306] In addition, they stated that plasma thiocyanate levels would not rise until there was prolonged usage and these concentrations were not a safe guide to free cyanide levels. They went on to recommend a total dose of sodium nitroprusside of 1.5 mg/kg,[306] one-half or less than the dose mentioned by Davies 1 year earlier.[298]

Although some authors have recommended reducing this dosage (1.5 mg/kg), the basic idea and dose range for short-term infusion has remained valid. With this dose in mind, and with the added warning to avoid progressive increases in sodium nitroprusside infusion rates if obvious resistance occurs, further fatalities have not been reported. It seems unwise to exceed the doses of 1.5 mg/kg for short-term administration, 0.5 mg/kg/h for prolonged use, or an infusion rate in excess of 10 $\mu$g/kg/min.[307] An initial infusion rate of 0.5–1.5 $\mu$g/kg/min has been used by many authors.[308]

We now know that sodium nitroprusside is rapidly distributed to a volume approximating the extracellular space and is cleared almost immediately by intraerythrocytic reactions with hemoglobin, resulting in a circulatory half-life of approximately 2 minutes. In a nonenzymatic reaction, one electron from the ferrous iron of oxyhemoglobin is transferred to the sodium nitroprusside molecule, making the sodium nitroprusside unstable and causing the release of all five cyanide ions in its structure.[162] The oxyhemoglobin, now with a ferric iron, becomes methemoglobin, and one cyanide ion combines with it to form cyanmethemoglobin. In an enzymatic reaction, the majority of the cyanide ions are converted to thiocyanate by thiosulfate sulfurtransferase, better known as rhodanese. This enzyme is present in mitochondria, found predominantly in the liver and kidneys, and requires cofactors of vitamin $B_{12}$ (hydroxocobalamin)

and thiosulfate. The thiocyanate formed is slowly excreted in the urine; the cyanocobalamin formed from the vitamin $B_{12}$ is rapidly excreted in the urine.[309] Any free cyanide ions remaining may combine with tissue cytochrome oxidase (Fig. 8– 10), inhibiting oxidative phosphorylation. Cyanide rapidly inhibits the electron transport system, decreases oxygen use, decreases $CO_2$ production via Krebs cycle inhibition, and increases anaerobic metabolites.

Greiss and associates[310] have shown that patients' response to an infusion of sodium nitroprusside must be carefully observed, particularly in the first 30 minutes. During that time the observer should monitor the infusion pump setting, blood pressure response, and arterial blood gases. Four distinct responses to a sodium nitroprusside infusion have been described[289,310] of which only the first is considered normal:

1. A good and relatively steady response to a low dose of sodium nitroprusside (less than 10 $\mu$g/kg/min)
2. A good response to sodium nitroprusside, but only at high levels (higher than 10 $\mu$g/kg/min)
3. Tachyphylaxis, usually apparent 30–60 minutes into the infusion.
4. Resistance, usually apparent 5–10 minutes after the start of an infusion. A desired hypotensive level cannot be reached, even with unsafe doses.

Each of the latter three response groups may be associated with increased $P\bar{v}O_2$, decreasing arterial to mixed venous oxygen content difference and metabolic acidosis. The addition of $\beta$-adrenergic blockers and/or an increasing concentration of an inhaled anesthetic agent may alleviate the problem of "apparent" tachyphylaxis, enabling the dose to be adjusted downward appropriately. On the other hand, sodium nitroprusside is not necessarily the drug needed or best suited in all cases.

Although the dose range is 0.5–10 $\mu$g/kg/min, the high rate should never be used for more than 10 minutes. At normal methemoglobin levels, the cyanide binding capacity of packed red cells is a little less than 200 $\mu$mol/L (5 mg/L), toxicity is seen at levels only slightly higher, and death has been noted at a level as low as 300 $\mu$mol/L (8 mg/L). A normal patient with a normal red blood cell mass of 35 mL/kg can buffer approximately

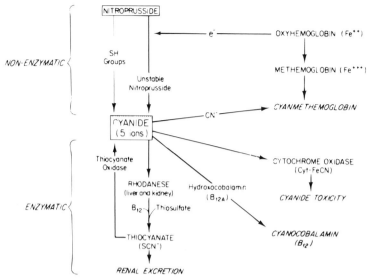

**Fig. 8–10.**   Metabolism of sodium nitroprusside. Modified from Tinker JH, Michenfelder JD: Sodium nitroprusside: pharmacology, toxicology and therapeutics. Anesthesiology 1976; 45:340, with permission.

175 mg/kg of cyanide; this amounts to less than 500 $\mu$g/kg of sodium nitroprusside, which is 35 mg/70 kg, that is, less than one ampule (50 mg) of sodium nitroprusside. Any infusion rate higher than 2 $\mu$g/kg/min will generate cyanide ion faster than the body can handle. The red blood cell cyanide-level assay is still a technically difficult one, and levels of cyanide in other body fluids are extremely hard to interpret. The current recommendation is to start at 0.3 $\mu$g/kg/min and then titrate slowly upward from there if needed.

The treatment of cyanide toxicity depends first on our knowledge of certain basic facts:

1. As previously indicated, cyanide levels are not rapidly, reliably, or readily available.
2. Metabolic acidosis, although an important indicator of toxicity, is not apparent immediately, that is, it may not appear until some time (perhaps 1 hour or more) after cyanide levels are already significantly elevated.
3. As indicated, the body cannot normally dispose of cyanide generated by a sodium nitroprusside infusion greater than 2 $\mu$g/kg/min.
4. Reasonable suspicion of cyanide toxicity seems to be an adequate indication for the initiation of treatment. In the awake patient clinical reports indicate nausea, vomiting, headache, tremor, dyspnea, fatigue, ataxia, muscle spasms, rigidity, angina-like symptoms, disorientation, psychotic behavior, convulsions, and cardiovascular collapse from cyanide. During anesthesia the signs,

in addition to the already mentioned tachyphylaxis, resistance, metabolic acidemia, and bright venous blood, include progressive hypotension with a narrowing pulse pressure and/or refractory hypotension unresponsive to the usual therapy.[61]

5. Cyanide's "poisoning" effect depends on its ability to interfere with the major pathway of high-energy phosphate production, aerobic metabolism. When the ferric iron ($Fe^{+++}$) of cytochromes is bound to cyanide, these cytochromes are unable to participate in oxidative metabolism. Many of these cells are able to use anaerobic pathways to provide for their energy needs but generate lactic acid, which is a progressive burden to the body. Other cells are unable to use this alternative metabolic pathway or cannot produce sufficient energy from it, and die hypoxic deaths. The combination of tissue hypoxia with normal or elevated $P\bar{v}O_2$ is the hallmark of cytotoxic hypoxia produced by cyanide.[61,162,311,312]

The best treatment for cyanide toxicity is prevention. Restricting the dose of sodium nitroprusside leads to lower amounts of free cyanide. Some investigators have attempted to convert liberated cyanide to less toxic forms prophylactically. Hydroxocobalamin (vitamin $B_{12a}$) was advocated to absorb free cyanide radicals and produce cyanocobalamin that could then be renally excreted.[297,313–315] This remains only a theoretical possibility. To be effective as an antitoxin, the hydroxocobalamin would have to be infused in very high doses, perhaps equimolar to the cyanide.[316,317] Problems associated with this use of vitamin $B_{12a}$ include lack of product in these amounts, excessive expense if it could be obtained, lack of cardiovascular stability, problems with storage and solubility of the product, and lack of proper toxicological testing. In addition, frequent or continuous doses would have to be given because the plasma half-life of hydroxocobalamin is only approximately 5 minutes as opposed to 10 hours for cyanide. The recommended dose is 50 mg/kg as a bolus, plus 100 mg/kg/h if needed.

Similar prophylaxis has been advocated in the past with the use of sodium thiosulfate, giving a mixed infusion accompanying the sodium nitroprusside.[312,316,317] If thiosulfate is present in a quantity at least three times larger than the cyanide, it can provide good protection and detoxification. During sodium nitroprusside therapy, most of the cyanide released is converted to thiocyanate via the rhodanese (thiosulfate sulfurtransferase) reaction with thiosulfate. If the endogenous supply of thiosulfate were exhausted, cyanide would begin to accumulate rather than thiocyanate.

In animal experiments, thiosulfate was reported to be relatively nontoxic with no adverse respiratory or hemodynamic changes; thiosulfate has an osmotic diuretic effect and is rapidly excreted by the kidneys. Thiocyanate, however, is cleared slowly by the kidneys and can accumulate during prolonged therapy, especially with renal failure (Fig. 8–11).[318] High concentrations of thiocyanate have been reported to cause weakness, hypoxia, nausea, muscle spasms, tinnitus, disorientation, and even psychosis—all symptoms similar to that seen with cyanide itself. Thiocyanate also interferes with the transport of iodine by the thyroid gland and could lead to hypothyroidism.[295]

What is the treatment if sodium nitroprusside is given and cyanide intoxication is suspected? The following steps have been advocated:

1. Stop the sodium nitroprusside infusion immediately
2. Administer 100% oxygen
3. Provide a buffer for cyanide to convert as much hemoglobin into methemoglobin as the patient

can tolerate with safety. The first step may be the use of amyl nitrite ampule pearls by inhalation for 15–30 seconds every minute. This is only a temporizing measure while the drug you really want, sodium nitrite, is being prepared as a 3% solution for intravenous use. If an intravenous line is accessible and if and when the sodium nitrite is available, the amyl nitrite is not needed. Sodium nitrite is given as 4–6 mg/kg (approximately 0.2 mL/kg) over 2–4 minutes. The nitrite will cause a fraction (perhaps 10%) of the hemoglobin to convert to methemoglobin by oxidizing the ferrous iron ($Fe^{++}$) to ferric iron ($Fe^{+++}$), thus shifting the equilibrium toward the relatively stable and nontoxic cyanmethemoglobin; some cyanide will then be released from cellular cytochrome oxidase. The nitrite may cause transient vasodilation and hypotension. A constant infusion of 5 mg/kg/h may be used if needed.

4. Provide a sulfur donor for the rhodanese enzyme system to work on. Sodium thiosulfate should be infused to provide the sulfhydryl radicals needed to form thiocyanate from cyanide. Cole and Vesey[319] reported on 30 patients receiving sodium nitroprusside. One-half were given thiosulfate as a small bolus injection immediately after the sodium nitroprusside was discontinued; they found an effective reduction in plasma and red cell cyanide concentrations in this group. They recommended 25 mL of 50% sodium thiosulfate by intravenous injection and the use of sodium bicarbonate as needed to correct any metabolic acidosis. Others had suggested a lower dose an intravenous bolus of 30 mg/kg followed by 60 mg/kg/h via continuous infusion.

5. The nitrite-thiosulfate regimen can be repeated, at half the original dose, in approximately 2 hours.

6. Cyanide also has a high affinity for cobalt. In severe cases, some authors advocate the use of dicobalt edetate[307,320,321] injected intravenously in a dose of 300 mg given slowly. This may, however, have more toxic side effects.[319,322]

The concept that cyanide is released in vivo has been challenged by the argument that cyanide detected after sodium nitroprusside is due to photodegradation of the sodium nitroprusside in vitro.[323] Thus, toxicity can be avoided if the solution is not exposed to light before or during its infusion. Others argue that the cyanide would still be released by metabolism after infusion.[324,325] Further in vitro work confirmed that exposure of sodium nitroprusside to light leads to rapid conversion

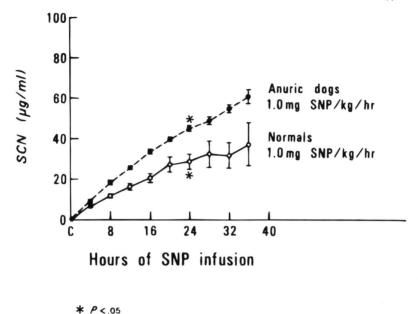

**Fig. 8–11.**  Plasma thiocyanate (SCN) concentrations are greater in anuric than normal dogs. From Tinker JH, Michenfelder JD: Increased resistance to nitroprusside-induced cyanide toxicity in anuric dogs. Anesthesiology 1980; 52:40, with permission.

to unstable ionic aquapentoferrocyanate, which readily releases free cyanide.[307] It was, however, also shown that polyvinyl chloride solution bags and administration sets adsorb much of the cyanide and decrease the amount reaching the patient. Also, solutions protected from light are stable (i.e., contain little or no free cyanide) for approximately 24 hours. A recent animal study[326] showed that the same metabolic consequences occurred when cyanide was given, as occurred when cyanide-free sodium nitroprusside was used; the only difference was that the onset of effect was delayed when the sodium nitroprusside was used. This demonstrates that sodium nitroprusside is broken down in vivo after administration. Thus, cyanide release cannot be prevented, but it can be reduced and diminished by excluding light from the sodium nitroprusside solution.[327]

## Nitroglycerin

Glyceryltrinitrate, also called trinitroglycerin or simply nitroglycerin, is an organic nitrate that was among the first vasodilators introduced into medical practice. After Sobrero's initial combination of nitric and sulfuric acids with glycerin-synthesized nitro-

glycerin in 1846, Hering and Davis prepared the first sublingual tablet in 1847 by dissolving the nitroglycerin in alcohol and absorbing it into a pellet of sugar.[328] Brunton[329] treated angina pectoris with inhalations of amyl nitrite in 1867, and Murrell[330] established nitroglycerin as appropriate therapy for angina in 1879.

The sublingual onset of nitroglycerin is, of course, very rapid (less than 3 minutes), but the duration is brief; the plasma half-life is only approximately 2 minutes because of rapid redistribution and equally rapid hepatic metabolism. Transdermal applications were introduced in the 1970s using an ointment or patch for prolonged therapy. Oral forms have been generally unsuccessful. Intramuscular therapy was first attempted in 1968,[331] but intravenous infusion superseded it quickly.[95,332]

Nitroglycerin acts primarily to relax the venous capacitance vessels, thus producing peripheral blood pooling. It may reduce the size of the heart and also reduce ventricular wall tension;[333] at higher doses, arterial smooth muscle may be relaxed. The mechanism of action is now thought to resemble that of sodium nitroprusside, with activation of guanylate cyclase and a subsequent increase in cyclic

GMP levels; this may lead to protein kinase activation, myosin dephosphorylation, and smooth muscle relaxation.[276]

The liver has a large capacity to metabolize nitroglycerin in a single rapid passage using the enzyme glutathione organic nitrate reductase. Nitroglycerin is transformed into 1,3 and 1,2-glyceryl dinitrate, glyceryl mononitrate, and inorganic nitrite, all of which are water-soluble weak vasodilators that are rapidly excreted in the urine.[334,335] Inorganic nitrite can convert oxyhemoglobin to methemoglobin, and methemoglobinemia was reported after in vitro incubation of blood with nitroglycerin, as well as from inorganic nitrate therapy.[336] Nonetheless, although intravenous nitroglycerin has been associated with a rise in methemoglobin levels,[241] even high concentrations of nitroglycerin have not been associated with significant elevations,[337] that is, there seems to be no clinical relevance.

Nitroglycerin has been shown to decrease ischemic damage to the myocardium with acute myocardial infarction, in contrast to sodium nitroprusside, which seemed to worsen the injury.[278,338] Nitrates relieve typical anginal pain, primarily due to a decrease in myocardial oxygen demand.[339] Nitrates have a selective dilating action on large coronary vessels, without significant impairment of autoregulation in the smaller vessels that constitute 90% of coronary vascular resistance.[340,341] The resultant improvement in blood flow seems preferentially distributed to subendocardial regions of the myocardium that are ischemic. This may account for some of the pain relief in Prinzmetal's angina. Nitroglycerin also decreases left ventricular filling pressure and may relieve pulmonary congestion in patients suffering from heart failure, especially after myocardial infarction. It is commonly used for the control of hypertension after coronary artery surgery.

Fahmy[52] promulgated the use of nitroglycerin for deliberate hypotension during anesthesia. Comparing it directly with sodium nitroprusside (Fig. 8–12), he found hypotension with nitroglycerin came on more gradually, was smoother, had less potential to produce severe hypotension, eliminated some of the peaks and valleys in blood pressure, and was a better systemic venodilator. At comparable systolic pressures, mean and diastolic pressures were higher with nitroglycerin; because

coronary perfusion depends on arterial diastolic blood pressure, nitroglycerin might be expected to better preserve myocardial perfusion.

Endrich and colleagues[342] studied microcirculatory changes during sodium nitroprusside and nitroglycerin-induced hypotension. They confirmed previous reports of severe tissue hypoxia in the liver and skeletal muscle of both humans and experimental animals during sodium nitroprusside therapy.[343] They found more favorable results with nitroglycerin, including tissue oxygenation that remained unaffected. They concluded that, from this particular standpoint, nitroglycerin might be preferable to sodium nitroprusside for deliberate hypotension.

Nitroglycerin is supplied commercially as a 0.05% solution, as for example, 5 mg in a 10-mL ampule. This can be diluted further to a 0.01% solution for infusion. The solution is administered from glass bottles or a rigid polyethylene infusion pack and tubing; it is not compatible with the standard polyvinylchloride infusion bags or tubing,[344] because the nitroglycerin loses its potency and is absorbed by prolonged contact with plastic tubing. The usual dose is from 1 to 10 $\mu$g/kg/min, although much larger doses have been used. Fahmy[52] reported using 4.7 $\mu$g/kg/min in his original report.

## Ganglionic Blockers

The clinically useful ganglionic blocking drugs produce blockade in the absence of stimulation and depolarization.[345] They are classified as competitive blocking drugs, implying that their mode of action is competition with acetylcholine for the nicotinic receptors found on the postjunctional membrane of the autonomic ganglia.[87] The effects of ganglion blockade are numerous because of the diverse nature and widespread distribution of the autonomic nervous system. Thus, in addition to the desired effect of hypotension, there may be undesirable side effects. The side effects are relatively insignificant after short-term intravenous use with the exception of cycloplegia and mydriasis, which may lead to confusion in a postoperative neurological assessment.[59] Most organs are reciprocally innervated by parasympathetic and sympathetic nerves, and the ultimate overall effect of autonomic block-

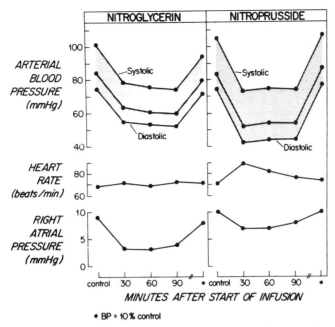

**Fig. 8–12.** Comparison of the effects of nitroglycerin and sodium nitroprusside on blood pressure, heart rate, and right atrial pressure when systolic arterial pressure is decreased to approximately 75 mm Hg. Note the higher diastolic pressure with nitroglycerin. From Fahmy NR, Almaz MG: Vasodilator drugs. In Stoelting RG, Barash PG, Gallagher TJ, eds, Advances in Anesthesia. Chicago, 1989, Year Book Medical Publishers Inc., vol. 6, p. 143, with permission.

ade depends on the predominance of one of these systems at the end organ in question.[215]

Pentolinium (Ansolysen) has not been commercially available in the United States since January 1977 when its manufacture and distribution ceased.[346] Because it was available as a powder with a long shelf life, however, numerous centers had sufficient private supplies to continue its use for a few more years. Pentamethylene bis 1-methylpyrollidinium hydrogen tartrate was first synthesized by Wien and Mason in 1953.[347] Enderby reported on its use for controlled hypotension in 1954,[23,24] and it soon become a favorite drug in the United Kingdom. It was used as an oral antihypertensive and was also found helpful in the treatment of peripheral vascular disease. The parenteral solution was 10 mg/mL in 10-mL vials. Many physicians used it intramuscularly or subcutaneously, whereas others gave it as a single intravenous bolus. Tinker[348] suggested an initial intravenous dose of 3 mg and the balance of a total dosage of 0.1–0.3 mg/kg given over 10 minutes. He reported a peak effect in 30 minutes and an extremely variable duration of action of 1–4 hours. Fahmy and Laver[97] also reported favor-

ably on the use of pentolinium. Salem and associates[53,98] reported on its effective use in pediatric patients. In addition to a great variation in sensitivity to the drug, it had an unusual tachyphylaxis; the first dose was often the only one effectively inducing hypotension.[215]

Trimethaphan camphorsulfonate (Arfonad) is a thiophanium derivative with the chemical name of d-3,4-(1',3'-dibenzyl-2'-keto-imidazolido)-1,2-trimethylenethiophanium d-camphorsulfonate, first described by Randall and colleagues in 1949.[25] It was introduced into clinical anesthesia practice in 1953 by Magill and others[28] in the United Kingdom and by Sadove and others (1953)[30] in the United States, contemporaneously with other investigators. Trimethaphan is a rapidly acting vasodilator that decreases blood pressure by decreasing the SVR. It differs from pentolinium by virtue of its rapidity of onset and by its evanescent action that requires continuous intravenous infusion.

The mechanisms of action of trimethaphan have been disputed over the years. The decrease in vascular resistance has been variably attributed to ganglionic blockade (venular plus arterial), histamine release, direct vasodilation, and, in higher doses, $\alpha$-adrenergic blockade. A 1951 study[349] found that large, even lethal, amounts of histamine could be released after intravenous trimethaphan in dogs. Intradermal tests also showed a typical wheal and flare in humans. Although histamine release seemed greater in animals, especially dogs, than in humans, histamine release in humans was confirmed by numerous investigators.[350-352] Later studies and clinical observations pointed to the conclusion that although histamine release does seem to occur in humans, particularly if rapid bolus injections are given, it does not play a significant role in the hemodynamic (hypotensive) effects of trimethaphan.[88] McCubbin and Page in 1952[26] found direct vasodilation and believed that neither histamine nor ganglionic blockade were of significance. Twenty-five years later,[353] a potent vasodilating property of trimethaphan in dogs was confirmed, but a variable degree of ganglionic blockade was also noted. A later study confirmed direct arterial vasodilation and also noted $\alpha$-adrenergic antagonism.[354]

Although heart rate, stroke volume, and CO are usually not altered with trimethaphan, CO may tend to decrease if the patient is in a head-up position or if right atrial pressures decrease significantly.[88] When vagal tone is initially high, tachycardia may ensue with trimethaphan. Knight and coworkers[195] corroborated the activation of the renin-angiotensin system by sodium nitroprusside as well as the sodium nitroprusside-induced release of catecholamines (Fig. 8–13). In contrast, trimethaphan-induced hypotension resulted in no activation of the renin-angiotensin system and less of an increase in circulating catecholamines. They stated that the autonomic response and production of hormones associated with sodium nitroprusside might prove detrimental and noted that in this study, as well as in a prior report,[355] there were patients who had a poor response to sodium nitroprusside. Two of their six patients receiving sodium nitroprusside in this study had an unsatisfactory surgical field at all times despite the use of propranolol and a mean arterial blood pressure of 40 mm Hg; none of the six patients receiving trimethaphan had similar findings. In addition, three of six sodium nitroprusside patients had significant postoperative bleeding, leading to wound hematomas and the need for multiple changes of wound dressings; none of the trimethaphan group had this problem.

In monkeys, trimethaphan was associated with decreases in cerebral blood flow without altering the cerebral metabolic rate for oxygen (Fig. 8–14).[238] In humans, trimethaphan, with an onset slower than that of sodium nitroprusside, may allow more time for autoregulation of cerebral blood flow to occur and result in a smaller increase of intracranial pressure.[143] Because ganglionic blockade generally spares the cerebral circulation, trimethaphan seldom increases intracranial pressure, but under abnormal circumstances of reduced intracranial compliance and altered cerebral autoregulation, trimethaphan could lead to an increase in intracranial pressure if it were infused rapidly. Cerebral ischemia has been reported[356] in dogs receiving trimethaphan when the mean arterial pressure is reduced under 55 mm Hg; a similar event has not been noted with other hypotensive agents. A 1971 article[357] studied 10 dogs during trimethaphan-induced hypotension to mean arterial pressures of 30–40 mm Hg, finding inadequate cerebral perfusion and a state of ischemia with anaerobic metabolism. Others had noted an isoelectric EEG at comparable blood pressures.[358] More recently, reduced spinal cord blood flow in dogs during trimethaphan hypotension was reported,[359] but the clinical significance of this for humans remains to be elucidated.

Randall and coworkers[25] pointed out that a very weak nondepolarizing neuromuscular blockade could be seen with trimethaphan, and this effect was later confirmed.[360,361] Deacock and Davis[361] reported that 2400 mg trimethaphan in vitro (a huge dose, far larger than any used clinically) could lead to neuromuscular blockade. They also stated that trimethaphan was not reversed by the administration of neostigmine, in contrast to Randall et al.'s original comment[25] that neostigmine could effectively counteract both the fall in blood pressure and block of ganglia produced by trimethaphan in animals. Eckenhoff[362] reported that apnea persisting for up to 3 hours was seen after the simultaneous use of succinylcholine and trimethaphan. Gasping respiration was noticed when the blood pressure was lowered too far.[363] In 1957, Tewfik[364]

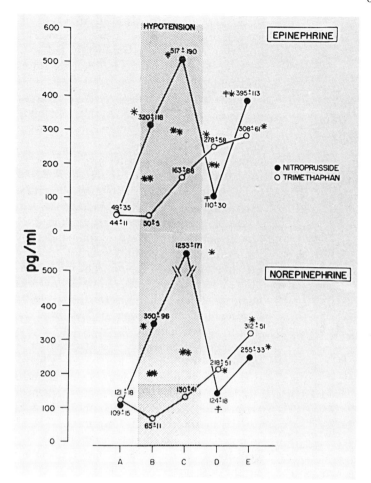

**Fig. 8–13.** Increased plasma concentrations of epinephrine and norepinephrine accompany hypotension induced by sodium nitroprusside but not by trimethaphan. From Knight PR, Lane GA, Hensinger RN, et al: Catecholamine and renin-angiotensin response during hypotensive anesthesia induced by sodium nitroprusside or trimethaphan camsylate. Anesthesiology 1983; 59: 248, with permission.

used 10–20 mg trimethaphan as a premedicant before electroconvulsive therapy and noted that the apnea after succinylcholine was prolonged for an average of 2 minutes in 9 of 10 patients when compared with an atropine premedication control. He postulated that trimethaphan was destroyed in vivo as well as in vitro by pseudocholinesterase.

Bentel and Ginsberg[365] previously stated that the fate of trimethaphan in the body was unknown, and Scurr and Wyman[366] could not determine any metabolic products. Gertner and associates[367] found they could recover only one-third of the injected quantity of trimethaphan from the urine, but this excreted drug was still biologically active. Both direct contact from the manufacturer in 1992 and a literature search to 1994 could reveal nothing more about possible metabolites, because the action of the drug commences and ceases so rapidly.

Deacock and Hargrove[368] agreed with Tewfik[364] that trimethaphan inhibits plasma cholinesterase, but there was still significant disagreement as to whether or not trimethaphan is a substrate for the enzyme. The possible hydrolysis of trimethaphan by plasma cholinesterase was discussed in 1977.[369] In 1978, Anton et al.[370] suggested that the brief duration of action of trimethaphan is not due to inactivation by plasma cholinesterase; this agreed with investigators who pointed out that trimethaphan is not an ester. A 1989 abstract seemed to confirm the 1978 study.[371] As yet, an exact metabolic pathway has not been clearly defined for trimethaphan. In clinical practice the argument is usually irrelevant because most patients having surgery requiring trimethaphan also require nondepolarizing muscle relaxants and receive either no succinylcholine or a single intubating dose early in the case. The literature suggests caution in

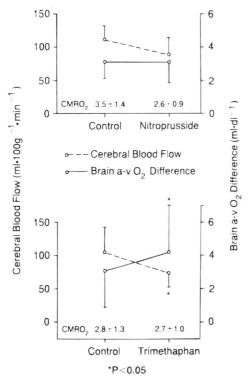

**Fig. 8–14.** Hypotension produced by trimethaphan, but not by sodium nitroprusside, reduces cerebral blood flow, whereas cerebral metabolic oxygen requirements, as reflected by an increased brain arterio-venous oxygen difference, remain unchanged. From Sivarajan M, Amory DW, McKenzie SM: Regional blood flows during induced hypotension produced by nitroprusside or trimethaphan in the rhesus monkey. Anesth Analg 1985; 64:759,[546] with permission.

the use of trimethaphan in patients likely to have a low pseudocholinesterase level (severe liver disease, severe malnutrition) or after excessively massive doses of succinylcholine.

Eckenhoff[362] reported finding significant delays in the recovery of blood pressure after the discontinuance of trimethaphan; some patients receiving succinylcholine took up to 3 hours to return to baseline. Payne[372] recorded delays of up to 2 hours, especially in the elderly. Green[215] postulated that the delays may be due to the phenomenon of a "baseline hypotension" from which blood pressure cannot be further reduced despite further doses of trimethaphan; this may lead to excessive doses being given, even though they seem ineffective. It was recommended that the infusion be slowed or stopped at intervals to assess the situation, waiting for a rise in the blood pres-

sure. Scott and others[99] studied circulatory effects of trimethaphan and made the observation that trimethaphan frequently led to a prolonged fall in pressure shortly after it was discontinued.

Trimethaphan is a white crystalline powder marketed in a 10-mL glass ampule containing 500 mg. It is given by intravenous infusion using a microdrip or preferably via a regulated infusion pump. The powder is to be kept refrigerated and carries an expiration time of 4 years. A freshly prepared solution should be used as needed and the remainder discarded; it is stable at room temperature for at least 24 hours. The usual dilution recommended by the manufacturer is a 0.1% solution (1 mg/mL) in 5% dextrose injection. The more common solutions of 5% dextrose in water, normal saline, or Ringer's solutions are also stable.[346] The reported rate of infusion varies from author to author. The product brochure advises that required infusion rates vary from 4 drops/min to over 100 drops/min. A literature search found 0.1–5 mg/min as an initial starting range, with titration to higher or lower doses as needed. Eckenhoff[362] advocated a maximum of 100 mg in the first 15 minutes and a total dose of no more than 1 g per patient. No totally satisfactory explanation for the dose limitation seems apparent, except for the potential of prolonged hypotension. Eckenhoff also noted that approximately 20% of his patients would not respond with satisfactory hypotension. All investigators agree that there is a marked variation in individual patient responsiveness and that supplemental agents may be needed. For some resistant or larger patients, many practitioners use a 0.2% concentration for infusion rather than 0.1%. Tachyphylaxis to the hypotensive effect may develop.

## Labetalol

Labetalol (5-[1-hydroxy-2-{(1-methyl-3-phenylpropyl) amino} ethyl] salicylamide monohydrochloride; Normodyne) is a dual product that is both a selective competitive $\alpha_1$ and nonselective competitive $\beta$-adrenoceptor antagonist. In humans, the ratios of $\alpha$-adrenergic to $\beta$-adrenergic blockade are estimated at approximately $1:3$ orally and $1:7$ intravenously. In animals, $\beta_2$-agonist activity has been detected and, in higher doses, a membrane stabilizing effect.[373–377]

Initial studies in animals demonstrated that labetalol was a more potent inhibitor of $\beta$ receptors than $\alpha$ receptors,[374] and a variety of in vitro and in vivo studies in animals demonstrated that labetalol was 1.5–4 times less potent than propranolol at $\beta$-adrenergic receptors and 6–10 times less potent than phentolamine at $\alpha$-adrenergic receptors.[374,378,379] The $\alpha$-adrenergic receptor blockade could produce capacitance and resistance vessel blockade, leading to a fall in arterial pressure, but the anticipated reflex increase in both heart rate and CO would be effectively prevented by the concurrent $\beta$-adrenergic blockade; occasional bradycardia was even reported to accompany a fall in blood pressure.[380] In human volunteers labetalol was found to reduce both systolic and diastolic blood pressures and to abolish tilt-induced tachycardia.[381] Similarly, in anesthetized patients labetalol reduced blood pressure via a large decrease in SVR and small decreases in heart rate and CO.[51,275]

Although primarily used orally for the treatment of hypertension,[382,383] it was also noted to be effective in the intravenous treatment of severe hypertension.[384,385] That prompted Scott and others[386] to use it for hypotensive anesthesia. They gave 25 mg labetalol intravenously to patients receiving halothane, finding a fall in blood pressure related to a decrease in SVR and a minimal decrease in CO. Kaufman[387] noted excellent dry surgical fields when labetalol was used. Multiple articles noted a seeming synergism in hypotension when labetalol was combined with a potent inhalational anesthetic agent.[380,386,387]

After intravenous administration, a fall in blood pressure is seen in 5 minutes,[388] but the elimination half-life is prolonged to approximately 4 hours; intravenous infusion of 0.5–1.0 mg/kg over a 10- to 20-minute period produced a maximal hypotensive response in 25–40 minutes.[389] After an infusion, the elimination half-life is approximately 5.5 hours, and the total body clearance is approximately 33 mL/kg/min.[390,391] Clinical experience has shown that a return toward baseline blood pressure usually takes only 15–45 minutes after the infusion ceases.[392] The elimination half-life is unchanged with decreased renal or hepatic function, but hepa-

tically impaired patients have a decreased first-pass metabolism and thus an increased bioavailability. Labetalol is metabolized mainly through conjugation to glucuronides, but there are no important active metabolites; metabolites are present in the plasma and then rapidly and virtually completely excreted in the urine and, via the bile, into the feces. Approximately 55–60% of a dose appears in the urine as conjugated or unchanged labetalol within 24 hours, and approximately 50% of the drug is bound to plasma proteins.

Fahmy and associates[275] compared labetalol with sodium nitroprusside and found them both useful agents for the induction of hypotension during enflurane anesthesia for orthopedic procedures. Labetalol was given as an incremental injection of 10–20 mg after a 20-mg bolus loading dose. A mean arterial pressure of 50–55 mm Hg was achieved in an average of 14 minutes; the average total dose was 156.5 mg (range 90–230 mg) given over 3–6 hours. The sodium nitroprusside infusion often led to significant increases in heart rate and CO, along with some instances of rebound hypertension; labetalol was judged to be superior because it caused none of these. Goldberg and others[392] also compared labetalol and sodium nitroprusside, this time during isoflurane anesthesia for laminectomy. Using 10-mg increments of labetalol every 10 minutes as needed, their goal was a mean pressure of 55–60 mm Hg and their results were similar to those of Fahmy and associates.[275] They agreed with Scott et al.[386] and Kaufman[387] that only small doses of labetalol are needed to help achieve hypotension; their mean total dose was only 29.37 $\pm$ 21.94 mg, and their duration was 223 $\pm$ 175 minutes. Sodium nitroprusside produced significant increases in both heart rate and shunt fraction that were not seen with labetalol.

Kanto and coworkers[391] described the use of labetalol with a technique of nitrous oxide and opioid. In contrast to the successful studies with any of the three potent inhalational anesthetic agents, they found higher doses of labetalol were required (up to 2 mg/kg) and there was difficulty achieving a satisfactory level of hypotension. Similarly, in a dog experiment with neurolept anesthesia,[393] a 15-mg/kg dose of labetalol could produce only a maximum 30% reduction in mean arterial pressure, and no further degree of hypotension could be achieved with any higher doses; CO did not change in this study. Another animal study found that cardiac depression in animals became significant above 20 mg/kg.[394]

After intravenous labetalol there is no increase in intracranial pressure even when intracranial compliance is reduced.[393] Added to the readily controlled hypotension and the lack of tachycardia, tachyphylaxis, or rebound hypertension, the avoidance of intracranial pressure increases is a distinct advantage in intracranial surgery.[395,396] Labetalol was also recommended to control blood pressure after neurovascular surgery for arteriovenous malformations or cerebrovascular aneurysms because of its effectiveness, as well as its lack of adverse action on intracranial pressure or cerebral perfusion pressure.

Because labetalol has $\beta$-adrenergic blocking activity, its effect on the respiratory system has been the subject of concern. In both healthy patients and asthmatics, labetalol did not decrease forced expiratory volume or peak expiratory flow rates.[397,398] Another study, however, found worsening of bronchoconstriction in asthmatics.[399]

Intravenous dosage in the literature has a wide range. Many authors now recommend an initial starting dose of 2.5 mg, followed by increments of 2.5–5.0 mg as needed to achieve the effect and pressure desired. Others use 10–20 mg as a loading dose and then 10-mg increments when indicated.

### $\beta$-Adrenergic Blockers

Simpson and others[400] prophylactically administered an oral $\beta$-adrenergic blocker 2 hours before induction in 30 patients scheduled for major middle ear surgery with a trimethaphan-sodium nitroprusside mixture for induced hypotension. They chose metoprolol as a pure $\beta_1$-adrenergic blocker with a rapid onset and brief duration in 20 cases and used oxprenolol, a $\beta$-adrenergic blocker with some intrinsic sympathomimetic activity and short duration, in the other 10 cases. Although the infusion rate of the hypotensive mixture was significantly reduced by the use of $\beta$-adrenergic blockers, they found an unacceptably high incidence of profound bradycardia after induction; 5 of 30 patients required intravenous atropine for heart rates less than 45 beats per minute. They believed that the routine use of

oral $\beta$-adrenergic blockers could not be justified.

Coad[401] reported on 20 patients premedicated with 100 mg oral labetalol 2 hours before surgery. A decrease in the total dose of sodium nitroprusside required was found, and no instances of bradycardia (heart rate less than 50 beats per minute) were noted.

### ESMOLOL

Propranolol has been the most widely recommended and used $\beta$-blocking agent for many years. It has been advocated to diminish the side effects of sodium nitroprusside, but its disadvantages are well known: a slow onset, a relatively slow recovery time, and a lack of adequate $\beta_1$-adrenergic antagonism. The last may be troublesome in patients with reactive airway disease, and the long duration could theoretically blunt the tachycardia that immediate postoperative hypovolemia or hypoxemia might produce. Esmolol hydrochloride is a recently introduced ultra-short-acting intravenous cardioselective $\beta$-adrenergic blocker with a very rapid onset and offset, having a half-life of 9.2 minutes. The drug seems to be safe to use even in the presence of hepatic or renal impairment; it is metabolized to an inactive metabolite primarily by esterases in the cytosol of erythrocytes.[402] It has been used to blunt some of the adverse physiological responses induced by deliberate hypotension. Esmolol can potentiate deliberate hypotension induced by another agent by diminishing or preventing the associated tachycardia and in larger doses can induce hypotension on its own. A third function described is the control of postoperative hypertension in coronary artery bypass patients. Compared with sodium nitroprusside, esmolol maintained the diastolic blood pressure and $PaO_2$ better; however, whereas sodium nitroprusside slightly increased the cardiac index, esmolol significantly decreased the index from 2.9 to 2.2 $L/min/m^2$. The esmolol was used as a titrated infusion at rates from 25 to 300 $\mu g/kg/min$.[403]

Ornstein and coworkers[404–406] reported on the use of esmolol to induce deliberate hypotension during isoflurane anesthesia. Esmolol was used as a bolus of 750 $\mu g/kg$, followed by an infusion at 100 $\mu g/kg/min$ for 4 minutes and then incremental increases in dose to a maximum of 300 $\mu$g/kg/min; sodium nitroprusside was added if needed for blood pressure control, whereas other patients received sodium nitroprusside alone. In clinical trials, esmolol had previously been noted to show a dose-related transient attenuation of the increases in heart rate, blood pressure, and rate-pressure product that can result from the stimulation of induction and surgery.[206,407–413] Ornstein and associates[406] found that esmolol was effective, safe, lacking in reflex tachycardia and significant rebound hypertension, and able, in conjunction with isoflurane, to produce a 30% reduction in blood pressure. Two of 15 esmolol patients were described as apparent titration failures, with inadequate reductions in their blood pressures.

Edmondson and colleagues[414] studied the effects produced when an esmolol infusion at rates of 200, 300, and 400 $\mu$g/kg/min was used to potentiate the hypotension induced by sodium nitroprusside during nitrous oxide-fentanyl anesthesia for radical intraabdominal urological surgery. Hypotension induced by sodium nitroprusside produced significant increases in heart rate. The addition of esmolol resulted in significant dose-dependent reductions in the sodium nitroprusside requirement for maintenance of the chosen blood pressure (mean arterial pressure 60 mm Hg) with a "profound potentiation" of sodium nitroprusside's hypotensive action; significant reductions in the heart rate and plasma levels of renin activity were achieved with all infusion rates of esmolol. At levels of 300 $\mu$g/kg/min or higher, there was a significant increase in $PaO_2$ and a decrease in plasma norepinephrine and epinephrine. Esmolol appeared to have a negative chronotropic effect on the heart, as well as the ability to inhibit the renin-angiotensin and catecholamine responses usually elicited by sodium nitroprusside-induced hypotension. Esmolol has been shown to depress both stroke volume and CO during general anesthesia in humans.[206,412,415] Although this negative inotropic effect of esmolol was also postulated in this study, it could not be documented. Ornstein and coworkers[416] also cautioned about the potential for profound myocardial depression with esmolol.

Fromme and coworkers[417] previously demonstrated no benefit from sodium nitroprus-

side-induced hypotension in orthognathic surgery. Blau and associates[418] found esmolol to be more effective than nitroprusside in reducing blood loss and achieving a drier surgical field for these procedures, with greater control of the blood pressure.

## Clonidine

Clonidine is an $\alpha_2$-adrenergic agonist synthesized in 1962 and subsequently noted to produce a lowering of blood pressure and bradycardia. Its antihypertensive action may be related to the stimulation of central postsynaptic $\alpha_2$ receptors combined with a negative feedback effect from peripheral $\alpha_2$ adrenoreceptors that inhibit catecholamine release. It also seems to inhibit renin release from the kidney and may decrease vasopressin release. In addition to its use as an antihypertensive, it has sedative properties used in alcohol, tobacco, and narcotic withdrawal programs. It also seems to produce analgesia, anxiolysis, and sedation sufficient to reduce the MAC for halothane anesthesia while maintaining hemodynamic stability.[419]

Clonidine, in a dose of 4–10 $\mu$g/kg given 2 hours before surgery as an oral premedicant, has been demonstrated to decrease opioid and isoflurane requirements by up to 60% intraoperatively[420,421] and to attenuate the sympathetically mediated tachycardia and hypertension commonly seen with intubation.[422] The antihypertensive action depends on the preexisting level of blood pressure and sympathetic tone; clonidine has little effect on the blood pressure in normotensive patients. Clonidine has also been shown to reduce the dose requirements for labetalol[423] and sodium nitroprusside (by up to 45%).[424,425] The main disadvantage of clonidine premedication has been a slightly delayed recovery from anesthesia.[421] Whether or not clonidine will prove useful as an adjunct in cases of deliberate hypotension has not yet been fully elucidated.

## Captopril

The induction of hypotension leads to a complex series of alterations in physiology. The renin-angiotensin system and sympathetic nervous system are altered, baroreceptor sensitivity may be altered,[198] and even the role of increased levels of vasopressin[426] has been studied. The activation of the sympathetic nervous system seems to be a contributor to the progressive resistance to sodium nitroprusside that is seen in some patients, as well as to the associated tachycardia and rebound hypertension.[192,193,427]

Renin is an enzyme that can be released from the juxtaglomerular cells of the kidney in response to multiple hormonal stimuli, including substances such as antidiuretic hormone and angiotensin II, increased plasma potassium, decreased renal perfusion, increased renal sympathetic nerve activity, renal humorally released catecholamines, and decreased plasma sodium.[428] Renin can convert an $\alpha_2$-globulin from the liver, angiotensinogen, to a decapeptide angiotensin I that is relatively inactive but is rapidly converted by the angiotensin-converting enzyme to the potent and active octapeptide angiotensin II; angiotensin-converting enzyme is present in the lungs and blood vessel walls and is also known as peptidyl dipeptidase. Angiotensin II can stimulate the release of aldosterone, can potentiate the release of and pressor response to norepinephrine, and can itself cause severe vasoconstriction.[429] Even low concentrations of angiotensin II, which lack effects on the blood pressure, can facilitate a calcium-dependent mechanism aiding the conversion of cholesterol to pregnenolone and thus stimulate synthesis and secretion of aldosterone from the adrenal cortex. Aldosterone acts on the kidney, causing retention of sodium and excretion of hydrogen and potassium ions.

Captopril is an oral angiotensin-converting enzyme inhibitor that blocks the angiotensin I to angiotensin II process and thereby diminishes the cardiovascular effects of the renin-angiotensin system.[209,430] Captopril causes an increased compliance of large arteries with systemic arteriolar dilatation, thus producing decreased vascular resistance and a decrease in systemic blood pressure.[430] Although the initial drop in pressure has been correlated with precaptopril plasma renin activity, this correlation is quickly lost. Cerebral and coronary blood flows, stroke volume, and CO all tend to be relatively stable and unchanged, whereas the heart rate may be slightly increased. Renal blood flow tends to increase, with a resultant natriuresis; aldosterone secretion[209] and pulmonary vascular pressures are both decreased. CO may actually increase if the patient is in heart failure, and the symptoms of failure may abate.[431] Severe hypotension may occur if the patient is hypovolemic, especially with the first dose.

Well-absorbed orally, captopril[432] reaches peak plasma levels in 30–90 minutes, is 65% bioavailable, has a half-life of 2 hours or less, and is primarily excreted by the kidneys with 50% being unchanged. Unfortunately, it has many side effects; among these are up to a 10% incidence of skin rash often accompanied by fever, joint pain and pruritus, altered to absent sense of taste in up to 7% of patients, headache, and vertigo. Hyperkalemia and a rise in creatinine levels have been noted in renally impaired or volume-depleted patients. In addition, proteinuria (1%) and neutropenia (0.3%) are reported. In patients with chronic obstructive pulmonary disease, cough and/or increasing dyspnea have also been noted, possibly secondary to a potentiation of the effects of kinins due to the captopril-induced inhibition of peptidyl dipeptidase.

Investigators have questioned how captopril could benefit patients during induced hypotension.[279] The first major report on the interaction of captopril and sodium nitroprusside came in 1981.[433] In awake volunteers, pretreatment with captopril led to an enhanced hypotensive response when sodium nitroprusside was used. Woodside and co-workers[434] showed that 3 mg/kg orally, given before transport to the operating room, significantly reduced the dose of sodium nitroprusside needed for the induction and maintenance of induced hypotension; this reduced sodium nitroprusside requirement led to reduced cyanide production, reduced blood cyanide levels, and a reduced potential for cyanide toxicity.

Porter and associates[435] did a similar study in 1988 but also added a comparison with intravenous nitroglycerin. They found no significant differences between their three techniques in terms of actual blood loss, effect on pulmonary function, or cardiovascular changes severe enough to lead to morbidity. Their target mean arterial pressure was 60–70 mm Hg, higher than in most other studies. Nitroglycerin was inadequate in several patients. With sodium nitroprusside alone, they found a significant degree of rebound hypertension with a postinfusion increase in mean arterial pressure. There was no significant reduction of sodium nitroprusside dosage when

3 mg/kg oral captopril was given 2 hours before induction. In addition, significant rebound hypertension also occurred in the captopril group; measurements were taken up to an average of 8.6 hours after the oral dose. Similarly, plasma renin activity in the captopril group was significantly higher than in the other two groups. It would appear that the lack of feedback inhibition of renin release by angiotensin II is the cause for renin level elevation.[434,435]

In the Porter study,[435] preinduction captopril did produce a slight reduction in mean arterial pressure preoperatively and a significant reduction after induction. Although there was no evidence of impaired perfusion, both Porter and Woodside raise the issue of potential detrimental effects in the elderly, hypovolemic patients, patients on antihypertensive medications, or patients with poor cardiovascular reserve. Captopril is not innocuous and must be used with caution.

## Nicardipine

Nicardipine is a dihydropyridine calcium channel blocker with potent systemic and coronary artery vasodilatory effects, without negative chronotropic, inotropic, or dromotropic effects.[436] Although its half-life is approximately 1 hour, accumulation during an infusion slows its elimination and increases the half-life to 4–8 hours. Commonly used for the treatment of hypertension, it was given by intravenous infusion to induce hypotension in a study comparing it with sodium nitroprusside.[437] The results were very similar, with both agents leading to systemic vasodilation, hypotension, tachycardia, and increased CO. In addition, both agents led to increases in plasma renin activity and catecholamine concentrations.

The disadvantage of nicardipine was its cumulative effect of persistent vasodilation, hypotension, and tachycardia that could prove detrimental in some patients. The authors conclude that nicardipine is not the ideal hypotensive agent because of its inability to promptly restore blood pressure toward normal when its infusion rate is reduced or stopped. In a follow-up study,[438] long-term nicardipine administration was given by infusion for $270 \pm 20$ minutes. Decreased pulmonary and SVR, decreased arteriovenous $O_2$ content difference, and increased cardiac index were found. There was an increasing effect of nicardipine with time, and prolonged hypotension persisted in spite of decreasing plasma levels of nicardipine.

## Fenoldopam

Fenoldopam is a dopamine-1 receptor antagonist representing a new class of investigational drugs. In a dog study it was shown to induce hypotension with a decrease in SVR. Unlike the reduction in renal blood flow often seen with sodium nitroprusside, a 30% decrease in blood pressure was accompanied by an 11% increase in renal blood flow. Human studies may follow.[439]

## Adenosine

Adenosine, a metabolic end product of adenosine triphosphate, is an endogenous vasodilator that has been implicated in local regulation of blood flow in a variety of tissues, most notably the myocardium.[440] Intravenous infusions of adenosine triphosphate have been used to induce hypotension, but this effect is apparently mediated by adenosine whose arterial concentration increases because of degradation of adenosine triphosphate in the blood.[441] Recently, exogenous adenosine itself has been used to induce hypotension in patients.[442–445] Intravenous infusion of adenosine causes arterial hypotension that is rapidly achieved, easily controlled, short-lived, and not accompanied by rebound hypertension when the infusion is discontinued.[443,446–448] There is no evidence of tachyphylaxis.

The hypotensive effect of adenosine is entirely due to a pronounced decrease in SVR, because CO remains either unchanged or increased.[443,446,449] Venous pressures are stable during adenosine-induced hypotension, suggesting that the venous segments of the circulation are less sensitive to adenosine-induced relaxation than are the arterial segments. In dogs, adenosine-induced hypotension is accompanied by decreases in heart rate, probably reflecting a direct depressive effect on the sinoatrial node.[448,449] Although in humans heart rate has been shown to increase, this increase is much smaller than that observed when other agents, for example, sodium nitroprusside, are used to induce hypotension;[443]

thus, $\beta$-adrenergic blocking drugs may not be needed to control heart rate during adenosine-induced hypotension. Adenosine causes dose-dependent changes in cardiac conduction from first degree A-V block to third degree A-V block and atrial flutter.[450,451] Hypotensive infusions of adenosine have a favorable influence on myocardial oxygen supply and demand balance in normal hearts, because blood flow is increased markedly via a potent coronary dilator effect, whereas afterload and heart rate, two major determinants of myocardial oxygen demand, are reduced.[448] However, in animal models of coronary stenoses, adenosine has been shown to cause diversion of flow away from flow-restricted myocardium to normally perfused myocardium, the "coronary steal phenomenon."[452] A similar pattern in humans leads to S-T segment changes suggestive of ischemia.[453] A follow-up study[454,455] also confirmed significant ST segment depression during adenosine administration even at low nonhypotensive infusion rates. A prolongation of atrioventricular condition time was also seen. This implies that adenosine may not be safe in patients with coronary insufficiency.

Direct application of adenosine causes relaxation of cerebral vasculature.[456] Local administration of adenosine into the carotid artery increased cerebral blood flow in baboons[457] and rabbits[458] but did not change cerebral blood flow in dogs and cats.[443,456] This was probably due to species differences in transport of adenosine across the blood-brain barrier and in the extracranial versus intracranial distribution of the carotid artery blood supply.[458] Cerebral blood flow was well maintained and cerebral oxygen demand was reduced (suggesting favorable cerebral oxygenation) when controlled hypotension was induced with adenosine in patients undergoing cerebral aneurysm surgery.[445]

Although the direct effect of adenosine is vasodilation in most tissues, it causes vasoconstriction when infused locally into the arterial supply of the kidney.[459] Adenosine-induced hypotension is associated with pronounced decreases in renal blood flow, glomerular filtration rate, and urine output.[443,447] This data was recently confirmed by Zall and associates,[454] who studied postcoronary artery surgery hypertension. Adenosine produced significant decreases in glomerular filtration rate,

urine output, and renal blood flow even at lower nonhypotensive doses. Thus, impairment of renal function must be considered a potential risk when adenosine is used for controlled hypotension,[450] and patients with impaired renal function should probably not receive adenosine. Adenosine inhibits renin release in the kidney and thus prevents the activation of the renin-angiotensin system,[449,460] which may explain the stable arterial blood pressure and lack of tachyphylaxis or rebound hypertension. One problem with adenosine has been difficulty in relating effects to the administered dosage; central venous administration has been advocated by some, because of the 30–50% rapid metabolism by red blood cells and the rapid reuptake of the balance.[461] One technique attempted to avoid the much larger doses needed peripherally has been to decrease uptake by pretreatment with dipyridamole.[462] It is still premature to conclude whether adenosine will gain wide acceptance as a hypotensive agent, but studies are continuing. Adenosine has not been approved for use as a hypotensive drug in the U.S.A.

## Urapidil

Urapidil is an antihypertensive agent that has been introduced into clinical practice in Europe. It appears to have a dual mode of action affecting both the 5-HT$_{1A}$ brain receptors and the peripheral $\alpha$-adrenergic receptors and produces vasodilation without significant sympathetic activation.[463] Cerebral blood flow, intracranial pressure, and intracranial compliance seem to be unaffected.[464,465] Rebound hypertension is not observed.[466] Only a moderate level of hypotension can be achieved with urapidil, and an increased dose does not achieve more hypotension. It is now being used in parts of Western Europe for hypotensive anesthesia as an adjunct to isoflurane.[467] Its future in the United States is uncertain.

## EFFECT OF DELIBERATE HYPOTENSION ON BLOOD LOSS

The issue of blood loss during deliberate hypotension has been controversial. Is loss truly diminished and, if so, by how much? Donald[468] points out that early literature was filled with enthusiastic clinical reports but often lacked substantiation for reputed claims.

He found only five studies in which actual blood loss measurements were made comparing the same operation, with or without hypotension, during the period up to 1966.[469-473] Some authors appeared to show a bias, seeking benefits from the technique, and in one case even commenting that they could not understand why their own results did not show a reduction in blood loss.[474] Donald[468] found no linear relationship between arterial pressure and blood loss but rather a "step-down" phenomenon leading to a distinct decrease in blood loss when systolic pressure was at levels of 80–100 mm Hg; no further blood loss reduction took place at lower pressures. Similarly, when blood pressure was deliberately reduced by 20–40 mm Hg, the blood loss was reduced significantly; further reductions were not beneficial. Although one other author reported similar findings,[475] the weight of evidence in the literature suggests otherwise, and most articles conclude that a 40–50% reduction in blood loss can be found, in a rather linear fashion, during deliberate hypotension.

Anderson and McKissock[476] first reported on the use of controlled hypotension for pediatric surgery in 1953. Goldstein in 1966[477] was among the first to suggest that hypotensive anesthesia might reduce the significant blood loss associated with scoliosis surgery. In a series of three articles in 1974,[53,60,478] induced hypotension in children and its applicability to surgery, including scoliosis, was discussed. The use of hypotensive anesthesia decreased the need for blood replacement and total blood loss by approximately 40% while reducing the operating time by approximately 30 minutes. The blood loss per level fused decreased from 337 to 223 mL, and the blood transfused decreased from 2.27 to 1.38 L. No complications directly related to the hypotensive technique were found. Although first reported in pediatric patients in 1953 and Anderson[479] in 1955, it was the 1974 articles by Salem and his associates[53,60,478] that led to the widespread use of deliberate hypotension for scoliosis surgery.

Enderby's[18] first report in 1950 demonstrated a significant benefit from hypotension in 26 of 35 patients. Boyan[480] followed that in 1953 with a report on hexamethonium in radical cancer surgery using systolics of 65–70 mm Hg, and leading to the clinical impression

of improved surgical fields and diminished blood loss, but this was not measured. Eckenhoff and Rich[473] published a better study on 231 patients for a variety of surgery and found an approximate 50% decrease in measured blood loss in the hypotensive group.

Deliberate hypotension has been used successfully for a great variety of surgical procedures (Table 8–1). For example, a 50% reduction in blood loss and transfusion was reported in radical cystectomy,[481] lienorenal shunts for portal hypertension,[482] retropubic prostatectomy,[471,483] radical retroperitoneal lymph node dissection,[484] pelvic floor surgery,[485] and "radical" surgical procedures.[268,486] Other reports include oral and maxillofacial surgery[487,488] and head and neck surgery[470,489,490] with 40% reductions in red cell loss; craniectomy in infants[217] where blood loss was decreased from 20 to 48%; middle ear surgery[491-494] where operating conditions were improved and bleeding was lessened though not measured; radical hysterectomy with pelvic lymphadenectomy[495] where operating time was shortened by 29%, blood loss lessened by 70%, and the percentage of patients requiring transfusion decreased from 81 to 11.5%; neurological,[496] plastic,[497] and gynecological surgeries,[498] all with improved conditions; radical mastectomy[469,499] with a decrease in blood loss of 50% in one study and a decrease in the transfusion rate of 75% in the other; and spinal surgical procedures including scoliosis and fusion[60,299,478,500-503] that generally show minor improvements in operating time (8–10%) but major decreases in blood loss (34–58%) and transfusions (28–45%).

Many studies have been published involving major orthopedic cases, particularly hip arthroplasty. Mallory[504] found decreases in blood loss of 55% for hip replacement and 40% in repeat hip replacement surgery, along with a reduction of 25% in operative time. Nelson and Bowen[505] studied 100 Jehovah's Witnesses having total hip replacement, all but 11 under sodium nitroprusside-induced hypotensive anesthesia. They found a 43% reduction in blood loss in first-time hip operations and a 30% reduction after previous hip surgery, as compared with a control group who were not Jehovah's Witnesses. Factors other than hypotension that aided in reducing blood loss included meticulous hemostasis in

**Table 8–6.   Blood loss with normotension versus hypotension**

| Author | Procedure | Normotension | Hypotension |
|---|---|---|---|
| Davis et al., 1974[540] | Total Hip Arthroplasty | 2250 | 1430 |
| Amaranath et al., 1975[239] | Total Hip Arthroplasty | 1753 | 1033 |
| Schaberg et al., 1976[487] | Oral-Facial Corrective Surgery | 456 | 256 |
| Thompson et al., 1978[174] | Total Hip Arthroplasty | 1183 | 326 |
| Vazeery & Lunde, 1979[541] | Total Hip Arthroplasty | 1038 | 212 |
| Eerola et al., 1979[542] | Total Hip Arthroplasty | 2336 | 730 |
| Diaz & Lockhart, 1979[217] | Craniectomy in Infancy | 133 | 72 |
| Barbier-Bohm et al., 1980[543] | Total Hip Arthroplasty | 900 | 320 |
| Qvist et al., 1982[544] | Total Hip Arthroplasty | 1909 | 809 |
| Malcolm-Smith & McMaster, 1983[545] | Harrington Rod | 1530 | 525 |
| Powell et al., 1983[495] | Radical Hysterectomy; Hysterectomy & Lymphadenectomy | 1133 | 331 |
| Lawhon et al., 1984[501] | Harrington Rod Insertion | 1559  (adults) (children) | 1037 801 |
| Patel et al., 1985[502] | Harrington Rod Insertion | 1540 | 1102 |
| Nelson & Bowen, 1986[505] | Total Hip Arthroplasty | 800 | 450 |
| Sood, 1987[482] | Splenectomy & Lienorenal Shunt | 1286 | 517 |
| Ting, 1988[503] | Scoliosis (Luque Rods) | 1822 | 1201 |

a well-planned surgical procedure involving careful technique; thus, even the 11 normotensive first-time patients showed a 35% reduction in blood loss. See Table 8–6 for studies of hypotension versus normotension.

Although surgical blood loss is usually decreased by deliberate hypotension, there are many exceptions in the literature.[46,366,417,474,485,506,507] The failures fall into different categories: (a) failure to achieve significant hypotension because of tachycardia, tachyphylaxis, resistance, an unwillingness to give more of the drug or drugs because of fear of complications, development of side effects or toxicity, and so on; (b) achievement of significant hypotension but with a nonlinear decrease in blood loss, that is, the amount of blood lost decreases but not as much as might have been predicted;[506] and (c) achievement of significant hypotension but without significant improvement of the surgical field and/or without a decrease in blood loss. The comment "for unexplained reasons, not all patients respond as predicted"[227] is an old but true observation. Scurr and Wyman[366] pointed out that good operating conditions did not always occur even when a satisfactory blood pressure was achieved; this view was repeated by Hellewell and Potts in 1966,[46] even with propranolol control of tachycardia.

A "wide range of bleeding is an invariable feature of all blood loss investigations."[485] Hercus and others[508] measured the blood lost during 412 major surgical procedures, finding wide ranges for prostatectomy (150–2750 mL), radical mastectomy (380–3200 mL), partial gastrectomy (200–1800 mL), and so on. Donald[485] states that "the significance of this universally observed wide range is that it demonstrates clearly that the causes of bleeding during surgery are unknown and largely uncontrollable . . . . The fact is that some patients, for unknown reasons, bleed to an inordinate degree during surgery, whilst others, in no way distinguishable from these, present a dry operating field to the surgeon." Others in the past have also noted and speculated on the causes of excessive surgical bleeding.[509,510] McGowan and Smith[511] also noted the same problem with blood loss measured during prostatectomy from 6 mL to over 2000 mL.

Is there something, some factor we cannot yet identify, that makes some patients bleed so little? Donald[468] asks this question, without an answer. In his experience comparable procedures show less blood loss when performed under local anesthesia than under general anesthesia. He speculates that general anesthesia may somehow interfere with some aspects of hemostasis, perhaps at the central nervous system level. In conclusion, we can say that despite occasionally conflicting articles, the preponderance of evidence and our own clinical experience indicate that well-controlled deliberate hypotension usually succeeds in reducing blood loss and transfusions by approximately 40–50%.

## MONITORING DURING DELIBERATE HYPOTENSIVE ANESTHESIA

Monitoring has improved with increasing sophistication, as in any other workplace. In addition, we have been subjected to increasing scrutiny and demands for safety from a plethora of sources, including the individual consumer, various governmental and consumer advocacy groups, the watchdog press and media, and our own specialty society committees. Standards of practice continue to evolve, and we have attempted to rethink and modify our techniques and attitudes appropriately.

Monitoring for deliberate hypotension involves all of the usual standard modalities common to current modern practice and then adds to these meticulously in specific situations.

### Temperature

Pharmaceutical agents used to deliberately induce hypotension may also contribute to an unwanted temperature reduction by virtue of vasodilatation and/or venodilatation and associated loss of heat. Temperature monitoring should be used from the beginning of the case. Esophageal temperature probes, frequently as part of an esophageal stethoscope monitor, are in common usage; skin temperature monitors have also become more accurate but are not as reliable. Additional causes of hypothermia include a cold operating room and the transfusion of cold blood. An extensive surgical incision with a large exposed surface may also lead to excessive heat loss. It is not uncommon to see a fall of 2 or 3° C during a major corrective procedure for scoliosis.[235] Among the reported adverse consequences of hypothermia are the accentuation of hypotension and the potentiation of nondepolarizing muscle relaxants.[512] Measures to prevent heat loss are often more effective than attempts to correct heat loss later in the case. These might include heat and moisture retaining filters, blood and fluid warmers, a warming mattress when possible, head covers, thermal blankets, warming the ambient air, and in-line heated humidifiers. The opposite situation, that of malignant hyperthermia, has of course also been noted, with Relton and others[513] reporting an increased association in patients undergoing scoliosis correction.

### Blood Loss Measurement

The current methods of estimating blood loss have not evolved significantly for many years. Often the surgeon's estimate, often inaccurate, is used, frequently underestimating blood loss by 50%.[487] The alternatives involve (*a*) measurement of suctioned blood, and the subtraction from it of measured irrigating solutions; (*b*) weighing of all sponges and laps while still wet, and the subtraction of the dry weight of such materials; (*c*) a visual estimation of blood loss on such laps and sponges, using clinical acumen and statistical approximations as an alternative to weighing; and (*d*) use of blood salvage apparatus, from which a blood loss estimate can be made.

Two facts should be kept in mind: the smaller the patient (and therefore the smaller the blood volume), the more critical is each milliliter of blood loss, and therefore the more vital are accurate measurements, and during deliberate hypotensive anesthesia, where autonomic controls may be blunted or absent, relatively small percentage differences in blood loss may produce critically significant differences in blood pressure. It is recommended that two intravenous lines should be used (at least one large bore) for these cases. A short-acting intravenous hypotensive agent may be preferable, because its discontinuance would lead to a more rapid return of blood pressure.

### Arterial Blood Pressure and Arterial Blood Gases

A historical summary of the development of blood pressure monitoring was published in 1985.[512] The standard method, a sphygmomanometer cuff used either with palpation or with the placement of a stethoscope over the brachial artery, is still widely accepted worldwide but is often inadequate when moment-to-moment control is necessary and may prove unreliable at low blood pressures.

The oscillometer or oscillotonometer is based on work by Pachon[514] and Boulitte[512] in France and by von Recklinghausen[512] in Germany. Their independent publications in the early years of this century were based on earlier work of Erlanger.[515] "The oscillometer is, in essence a pulse wave monitor which gives an estimate of blood pressure by measuring the pressure required inside a cuff to obliterate the wave and displaying this pressure wave as oscillations on a dial."[512] The system in use today depends on a double cuff devised by Gallavardin in 1922.[516] Automated oscillometers have been in use for many years.

All noninvasive automated blood pressure monitors in use today are vastly improved from those introduced in the 1960s; those units suffered from extreme sensitivity to cuff contact, very slow cycling times, and extreme unreliability at low blood pressures. Current units are less likely to give false information based on contact but may do so nonetheless; they are more reliable at sensing down to lower blood pressures but still suffer from the time required for the inflation-deflation sensing cycle that may take 30–60 seconds. "Therefore arterial cannulation is essential for long surgical procedures, when excessive blood loss is anticipated, in critically ill patients, when the procedure is done with the patient in the prone position, and when profound hypotension is necessary."[61]

The indwelling arterial cannula serves numerous purposes in addition to the instantaneous detection of blood pressure changes; arterial blood gases are, for example, an essential element in the management of deliberate hypotension, facilitating the early diagnosis of malignant hyperthermia, cyanide toxicity, altered ventilatory status, and so on. Visual display of the tracing may also aid in the recognition of myocardial dysfunction or hypovolemia. Direct arterial access also allows easier blood sampling for the measurement of hematocrit, electrolytes, and glucose levels in addition to the blood gases.

The most common site is a radial artery; to avoid the potential for ischemia or gangrene, which could result if thrombosis occurred, Allen's test for adequacy of collateral blood supply is performed. Other potential sites include the dorsalis pedis or posterior tibial, brachial, or femoral or even temporal arteries. One study indicates that the dorsalis pedis overestimates blood pressure when sodium nitroprusside is used as the hypotensive agent but underestimates it when isoflurane is used for hypotension.[517]

Recently, an attempt was made to introduce a new noninvasive blood pressure monitor that provides continuous measurement and waveform display with the use of a finger cuff (Finapres).[518] Although reliable in many patients, large discrepancies were reported in some measurements between arterial pressure and pressure recorded at the finger. No predictability as to patient or circumstance leading to unreliability was noted. Arterial pressure monitoring remains the "gold standard."

## POSTOPERATIVE CARE

The patient receiving deliberate hypotension deserves and requires more skilled supervision postoperatively than the average case. Postoperative care really is initiated in the operating room, as the anesthesiologist begins to awaken the patient after slowly allowing the blood pressure to rise toward normal and after ascertaining the results of the final set of arterial blood gases and hematocrit. If the endotracheal tube is to be kept in, it must be resecured skillfully, particularly if the patient has been in the prone or lateral position where secretions may have loosened the previously placed adhesive tape. The decision to extubate should be made thoughtfully and carefully, and the patient transferred only when the airway is guaranteed. Sudden jerking and bouncing movements of the patient are best avoided because of the potential for hypotension to develop.

Pain management may require an initial period of conservatism, where drugs are given in reduced doses until both respiratory and hemodynamic stability are assured. Patient-controlled analgesia has become a popular modality for pain control postoperatively. Incremental intravenous narcotics, continuous infusions of narcotics from a patient-controlled analgesia unit, intramuscular analgesics, epidural catheter infusions, and intrapleural catheters are all potentially useful techniques to be considered.

Care is needed in reestablishing fluid balance and equilibrium after some of the major procedures using deliberate hypotension. Many physicians like to keep their patients relatively "dry" intraoperatively to facilitate hypotensive technique; others believe in fluid loading to avoid sudden untoward drops in blood pressure. In either case, blood loss, fluid shifting, third-space losses, and the use of a "cell-saver" type device for suctioning blood off the surgical field with the potential for autologous reinfusion all may contribute to uncertainty about the patients current volume status, and this in turn may lead to potential vascular instability. Serial monitoring of hemoglobin/hematocrit, electrolytes, arterial blood gases, and urine output may all be beneficial, and a central line is sometimes helpful.

It is of more than just historical interest to recall that Larson,[59] when reviewing reported deaths from 1958 to 1963 in which induced hypotension seemed implicated, found that 97% of these deaths occurred in the postoperative period.

## POSTOPERATIVE HEMORRHAGE

Many clinicians have expressed a concern about the possibility of postoperative bleeding upon discontinuation of the hypotensive technique. Rebound hypertension, previously discussed, certainly can occur, especially with sodium nitroprusside; nonetheless, the incidence of this becoming a significant factor is extremely small, particularly with our increased recognition, understanding, and prophylaxis against the problem.

There seems to be no clear evidence linking postoperative bleeding and the prior performance of induced hypotension. Salem and El-Etr[519] suggested performing the following steps whenever hypotension has been deliberately used:

1. Allow a slow, gradual, gentle return of blood pressure
2. Do not use vasopressors
3. Return the pressure toward normal early enough in the closure that all bleeding sites are visible and hemostasis can be obtained
4. Apply pressure dressings whenever and wherever possible
5. Attempt to minimize coughing and straining during the emergence, extubation, and immediate postanesthetic period.

## COMPLICATIONS ASSOCIATED WITH DELIBERATE HYPOTENSION

The true incidence of complications associated with the use of deliberate hypotension is unknown, despite numerous, albeit sometimes conflicting, reports in the literature. During the earlier years of the technique, errors in patient selection and anesthetic management, along with a deficiency of proper monitoring, led to a potential lack of safety. Davidson[520] and Shackleton[34] each raised some questions, and Enderby in 1952[521] reported on two deaths from cardiac arrest during the first 250 cases of deliberate hypotension; Gillan[522] noted two cases of unilateral blindness after hexamethonium deliberate hypotension but could not distinguish the relative contribution of the hypotension versus pressure placed on the eye. Other early reports of complications included amaurosis from two additional authors,[523,524] EEG changes,[525] diminished renal blood flow and urine production,[526] and the occurrence of thrombosis of major blood vessels during the postoperative period.[527]

Hampton and Little[32] sent a questionnaire to members of the Association of Anaesthetists of Great Britain and Ireland, and the results were published in 1953; simultaneously, a similar questionnaire was sent to Diplomates of the American Board of Anesthesiology and those results were also reported.[31] Both studies were uncontrolled retrospective reports done through the mail that provided statistics but attempted no explanation for the findings. Nonetheless, these two reports "almost caused the abolition of deliberate hypotension,"[528] at least in the United States. Little[529] subsequently published a 1955 article and a 1956 book on controlled hypotension.

The American study included 144 anesthesiologists and 6805 patients and was flawed by "improper wording of certain questions" that gave some data of "no statistical value."[31] The British study[32] included 178 anesthetists and 21,125 hypotensive anesthetics. The mortality rate was 0.34% overall (96 deaths in 27,930 cases combining the two surveys) or 1 in 291, but the complication rate was 1 in 31 cases or 3.2%.[529] Among the complications reported, those related to the central nervous system were among the most common; these included cerebrovascular accidents, blurring of vision, delayed awakening, and dizziness. Other complications included oliguria, reactionary hemorrhage, and retinal thrombosis. Although some anesthesiologists now abandoned the technique as too dangerous, others believed the high complication rate was not necessarily a true reflection of the hypotension but condemned either the study and/or the inexperience of the practitioners who had committed errors of judgement and technique. "Seldom has the pendulum swung so quickly or so violently from the one extreme of enthusiastic uncritical reception, to that of biased, prejudiced and equally uncritical opposition."[1] The reaction to abandon the technique was perhaps even more evident in the United States, for the studies that showed a mortality rate of 1 in 459 in the Great Britain study revealed a mortality rate of 1 in 136 in the United States. Little[529] notes that deliberate hypotension was viewed as "a menace to humanity" and concluded that "the profound dangers of induced hypotension dictate that the use of these techniques be restricted to those cases in which they are potentially life-saving." Beecher and Todd[530] revealed an overall mortality rate of only 1 in 1560, a far less ominous statistic.

The next major study was that of Enderby,[45,497] covering 9107 hypotensive anesthetics during the period 1950–1960; this report was, according to the author himself, "the first presentation of a series large enough to make an analysis of value and to demonstrate unequivocally that hypotension could be practiced safely."[1] There were nine deaths in the series, for a rate of 1 in 1000 or 0.1%. In a follow-up,[237,531] now covering 20,558 hypotensive anesthetics from 1950 to 1979, Enderby found only 10 deaths, yielding a mortality of 1 in 2055 or 0.05%; of the 10, 5 were definitely not attributable to the hypotensive technique, thus yielding a true rate of only 5 per 20,558 or 1 per 4111 (or 0.025%). The majority of these cases were done in the "head-up tipped" position with blood pressures at heart level held between 50 and 100 mm Hg, but 78% of these had pressures between 60 and 80 mm Hg. The majority of the cases were head and neck and only American Society of Anesthesiologist's physical status I and II patients were selected. With 60 as the lowest acceptable pressure, Enderby felt comfortable in saying that a hypotensive anesthetic should be considered as safe as a normotensive anesthetic.

Eckenhoff and Rich[473] published their experiences with 231 patients, of whom 115 received deliberate hypotension. No deaths related to the use of hypotension occurred, and there was a significant reduction in blood loss. They believed the prior studies of Hampton and Little[31,32] were tainted by an improper choice of both patients and anesthetic agents, inadequate pulmonary ventilation, inadequate monitoring, a failure to elevate the operative site when feasible, and an excessive concentration on achieving a low blood pressure number. Hampton himself, in a discussion attached to the Eckenhoff and Rich article, notes that many of the earlier reports included the use of large doses of hexamethonium, which sometimes led to precipitous and often prolonged hypotension. "Induced hypotension was not always synonymous with controlled hypotension." Hampton praised the use of halothane and the newer ganglionic blocking agents; admonished anesthesiologists to maintain careful and detailed monitoring on a continuous basis, including the immediate postoperative period; reminded us that complications seemed minimal if the systolic blood pressure remained at 80 mm Hg or higher; and noted his approval of the use of reduced bleeding as the endpoint rather than preselecting an actual number value for blood pressure.[473]

Salem and others[256] published a five-institution collaborative retrospective study covering the period from 1965 to 1975 that looked at complications related to deliberate hypotension. The complications noted seemed to fall into a group of categories: uncontrolled and severe fall in blood pressure, which sometimes led to cardiac arrest; neurological deficits; reactionary hemorrhage; and failures in technique. The latter category, faulty technique, was determined to be causative in the majority of complications. Among the technical errors were excessive rapidity of hypotensive onset and/or maintaining this hypotension for an excessive duration, extremes of head-up tilt, underestimating the blood loss, hypoxemia, hypocapnia, the failure to detect early warning signs, inappropriate pharmacological usage, and inappropriate patient selection.

Nonfatal complications are, of course, more common, with Hampton and Little[31] reporting an incidence of 3.3%. The major concerns have been central nervous system and renal complications, and a 1974 article reported on two incidents of cerebral damage,[223] one being hemiplegia after surgery and the other a failure to awaken. Retinal thrombosis was found in 3 of 27,930 cases summarized by Little.[529] One case of cerebral artery thrombosis was noted in 50 cases of induced hypotension,[532] but in 1000 cases in another study there were no cerebral complications.[498] A 1988 report[533] looked prospectively at 52 operations performed on 43 patients for correction of scoliosis using deliberate hypotension. Renal function proved to be unaffected in all patients, and spinal cord function was likewise unimpaired. It was suggested that avoidance of water and sodium depletion with maintenance of circulating volume was important to protect renal perfusion.

From the data currently available it appears that improvements in our anesthetic practice have made deliberate hypotension safe, provided we are restricting ourselves to lowering the mean blood pressure to the range of 50–65 mm Hg and looking at relatively healthy young patients.[227] Miller[227] states, however, that patients with underlying major organ dysfunction may be at higher risk for the development of complications.

## CONTRAINDICATIONS

Although authors may disagree about some of the disorders, diseases, and abnormalities that constitute contraindications to the use of deliberate hypotension, the following list is a representative sampling of opinions in the literature.[55,61]

1. Lack of an anesthesiologist with sufficient knowledge and experience with the technique.
2. Neonates and infants, except for specific indications.
3. Children with known cardiac shunts. A decrease in SVR can potentially produce a sudden and severe increase in right to left shunting and concomitant hypoxemia.[534]
4. Severe hypertension. In 1960 it was suggested that hypertensive patients could be done safely, provided that systolic blood pressure be kept at 80 mm Hg.[535,536]
5. Patients with sickle cell disease. Those with "trait" who have relatively normal hemoglobin/hematocrit values and a negative history of "crisis" can probably be done safely. In the disease state, a decrease in CO can lead to a decrease in $P\bar{v}O_2$ below a critical level of 30 mm Hg and thus a "crisis" can be initiated.[537]

6. A patient with significant anemia and/or significant hypovolemia.
7. Renal artery stenosis or significant abnormalities in renal function.
8. Hepatic impairment with elevated liver function tests.
9. Polycythemia and hypotension may lead to an increase in sludging and a greater risk of thrombosis.
10. Cerebrovascular accident or the presence of known cerebral artery stenosis.
11. Severe coronary artery disease, especially a recent myocardial infarction, and/or heart failure.
12. Severe respiratory insufficiency and/or a major reduction in the delivery of oxygen.
13. The use of ganglionic blockers is controversial in patients with narrow-angle glaucoma because of the associated pupillary dilatation.

In Larson's 1964 article,[59] virtually any and all systemic diseases seemed to be absolute contraindications to the use of induced hypotension, and some patients were denied the benefits of the technique. By contrast, we have very few, if any, absolute contraindications in modern practice, and most of the former absolutes are now considered to be only "relative" contraindications.

## SUMMARY

"Hypotension must only be induced in the honest belief that some good to the patient will accrue."[59] This is a "truth" that remains with us today. Deliberate or induced hypotension seems to be an effective method to decrease blood loss and the need for transfusion, while providing a clearer surgical field. There are a multiplicity of pharmaceutical agents and techniques that have been used or attempted, but in most cases the level of blood pressure and/or CO and the smoothness of its maintenance are the crucial determinants. "Skilled anesthesia, technical competence, and constant vigilance are essential prerequisites for the safe conduct of hypotensive techniques."[255] Among the factors that may improve safety and outcome are the establishment of a secure airway, avoidance of severe hypocapnia, careful patient screening and selection, a gradual onset and offset of hypotension with scrupulous monitoring, insertion of an arterial line with liberal drawing of blood gases and a relatively high $FIO_2$ as needed, setting realistic and safe goals for the level of blood pressure desired consistent with the surgical requirements, but remaining cognizant that what is important is the dry surgical field and good postoperative care. In the young healthy patient population, for example the teenager with idiopathic scoliosis, the complication rate is very low, whereas in the infirm elderly the risk may be increased.

The cost-effectiveness of this technique and its potential for saving lives commend it to our attention and demand that we continue our efforts to make it safe, effective, and accepted. In 1978, Aach et al.[538] stated that 300 deaths directly related to the transfusion of blood occur annually and that 3% of patients who receive from one to five units of blood will contract viral hepatitis. Based on a 1982 survey of total hip arthroplasty, in the United States alone, more than 100,000 hip replacements are performed annually.[539] Because the average hip arthroplasty patient receives two units of blood in the course of their hospitalization,[505] at a cost of approximately $300, there is a potential cost savings of $30,000,000 with deliberate hypotension for this procedure. In addition, these 100,000 patients (probably more in 1995 than in 1982) could theoretically turn into 3000 new cases of viral hepatitis annually, with the attendant costs and risks of morbidity and mortality. Add to that the newer and even more dramatic potential for the transmission of the human immunodeficiency virus and the acquired immunodeficiency syndrome and you have compelling reasons for any procedure that can decrease the transfusion of blood.

Deliberate hypotension is a challenging technique with low risk, when properly performed by a trained professional, and potentially significant immediate (decreased bleeding in the operative site, improved exposure, decreased operating time, decreased need for transfusion with decreased costs) and long-term (decreased risk of hepatitis and acquired immunodeficiency syndrome) benefits. It is a technique worth learning and using as part of our armamentarium.

## REFERENCES

1. Enderby GEH: Historical review of the practice of deliberate hypotension. In: Enderby GEH, ed, Hypotensive Anaesthesia. London, 1985, Churchill Livingstone.
2. Leigh JM: The history of controlled hypotension. Br J Anaesth 1975; 47:745.
3. Pitkin GP: Controllable spinal anaesthesia. Am J Surg 1928; 5:537.
4. Cushing H: Tumors of the nervus acusticus. Philadelphia, 1917, W.B. Saunders.
5. Cottrell JE: Is deliberate hypotension a useful clinical technique in 1987? ASA Refresher Course Lectures 1987; #331.
6. Kohlstaedt KG, Page IH: Haemorrhagic hypotension and its treatment by intra-arterial and intravenous infusion of blood. Arch Surg 1943; 47:178.
7. Gardner WJ: The control of bleeding during operation by induced hypotension. JAMA 1946; 132:572.
8. Bilsland WL: Controlled hypotension by arteriotomy in intracranial surgery. Anaesthesia 1951; 6:20.
9. Griffiths HWC, Gillies J: Thoracolumbar splanchnicectomy and sympathectomy: anaesthetic procedure. Anaesthesia 1948; 3:134.
10. Bromage PR: Vascular hypotension in 107 cases of epidural analgesia. Anaesthesia 1951; 6:26.
11. King H: Curare alkaloids. I. Tubocurarine. Chem Soc 1935; 57:1381.
12. Acheson GH, Moe GK: The action of tetraethylammonium ion in the mammalian circulation. J Pharmacol Exp Ther 1946; 87:220.
13. Acheson GH, Pereira SA: The blocking effect of tetraethylammonium ion on the superior cervical ganglion of the cat. J Pharmacol Exp Ther 1946; 87:273.
14. Barlow RB, Ing HR: Curare-like action of polymethylene bisquaternary ammonium salts. Nature 1948; 161:718.
15. Paton WDM, Zaimis EJ: Curare-like action of polymethylene bisquaternary ammonium salts. Nature 1948; 161:718.
16. Paton WDM, Zaimis EJ: Clinical potentialities of certain bisquaternary salts causing neuromuscular and ganglionic block. Nature 1948; 162:810.
17. Organe GSW, Paton WDM, Zaimis EJ: Preliminary trials of bistrimethylammonium decane and pentane diiodide (C10 and C5) in man. Lancet 1949; 1:21.
18. Enderby GEH: Controlled circulation with hypotensive drugs and posture to reduce bleeding in surgery. Preliminary results with pentamethonium iodide. Lancet 1950; 1:1145.
19. Scurr CF: Reduction of haemorrhage in the operative field by the use of pentamethonium iodide: a preliminary report. Anesthesiology 1951; 12:253.
20. Barnett AJ: Comparison of pentamethonium and hexamethonium bromide. Lancet 1951; 1:1415.
21. Enderby GEH, Armstrong-Davison MH, Boyes KF, et al: Discussion on the use of hypotensive drugs in surgery. Proc R Soc Med 1951; 44:829.
22. Enderby GEH, Pelmore JF: Controlled hypotension and postural ischaemia to reduce bleeding in surgery. Lancet 1951; 1:663.
23. Enderby GEH: Postural ischaemia and blood pressure. Lancet 1954; 2:1097.
24. Enderby GEH: Pentolinium tartrate in controlled hypotension. Lancet 1954; 2:1097.
25. Randall IO, Peterson WG, Lehmann G: The ganglionic-blocking action of thiophanium derivatives. J Pharmacol Exp Ther 1949; 97:48.
26. McCubbin JW, Page JH: Nature of the hypotensive action of a thiophanium derivative (RO2-2222) in dogs. J Pharmacol Exp Ther 1952; 105:437.
27. Sarnoff SJ, Goodale WT, Sarnoff L: Graded reduction of arterial pressure in man by means of a thio-

phanium derivative (RO 2-2222). Circulation 1952; 6:63.

28. Magill IW, Scurr CF, Wyman JB: Controlled hypotension by a thiophanium derivative. Lancet 1953; 1:219.

29. Nicholson MJ, Sarnoff SJ, Crehan JP: Intravenous use of a thiophanium derivative (Arfonad–RO 2-2222). Anesthesiology 1953; 14:215.

30. Sadove MS, Wyant GM, Gleave G: Controlled hypotension: study of Arfonad (RO 2-2222). Anaesthesia 1953; 8:175.

31. Hampton LJ, Little DM: Complications associated with the use of "controlled hypotension" in anesthesia. Arch Surg 1953; 67:549.

32. Hampton LJ, Little DM: Results of a questionnaire concerning controlled hypotension in anesthesia. Lancet 1953; 1:1299.

33. Rollason WN: Anesthesia and the "bloodless" field. Anesth Analg 1953; 32:289.

34. Shackleton RPW: The reduction of surgical haemorrhage—some observations on controlled hypotension with methonium compounds. Br Med J 1951; 1:1054.

35. Organe GSW: Hypotensive anaesthesia. Anesth Analg 1953; 32:19.

36. Saunders JW: Negative pressure device for controlled hypotension. Lancet 1952; 1:1286.

37. Brown AS, Horton JM: Elective hypotension with intracardiac pacemaking for the operative management of ruptured intracranial aneurysms. Acta Anaesthesiol Scand Suppl 1966; 23:665.

38. Dimant S, Piper CA, Murphy TO: Pacemaker-controlled hypotension in surgery. Surgery 1967; 62:663.

39. Enderby GEH: Posture, respiration et hypotension controlee. Cah Anesthiol 1957; 5:189.

40. Johnstone MA: Human cardiovascular response to fluothane anaesthesia. Br J Anaesth 1956; 28:392.

41. Raventos J: The action of fluothane on the autonomic nervous system. Helv Chir Acta 1961; 28:358.

42. Enderby GEH: Halothane and hypotension. Anaesthesia 1960; 15:25.

43. Moraca PP, Bitte EM, Hale DE, et al: Clinical evaluation of sodium nitroprusside as a hypotensive agent. Anesthesiology 1962; 23:193.

44. Hale DE, Moraca PP, Bitte EM: Clinical evaluation of sodium nitroprusside as a hypotensive agent in renal angiography. Abstr 2nd World Congr Anaesth, Toronto, 1961.

45. Enderby GEH: A report on mortality and morbidity following hypotensive anesthetics. Br J Anaesth 1961; 33:109.

46. Hellewell J, Potts MW: Propranolol during controlled hypotension. Br J Anaesth 1966; 38:794.

47. Johnstone MA: Propranolol (Inderal) during halothane anaesthesia. Br J Anaesth 1966; 38:516.

48. Hewitt PB, Lord PW, Thornton HL: Propranolol in hypotensive hypotension. Anaesthesia 1967; 22:82.

49. Enderby GEH: Effects of propranolol on bleeding during plastic surgical operations. Proc 3rd Asian and Australasian Congr Anaesth, Canberra, 1970, Butterworths (Sydney).

50. Salem MR, Ivankovic AD: The place of beta adrenergic blocking drugs in the deliberate induction of hypotension. Anesth Analg 1970; 49:427.

51. Scott DB, Buckley FP, Littlewood DG, et al: Circulatory effects of labetalol during halothane anaesthesia. Anaesthesia 1978; 33:145.

52. Fahmy NR: Nitroglycerin as a hypotensive drug during general anesthesia. Anesthesiology 1978; 49:17.

53. Salem MR, Wong AY, Bennett EJ, et al: Deliberate hypotension in infants and children. Anesth Analg 1974; 53:975.

54. Salem MR: Therapeutic uses of ganglionic blocking drugs. Int Anesthesiol Clin 1978; 16:171.

55. Fahmy NR: Indications and contraindications for deliberate hypotension with a review of its cardiovascular effects. Int Anesthesiol Clin 1979; 17:175.

56. Lam AM: Induced hypotension. Can Anaesth Soc J 1984; 31:S56.

57. Sollevi A: Hypotensive anesthesia and blood loss. Acta Anaesthesiol Scand Suppl 1988; 89:39.

58. Petrozza PH: Induced hypotension. Int Anesthesiol Clin 1990; 28:223.

59. Larson AG: Deliberate hypotension. Anesthesiology 1964; 25:682.

60. Bennett EJ, Salem MR, Sakul SP, et al: Induced hypotension for spinal corrective procedures. Middle East J Anesthesiol 1974; 4:177.

61. Salem MR, Bikhazi GB: Hypotensive anesthesia. In: Motoyama EA, Davis PJ, eds, Smith's Anesthesia for Infants & Children, 5 ed. St. Louis, 1990, C. V. Mosby.

62. Glenn WWL, Hampton LJ, Goodyer AVN: The use of controlled hypotension in large blood vessel surgery. Arch Surg 1954; 86:1.

63. Dalal FY, Bennett EJ, Salem MR, et al: Anaesthesia for coarctation. A new classification for rational anaesthetic management. Anaesthesia 1974; 29:704.

64. Chiu CJ, Shaftan GW, Dennis C: Control of experimental hemorrhage with Arfonad. J Trauma 1965; 5:392.

65. Boba A, Converse JG: Ganglionic blockade in the management of acute massive hemorrhage: a 10 year appraisal. Anesth Analg 1967; 46:211.

66. Hopkins RW, Fratianne RB, Abrams JS, et al: Controlled hypotension for uncontrolled hemorrhage. Arch Surg 1967; 95:517.

67. Salem MR, El-Etr AA, Rattenborg CC: Deliberate hypotension for the management of threatening hemorrhage. Anesthesiology 1968; 29:155.

68. Longnecker DE: The microvascular response to hypotensive drugs. In: Enderby GEH, ed, Hypotensive Anaesthesia. London, 1985, Churchill Livingstone.

69. Vane JR, Anggard EE, Botting RM: Regulatory functions of the vascular endothelium. N Engl J Med 1990; 323:27.

70. Jaffe EA: Biology of Endothelial Cells. The Hague, 1984, Maritnus Nijhoff Publishers.

71. Forsberg EJ, Feuerstein G, Shohami E, et al: Adenosine triphosphate stimulates inositol phospholipid metabolism and prostacyclin formation in adrenal medullary endothelial cells by means of $P_2$-purinergic receptors. Proc Natl Acad Sci U S A 1987; 84:5630.

72. Bhagyalakshmi A, Frangos JA: Mechanism of shear-induced prostacyclin production in endothelial cells. Biochem Biophys Res Commun 1989; 158:31.

73. Longmore DB, Bennett JG, Hoyle PM, et al: Prostacyclin administration during cardiopulmonary bypass in man. Lancet 1981; 1:800.

74. Jones DK, Higenbottam TW, Wallwork J: Treatment of primary pulmonary hypertension with intravenous epoprostenol (prostacyclin). Br Heart J 1987; 57:270.

75. Furchgott RF, Zawadzki JV: The obligatory role of endothelial cells in the relaxation of arterial smooth muscle by acetylcholine. Nature 1980; 288:373.

76. Ignarro LJ, Wood KS, Byrns RE: Pharmacological and biochemical properties of EDRF: evidence that EDRF is closely related to nitric oxide (NO) radical (Abstract). Circulation 1986; 74(suppl II):II-287.

77. Furchgott RF, Khan MT, Jothianandan D: Evidence supporting the proposal that endothelium-derived relaxing factors in nitric oxide (Abstract). Thromb Res Suppl 1987; 7:5.

78. Kelm N, Schrader J: Control of coronary vascular tone by nitric oxide. Circ Res 1990; 66:1561.

79. Palmer RMJ, Ferridge AG, Moncada S: Nitric oxide release accounts for the biological activity of endothelium-derived relaxing factor. Nature 1987; 327:524.

80. Rees DD, Palmer RM, Hodson HF, et al: A specific inhibitor of nitric oxide formation from L-arginine attenuates endothelium-dependent relaxation. Br J Pharmacol 1989; 96:418.

81. Garthwaite J, Charles SL, Chess-Williams R: Endothelium-derived relaxing factor release on activation of NMDA receptors suggests role as intercellular messenger in the brain. Nature 1988; 336:385.

82. Salvemini D, de Nucci G, Gryglewski RJ, et al: Human neutrophils and nonnuclear cells inhibit platelet aggregation by releasing nitric oxide-like factor. Proc Natl Acad Sci USA 1989; 86:6328.

83. Moncada S, Palmer RMJ, Higgs: Nitric oxide: physiology, pathophysiology, and pharmacology. Pharmacol Rev 1991; 43:110.

84. Rees DD, Palmer RMJ, Moncada S: Role of endothelium-derived nitric oxide in regulation of blood pressure. Proc Natl Acad Sci U S A 1989; 86:3375.

85. Holtz J, Forstermann U, Pohl U, et al: Flow-dependent, endothelium-mediated dilation of epicardial coronary arteries in conscious dogs: effects of cyclooxygenase inhibition. J Cardiovasc Pharmacol 1984; 6:1161.

86. Bassenge E, Busse R: Endothelial modulation of coronary tone. Prog Cardiovasc Dis 1988; 30:349.

87. Taylor P: Ganglionic stimulating and blocking drugs. In: Gilman AG, Goodman LS, Rall TW, et al, eds, The Pharmacological Basis of Therapeutics, 7 ed. New York, 1985, Macmillan Publishing Co., p 215.

88. Fahmy NR, Soter NA: Effects of trimethaphan on arterial blood histamine and systemic hemodynamics in humans. Anesthesiology 1985; 62:562.

89. Needleman P, Jakschik B, Johnson EM: Sulfhydryl requirements for relaxation of vascular smooth muscle. J Pharmacol Exp Ther 1973; 187:324.

90. Robinson BF, Collier JG: Vascular smooth muscle: correlations between basic properties and responses of human blood vessels. Br Med Bull 1979; 35:305.

91. Katsuki AW, Arnold W, Mittal C, et al: Stimulation of guanylate cyclase by sodium nitroprusside, nitroglycerin, and nitric oxide in various tissue preparations and comparison to the effects of sodium azide and hydroxylamine. J Cyclic Nucleotide Res 1977; 3:23.

92. Longnecker DE, Creasy RA, Ross DC: A microvascular site of action of sodium nitroprusside in striated muscle of the rat. Anesthesiology 1979; 50:111.

93. Armstrong PW, Walker DC, Burton JR, et al: Vasodilator therapy in acute myocardial infarction: a comparison of sodium nitroprusside and nitroglycerin. Circulation 1975; 52:1118.

94. Gerson JI, Allen FB, Seltzer JL, et al: Arterial and venous dilation by nitroprusside and nitroglycerin—is there a difference? Anesth Analg 1982; 61:256.

95. Kaplan JA, Dunbar RW, Jones EL: Nitroglycerin infusion during coronary artery surgery. Anesthesiology 1976; 45:14.

96. Yaster M, Simmons RJ, Tolo VT, et al: A comparison of nitroglycerin and nitroprusside for inducing hypotension in children: a double-blind study. Anesthesiology 1986; 65:175.

97. Fahmy NR, Laver MB: Hemodynamic response to ganglionic blockade with pentolinium during $N_2O$-halothane anesthesia in man. Anesthesiology 1976; 44:6.

98. Salem MR, Toyama T, Wong AY, et al: Haemodynamic responses to induced arterial hypotension in children. Br J Anaesth 1978; 50:489.

99. Scott DB, Stephens GW, Marshall RC, et al: Circulatory effects of controlled arterial hypotension with trimethaphan during nitrous oxide/halothane anaesthesia. Br J Anaesth 1972; 44:523.

100. Styles M, Coleman AJ, Leary WP: Some hemodynamic effects of sodium nitroprusside. Anesthesiology 1973; 38:173.

101. Strunin L: Organ perfusion during controlled hypotension. Br J Anaesth 1975; 47:793.

102. Lassen NA, Christensen MS: Physiology of cerebral blood flow. Br J Anaesth 1976; 48:719.

103. Green DW: Cardiac and cerebral complications of deliberate hypotension. In: Enderby GEH, ed, Hypotensive Anaesthesia. London, 1985, Churchill Livingstone.

104. Kety S, King B, Horvath SM, et al: The effect of acute reduction in blood pressure on the cerebral circulation of hypertensive patients. J Clin Invest 1950; 29:402.

105. Finnerty FA Jr, Witkin L, Fazekas JF: Cerebral hemodynamics during cerebral ischemia induced by acute hypotension. J Clin Invest 1954; 33:1227.

106. Strandgaard S, Olesen J, Skinhof E, et al: Autoregulation of brain circulation in severe arterial hypertension. Br Med J 1973; 1:507.

107. Strandgaard S: Autoregulation of cerebral blood flow in hypertensive patients. Circulation 1976; 53:720.

108. Howat DDC: Induced hypotension in the elderly patient. Proc 6th Eur Congr Anaesth, London, 1982, Academic Press, Grune & Stratton, p. 221.

109. Hoffman WE, Bergman S, Miletich DJ, et al: Regional vascular changes during hypotensive anesthesia. J Cardiovasc Pharmacol 1982; 4:310.

110. Hoffman WE, Miletich DJ, Albrecht RF: Cerebrovascular response to hypotension: effect of antihypertensive therapy. Anesthesiology 1982; 57:A36.

111. Hernandez MJ, Brennan RW, Bowman GS: Autoregulation of cerebral blood flow in the newborn dog. Brain Res 1980; 184:199.

112. Rogers MC, Nugent SK, Traystman RJ: Control of cerebral circulation in the neonate and infant. Crit Care Med 1980; 8:570.

113. Fieschi C, Battistini N, Bedushi A, et al: Regional cerebral blood flow and intraventricular pressure in

acute head injuries. J Neurol Neurosurg Psychiatry 1974; 37:1378.

114. Heilbrun MP, Oleson J, Lassen NA: Regional cerebral blood flow studies in subarachnoid hemorrhage. J Neurosurg 1972; 37:36.

115. Palvolgyi R: Regional cerebral blood flow in patients with intracranial tumors. J Neurosurg 1969; 31:149.

116. Farhat SM, Schneider RC: Observations on the effects of systemic blood pressure on intracranial circulation in patients with cerebrovascular insufficiency. J Neurosurg 1967; 27:441.

117. Donegan J: Anesthesia for patients with ischemic cerebrovascular disease. ASA Refresher Course Lectures 1981; #123.

118. Harp JR, Wollman H: Cerebral metabolic effects of hyperventilation and deliberate hypotension. Br J Anaesth 1973; 45:256.

119. Astrup J, Symon L, Brauston NM, et al: Cortical evoked potentials and extracellular $K^+$ and $H^+$ and critical levels of brain ischemia. Stroke 1977; 8:51.

120. Anderson JA: Deliberate hypotensive anesthesia for orthognathic surgery: controlled pharmacologic manipulation of cardiovascular physiology. Int J Adult Orthodon Orthognath Surg 1986; 1:133.

121. Lerman J: Special techniques: acute normovolemic hemodilution, controlled hypotension, and controlled hypothermia. In: Gregory GA, ed, Pediatric Anesthesia, 2 ed. New York, 1989, Churchill Livingstone.

122. Magness A, Yashon D, Locke G, et al: Cerebral function during trimethaphan induced hypotension. Neurology 1973; 23:506.

123. Cottrell JE, Van Aken H, Gupta B, et al: Induced hypotension. In: Cottrell JE, Turndorf H, eds, Anesthesia and Neurosurgery. St. Louis, 1986, C. V. Mosby.

124. Michenfelder JD, Sundt TM Jr: The effect of $PaCO_2$ on the metabolism of ischemic brain in squirrel monkeys. Anesthesiology 1973; 38:445.

125. Rudehill A, Gordon E, Sundqvist K, et al: A study of ECG abnormalities and myocardial specific enzymes in patients with subarachnoid hemorrhage. Acta Anaesthesiol Scand 1982; 26:334.

126. Eckenhoff JE, Enderby GEH, Larson A, et al: Pulmonary gas exchange during deliberate hypotension. Br J Anaesth 1963; 35:750.

127. Salem MR, Kim Y, Shaker MH: The effect of alteration of inspired oxygen concentration on jugular-bulb oxygen tension during deliberate hypotension. Anesthesiology 1970; 33:358.

128. Salem MR, Ivankovic AD, Shaker MH: Safety factors in deliberately induced hypotension. Middle East J Anesthesiol 1971; 3:107.

129. Levin RM, Zadigian ME, Hall SC: The combined effect of hyperventilation and hypotension on cerebral oxygenation in anaesthetized dogs. Can Anaesth Soc J 1980; 27:264.

130. Harper AM, Glass HI: Effects of alterations in the arterial $CO_2$ tension on the blood flow through the cerebral cortex at normal and low arterial blood pressure. J Neurol Neurosurg Psychiatry 1965; 28:449.

131. Gregory P, Ishikawa T, McDowall DG: $CO_2$ responses of the cerebral circulation during drug-induced hypotension in the cat. J Cereb Blood Flow Metab 1981; 1:195.

132. Artru AA: Cerebral vascular responses to hypocapnia during nitroprusside-induced hypotension. Neurosurgery 1985; 16:468.

133. Artru AA: Partial preservation of cerebral vascular responsiveness to hypocapnia during isoflurane-induced hypotension in dogs. Anesth Analg 1986; 65:660.

134. Artru AA, Colley PS: Cerebral blood flow response to hypocapnia during hypotension. Stroke 1984; 15:878.

135. McDowall DG: Cerebral circulation during induced hypotension. In: Enderby GEH, ed, Hypotensive Anaesthesia. London, 1985, Churchill Livingstone.

136. Artru AA: Cerebral metabolism and the electroencephalogram during hypocapnia plus hypotension induced by sodium nitroprusside or trimethaphan in dogs. Neurosurgery 1986; 18:36.

137. Artru AA: Cerebral metabolism and EEG during combination of hypocapnia and isoflurane-induced hypotension in dogs. Anesthesiology 1986; 65: 602.

138. Artru AA, Wright K, Colley PS: Cerebral effects of hypocapnia plus nitroglycerin-induced hypotension in dogs. J Neurosurg 1986; 64:924.

139. Newberg LA, Michenfelder JD: Cerebral protection by isoflurane during hypoxemia or ischemia (Abstract). Anesthesiology 1982; 57:A335.

140. Newberg LA, Milde JH, Michenfelder JD: Systemic and cerebral effects of isoflurane-induced hypotension in dogs. Anesthesiology 1984; 60:541.

141. Ivankovich AD, Miletich DJ, Albrecht RF, et al: Sodium nitroprusside and cerebral blood flow in the anesthetized and unanesthetized goat. Anesthesiology 1976; 44:21.

142. Stullken EH, Sokoll MD: Intracranial pressure changes during hypotension and subsequent vasopressor therapy in anesthetized cats. Anesthesiology 1975; 42:425.

143. Turner JM, Powell D, Gibson RM, et al: Intracranial pressure changes in neurosurgical patients during hypotension induced with sodium nitroprusside or trimetaphan. Br J Anaesth 1977; 49:419.

144. Cottrell JE, Patel K, Turndorf H, et al: Intracranial pressure changes induced by sodium nitroprusside in patients with intracranial mass lesions. J Neurosurg 1978; 48:329.

145. Rogers MC, Hamburger C, Owen K, et al: Intracranial pressure in the cat during nitroglycerin-induced hypotension. Anesthesiology 1979; 51:227.

146. Stoelting RG: Peripheral vasodilators. In: Stoelting RG, ed, Pharmacology and Physiology in Anesthetic Practice, 2 ed. Philadelphia, 1991, J.B. Lippincott Co.

147. Marsh ML, Aidinis SJ, Naughton KVH, et al: The technique of nitroprusside administration modifies the intracranial pressure response. Anesthesiology 1979; 51:538.

148. Singler RC: Special techniques: deliberate hypotension, hypothermia, and acute normovolemic hemodilution. In: Gregory GA, ed, Pediatric Anesthesia. New York, 1983, Churchill Livingstone, vol. 2, p. 553.

149. Dias PR, Andrew DS, Romanes GJ: Effect on the intraocular pressure of hypotensive anesthesia with intravenous trimethaphan. Br J Ophthalmol 1982; 66:721.

150. Beare RY: Indications for hypotensive anaesthesia.

In: Enderby GEH, ed, Hypotensive Anaesthesia. London, 1985, Churchill Livingstone.

151. Morrison JD, Mirakhur RK, Craig HJL: Intraocular Pressure, Anesthesia for Eye, Ear, Nose and Throat Surgery. Edinburgh, 1985, Churchill Livingstone, pp. 151–164.

152. Miller ED Jr: Deliberate hypotension. In: Miller RD, ed, Anesthesia, 2 ed. New York, 1986, Churchill Livingstone.

153. Naumann GOH, Eisert S, Gieler J, et al: Controlled hypotension by sodium-nitroprusside in general anaesthesia for difficult intraocular surgery (preliminary report). Klin Monatsbl Augenheilkd 1977; 170:922.

154. Constable IJ, Chester GH, Horne R, et al: Human chorioretinal biopsy under controlled systemic hypotensive anaesthesia. Br J Ophthalmol 1980; 64: 559.

155. Jantzen JP, Hennes HJ, Rochels R, et al: Deliberate arterial hypotension does not reduce intraocular pressure in pigs. Anesthesiology 1992; 77:536.

156. Feigl EO: Coronary physiology. Physiol Rev 1983; 1:205.

157. Simpson P, Bellamy D, Cole D: Electrocardiographic studies during hypotensive anaesthesia using sodium nitroprusside. Anaesthesia 1976; 31: 1172.

158. Manninen P, Lam A, Gelb A: Electrocardiographic changes during and after isoflurane-induced hypotension for neurovascular surgery. Can J Anaesth 1987; 34:549.

159. Rollason WN, Hough JM: Some electrocardiographic studies during hypotensive anaesthesia. Br J Anaesth 1959; 31:66.

160. Rollason WN, Hough JM: A re-examination of some electrocardiographic studies during hypotensive anaesthesia: the effect of rate of fall of blood pressure. Br J Anaesth 1969; 41:985.

161. Larson CP, Mazze RI, Cooperman LH, et al: Effects of anesthetics on cerebral, retinal, renal, and splanchnic circulations: recent developments. Anesthesiology 1974; 41:169.

162. Tinker JH, Michenfelder JD: Sodium nitroprusside: pharmacology, toxicology and therapeutics. Anesthesiology 1976; 45:340.

163. Moyer JH, Moris G, Selbert RA: Renal function during controlled hypotension with hexamethonium and following norepinephrine. Surg Gynecol Obstet 1955; 100:27.

164. Behnia R, Martin A, Koushanpour E, et al: Trimethaphan-induced hypotension: effect on renal function. Can Anaesth Soc J 1982; 29:581.

165. Behnia R, Siqueira EB, Brunner EA: Sodium nitroprusside-induced hypotension: effect on renal function. Anesth Analg 1978; 57:521.

166. Bagshaw RJ, Cox RH, Campbell KB: Sodium nitroprusside and regional arterial haemodynamics in the dog. Br J Anaesth 1977; 49:735.

167. Leighton KM, Bruce C, Macleod BA: Sodium nitroprusside-induced hypotension and renal blood flow. Can Anaesth Soc J 1977; 24:637.

168. Dong WK, Bledsoe SW, Eng DY, et al: Profound arterial hypotension in dogs: brain electrical activity and organ integrity. Anesthesiology 1983; 58:61.

169. Mazze RI, Cousins MJ, Barr GA: Renal effects and metabolism of isoflurane in man. Anesthesiology 1974; 40:536.

170. Lessard MR, Trepanier CA, Brochu JG, et al: Effects of isoflurane-induced hypotension on renal function and hemodynamics. Can J Anaesth 1990; 37:S42.

171. Bastron RD, Kaloyanides GJ: Effects of sodium nitroprusside on function in the isolated and intact dog kidney. J Pharmacol Exp Ther 1972; 181:244.

172. Birch AA, Boyce WH: Changes in renal blood flow following sodium nitroprusside in patients undergoing nephrolithotomy. Anesth Analg 1977; 56:102.

173. Ohmura A, Wong KC, Pace NL, et al: Effect of halothane and sodium nitroprusside on renal function and autoregulation. Br J Anaesth 1982; 54: 103.

174. Thompson GE, Miller RD, Stevens WC, et al: Hypotensive anesthesia for total hip arthroplasty: a study of blood loss and organ function (brain, heart, liver, and kidney). Anesthesiology 1978; 48:91.

175. McDougal WS: Renal perfusion/reperfusion injuries. J Urol 1988; 140:1325.

176. Lessard MR, Trepanier CA: Renal function and hemodynamics during prolonged isoflurane-induced hypotension in humans. Anesthesiology 1991; 74: 860

177. Gelman S: Anesthesia and the liver. In: Barash PG, Cullen BF, Stoelting RK, eds, Clinical Anesthesia. Philadelphia, 1989, J. B. Lippincott Co.

178. Richardson PDI: Physiologic regulation of the hepatic circulation. Fed Proc 1982; 41:2111.

179. Gelman S, Ernst EA: Hepatic circulation during sodium nitroprusside infusion in the dog. Anesthesiology 1978; 49:182.

180. Conzen PF, Hobbhahn J, Goetz AE, et al: Splanchnic oxygen consumption and hepatic surface oxygen tensions during isoflurane anesthesia. Anesthesiology 1988; 69:463.

181. Gelman S, Longnecker D: Isoflurane and hepatic oxygenation. Anesthesiology 1988; 69:639.

182. Epstein RM, Wheeler HO, Frumin MJ, et al: The effect of hypercapnea on estimated hepatic blood flow, circulating splanchnic blood volume and hepatic sulfobromophthalein clearance during general anesthesia in man. J Clin Invest 1961; 40:592.

183. Epstein RM, Deutsch S, Cooperman LH, et al: Splanchnic circulation during halothane anesthesia and hypercapnea in normal man. Anesthesiology 1968; 27:654.

184. Cooperman LH, Warden JC, Price HL: Splanchnic circulation during nitrous oxide anesthesia and hypocarbia in normal man. Anesthesiology 1968; 29: 254.

185. Salem MR: Pulse-rate changes in elderly patients during deliberate hypotension. Anesthesiology 1969; 30:329.

186. Salem MR, Ivankovic AD: Management of phentolamine resistant phaeochromocytoma by beta-adrenergic blockade. Br J Anaesth 1969; 41:1087.

187. Wildsmith JAW, Marshall RL, Jenkinson JL, et al: Haemodynamic effects of sodium nitroprusside during nitrous oxide/halothane anaesthesia. Br J Anaesth 1973; 45:71.

188. Merrifield AJ, Blundell MD: Toxicity of sodium nitroprusside. Br J Anaesth 1974; 46:324.

189. McDowall DG, Keaney NP, Turner JM, et al: The toxicity of sodium nitroprusside. Br J Anaesth 1974; 46:327.

190. Adams AP: Techniques of vascular control for de-

liberate hypotension during anaesthesia. Br J Anaesth 1975; 47:777.

191. Fahmy NR, Mihelakos PT, Battit GE, et al: Propranolol prevents hemodynamic and humoral events after abrupt withdrawal of nitroprusside. Clin Pharmacol Ther 1984; 36:470.

192. Miller ED Jr, Ackerly JA, Vaughan ED Jr, et al: The renin-angiotensin system during controlled hypotension with sodium nitroprusside. Anesthesiology 1977; 47:257.

193. Rawlingson WAL, Loach AB, Benedict CR: Changes in plasma concentration of adrenaline and noradrenaline in anaesthetized patients during sodium nitroprusside-induced hypotension. Br J Anaesth 1978; 50:937.

194. Khambatta HJ, Stone JG, Kahn E: Propranolol alters renin release during nitroprusside induced hypotension and prevents hypertension on discontinuation of nitroprusside. Anesth Analg 1981; 60:569.

195. Knight PR, Lane GA, Hensinger RN, et al: Catecholamine and renin-angiotensin response during hypotensive anesthesia induced by sodium nitroprusside or trimethaphan camsylate. Anesthesiology 1983; 59:248.

196. Knight PR, Lane GA, Nicholls MG, et al: Hormonal and hemodynamic changes induced by pentolinium and propranolol during surgical correction of scoliosis. Anesthesiology 1980; 53:127.

197. Chen RY, Matteo RS, Fan F-C, et al: Baroreflex sensitivity and induced hypotension. Anesthesiology 1979; 51:574.

198. Chen RY, Matteo RS, Fan F-C, et al: Resetting of baroreflex sensitivity after induced hypotension. Anesthesiology 1982; 56:29.

199. Packer M, Meller J, Medina J, et al: Rebound hemodynamic events after the abrupt withdrawal of nitroprusside in patients with severe chronic heart failure. N Engl J Med 1979; 301:1193.

200. McDonald FD, Thiel G, Wilson DR, et al: The prevention of acute renal failure in the rat by long-term saline loading: a possible role of the renin-angiotensin axis. Proc Soc Exp Biol Med 1969; 131:610.

201. Giese J: Renin, angiotensin, hypertensive vascular damage: a review. Am J Med 1973; 55:315.

202. Gavras H, Kremer D, Brown JJ, et al: Angiotensin and norepinephrine induced myocardial lesions: experimental and clinical studies in rabbits and man. Am Heart J 1975; 89:321.

203. MacDonald AG, Ingram CG, McNeill RS: The effect of propranolol on airway resistance. Br J Anaesth 1967; 39:919.

204. Sum CY, Yacobi A, Katzinel R, et al: Kinetics of esmolol, an ultra-short-acting beta blocker, and of its major metabolite. Clin Pharmacol Ther 1983; 34:427.

205. Gold MI, Brown MS, Selem JS: The effect of esmolol on hemodynamics after ketamine induction and intubation. Anesthesiology 1984; 61:A19.

206. Menkhaus PG, Reves JG, Kissin I, et al: Cardiovascular effects of esmolol in anesthetized humans. Anesth Analg 1985; 64:327.

207. Stephen GW, Davie IT, Scott DB: Haemodynamic effects of beta adrenoceptor blocking drugs during nitrous oxide/halothane anaesthesia. Br J Anaesth 1971; 43:320.

208. Delaney TJ, Miller ED Jr.: Rebound hypertension after sodium nitroprusside prevented by saralasin in rats. Anesthesiology 1980; 52:154.

209. Fahmy NR, Gavras HP: Impact of captopril on hemodynamic and hormonal effects of nitroprusside. J Cardiovasc Pharmacol 1985; 7:869.

210. Felisch M, Noack EA: Correlation between nitric oxide formation during degradation of organic material and activation of guanylate cyclase. Eur J Pharmacol 1987; 139:19.

211. MacRae WR, Wildsmith JAW, Dale BAB: Induced hypotension with a mixture of sodium nitroprusside and trimethaphan camsylate. Anaesthesia 1981; 36:312.

212. Wildsmith JAW, Sinclair CJ, Thorn J, et al: Haemodynamic effects of induced hypotension with a nitroprusside-trimethaphan mixture. Br J Anaesth 1983; 55:381.

213. Fahmy NR: Nitroprusside vs. a nitroprusside-trimethaphan mixture for induced hypotension: hemodynamic effects and cyanide release. Clin Pharmacol Ther 1985; 37:264.

214. Nakazawa K, Taneyama C, Benson KT, et al: Mixtures of sodium nitroprusside and trimethaphan for induction of hypotension. Anesth Analg 1991; 73:59.

215. Green DW: Techniques for deliberate hypotension: pharmacological blockade. In: Enderby GEH, ed, Hypotensive Anaesthesia. London, 1985, Churchill Livingstone, p. 109.

216. Patel H: Experience with the cerebral function monitor during deliberate hypotension. Br J Anaesth 1981; 53:639.

217. Diaz JH, Lockhart CH: Hypotensive anaesthesia for craniectomy in infancy. Br J Anaesth 1979; 51:233.

218. Eger EI Jr, Smith NT, Stoelting RK, et al: Cardiovascular effects of halothane in man. Anesthesiology 1970; 32:396.

219. Stevens WC, Cromwell TH, Halsey MJ, et al: The cardiovascular effects of a new inhalation anesthetic, forane, in human volunteers at constant arterial carbon dioxide tension. Anesthesiology 1971; 35:8.

220. Calverley RK, Smith NT, Jones CW, et al: Ventilatory and cardiovascular effects of enflurane anesthesia during spontaneous ventilation in man. Anesth Analg 1978; 57:610.

221. Merin RG: Are the myocardial, functional, and metabolic effects of isoflurane really different from those of halothane and enflurane? Anesthesiology 1981; 55:398.

222. Merin RG: Effects of inhalation anesthetics on the cardiovascular system. ASA Refresher Course Lectures 1987; #136.

223. Prys-Roberts C, Lloyd JW, Fisher A, et al: Deliberate profound hypotension induced with halothane. Studies of haemodynamics and pulmonary gas exchange. Br J Anaesth 1974; 46:105.

224. Lowe HJ, Feingold A, Hagler KS: Unusual cardiovascular stability during deep halothane anesthesia. Anesthesiology 1969; 30:471.

225. Lam AM, Gelb AW: Cardiovascular effects of isoflurane-induced hypotension for cerebral aneurysm surgery. Anesth Analg 1983; 62:742.

226. Maktabi M, Warner D, Sokoll M, et al: Comparison of nitroprusside, nitroglycerin and deep isoflurane anesthesia for induced hypotension. Neurosurgery 1986; 19:350.

227. Miller ED Jr: Deliberate hypotension. In: Miller

RD, ed, Anesthesia, 3 ed. New York, 1990, Churchill Livingstone.

228. Shapiro HM, Marshall LF: Intracranial pressure responses to PEEP in head-injured patients. J Trauma 1978; 18:254.

229. Luce JM, Huseby JS, Kirk W, et al: Mechanisms by which positive end expiratory pressure increases cerebrospinal fluid pressure in dogs. J Appl Physiol 1982; 52:231.

230. Nimmagadda U, Joseph NJ, Salem MR, et al: Positive end-expiratory pressure increases intraocular pressure. Crit Care Med 1991; 19:796.

231. Eckenhoff JE, Enderby GEH, Larson A, et al: Human cerebral circulation during deliberate hypotension and head-up tilt. J Appl Physiol 1963b; 18: 1130.

232. Berry AJ: Respiration support and renal function. Anesthesiology 1981; 55:655.

233. Relton JES: Anesthesia in the original correction of scoliosis. In: Riseborough EJ, Herndon JH, ed, Scoliosis and Other Deformities of the Axial Skeleton. Boston, 1975, Little, Brown & Co.

234. Rao TLK, Jacobs K, Salem MR, et al: Deliberate hypotension and anesthetic requirements of halothane. Anesth Analg 1981; 60;513.

235. Salem MR, Klowden AJ: Anesthesia for pediatric orthopedic surgery. In: Gregory GA, ed, Pediatric Anesthesia, 3 ed. New York, 1994, Churchill Livingstone.

236. Didier EP, Clagett OT, Theye RA: Cardiac performance during controlled hypotension. Anesth Analg 1965; 44:379.

237. Enderby GEH: Safe hypotensive anaesthesia. In: Enderby GEH, ed, Hypotensive Anaesthesia. London, 1985, Churchill Livingstone.

238. Sivarajan M, Amory DW, Everett GB, et al: Blood pressure, not cardiac output, determines blood loss during induced hypotension. Anesth Analg 1980; 59:203.

239. Amaranath L, Cascorbi HF, Singh-Amaranath AV, et al: Relation of anesthesia to total hip replacement and control of operative blood loss. Anesth Analg 1975; 54:641.

240. Lawson NW, Thompson DS, Nelson CL, et al: Sodium nitroprusside induced hypotension for supine total hip replacement. Anesth Analg 1976; 55:654.

241. Aveling W, Verner IR: Profound hypotension with intravenous nitroglycerin. In: Robinson BF, Kaplan JA, ed, The International Symposium on the Clinical Use of Tridil, Intravenous Nitroglycerin. Oxford, 1981, Medicine Publishing Foundation Symposium Series, p. 35.

242. Bramwell RG, Aveling W, Verner IR: NTG and profound hypotension (Letter). Br J Anaesth 1985; 58:247.

243. Guggiari M, Dagreou F, Lienhart A, et al: Use of nitroglycerine to produce controlled decreases in mean arterial pressure to less than 50 mm Hg. Br J Anaesth 1985; 57:142.

244. Pffeiderer T: Sodium nitroprusside, a very potent platelet disaggregating substance. Acta Univ Carol [Med Monogr] (Praha) 1972; 53:247.

245. Mehta P, Mehta J, Miale TD: Nitroprusside lowers platelet count. N Engl J Med 1978; 299:1134.

246. Saxon A, Kattlove HE: Platelet inhibition by sodium nitroprusside. Blood 1976; 47:957.

247. Hines R, Barash PG: Infusion of sodium nitroprus-

side induces platelet dysfunction. Anesthesiology 1989; 70:611.

248. Lichtenthal PR, Rossi EC, Louis G, et al: Dose-related prolongation of the bleeding time by intravenous nitroglycerin. Anesth Analg 1985; 64:30.

249. Ring T, Knudsen F, Kristensen SD, et al: Nitroglycerin prolongs the bleeding time in healthy males. Thromb Res 1983; 29:553.

250. Schror KS, Grodzinska L, Darius H: Stimulation of coronary vascular prostacyclin and inhibition of human platelet thromboxane $A_2$ after low-dose nitroglycerin. Thromb Res 1981; 23:59.

251. Levin RI, Jaffe EA, Weksler BB, et al: Nitroglycerin stimulates synthesis of prostacyclin by cultured human endothelial cells. J Clin Invest 1981; 67: 762.

252. Fitzgerald GA, Friedman LA, Miyamore L, et al: A double blind placebo controlled crossover study of prostacyclin in man. Life Sci 1979; 25:665.

253. Ubatuba FA, Moncada S, Vane JR: The effect of prostacyclin ($PGI_2$) on platelet behaviour, thrombus formation in vivo, and bleeding time. Thromb Haemost 1979; 41:425.

254. Hines R: Preservation of platelet function during trimethaphan infusion. Anesthesiology 1990; 72: 834.

255. Salem MR: Deliberate hypotension is a safe and accepted anesthetic technique. In: Eckenhoff JE, ed, Controversy in Anesthesiology. Philadelphia, 1979, W.B. Saunders.

256. Salem MR, Bennett EJ, Rao TLK, et al: An examination of complications related to hypotensive anesthesia (Abstract). Proc Am Soc Anesthesiol Annual Meeting, 1976.

257. Schallek W, Walz D: Effects of drug-induced hypotension on the electroencephalogram of the dog. Anesthesiology 1954; 15:673.

258. Wiederholt WC, Locke GE, Yashon D: Hypotension and its effect on the E.E.G. activity in the dog. Neurology 1972; 22:717.

259. Stone JG, Khambatta HJ, Matteo RS: Pulmonary shunting during anesthesia with deliberate hypotension. Anesthesiology 1976; 45:508.

260. Casthely PA, Lear S, Cottrell JE, et al: Intrapulmonary shunting during induced hypotension. Anesth Analg 1982; 61:231.

261. Don HF, Wabha WM, Craig DB: Airway closure, gas trapping, and functional residual capacity during anesthesia. Anesthesiology 1972; 36:533.

262. Sykes MK, Loh L, Seed RF, et al: The effect of inhalational anaesthesia on hypoxic pulmonary vasoconstriction and pulmonary vascular resistance in the perfused lungs of the dog and cat. Br J Anaesth 1972; 44:776.

263. Benumof JF, Wahrenbrock EA: Blunted hypoxic pulmonary vasoconstriction by increased lung vascular pressure. J Appl Physiol 1975; 38:846.

264. Kelman GR, Nunn JF, Prys-Roberts C, et al: The influence of cardiac output on arterial oxygenation. Br J Anaesth 1967; 39:450.

265. Kirby RB, Smith RA: An overview of anesthesia and critical care medicine. In: Miller RD, ed, Anesthesia, 2 ed. New York, 1986, Churchill Livingstone.

266. Philbin DM, Sullivan SF, Bowman FO, et al: Postoperative hypoxemia: contribution of the cardiac output. Anesthesiology 1970; 32:136.

267. Cheney FW, Colley PS: The effect of cardiac output

on arterial blood oxygenation. Anesthesiology 1980; 52:496.

268. Robinson JS: Hypotension without hypoxia. Int Anesthesiol Clin 1967; 5:467.

269. Jacobs HK, Lieponis JV, Bunch WH, et al: The influence of halothane and nitroprusside on canine spinal cord hemodynamics. Spine 1982; 7:35.

270. Askrog VF, Pender JW, Eckenhoff JE: Changes in physiological dead space during deliberate hypotension. Anesthesiology 1964; 25:774.

271. Khambatta HJ, Stone JG, Matteo RS: Effect of sodium nitroprusside-induced hypotension on pulmonary deadspace. Br J Anaesth 1982; 54:1197.

272. Salem MR, Paulissian R, Joseph NJ, et al: Effect of deliberate hypotension on arterial to peak expired carbon dioxide tension difference (Abstract). Anesth Analg 1988; 67:S194.

273. Playfair L: On the nitroprusside: a new class of salts. London, 1849, Taylor.

274. Taylor TH, Styles M, Lamming AJ: Sodium nitroprusside as a hypotensive agent in general anaesthesia. Br J Anaesth 1970; 42:859.

275. Fahmy NR, Bottros MR, Charchaflieh J, et al: A randomized comparison of labetalol and nitroprusside for induced hypotension. J Clin Anesth 1989; 1:409.

276. Rapoport RM, Murad F: Agonist-induced endothelium-dependent relaxation in rat thoracic aorta may be mediated through cGMP. Circ Res 1983; 52:352.

277. Becker LC: Conditions for vasodilator-induced coronary steal in experimental myocardial ischemia. Circulation 1978; 57:1103.

278. Chiariello M, Gold HK, Leinbach RC, et al: Comparison between the effects of nitroglycerin and nitroprusside on ischemic injury during acute myocardial infarction. Circulation 1976; 54:766.

279. Fahmy NR: Impact of oral captopril or propranolol on nitroprusside-induced hypotension (Abstract). Anesthesiology 1984; 61:A41.

280. Chatterjee K, Parmley WW: Vasodilator therapy for acute myocardial infarction and chronic congestive heart failure. J Am Coll Cardiol 1983; 1:133.

281. Hermann L: Über die Wirkung des Nitroprussidnatriums. Arch Ges Physiol 1886; 39:419.

282. Johnson CC: Mechanisms of actions and toxicity of nitroprusside. Proc Soc Exp Biol Med 1928; 26:102.

283. Johnson CC: The actions and toxicity of sodium nitroprusside. Arch Int Pharmacodyn Ther 1929; 35:489.

284. Lazarus-Barlow P, Norman BM: Fatal cases of poisoning with sodium nitroprusside (Correspondence). Br Med J 1941; 1:407.

285. Page IH, Corcoran AC, Dustan HP, et al: Cardiovascular actions of sodium nitroprusside in animals and hypertensive patients. Circulation 1955; 11:188.

286. Page IH: Treatment of essential and malignant hypertension. JAMA 1951; 147:1311.

287. Gifford RW: Current practices in general medicine: treatment of hypertensive emergencies including use of sodium nitroprusside. Proc Mayo Clin 1959; 34:387.

288. Gifford RW: Hypertensive emergencies and their treatment. Med Clin North Am 1961; 45:441.

289. Ivankovich AD, Miletich DJ, Tinker JH: Sodium nitroprusside: metabolism and general considerations. Int Anesthesiol Clin 1978; 16:1.

290. Bitte EM, Hale DE: Controlled hypotension in anaesthesia and surgery. In: Hale DE, ed, Anaesthesiology, 2 ed. London, 1963, Blackwell Scientific Publishers, p. 711.

291. Jones GOM, Cole P: Sodium nitroprusside as a hypotensive agent. Br J Anaesth 1968; 40:804.

292. Schiffmann H, Fuchs P: Controlled hypotension effected by sodium nitroprusside. Acta Anaesthesiol Scand 1966; 23:704.

293. Ahearn DI, Grim CE: Treatment of malignant hypertension with sodium nitroprusside. Arch Intern Med 1974; 133:187.

294. Koch-Weser J: Vasodilator drugs in the treatment of hypertension. Arch Intern Med 1974; 133:1017.

295. Nourok DS, Glassock RJ, Solomon DH, et al: Hypothyroidism following prolonged sodium nitroprusside therapy. Am J Med Sci 1964; 248:129.

296. Mani MK: Nitroprusside revisited. Br Med J 1971; 3:407.

297. Vesey CJ, Cole PV, Linnell JC, et al: Some metabolic effects of sodium nitroprusside in man. Br Med J 1974; 2:140.

298. Davies DW, Kadar D, Steward DJ, et al: A sudden death associated with the use of sodium nitroprusside for induction of hypotension during anaesthesia. Can Anaesth Soc J 1975; 22:547.

299. Smith RP, Kruszyna H: Nitroprusside produces cyanide poisoning via a reaction with hemoglobin. J Pharmacol Exp Ther 1974; 191:557.

300. MacRae WR, Owen M: Severe metabolic acidosis following hypotension induced with sodium nitroprusside. Br J Anaesth 1974; 46:795.

301. Davies DW, Greiss L, Steward DJ, et al: Sodium nitroprusside in children: observations on metabolism during normal and abnormal responses. Can Anaesth Soc J 1975; 22:553.

302. Jack RD: Toxicity of sodium nitroprusside. Br J Anaesth 1974; 46:952.

303. Dreisbach RH: Handbook of Poisoning: Diagnosis and Treatment. Los Altos, CA, 1971, Lange Medical Publications, p. 218.

304. Vesey CJ, Cole PV, Simpson PJ: Sodium nitroprusside in anaesthesia. Br Med J 1975; 3:229.

305. Vesey CJ, Cole PV: Nitroprusside and cyanide. Br J Anaesth 1975; 47:115.

306. Vesey CJ, Cole PV, Simpson PJ: Cyanide and thiocyanate concentrations following sodium nitroprusside infusion in man. Br J Anaesth 1976; 48:651.

307. Verner IR: Direct acting vasodilators. In: Enderby GEH, ed, Hypotensive Anaesthesia. London, 1985, Churchill Livingstone.

308. Palmer RF, Lassiter KD: Sodium nitroprusside. N Engl J Med 1975; 293:294.

309. Fahmy NR: Consumption of vitamin $B_{12}$ during sodium nitroprusside administration in humans. Anesthesiology 1981; 54:305.

310. Greiss L, Tremblay NAG, Davies DW: The toxicity of sodium nitroprusside. Can Anaesth Soc J 1976; 23:480.

311. Michenfelder JD: Cyanide release from sodium nitroprusside in the dog. Anesthesiology 1977; 46:196.

312. Michenfelder JD, Tinker JH: Cyanide toxicity and thiosulfate protection during chronic administration of sodium nitroprusside in the dog: correlation with a human case. Anesthesiology 1977; 47:441.

313. Posner MA, Tobey RE, McElroy H: Hydroxoco-balamin therapy of cyanide intoxication in guinea pigs. Anesthesiology 1976; 44:157.

314. Posner MA, Rodkey FL, Tobey RE: Laboratory report: nitroprusside-induced cyanide poisoning: antidotal effect of hydroxocobalamin. Anesthesiology 1976; 44:330.

315. Cottrell JE, Casthely P, Brodie JD, et al: Prevention of nitroprusside-induced cyanide toxicity with hydroxocobalamin. N Engl J Med 1979; 298:809.

316. Ivankovich AD, Braverman B, Kanuru RP, et al: Cyanide antidotes and methods of their administration in dogs. Anesthesiology 1980; 52:210.

317. Schulz V: Blood cyanide produced by long-term therapy with sodium nitroprusside. Br J Anaesth 1986; 58:247.

318. Tinker JH, Michenfelder JD: Increased resistance to nitroprusside-induced cyanide toxicity in anuric dogs. Anesthesiology 1980; 52:40.

319. Cole PV, Vesey CJ: Sodium thiosulphate decreases blood cyanide concentrations after the infusion of sodium nitroprusside. Br J Anaesth 1987; 59:531.

320. Bryson DD: Cyanide poisoning. Lancet 1978; 1:92.

321. Lancet 1977: Which antidote for cyanide? Lancet 1977; 2:1167.

322. Dodds C, McKnight C: Cyanide toxicity after immersion and the hazards of dicobalt edetate. Br Med J 1985; 291:785.

323. Bissett WIK, Butler AR, Glidewell C, et al: Sodium nitroprusside and cyanide release: reasons for reappraisal. Br J Anaesth 1981; 53:1015.

324. Smith RP, Kruszyna H, Kruszyna R: Cyanide release from nitroprusside. Br J Anaesth 1982; 54:1145.

325. Vesey CJ, Cole PV, Simpson PJ: Sodium nitroprusside and cyanide release. Br J Anaesth 1982; 54:791.

326. Norris JC, Hume AS: *In vivo* release of cyanide from sodium nitroprusside. Br J Anaesth 1987; 59:236.

327. Ikeda S, Schweiss JF, Frank PA, et al: *In vitro* cyanide release from sodium nitroprusside. Anesthesiology 1987; 66:381.

328. Munch JC, Petter HH: The story of glyceryl trinitrate. J Am Pharm Assoc 1965; 5:494.

329. Brunton TL: Use of nitrite of amyl in angina pectoris. Lancet 1867; 2:97.

330. Murrell W: Nitroglycerin as a remedy for angina pectoris. Lancet 1879; 1:80.

331. Viljoen JF: Anaesthesia for internal mammary implant surgery. Anaesthesia 1968; 23:515.

332. Viljoen JF, Gindi MY: Anesthesia for coronary artery surgery. Surg Clin North Am 1971; 51:1081.

333. Kaplan JA, Finlayson DC, Woodward S: Vasodilator therapy after cardiac surgery: a review of the efficacy and toxicity of nitroglycerin and nitroprusside. Can Anaesth Soc J 1980; 27:154.

334. Needleman P, Hunter FE Jr: The transformation of glyceryl trinitrate and other nitrates by glutathione-organic nitrate reductase. Mol Pharmacol 1965; 1:77.

335. Needleman P, Lang S, Johnson EM: Organic nitrates: relationship between biotransformation and rational angina pectoris therapy. J Pharmacol Exp Ther 1972; 181:489.

336. Fibuch EE, Cecil WT, Reed WA: Methemoglobin-emia associated with organic nitrate therapy. Anesth Analg 1979; 58:521.

337. Hussum B, Lindeburg T, Jacobsen E: Methemoglobin formation after nitroglycerin infusion. Br J Anaesth 1982; 54:571.

338. Epstein SE, Kent KM, Goldstein RE, et al: Reduction of ischemic injury by nitroglycerin during acute myocardial infarction. N Engl J Med 1975; 292:29.

339. Greenberg H, Dwyer EM, Jameson AG, et al: Effects of nitroglycerin on the major determinants of myocardial oxygen consumption. Am J Cardiol 1975; 36:426.

340. Flaherty JT: Beneficial haemodynamic effects of intravenous nitroglycerin in patients with acute myocardial infarction complicated by congestive failure. In: Robinson BF, Kaplan JA, ed, The International Symposium on the Clinical Use of Tridil, Intravenous Nitroglycerin. Oxford, 1981, Medicine Publishing Foundation Symposium Series.

341. Brown BG: Response of normal and diseased epicardial coronary arteries to vasoactive drugs: quantitative arteriographic studies. Am J Cardiol 1985; 56:23E.

342. Endrich B, Franke N, Peter K, et al: Induced hypotension: action of sodium nitroprusside and nitroglycerin on the microcirculation. Anesthesiology 1987; 66:605.

343. Hauss J, et al: Die kontrollierte hypotension mit natriumnitroprussid. Herz 1978; 10:379.

344. Cote DD, Torchie MG: Nitroglycerin absorption by polyvinyl chloride seriously interferes with its clinical use. Anesth Analg 1982; 61:541.

345. Paton WDM, Zaimis EJ: Paralysis of autonomic ganglia by methonium salts. Br J Pharmacol 1951; 6:155.

346. Klowden AJ, Ivankovich AD, Miletich DJ: Ganglionic blocking drugs: general considerations and metabolism. Int Anesthesiol Clin 1978; 16:113.

347. Wien R, Mason DEJ: Pharmacology of M and B 2050. Lancet 1953; 1:454.

348. Tinker JH: Prevention of blood loss: hypotensive techniques. ASA Annual Refresher Course Lectures, 1978, #205A.

349. Mitchell R, Newman PJ, Macgillivray D, et al: Evaluation of histamine liberator activity, illustrated by a thiophanium compound, RO 2-2222. Fed Proc 1951; 10:325.

350. Holman J, Goth A: Histamine release in human skin and effect of cortisone. Fed Proc 1952; 11:358.

351. Payne JP: Histamine release during controlled hypotension with Arfonad. Proc World Congr Anaesthesiol, Minneapolis, 1955, Burgess, pp. 180.

352. Larson AG: A new technique for inducing controlled hypotension. Lancet 1963; 1:128.

353. Wang HH, Liu LMP, Katz RL: A comparison of the cardiovascular effects of sodium nitroprusside and trimethaphan. Anesthesiology 1977; 46:40.

354. Harioka T, Hatano Y, Mori K, et al: Trimethaphan is a direct arterial vasodilator and an α-adrenoceptor antagonist. Anesth Analg 1984; 63:290.

355. Jones RM, Hantter CB, Knight PR: Use of pentolinium in postoperative hypertension resistant to sodium nitroprusside. Br J Anaesth 1981; 53:1151.

356. Michenfelder JD, Theye RA: Canine systemic and cerebral effects of hypotension induced by hemor-

rhage, trimethaphan, halothane, or nitroprusside. Anesthesiology 1977; 46:188.

357. Locke GE, Yashon D, Hunt WE: Cerebral tissue lactate in trimethaphan-induced hypotension. Am J Surg 1971; 122:818.

358. Wiederholt WC, Locke GE, Yashon D: Cerebral electrical activity in profound trimethaphan induced hypotension and haemorrhagic shock with and without carotid ligation in the dog. Neurology 1971; 21:402.

359. Wilton NC, Tait AR, Kling TF Jr, et al: The effect of trimethaphan-induced hypotension on canine spinal cord blood flow: measurement at different cord levels using radiolabelled microspheres. Spine 1988; 13:490.

360. Payne JP: The influence of mecamylamine on the action of certain other ganglion blocking agents. Br J Anaesth 1957; 29:358.

361. Deacock AR, Davis TDW: The influence of certain ganglion blocking agents on neuromuscular transmission. Br J Anaesth 1958; 30:217.

362. Eckenhoff JE: The use of controlled hypotension for surgical procedures. Surg Clin North Am 1955; 45:1579.

363. Hunter AR: Arfonad. Liverpool Soc Anesthesiol, 1954, Liverpool.

364. Tewfik GI: Trimethaphan: its effect on the pseudo-cholinesterase level of man. Anaesthesia 1957; 12:326.

365. Bentel H, Ginsberg H: The use of Arfonad in the production of controlled hypotension. S Afr Med J 1954; 28:827.

366. Scurr CF, Wyman JP: Controlled hypotension with Arfonad. Lancet 1954; 1:338.

367. Gertner SB, Little DM Jr, Bonnycastle DD: Urinary excretion of Arfonad by patients undergoing controlled hypotension during surgery. Anesthesiology 1955; 16:495.

368. Deacock AR, Hargrove RL: The influence of certain ganglionic blocking agents on neuromuscular transmission. Br J Anaesth 1962; 34:357.

369. Sklar GS, Lanks KW: Effects of trimethaphan and sodium nitroprusside on hydrolysis of succinylcholine in vitro. Anesthesiology 1977; 47:31.

370. Anton AH, Czinn S, Jazwa J, et al: Trimetaphan camsylate (Arfonad) and human plasma cholinesterase. Res Commun Chem Pathol Pharmacol 1978; 22:375.

371. Alston TA, deBros FM: Trimethaphan is not inactivated by pseudocholinesterase (Abstract). Anesthesiology 1989; 71:A268.

372. Payne JP: Ganglionic blockade. In: Gray TC, Nunn JF, eds, General Anaesthesia, 3 ed. New York, 1971, Appleton-Century-Crofts, p. 647.

373. Richards DA, Turner P: Labetalol symposium. Proceedings of the first symposium on labetalol. Tourquay. England, April, 1976. Br J Clin Pharmacol 1976; 3:S681.

374. Richards DA, Tuckman J, Prichard BNC: Assessment of α- and β-adrenoceptor blocking action of labetalol. Br J Clin Pharmacol 1976; 3:849.

375. Proceedings of the second symposium on labetalol, London, March, 1979. Br J Clin Pharmacol 1979; 8:89S.

376. Vanhoutte PM: Combined α- and β-adrenergic blockade in the treatment of hypertension: myth or reality. J Cardiovasc Pharmacol 1981: 3:S1.

377. Richards DA, Robertson JIS, Prichard BNC: Proceedings of the third symposium on labetalol. Ven-

ice, Italy, June, 1981. Br J Clin Pharmacol 1982; 13:S5.

378. Farmer JB, Kennedy I, Levy GP, et al: Pharmacology of AH5158. A drug which blocks both alpha and beta-adrenoceptors. Br J Pharmacol 1972; 45:660.

379. Blakely AGH, Summers RJ: The pharmacology of labetalol, an alpha and beta adrenoceptor blocking agent. Gen Pharmacol 1978; 9:399.

380. Cope DHP, Crawford MC: Labetalol in controlled hypotension. Administration of labetalol when adequate hypotension is difficult to achieve. Br J Anaesth 1979; 51:359.

381. Richards DA, Prichard BNC, Boakes AJ, et al: The pharmacological basis for the antihypertensive effects of intravenous labetalol. Br Heart J 1977; 39:99.

382. Prichard BNC, Thompson FO, Boakes AJ, et al: Some haemodynamic effects of compound AH 5158 compared with propranolol, propranolol and hydralazine and diazoxide: the use of AH 5158 in the treatment of hypertension. Clin Sci Mol Med 1975; 48:97.

383. Prichard BNC, Boakes AJ: Labetalol in long-term treatment of hypertension. Br J Clin Pharmacol 1976; 3S:743.

384. Agabiti-Rosei E, Trust PM, Brown JJ, et al: Intravenous labetalol in severe hypertension. Lancet 1975; 2:1093.

385. Cummings AMM, Brown JJ, Fraser R, et al: Blood pressure reduction by incremental infusion of labetalol in patients with severe hypertension. Br J Clin Pharmacol 1979; 8:359.

386. Scott DB, Buckley FP, Drummond GB, et al: Cardiovascular effects of labetalol during halothane anaesthesia. Br J Clin Pharmacol 1976; 3(suppl 3):817.

387. Kaufman L: Use of labetalol during hypotensive anaesthesia and in the management of phaeochromocytoma. Br J Clin Pharmacol 1979; 8:229S.

388. Cohn JN, Mehta J, Francis GS: A review of the haemodynamic effects of labetalol in man. Br J Clin Pharmacol 1982; 13:19S.

389. Larochelle P, Hamet P, Hoffman B, et al: Labetalol in essential hypertension. J Cardiovasc Pharmacol 1980; 2:751.

390. Martin LE, Hopkins R, Bland R: Metabolism of labetalol by animals and man. Br J Clin Pharmacol 1976; 3(suppl 3):695.

391. Kanto J, Pakkanen A, Allonen H, et al: The use of labetalol as a moderate hypotensive agent in otological operations—plasma concentrations after intravenous administration. Int J Clin Pharmacol Ther Toxicol 1980; 18:191.

392. Goldberg ME, McNulty SE, Azad SS, et al: A comparison of labetalol and nitroprusside for inducing hypotension during major surgery. Anesth Analg 1990; 70:537.

393. Van Aken H, Puchstein C, Schweppe ML, et al: Effect of labetalol on intracranial pressure in dogs with and without intracranial hypertension. Acta Anaesthiol Scand 1982; 26:615.

394. Brittain RT, Levy GP: A review of the animal pharmacology of labetalol. A combined alpha and beta adrenoceptor blocking drug. Br J Clin Pharmacol 1976; 3(suppl):681.

395. Carswell DJ, Varkey GP, Drake CG: Labetalol for controlled hypotension in surgery for intracranial

aneurysm (Abstract). Can Anaesth Soc J 1981; 28: 505.

396. Orlowski JP, Shiesley D, Vidt DG, et al: Labetalol to control blood pressure after cerebrovascular surgery. Crit Care Med 1988; 16:765.

397. Skinner C, Gaddie J, Palmer KNV: Comparison of intravenous AH 5158 (labetalol) and propranolol in asthma. Br Med J 1975; 2:59.

398. Richards DA, Woodings EP, Maconochie JG: Comparison of the effects of labetalol and propranolol in healthy men at rest and during exercise. Br J Clin Pharmacol 1977b; 4:15.

399. Jackson SHD, Beaver DG: Comparison of the effects of single doses of albuterol and labetalol on airway obstruction in patients with hypertension and asthma. Br J Clin Pharmacol 1983; 15:553.

400. Simpson DL, MacRae WR, Wildsmith JAW, et al: Acute beta-adrenoceptor blockade and induced hypotension. Anaesthesia 1987; 42:243.

401. Coad NR: Beta blockade and nitroprusside (Letter). Anaesthesia 1987; 42:1022.

402. Turlapaty P, Laddu A, Murthy VS, et al: Esmolol: a titrable short-acting intravenous beta blocker for acute critical care settings. Am Heart J 1987; 114: 866.

403. Gray RJ, Azad SS, Cantillo J, et al: Use of esmolol in hypertension after cardiac surgery. Am J Cardiol 1985; 56:49F.

404. Ornstein E, Matteo RS, Weinstein JA, et al: The use of esmolol for deliberate hypotension (Abstract). Anesthesiology 1986; 65:A575.

405. Ornstein E, Matteo RS, Weinstein JA, et al: A randomized controlled trial of esmolol for deliberate hypotension (Abstract). Anesthesiology 1987; 67: A423.

406. Ornstein E, Matteo RS, Weinstein JA, et al: A controlled trial of esmolol for the induction of deliberate hypotension. J Clin Anesth 1988; 1:31.

407. Anderson W, Brindle F, Liu P, et al: Effect of esmolol on heart rate and blood pressure during intubation in relatively healthy patients (Abstract). Anesthesiology 1985; 63:A104.

408. Elbert J, Gelman S, Coverman S, et al: Effect of esmolol on the heart rate and blood pressure response during endotracheal intubation (Abstract). Anesthesiology 1985; 63:A63.

409. Cucchiara RF, Benefiel DJ, Matteo RS, et al: Evaluation of esmolol in controlling increases in heart rate and blood pressure during endotracheal intubation in patients undergoing carotid endarterectomy. Anesthesiology 1986: 65:528.

410. Girard D, Shulman BJ, Thys DM, et al: The safety and efficacy of esmolol during myocardial revascularization. Anesthesiology 1986; 65:157.

411. Gold MI, Brown MS, Coverman S, et al: Heart rate and blood pressure effects of esmolol after ketamine induction and intubation. Anesthesiology 1986; 64:718.

412. Newsome LR, Roth JV, Hug CC, et al: Esmolol attenuates hemodynamic responses during fentanyl-pancuronium anesthesia for aortocoronary bypass surgery. Anesth Analg 1986; 65:451.

413. Harrison L, Ralley FE, Wynands JE, et al: The role of an ultra short-acting adrenergic blocker (esmolol) in patients undergoing coronary artery bypass surgery. Anesthesiology 1987; 66:413.

414. Edmondson R, Del Valle O, Shah N, et al: Esmolol for potentiation of nitroprusside-induced hypotension: impact on the cardiovascular, adrenergic, and

renin-angiotensin systems in man. Anesth Analg 1989; 69:202.

415. Gorczynski RJ: Basic pharmacology of esmolol. Am J Cardiol 1986; 56:3f.

416. Ornstein E, Young WL, Ostapkovich N, et al: Deliberate hypotension in patients with intracranial arterio-venous malformations: esmolol compared with isoflurane and sodium nitroprusside. Anesth Analg 1991; 72:639.

417. Fromme GA, MacKenzie RA, Gould AB, et al: Controlled hypotension of orthognathic surgery. Anesth Analg 1986; 65:683.

418. Blau WS, Kafer ER, Anderson JA: Esmolol is more effective than sodium nitroprusside in reducing blood loss during orthognathic surgery. Anesth Analg 1992; 75:172.

419. Bloor BC, Flacke WE: Reduction in halothane anesthetic requirement by clonidine. An alpha-adrenergic agonist. Anesth Analg 1982; 61:741.

420. Woodcock TE, Millard RK, Dixon J, et al: Clonidine premedication for isoflurane-induced hypotension. Br J Anaesth 1988; 60:388.

421. Maroof M, Khan RM, Bhatti TH: Clonidine premedication for induced hypotension with total intravenous anaesthesia for middle ear microsurgery. Can J Anaesth 1994; 41:164.

422. Maze M, Segal IS, Bloor BC: Clonidine and other alpha 2 adrenergic agonists: strategies for the rational use of these novel anesthetic agents. J Clin Anesth 1988; 1:146.

423. Toivonen J, Kaukinen S: Clonidine premedication: a useful adjunct in producing deliberate hypotension. Acta Anaesthesiol Scand 1990: 34:653.

424. Bloor BC, Finander LS, Flacke WE, et al: Effect of clonidine on sympathoadrenal response during sodium nitroprusside hypotension. Anesth Analg 1986; 65:469.

425. Ghignone M, Calvillo O, Caple S, et al: Clonidine reduces the dose requirement for nitroprusside induced hypotension (Abstract). Anesthesiology 1986; 65:A51.

426. Zubrow AB, Daniel SS, Stark RI, et al: Plasma renin, catecholamine and vasopressin during nitroprusside-induced hypotension in ewes. Anesthesiology 1983; 58:245.

427. Fahmy NR, Sunder N, Moss J, et al: Tachyphylaxis to nitroprusside. Role of the renin-angiotensin system and catecholamines in its development (Abstract). Anesthesiology 1979; 51:S72.

428. Davis JO, Freeman RH: Mechanisms regulating renin release. Physiol Rev 1976; 56:1.

429. Fahmy NR, Almaz MG: Vasodilator drugs. In: Stoelting RG, Barash PG, Gallagher TJ, eds, Advances in Anesthesia. Chicago, 1989, Year Book Medical Publishers Inc., vol. 6.

430. Vidt DG, Bravo EL, Fouad FM: Captopril. N Engl J Med 1982; 306:214.

431. Turini GA, Bribic M, Brunner HR, et al: Improvement of chronic congestive heart failure by oral captopril. Lancet 1979; 1:1213.

432. Kripalani KJ, McKinstry DN, Singhvi SM, et al: Disposition of captopril in normal subjects. Clin Pharmacol Ther 1980; 27:636.

433. Jennings GL, Gelman JS, Stockigt JR, et al: Accentuated hypotensive effect of sodium nitroprusside in man after captopril. Clin Sci 1981; 61:521.

434. Woodside J, Garner L, Bedford RF, et al: Captopril reduces the dose requirement for sodium nitroprus-

side induced hypotension. Anesthesiology 1984; 60:413.

435. Porter SS, Asher M, Fox DK: Comparison of intravenous nitroprusside, nitroprusside-captopril, and nitroglycerin for deliberate hypotension during posterior spine fusion in adults. J Clin Anesth 1988 1:87.

436. Frishman WH: New therapeutic modalities in hypertension: focus on a new calcium antagonist—nicardipine. J Clin Pharmacol 1987; 29:481.

437. Bernard JM, Pinaud M, François T, et al: Deliberate hypotension with nicardipine or nitroprusside during total hip arthroplasty. Anesth Analg 1991; 73: 341.

438. Bernard JM, Passuti N, Pinaud M: Long term hypotensive technique with nicardipine and nitroprusside during isoflurane anesthesia for spinal surgery. Anesth Analg 1992; 75:179.

439. Aronson S, Goldberg LI, Roth S, et al: Preservation of renal blood flow during hypotension induced with fenoldopam in dogs. Can J Anaesth 1990; 37: 380.

440. Berne RM: The role of adenosine in the regulation of coronary blood. Circ Res 1980; 47:807.

441. Sollevi A, Lagerkranser M, Andreen M, et al: Relationship between arterial and venous adenosine levels and vasodilation during ATP- and adenosine-infusion in dogs. Acta Physiol Scand 1984; 120: 171.

442. Sollevi A, Lagerkranser M, Irestedt L, et al: Controlled hypotension with adenosine in cerebral aneurysm surgery. Anesthesiology 1984; 61:400.

443. Sollevi A: Cardiovascular effects of adenosine in man: possible clinical implications. Prog Neurobiol 1986; 27:319.

444. Owall A, Jarnberg P-O, Brodin L-A, et al: Effect of adenosine-induced hypotension in myocardial hemodynamics and metabolism in fentanyl anesthetized patients with peripheral vascular disease. Anesthesiology 1988; 68:416.

445. Lagerkranser M, Bergstrand G, Gordon E, et al: Cerebral blood flow and metabolism during adenosine-induced hypotension in patients undergoing cerebral aneurysm surgery. Acta Anaesthesiol Scand 1989; 33:15.

446. Kassel NF, Boarini DJ, Olin JJ, et al: Cerebral and systemic circulatory effects of arterial hypotension induced by adenosine. J Neurosurg 1983; 58:69.

447. Crystal GJ, Rooney MW, Salem MR: Regional hemodynamics and oxygen supply during isovolemic hemodilution alone and in combination with adenosine-induced controlled hypotension. Anesth Analg 1988; 67:211.

448. Crystal GJ, Rooney MW, Salem MR: Myocardial blood flow and oxygen consumption during isovolemic hemodilution alone and in combination with adenosine-induced controlled hypotension. Anesth Analg 1988; 67:539.

449. Lagerkranser M, Irestedt L, Sollevi A, et al: Central and splanchnic hemodynamics in the dog during controlled hypotension with adenosine. Anesthesiology 1984; 60:547.

450. Zall S, Eden E, Winso I, et al: Controlled hypotension with adenosine or sodium nitroprusside during cerebral aneurysm surgery: effects on renal hemodynamics, excretory function, and renin release. Anesth Analg 1990; 71:631.

451. Taneyama C, Goto H, Benson KT, et al: Vagal involvement in the action of exogenous adenosine triphosphate on reflex sympathetic nerve activity. Anesth Analg 1991; 72:351.

452. Patterson RE, Kirk ES: Coronary steal mechanisms in dogs with one-vessel occlusion and other arteries normal. Circulation 1983; 67:1009.

453. Zall S, Milocco I, Ricksten SE: Effects of adenosine on myocardial blood flow and metabolism after coronary artery bypass surgery. Anesth Analg 1991; 73:689.

454. Zall S, Milocco I, Ricksten SE: Effects of adenosine on renal function and central hemodynamics after coronary artery bypass surgery. Anesth Analg 1993; 76:493.

455. Zall S, Kirno K, Milocco I, Ricksten SE: Vasodilation with adenosine or sodium nitroprusside after coronary artery bypass surgery: a comparative study on myocardial blood flow and metabolism. Anesth Analg 1993; 76:498.

456. Berne RM, Winn R, Rubio R: The local regulation of cerebral blood flow. Cardiovasc Res 1981; 24: 243.

457. Forrester T, Harper AM, McKenzie ET, et al: Effect of adenosine triphosphate and some derivatives on cerebral blood flow and metabolism. J Physiol 1979; 296:343.

458. Heistad DD, Marcus ML, Gourley JK, et al: Effect of adenosine and dypyridamole on cerebral blood flow. Am J Physiol 1981; 240:H775.

459. Tagawa H, Vander AJ: Effects of adenosine compounds on renal function and renin secretion in dogs. Circ Res 1970; 26:327.

460. Lagerkranser M, Sollevi A, Irestedt L, et al: Renin release during controlled hypotension with sodium nitroprusside, nitroglycerine and adenosine: a comparative study in the dog. Acta Anaesthesiol Scand 1985; 29:45.

461. Nyberg G: Effects of adenosine (Letter). Anesth Analg 1993; 76:672.

462. Khambatta HJ, Stone JG, Kaus SJ: Agents: vasodilators. Probl Anesth 1993; 7:57.

463. Kolassa N, Beller KD, Sanders KH: Evidence for the interaction of urapidil with 5-$HT_{1A}$ receptors in the brain leading to a decrease in blood pressure. Am J Cardiol 1989; 63:36c.

464. Puchstein C, Van Aken H, Anger C, et al: Influence of urapidil on intracranial pressure and intracranial compliance in dogs. Br J Anaesth 1983; 55:443.

465. Anger C, Van Aken H, Feldhaus P, et al: Permeation of the blood-brain barrier by urapidil and its influence on intracranial pressure in man in the presence of compromised intracranial dynamics. J Hypertens 1988; 6:S63.

466. Sicking K, Puchstein C, Van Aken H: Blutdrucksenkung mit Urapidil: Einfluss auf die Hirndurchblutung. Anesth Intensivmed 1986; 27:147.

467. Van Aken H, Van Hemelrijck J: Deliberate hypotension. IARS Review Course Lectures, 1993; #20.

468. Donald JR: Induced hypotension and blood loss during surgery. J R Soc Med 1982; 75:149.

469. Safar P: A study of deliberate hypotension in anesthesia with special consideration of surgical blood loss in comparable groups of normotensive and hypotensive anesthesia. Surgery 1955; 37:1002

470. Ditzler JW, Eckenhoff JE: A comparison of blood loss and operative time in certain surgical procedures completed with and without controlled hypotension. Ann Surg 1956; 143:289.

471. Bodman RI: Blood loss during prostatectomy. Br J Anaesth 1959; 31:484.

472. Bruce AW, Zorab J, Still B: Blood loss in prostatic surgery. Br J Urol 1960; 32:422.

473. Eckenhoff JE, Rich JC: Clinical experiences with deliberate hypotension. Anesth Analg 1966; 45:21.

474. Thorud T, Lund I, Holme I: The effect of anaesthesia on intraoperative and postoperative bleeding during abdominal prostatectomies: a comparison of neurolept anaesthesia, halothane anaesthesia, and epidural anaesthesia. Acta Anaesthesiol Scand Suppl 1975; 57:83.

475. Urquhart-Hay D, Marshall NG, Marsland JM: Comparison of epidural and hypotensive anaesthesia in open prostatectomy. Series 2. N Z Med J 1969; 70:223.

476. Anderson SM, McKissock W: Controlled hypotension with Arfonad in neurosurgery with special reference to vascular lesions. Lancet 1953; 2:754.

477. Goldstein LA: Surgical management of scoliosis. J Bone Joint Surg [Am] 1966; 48A:167.

478. McNeill TW, DeWald RL, Kuo KN, et al: Controlled hypotensive anesthesia in scoliosis surgery. J Bone Joint Surg [Am] 1974; 56A:1167.

479. Anderson SM: Controlled hypotension with Arfonad in paediatric surgery. Br Med J 1955; 2:103.

480. Boyan CP: Hypotensive anesthesia for radical pelvic and abdominal surgery. Arch Surg 1953; 67:803.

481. Ahlering TE, Henderson JB, Skinner DG: Controlled hypotensive anesthesia to reduce blood loss in radical cystectomy for bladder cancer. J Urol 1983; 129:953.

482. Sood S, Jayalaxmi TS, Vijayaraghavan S, et al: Use of sodium nitroprusside induced hypotensive anaesthesia for reducing blood loss in patients undergoing lienorenal shunts for portal hypertension. Br J Surg 1987; 74:1036.

483. Boreham P: Retropubic prostatectomy with hypotensive anaesthesia. Proc Roy Soc Med 1964; 57: 1181.

484. Stirt JA, Korn EL, Reynolds RC: Sodium nitroprusside-induced hypotension in radical thoraco-abdominal dissection of retroperitoneal lymph nodes. Br J Anaesth 1980; 52:1045.

485. Donald JR: The effect of anaesthesia, hypotension and epidural analgesia on blood loss in surgery for pelvic floor repair. Br J Anaesth 1969; 41:155.

486. Mannheimer WH, Keats AS, Chamberlain JA: Safety in hypotensive anaesthesia. Surgery 1963; 54:883.

487. Schaberg SJ, Kelly JF, Terry BC, et al: Blood loss and hypotensive anesthesia in oral facial corrective surgery. J Oral Surg 1976; 34:147.

488. Chan W, Smith DE, Ware WH: Effects of hypotensive anesthesia in anterior maxillary osteotomy. J Oral Surg 1980; 38:504.

489. Condon HA: Deliberate hypotension in ENT surgery. Clin Otolaryngol 1979; 4:241.

490. Ward CF, Alfery DD, Saidman LJ, et al: Deliberate hypotension in head and neck surgery. Head Neck Surg 1980; 2:185.

491. Deacock AR: Aspects of anaesthesia for middle ear surgery and blood loss during stapedectomy. Proc Roy Soc Med 1971; 64:44.

492. Holmes F: Bloodless operating field in middle ear surgery. A review of 138 cases of induced hypotension with hexamethonium bromide ($C_6$). J Laryngol Otol 1961; 75:248.

493. Kerr AR: Anaesthesia with profound hypotension for middle ear surgery. Br J Anaesth 1977; 49:447.

494. Saarnivaara L, Brander P: Comparison of three hypotensive anaesthetic methods for middle ear microsurgery. Acta Anaesthesiol Scand 1984; 28:435.

495. Powell JL, Mogelnicki SR, Franklin EW III, et al: A deliberate hypotensive technique for decreasing blood loss during radical hysterectomy and pelvic lymphadenectomy. Am J Obstet Gynecol 1983; 147:196.

496. Geevarghese KP: Induced hypotension and its application in neurological surgery. Int Anesthesiol Clin 1977; 15:195.

497. Enderby GEH: Hypotensive anaesthesia in plastic surgery. Br J Plastic Surg 1961; 14:41.

498. Linacre JL: Induced hypotension in gynaecological surgery. Br J Anaesth 1961; 33:45.

499. Moersch RN, Patrick RT, Clagett OT: The use of hypotensive anesthesia in radical mastectomy. Ann Surg 1960; 152:911.

500. Grundy BL, Nash CL, Brown RH: Deliberate hypotension for spinal fusion (Abstract). Anesthesiology 1979; 51:S78.

501. Lawhon SM, Kahn A III, Crawford AH, et al: Controlled hypotensive anesthesia during spinal surgery. Spine 1984; 9:450.

502. Patel NJ, Patel BS, Paskin S, et al: Induced moderate hypotensive anesthesia for spinal fusion and harrington-rod instrumentation. J Bone Joint Surg [Am] 1985; 67A:1384.

503. Ting MC, Ng DHF, Hsu JC, et al: Hypotensive anesthesia for spinal fusion and Luque spinal segmental instrumentation. Anesth Sinica 1988; 26:427.

504. Mallory TH: Hypotensive anesthesia in total hip replacement. JAMA 1973; 224:248.

505. Nelson CL, Bowen WS: Total hip arthroplasty in Jehovah's Witnesses without blood transfusion. J Bone Joint Surg [Am] 1986; 68A:350.

506. Donald JR: Epidural anaesthesia, induced hypotension and blood loss during surgery. Acta Anaesthesiol Scand 1983; 27:91.

507. Simpson DA, Ireland J: Hypotensive and normotensive anaesthesia in total hip replacement: a comparative study. Br J Clin Pract 1983; 37:16.

508. Hercus VM, Reeve TS, Tracey GD, et al: Blood loss during surgery. Br Med J 1961; 2:1467.

509. Gillies J: Anaesthetic factors in the causation and prevention of excessive bleeding during surgical operations. Ann R Coll Surg Engl 1950; 7:204.

510. Moir DD: Blood loss during major vaginal surgery. Br J Anaesth 1968; 40:233.

511. McGowan SW, Smith GFN: Anaesthesia for transurethral prostatectomy. Anaesthesia 1980; 35:847.

512. Enderby DH: Monitoring hypotensive anaesthesia blood pressure and other systems. In: Enderby GEH, ed, Hypotensive Anaesthesia. London, 1985, Churchill Livingstone.

513. Relton JES, Creighton RE, Johnston AE, et al: Hyperpyrexia in association with general anaesthesia in children. Can Anaesth Soc J 1966; 13:419.

514. Pachon V: Oscillomètre sphygmométrique a grande sensibilité et a sensibilité constante. Comptes Rendues des Séances de la Société de Biologie (Paris) 1909; 66:776.

515. Erlanger J: A new instrument for determining the minimum and maximum blood pressures in man. Johns Hopkins Hosp Rep 1904; 7:53.

516. Gallavardin L: Sur un nouveau brassard sphygmomanometrique. La Presse Med 1922; 9:766.

517. Abou-Madi M, Lenis S, Archer D, et al: Compari-

son of direct blood pressure measurements at the radial and dorsalis pedis arteries during sodium nitroprusside- and isoflurane-induced hypotension. Anesthesiology 1986; 65:692.

518. Gibbs NM, Larach DR, Derr JA: The accuracy of Finapres noninvasive mean arterial pressure measurements in anesthetized patients. Anesthesiology 1991; 74:647.

519. Salem MR, El-Etr AA: Management of hemorrhage following induced hypotension. Anesthesiology 1967; 28:1104.

520. Davidson AHM: Discussion on the use of hypotensive drugs in surgery. Proc Roy Soc Med 1951; 55: 942.

521. Enderby GEH: Hypotensive anaesthesia in surgery. Ann R Coll Surg Engl 1952; 11:310.

522. Gillan JG: Two cases of unilateral blindness following anesthesia with vascular hypotension. Can Med Assoc J 1953; 69:294.

523. Goldsmith AJB, Hewer AJH: Unilateral amaurosis with partial recovery after using hexamethonium iodide. Br Med J 1952; 2:759.

524. Bozza Marrubini L, Celotti M, Frera C: Amaurosi unilaterale permanente dopo ipotensione controllata. Chirurgie 1953; 8:454.

525. Bromage PR: Some electroencephalographic changes associated with induced vascular hypotension. Proc Roy Coll Med 1953; 46:919.

526. Wakim KG: Certain cardiovasculorenal effects of hexamethonium. Am Heart J 1955; 50:435.

527. Association of Anaesthetists' Committee Report: Death associated with anaesthesia: cases in which hypotension has been used. Anaesthesia 1953; 8: 263.

528. Eckenhoff JE: Deliberate hypotension (Editorial). Anesthesiology 1978; 48:87.

529. Little DM: Induced hypotension during anesthesia and surgery. Anesthesiology 1955; 16:320.

530. Beecher HK, Todd DP: A study of the deaths associated with anesthesia and surgery, based on a study of 599,548 anesthetics in 10 institutions 1948–1952 inclusive. Ann Surg 1954; 140:2.

531. Enderby GEH: Hypotensive anaesthesia. In: Grey TC, Nunn JF, Utting JE, eds, General Anaesthesia, 3 ed. London, 1980, Butterworths, p. 1149.

532. Way GL, Clarke HL: An anaesthetic technique for prostatectomy. Lancet 1959; 2:888.

533. Rylance PB, Carli F, McArthur SE, et al: The effect of induced hypotension and tissue trauma on renal function in scoliosis surgery. J Bone Joint Surg [Br] 1988; 70B:127.

534. Laver MB, Bland JHL: Anesthetic management of the pediatric patient during open-heart surgery. Int Anesthesiol Clin 1975; 13:143.

535. Rollason WN, Hough JM: A study of hypotensive anaesthesia in the elderly. Br J Anaesth 1960; 32: 276.

536. Rollason WN, Hough JM: Is it safe to employ hypotensive anaesthesia in the elderly? Br J Anaesth 1960; 32:286.

537. Bennett EJ, Dalal FY: Haemoglobin S and its clinical application. In: Payne JP, Hill DW, eds, Oxygen Measurement in Biology and Medicine. London, 1975, Butterworths.

538. Aach RD, Lander JJ, Sherman LA, et al: Transfusion-transmitted viruses: interim analysis of hepatitis among transfused and non-transfused patients. In: Vyas GN, Cohen SN, Schmid R, eds, Viral Hepatitis: A Contemporary Assessment of Etiology, Epidemiology, Pathogenesis, and Prevention. Philadelphia, 1978, Franklin Institute Press, pp. 383–396.

539. Melton EJ III, Stauffer RN, Chao EYS, et al: Rates of total hip arthroplasty. A population-based study. N Engl J Med 1982; 307:1242.

540. Davis NJ, Jennings JJ, Harris WH: Induced hypotensive anesthesia for total hip replacement. Gen Orthop 1974; 101:93.

541. Vazeery AK, Lunde O: Controlled hypotension in hip joint surgery. Acta Orthop Scand 1979; 50:433.

542. Eerola R, Eerola M, Kaukinen L, et al: Controlled hypotension and moderate haemodilution in major hip surgery. Ann Chir Gynaecol 1979; 69:109.

543. Barbier-Böhm G, Desmonts JM, Couderc E, et al: Comparative effects of induced hypotension and normovolaemic haemodilution on blood loss in total hip arthroplasty. Br J Anaesth 1980; 52:1039.

544. Qvist TF, Skovsted P, Bredgaard Sörensen M: Moderate hypotensive anaesthesia for reduction of blood loss during total hip replacement. Acta Anaesthesiol Scand 1982; 26:351.

545. Malcolm-Smith NA, McMaster MJ: The use of induced hypotension to control bleeding during posterior fusion for scoliosis. J Bone Joint Surg [Br] 1983; 65B:255.

546. Sivarajan M, Amory DW, McKenzie SM: Regional blood flows during induced hypotension produced by nitroprusside or trimethaphan in the rhesus monkey. Anesth Analg 1985; 64:759.

# 9

# BLOOD SALVAGE TECHNIQUES

*Ninos J. Joseph, Judith Kamaryt, and Robert Paulissian*

## HISTORICAL ASPECTS OF BLOOD SALVAGE

"It has always seemed illogical to throw away a patient's blood and then institute a frantic search for a donor to supply blood, for even though the blood is of the same type and is compatible, still we know that a severe reaction sometimes follows."
Lilian K. P. Farrar, M.D., 1923

The inability to safely match and store blood and the improbable availability of a compatible donor during acute hemorrhage or emergency surgery provided the earliest impetus for blood salvage.[1–8] Although the first reported blood transfusion was performed in the early 17th century, the widespread use of allogeneic blood transfusion was impeded for various reasons. First, the 17th century physician, believing that blood contained factors that affected psychological status but failing to alter personality traits by blood transfusion, became disillusioned with the technique. Furthermore, because the distinction between human and animal blood was not then appreciated, the substitution of animal blood (usually lamb's blood) often resulted in severe transfusion reactions. Finally, even when human blood was used, numerous fatalities resulted because the identification of specific blood types and antigens had as yet not occurred. Thus, by the mid-17th century, blood transfusion had fallen into disfavor and ceased to be practiced.[9]

In the early 19th century, Dr. James Blundell's interest in blood transfusion was prompted when a patient died of an uncontrollable uterine hemorrhage despite vigorous medical attention. He concluded that immediate blood transfusion was the only therapy that might have saved the patient. Interested in reviving blood transfusion as a clinical practice, Blundell performed a series of 10 experiments designed to assess the "fitness" of shed blood, if returned promptly to the circulation by syringe, in resuscitating dogs after exsanguination. In the second experiment of this series, he determined that if shed blood was captured and reinfused before coagulation and without the introduction of air, complete recovery was probable. Unknowingly, he reported the first recognized example of autotransfusion of salvaged blood.[10] Blundell continued his work over the next several years and made considerable contributions to the revival of allogeneic blood transfusion.[10–13] By the end of the 19th century, allogeneic blood transfusion had become an accepted therapeutic modality.[9]

When confronted with a similar situation as was Blundell (postpartum hemorrhage) and lacking an acceptable donor, Highmore[1] in 1874 regretted the loss of a large quantity of shed blood, which he described as "several pounds of blood in a vessel and in the bed." He resolved that on the next case of hemorrhage he would capture and reinfuse this shed blood. In addition to the collection of shed blood, he also suggested "defibrinating" (by agitation with a glass rod) and warming (in a water bath) the blood before reinfusion. Several years later, the first two documented accounts of blood salvage in humans were reported from the Royal Infirmary, Edinburgh, Scotland.[2,3] In both cases, above-knee amputations were performed under chloroform anesthesia. Blood was collected from the amputated limbs and from the stumps during closure and drained into a basin containing a 5% solution of phosphate of soda. The mixtures of shed blood and phosphate solution were then reinfused to the patients through exposed and cannulated femoral veins in the stumps before closure of the wounds. In both instances, the patients survived and fully recovered from surgical procedures in which the outcome would normally have been doubtful because of excessive blood loss.

Although blood salvage was originally suggested and practiced in the United Kingdom, its first widespread use appeared in Germany

during World War I. The first German report was by Thies in 1914.[4] He reported the successful autotransfusion of salvaged blood in three patients with ruptured ectopic pregnancies. During the next 8 years as many as 164 reported cases of autotransfusion appeared in the European literature, all but four being German.[14,15] The majority of these cases (118) were ruptured ectopic pregnancies.[4,16–32] Other surgical procedures included ruptured spleen or liver (13),[22,30,33–39] spinal cord or intracranial injury (6),[40–42] hemothorax (1),[5] and other unspecified cases (27).[16,18,23,29,43] The overall mortality from this early experience with autotransfusion of salvaged blood was 8.5%, and posttransfusion reactions occurred in 4% of the surviving patients.[14,15] This extensive experience with blood salvage yielded much information that was helpful to later attempts at autotransfusion: (a) autotransfusion of salvaged blood was a safe procedure, although reactions occur in a limited number of patients; (b) blood should be reinfused immediately, and sodium citrate or dilution with normal saline was often unnecessary, especially with salvaged hemothorax blood, which remains uncoagulated for extended periods of time; (c) blood may be expressed from soaked gauze or sponges; (d) blood can be filtered through layers of gauze before reinfusion to remove gross clots (Fig. 9–1); and (e) contaminated blood should not be reintroduced into the circulation.

The first report of blood salvage in the United States, and an early example of blood salvage for elective surgery, was by Lockwood in 1916.[44] After excision of an enlarged and very vascular spleen, Lockwood noted that approximately 1 L of blood escaped into a sterile basin after unclamping of the vessels. A surgical colleague suggested that this blood might be reinfused. They were able to salvage 750 mL, and after filtration, defibrination, and dilution with normal saline, they reinfused this blood. In a second procedure, Lockwood was able to express 500 mL of blood from an excised spleen, which was later reinfused. By the 1930s autotransfusion was well established in the North American medical literature. Reports included autotransfusion for major abdominal,[6,7,44,45] thoracic,[8,46] neurosurgical,[47] and gynecological[6,48,49] surgeries. In 1943,

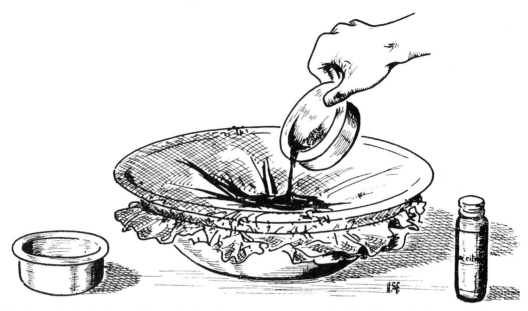

**Fig. 9–1.** The lack of appropriate medical equipment and access to banked blood in developing nations often force physicians to apply simple but crude methods. Shed blood is scooped from the field and filtered through several layers of gauze into a basin. Blood is then drawn into a syringe for reinfusion. From Lawson JB, Stewart DB: Obstetrics and Gynecology in the Tropics and Developing Nations. London, 1967, Edward Arnold (Publishers) LTD, p. 376, with permission.

Griswold and Ortner[50] reported on a series of 100 patients over a 10-year period; these included ruptured ectopic pregnancies, penetrating wounds to the thorax, nonpenetrating wounds of the abdomen, and penetrating wounds of the abdomen with and without perforation of a hollow viscus.

The adaptation of aspiration apparatus for the evacuation of shed blood from body cavities was initially reported by White in 1923.[45] Before this time, shed blood was collected by such inefficient means as ladling, syringe aspiration, or soaked sponges. The suction wand, with carefully controlled vacuum, proved less damaging to formed blood elements and was so much more efficient that harvest of salvaged blood often exceeded that which could not be immediately reinfused.[47,50] Hesitating to dispose of unused blood, White,[45] as early as 1923, suggested refrigerated storage of this blood for later use on the same patient or as allogeneic blood.

By the 1940s, events were taking place in the United States and around the world that were to have far-reaching effects on the auto-transfusion of salvaged blood. The introduction of citrate anticoagulation[51–54] and the utility of refrigerated storage[55] completely transformed the practice of blood transfusion. Institutionalized blood banks, both military[56,57] and civilian,[58,59] were able to provide much of the blood necessary for treatment of casualties during World War II.

As a consequence of the ready availability of typed allogeneic banked blood, interest in blood salvage techniques began to decline.[60] Blood salvage appears to have been nearly abandoned as a clinical practice through the late 1940s and 1950s.[61] This occurred despite the knowledge that although allogeneic blood was screened, typed, and compatibility tested with recipient blood before transfusion, disease transmission[45,50] or transfusion reactions[6,50] were not always avoided.

The 1960s brought a resurgence of interest in blood conservation techniques. The ever-increasing demands for allogeneic banked blood began to strain blood-banking resources. Despite the apparent success of civilian blood banking in the late 1930s, acute shortages of banked blood and blood components were felt as early as 1943. Griswold and Ortner[50] noted that a disproportionate number of patients died on the operating table or shortly after operation because of tardy or inadequate replacement of the lost circulating blood volume. They reasoned that the time lost in cross matching blood and plasma from the blood bank often proved fatal and that the blood supply of the correct type was too often insufficient to provide for the needs of patients who had lost large amounts of blood.[50] Ferrara[62] was disturbed that the limited supply of banked whole blood often resulted in cancellation of elective surgical procedures, particularly operations for cancer. Furthermore, the considerable advances made in surgical and anesthetic techniques and technology after World War II led to the development of new and more extensive surgical procedures. The demands for blood for cardiovascular, radical cancer, and trauma surgeries frequently exceeded donor reserves in some communities.[60,63] Finally, patients with rare blood types proved difficult or impossible to perfectly cross match and thus often faced long delays or cancellation of surgery until compatible (or near compatible) blood was located. Many of the blood shortages described did not merely represent inadequate allogeneic blood collection but frequently resulted from wastage of valuable stores by inefficient transfusion practices.[60,64,65]

War in southeast Asia (1963–1973) placed further demands for blood and provided a major impetus for the resurgence of interest in blood salvage as well as other blood conservation techniques.[60,66–68] Blood stores, sometimes insufficient for civilian needs, were further taxed by the increasing numbers of casualties resulting from escalating involvement of United States servicemen. Thus, the U.S. Department of Defense, citing the excellent results of autotransfusion practiced during World War I, became a key proponent and a primary financier of research in blood salvage techniques.[69]

It was at this time that other blood conservation measures were being investigated. The first autologous predeposit program was instituted at Augustana Hospital in Chicago, Illinois.[70] First demonstrated in 1921 by Grant,[52] autologous predeposit was at that time limited by the lack of proper blood-banking facilities and preservation methodology (see Chapter 6: Preoperative Autologous Blood Donation). Another source of salvaged blood, although not autologous, was being investigated. In 1960, Tarasov[71] presented experiences with cadaveric blood transfusion over a 30-year period in the former U.S.S.R.

Cadaveric blood transfusion was originally demonstrated in the dog by Shamor in 1928 and then used experimentally in humans by Yudin throughout the early 1930s.[72] By the 1960s, this potential source of large quantities of allogeneic blood was largely ignored except at the Sklifossovsky Institute in Moscow where Yudin had originally done his pioneering work.[73] Sporadic reports of cadaveric blood transfusion did appear in the western literature, but this source of blood has yet to be exploited because of an aura of "untouchability" connected with corpse blood.[74,75] It has been speculated that the development of cadaveric organ banking, for example, eye, skin, and bone, may lead to a resurgence in interest in cadaveric blood salvage techniques.[76] Today, however, it seems doubtful that any interest that ever existed in cadaveric blood salvage remains.

The modern era of blood salvage began in 1970 with the introduction of the first commercially available autotransfusion apparatus. Introduced as the Bentley Autotransfusion System (ATS100, Bentley Laboratories, Santa Ana, CA), this device was a modified version of a design extensively field-tested during hostilities in southeast Asia.[66,77–79] Functionally similar to the cardiotomy suction apparatus used during cardiopulmonary bypass, many of the components were borrowed from Bentley's early bypass technology. The system (Fig. 9–2) consisted of one (or two) suction wands and in-flow tubing for aspiration of shed blood from the surgical site. The distal end of the in-flow tubing was mounted into a roller pump that provided the necessary suction. The tubing terminated in a collection chamber (a modified cardiotomy reservoir). Blood return to the patient was through an intravenous line returning from the chamber to a venous cannulation site. A 125-$\mu$m filter was interposed into the out-flow tubing to trap clots, bits of tissue, and particulate. Reinfusion of salvaged blood was controlled by regulating compressed air pressure in the collection chamber. A maximal reinfusion flow rate of 600 mL/min was possible. Anticoagulation was accomplished by priming the collection reservoir with lactated Ringer's solution containing 3000 units/L heparin and occasional flushing of the in-flow tubing with heparinized solution.[80,81] Unfortunately, troubles plagued this machine from the incep-

**Fig. 9–2.** The Bentley Autotransfusion System, model ATS-100, consists of an aspirating unit that is activated by a roller pump (a), a reservoir (b) that contains a crude filter (c), an air exit vent (d) at the apex of the reservoir that permits variable control of intracavitary pressure, and two delivery systems (e), each fitted with a standard blood transfusion filter. There is an additional vent (f) at the apex of the reservoir that permits admixture and the addition of agents. From Klebanoff G: Intraoperative autotransfusion with the Bentley ATS-100. Surgery 1978; 84:708, with permission.

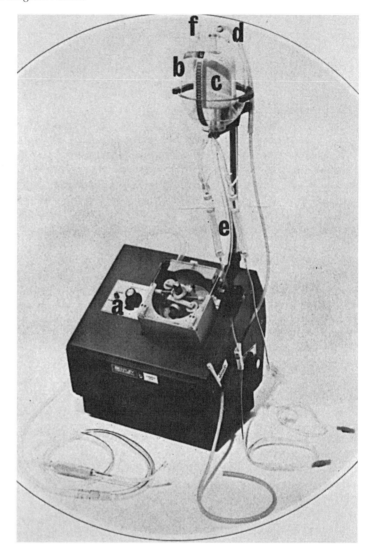

tion. Red blood cell (RBC) and platelet destruction, dilution or consumption of coagulation factors, and incidences of disseminated intravascular coagulation (DIC) were blamed on the suction apparatus, roller pump, insufficient anticoagulation, and inadequate filtration. Finally, several incidents of venous air embolism related to the use of the Bentley ATS100 were reported.[80–82] Although many of the problems encountered were resolved or traced to human error, this system was eventually withdrawn from the market by the manufacturer.[61,68]

In 1976, Noon and associates[83] developed a new autotransfusion device that encompassed major improvements over the Bentley ATS100 design. The major points included improved mixing of anticoagulant and blood, the use of controlled wall suction rather than a roller pump for aspiration, and, most importantly, gravity reinfusion to the patient rather than by air pressurization, greatly reducing the risk of air embolism. Noon and coworkers' original design was eventually merged with prototypes from Sorensen Research Corporation (Salt Lake City, UT) and finally marketed as the Sorensen Autotransfusion System (Fig. 9–3).[84] Today, filtration salvage systems are still being used intraoperatively. However, their primary use is in the emergency department and for postoperative wound drainage.

At about this same time, several manufacturers were actively working on an alternative

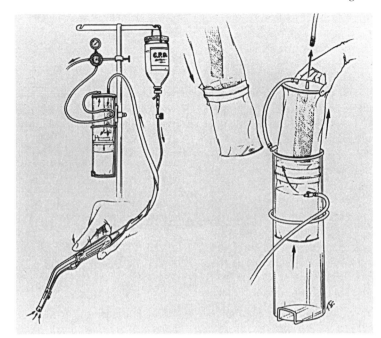

**Fig. 9–3.** The Sorenson Receptal Autotransfusion System. *Left:* The system of autotransfusion is assembled and ready for intraoperative collection of autologous blood. *Right:* Removal of reservoirs to be prepared for autotransfusion and their immediate replacement with a new sterile set are demonstrated. From Noon GP, Solis T, Natalson EA: A simple method of intraoperative autotransfusion. Surg Gynecol Obstet 1976; 143:65, with permission.

to filtration autotransfusion systems. Blood salvaged by these systems was processed by centrifugation and washing and resulted in a product that resembled packed RBCs. Such technology had been used since the 1960s in hospitals and regional blood centers for deglycerolizing blood in frozen storage after thawing.[85] Processing of salvaged blood removes virtually all debris and contaminants, plasma, proteins, and clotting factors.[87] More advanced versions of these cell processors are now capable of performing plasmapheretic separation of platelet-rich and platelet-poor plasma, as well as packed RBCs.[87–89] Intraoperative hemofiltration is currently being used for the maintenance of a desired hematocrit (HCT) during extracorporeal circulation and for hemoconcentration of dilute residual oxygenator contents at the conclusion of extracorporeal circulation[90,91] (see Chapter 12: Blood Conservation in Special Situations: Cardiac Surgery).

The development of these intraoperative autotransfusion devices was accompanied by devices for use outside the operating theater. Filtration systems were devised for drainage of chest blood from traumatic hemothoraces

and for after cardiac surgery.[61,92–94] The cumbersome size and high degree of sophistication of blood processing devices usually limited their use to the operating room. Recent advances in blood processor technology, however, have resulted in highly automated more compact "transportable" blood processors that can be used at the patient bedside. Thus, blood salvage has been extended to the postanesthesia recovery and intensive care units and exported to the emergency department.

As the 21st century approaches, the future of blood salvage, as well as all blood conservation techniques, appears to be linked to the development of oxygen-carrying blood substitutes[95] (see Chapter 10: Blood Substitutes). A safe and effective blood substitute with a long shelf-life that can reversibly bind oxygen under physiological conditions would probably render some blood salvage procedures unnecessary.

## CURRENT RATIONALE FOR BLOOD SALVAGE
### Advantages of Blood Salvage

Normally, the circulating RBC mass is abundantly capable of providing the oxygen requirements of the body. Small to moderate blood loss can be replaced with cell-free solutions (colloids or crystalloids).[96] However, anemia resulting from moderate to massive blood loss, decreasing the oxygen-carrying capacity to a level near or below the metabolic requirements of the body, must be corrected if ischemia to the tissues is to be avoided. This anemia is corrected with an RBC transfusion. Traditionally, the source of these RBCs has been banked allogeneic blood, a finite commodity becoming increasingly difficult to maintain in adequate quantities. Autologous blood provides an attractive alternative source of RBCs. Because predonation of autologous blood is not always a viable option or cannot always provide blood in sufficient quantity (see Chapter 6: Preoperative Autologous Blood Donation), the salvage of shed blood has become an important source of blood.

Practically, only the advanced industrialized countries can meet the needs for blood in surgery today. Most developing nations have inadequate blood-banking facilities and unreliable donor recruitment.[97] Moreover, in these countries, endemic diseases such as malaria are very common, as well as a chronic state of malnutrition and anemia, render a major part of the population unable to donate blood.[68] In such cases, salvaged blood may often be the only blood available. Blood salvage must often be accomplished by using techniques not surprisingly similar to those used at the turn of the century for lack of resources and modern technology (Figure 9–1).[98–102]

The major advantage of blood salvage is the immediate availability of type-specific, compatible, normothermic blood without the risk of disease transmission or isoimmunization and a marked reduction almost to the point of absence in febrile, allergic, graft-versus-host, and hemolytic problems that are seen concomitantly or after the transfusion of allogeneic blood.[68] Because salvaged blood usually does not require handling, transport, typing, or compatibility and disease testing, technical errors from handling are substantially eliminated.[103] Salvaged blood is normothermic and thus precludes hypothermia induced by the administration of room temperature or refrigerated blood.[104] Normothermic blood also eliminates the need for passage through a blood warmer, because

**Table 9–1.  Advantages of Blood Salvaging Techniques**

Lack of disease transmission or alloimmunization

Avoidance of transfusion reactions

Source of compatible blood for patient with multiple alloantibodies

Technical errors associated with procurement, compatibility testing, handling, and labeling avoid

Useful source of readily available compatible blood during periods of rapid blood loss

Reduction in demands on allogeneic blood supply

Psychological benefit to recipient

Sometimes avoids religious objections to allogeneic blood transfusion

Avoidance or modification of any immunosuppressive effects of transfusion

Can be used in combination with other blood conservation techniques

Modified from the Guidelines for blood salvage and reinfusion in surgery and trauma. Arlington, 1990, American Association of Blood Banks.

most blood warmers often limit the rate of reinfusion.[105] Biochemically, salvaged blood may be superior to stored bank blood in that levels of $2',3'$- diphosphoglycerate (2,3-DPG), adenosine triphosphate are significantly above even 4-day-old banked blood[106] and complications of metabolic acidosis, hypocalcemia, and hyperkalemia are avoided (Table 9–1).[65]

## Indications for Blood Salvage

Blood salvage is routinely used intraoperatively for a variety of emergency and elective surgical procedures and has led to significant decrease or elimination of allogeneic blood transfusion.[64,107–109] Extending blood salvage to the postoperative period and the emergency room can result in additional reductions in allogeneic blood usage. Of the two types of blood salvage (filtration and blood processing), blood processing is most widely used intraoperatively, whereas filtration is used intraoperatively but primarily in the emergency room and postoperatively.[103,110–117] This is essentially due to logistical factors, such as the highly sophisticated instrumentation, high cost, availability of a trained operator, and slower recycling time involved with the use of cell processors. Blood salvage by filtration is significantly less expensive, requires less setup time without the need of extensive training, and blood is immediately available because processing time is eliminated. The introduction of more portable and easier to use cell processors has led to increased use of cell processors in emergency departments, intensive care units, and recovery rooms.

## INDICATIONS FOR INTRAOPERATIVE BLOOD SALVAGE

The salvage and reinfusion of blood lost during surgery is the most common form of autologous blood transfusion, because it can provide large volumes of autologous blood rapidly without the limitations of preoperative autologous blood donation or acute normovolemic hemodilution.[118]

The presence of any of the following criteria may be indications for intraoperative blood salvage: (*a*) anticipated blood loss of 20% or more of the patient's estimated blood volume; (*b*) blood would ordinarily be cross matched for the proposed procedure or patient; (*c*) more than 10% of patients undergoing the procedure require transfusion; and (*d*) the mean transfusion requirement for the procedure exceeds one unit (Table 9–2).[119]

It is generally recognized that some blood salvage technique is indicated if the anticipated blood loss is more than 1000–1500 mL in the adult surgical patient.[109,120–123] When some uncertainty exists as to the extent of blood loss or the possibility of contamination, it may be more cost efficient to set up only suction and anticoagulated collection apparatus in advance. The blood processor can be quickly set up if blood loss in sufficient quantities is salvaged. The decision to autotransfuse or discard the salvaged blood can be made during the procedure.[119]

**Table 9–2.  Indications for Intraoperative Blood Salvage**

Anticipated blood loss ≥20% estimated blood volume

Blood would ordinarily be cross matched to patient or procedure

≥10% of patients undergoing the procedure require transfusion

Mean transfusion requirement for the procedure exceeds one unit

Patients who cannot be transfused with allogeneic blood (rare blood types, lack of stored, compatible blood, religious beliefs)

## Blood Salvage in Infants and Children

Blood salvage has been effectively used in children. Orthopedic procedures, orthotopic liver transplantation, and surgical correction of congenital cardiovascular anomalies in infants and children are often accompanied with significant blood loss and thus warrant blood salvage techniques.[124–126] The maximum allowable blood loss should be calculated by using an accurate preoperative hemoglobin or HCT. Perioperative blood loss estimates should include blood withdrawn for laboratory analysis. When blood loss of greater than 20% of the estimated blood volume is anticipated, blood salvage techniques are appropriate in older children. In younger children and infants (weighing < 10 kg) blood salvage becomes less practical, unless blood loss is expected to be massive (1–1.5 times the blood volume).[127] Although the efficiency of the modern blood salvage apparatus has improved over the years, even pediatric salvage equipment often requires blood losses greater than can be tolerated in the infant. Considering average RBC yield per milliliter of blood lost is between 50 and 70%, an anticipated blood loss of over 700 mL has been suggested.[124,125] Because the loss of even small amounts of blood in the infant can significantly reduce oxygen-carrying capacity, blood salvage can usually only supplement allogeneic blood transfusion. When RBC harvest through blood salvaging is inadequate, minimal-exposure allogeneic transfusion (blood components collected from a limited number of donors) and the use of pediatric packs (multiple 50- to 100-mL units derived from a single adult allogeneic donation) have been advocated.[128,129] Minimal-exposure allogeneic blood products reduce the risk of alloimmunization, particularly important in infants and children with rare blood types, congenital abnormalities requiring future blood product transfusion during surgical correction, sickle cell anemia, and hemophilia, in whom alloimmunization may complicate future blood transfusions

## INDICATIONS FOR POSTOPERATIVE BLOOD SALVAGE

Blood salvage in the postoperative period is almost exclusively used after cardiac, thoracic, and vascular procedures and orthopedic procedures for joint replacement and major spinal operations.[112,130–133] Because wound drainage devices are almost always used after these procedures, it has been a relatively simple matter to substitute collection canisters suitable for autotransfusion of salvaged blood should it be later desired. Blood salvaged from serous cavities or orthopedic wounds can be autotransfused if free of significant hemolysis, contamination, or clots and should not be allowed to stand in a collection chamber for more than 4–6 hours.[99,107,123,134,135]

Postoperative blood salvage is not widespread. Although some institutions routinely use postoperative blood salvage, others may reserve its use to only those patients in whom substantial postoperative bleeding is anticipated, in patients expressly desiring alternatives to allogeneic blood, when allogeneic blood is difficult to obtain, or in patients whose religious beliefs disallow allogeneic blood transfusion. The main reason appears to be a hesitancy to transfuse unwashed blood, although most data do not support such a position.[120,136,137] Cell-washing systems have been used in the postanesthesia care and intensive care units with some success and are becoming increasingly common.[137,138] The appearance of cell processors in the postsurgical unit has been limited because of the high cost of these devices and the need for trained personnel to operate them. Alternately, blood salvaged by filtration can be transported to the blood bank for processing before reinfusion. This process is more troublesome, time-consuming, expensive, and increases risks because the blood leaves the vicinity of the patient.

## INDICATIONS FOR BLOOD SALVAGE IN THE EMERGENCY ROOM

Indications for the use of blood salvage in the emergency room include (*a*) blunt or penetrating chest trauma with an acute chest tube loss of 1500 mL or more[107,134]; (*b*) patients requiring immediate transfusion in whom no allogeneic blood is available because of the urgency of the situation, blood bank shortages, or a difficult cross match—in such patients autotransfusion has been used regardless of the type of injury or degree of contamination[107]; (*c*) patients requiring immediate thoracotomy or sternotomy; (*d*) as a supplement to massive allogeneic blood transfusion; and (*e*) for patients who cannot be transfused with allogeneic blood (rare blood types, lack of stored compatible blood, or religious beliefs).[65,105,117]

# DISADVANTAGES, COMPLICATIONS, AND CONTRAINDICATIONS FOR BLOOD SALVAGE

## Disadvantages and Complications of Blood Salvage

The principle disadvantages of blood salvage may include the high cost of blood salvage technology (primarily cell processing), the quality of salvaged blood, the utility of blood salvage during massive blood loss, the possibility of inadvertent infusion of contaminated salvaged blood, and the inability of these techniques to completely avoid allogeneic blood transfusion (Table 9–3).

The utility of blood salvage is often dependant on the rate of blood loss, the salvage harvest, the quality of the infusate, and the rate of reinfusion. Massive hemorrhage is defined as blood loss in excess of 15 units of blood in the adult and 1–1.5 times the blood volume in the pediatric patient. Despite meticulous attention, blood salvaging yields only a portion of the shed RBCs, because some blood is invariably lost to drapes and sponges or is inaccessible to suction, and many RBCs

**Table 9–3.  Potential Complications of Blood Salvage**

Erythrocytes
　Hemoglobinemia
　Shortened survival
　Procoagulant membrane debris
Platelets
　Quantitative, qualitative defects
　Procoagulant aggregates
Clotting factors
　Depletion
　Procoagulant activation
Inadvertent transfusion
　Fat globules and denatured plasma lipoproteins
　Tissue debris (bone, cartilage, marrow)
　Air
　Heparin
　Bone cement
　Bacteria
　Tumor cells
　Amniotic fluid
Uncertain perioperative drug metabolism

Modified from Eisenstaedt RS: Operative red cell salvage and auto-transfusion. Transfu Sci 1989; 10:185, with permission.

are trapped in clots, filters, or are lost or damaged during aspiration and processing. Furthermore, salvaging (by filtration or cell processing) may alter the chemical and hematological constituents of blood, particularly after the loss and replacement of several blood volumes. In such cases, specific component therapy may be required to replace lost cellular elements, coagulation factors, and reestablish electrolyte balance.

The discontinuous collection-reinfusion nature and limited capacity of filtration and cell processors decreased their effectiveness during periods of massive blood loss.[83,139] Although improvements in capacity and processing speed have been incorporated in more recent technology, delays in reinfusion resulting from processing (filtration or washing/centrifugation) often necessitate the rapid infusion of allogeneic blood by using a high-volume rapid-infusion device. For this purpose, rapid-infusion devices capable of infusing warmed fluids at rates greater than 250 mL/min have been introduced (see Chapter 1: Principles of Blood Transfusion).

Compliment-induced granulocyte aggregation has been reported as a mechanism to explain noncardiogenic pulmonary edema and complement cascade activation by autotransfusion of salvaged blood.[140] Bengston and colleagues[141] showed elevations in both C3a and C5a fragments in postoperative wound drainage, although no patient developed clinical effects. Other sources of compliment activation can be traced to nylon, cellophane, silicone polymer, possible components of blood salvage apparatus, and endotoxin contamination.[142] Bland and associates[143] have demonstrated the high incidence of endotoxin contamination in blood salvaged from open chest during cardiac surgery.

## CONTRAINDICATIONS FOR BLOOD SALVAGE

The contraindications for the use of blood salvage all appear to be controversial as to whether absolute or relative. Table 9–4 lists some suggested contraindications. All of the suggested contraindications (except for its use in some Jehovah's Witness patients) are related to altered characteristics of salvaged blood that may potentially be deleterious. The word "potentially" should be emphasized,

**Table 9–4. Potential Contraindications of Blood Salvage**

Extravasated blood over 6 hours old
Suspected or confirmed enteric contamination
Suspected or confirmed malignant cell contamination
In the presence of amniotic fluid contamination (cesarean section)
Sickle cell anemia patients
Hemolyzed blood
Some Jehovah's Witness patients
In the presence of certain hemostatic substances
In the presence of some wound-sterilizing substances
Surgical excision of pheochromocytoma tumors
Patients with positive viral antigen markers

because data supporting these assumptions are either nonexistent or inconclusive.

A possible contraindication that should be seriously considered is the use of blood salvage techniques in patients positive for the acquired immunodeficiency virus or hepatitis B surface antigen. In these situations, the benefit to the patient should be weighed against the potential risks posed to staff handling such blood.[118,144]

## ADMINISTRATIVE ASPECTS OF BLOOD SALVAGE

Perioperative blood salvage is an important aspect of a comprehensive blood conservation program. However, cell-processing technology is expensive, and therefore the need for this service must be carefully considered before the initiation of such a program. Establishment of an effective program is much easier if physicians are enthusiastic. Special effort must be made to educate and inform the uninterested as well. Finally, the type of technology purchased should be based on specific requirements of the institution.[123]

A qualified individual (preferably a physician) should assume responsibility for the program. This selected individual should be (or become) knowledgeable concerning blood salvage devices, prepare protocols, and direct the training of personnel. Surgeons, anesthesiologists, transfusion medicine specialists, and hematologists are particularly suited for such duty. The transfusion committee (or its equivalent) should oversee all aspects of such a program. Their responsibilities should include approving protocols for autologous transfusion and reviewing utilization of autologous blood or blood products, as well as of the service in general.[123]

Protocols defining accepted procedures; hours of service; procedure scheduling; qualifications of the operators; equipment maintenance; and labeling, handling, and storage of autologous blood should be written by the administrator of the service and approved by the transfusion committee. Care and maintenance of equipment should be in accordance with the manufacturers recommendations and records must be maintained. Cleaning procedures and sterile technique should conform to those recommended by the institutional infection control committee. It is strongly recommended that a log of all procedures be kept. This log can be important when auditing usage of the service. Information should include date, patient name, hospital identification number, operative procedure, surgeon, anesthesiologist, time of procedure, amount of blood salvaged and reinfused, type and amount of anticoagulant, operator's name, pertinent laboratory studies, and any complications. Logging of unit or lot numbers of disposable items can be valuable in cases of infection. The use of blood salvage techniques should be noted in the patient chart along with other appropriate information.

Blood leaving the immediate vicinity of the patient (for further processing in the blood bank and so on) should be conspicuously labeled and identified to prevent mishandling.[114] Often any blood received by the blood bank must be ABO and Rh typed before return to the patient. Blood salvaged outside the operating room requires similar documentation.

The autologous program should be included in the hospital's quality assurance program. Mechanisms for review of protocols, usage, product quality, equipment performance and maintenance schedules, and adherence to protocols should be included. Both patient-specific chart reviews and program-wide reviews are recommended.[118,123,145]

## Costs

The initial purchase price of a cell processor is high. Depending on the degree of automation and capability of performing various additional functions (e.g., sequestration of plate-let-rich plasma), the initial cost of a cell processor may vary between $20,000 and $40,000. There are two approaches to obtaining blood salvage equipment. First, the equipment can be purchased outright, or in some circumstances a contractual arrangement can be entered with the distributor whereby the equipment is provided either by lease agreement or free of charge with the understanding that a specified number of disposable processing sets will be purchased (usually at an inflated cost) over a period of time. When blood processing equipment requiring the presence of trained personnel is used, that operator is usually provided by the institution. This individual is responsible for assembling the apparatus, selecting cycling parameters, regulating the amount of anticoagulant, changing solution and waste bags, and monitoring and documenting all aspects of the procedure.[119] In some areas, a regional blood center or private company will offer this service. In this case, the institution is charged for the service as determined either by type of case, by hourly charge, or by some combination of the two. In determining the cost of providing blood salvage, several factors must be considered. Besides the allocated cost of the capital equipment, the costs of the collection reservoir, disposable processing software, consumable supplies (anticoagulant, wash solutions, reinfusion bags), and personnel must be considered. Of course, the cost of the first unit will be the most expensive, with succeeding units considerably less expensive (until exhaustion of software and consumable supplies).

The allocated cost of the capital equipment (cell processor) can be calculated by adding the initial purchase price (less residual or scrap value) to the anticipated cost of service and maintenance over its useful life and, in some accounting systems, the anticipated cost of replacement, divided by the anticipated usage. In a calculation of the cost-effectiveness, this calculated cost must be compared with the total cost of administering allogeneic blood.

Cost analyses have shown that when blood loss ordinarily requires the transfusion of two or more units of blood, blood salvaging becomes economically feasible.[110,146] In a careful examination of cost-effectiveness of routine blood salvaging during coronary artery surgery, Nightingale and associates[109] found that although intraoperative (by cell processing) and postoperative mediastinal (filtration) blood salvage maneuvers decreased allogeneic blood requirements, only mediastinal drainage collection and reinfusion was related to a net decrease in costs. However, these data do not reflect the reduction in risks, as compared with the transfusion of allogeneic blood. The economic benefit from reduction of transfusion-related complications are probably significant, although difficult to estimate.[80,81,147] Although the hardware can be expensive, the per patient cost is reduced by use of the same software for the transfusion of multiple units.

## Personnel

Recent American Association of Blood Banks (AABB) guidelines[123] emphasized the importance of trained and dedicated (without other concurrent duties) operators of intraoperative blood salvage equipment. The use of these instruments (primarily cell processors) should not be casually delegated to members of the surgical or anesthesia team caring for the patient.[123] This is especially important when blood salvage schemes include automated or continuous direct reinfusion of salvaged blood (e.g., Jehovah's Witnesses or intraoperative platelet sequestration). Although cost efficiency may dictate heaping other duties and responsibilities on the operator of blood salvage equipment, this inclination should be avoided.[148,149]

Stemming from their extensive experience with extracorporeal circuits, cardiotomy suction, and early experience with blood salvage technology, perfusionists emerge as the likeliest candidates to provide these services. However, perfusionists are not available in all institutions or may be otherwise unable to provide services outside cardiac procedures.[148] Hence, other personnel (either hospital-based or outside contractors) such as anesthesiologists, nurse anesthetists, operating room/anesthesia nurses or technicians, regional or local blood bank technologists, and transfusion or intravenous therapy nurses have been used.[148,150] The most effective use of personnel will vary with the type of institution and the volume and character of the surgical practice.[118]

Until recently, the use of cell processors outside the operating room has been limited.

Although newer less-expensive "transportable" blood processors are now becoming available, filtration systems are still extensively used in these areas. These are much simpler to use, requiring minimal training of existing personnel. High nurse's acceptance of filtration devices has popularized their use of blood salvage techniques in these areas.[151,152] This probably stems from similarities in function and equipment to traditional methods of treatment of hemothoraces and postoperative wound drainage.

## BLOOD SALVAGE APPARATUS

Currently available blood salvage technology can be divided into two types: filtration and cell processors.

### Filtration

Blood salvage by filtration is based on the tenet that the mere extravasation of blood does not render that blood unfit for reinfusion provided coagulation, contamination, and significant hemolysis are prevented. Shed blood is altered only by filtration (typical filter sizes of 170 $\mu$m during collection and 20–50 $\mu$m during reinfusion) and the addition of anticoagulant, if required. Lacking sophisticated technology, blood salvage has been accomplished by variants of this principle since first reported in 1888. Various filtration systems are available today that differ slightly depending on the route of administration of anticoagulant, intraoperative or postoperative usage, portability, and direct versus indirect reinfusion.

Blood is collected in a reservoir ranging in size between 500 and 3000 mL (Fig. 9–4). This reservoir can be divided into two chambers separated by a course mesh filter (150–180 $\mu$m) or a single chamber with a course mesh filter incorporated into the inlet. A regulated vacuum source is connected to the reservoir, and negative pressure is limited to below $-150$ mm Hg (and as low as $-30$ to $-50$ mm Hg) to prevent damage to formed blood elements. Foaming inside the reservoir is prevented by the presence of a defoaming material either inside the chamber or a coating on the course filter. When the patient is not systemically heparinized anticoagulant must be added to either the reservoir before collection of blood or administered through the use

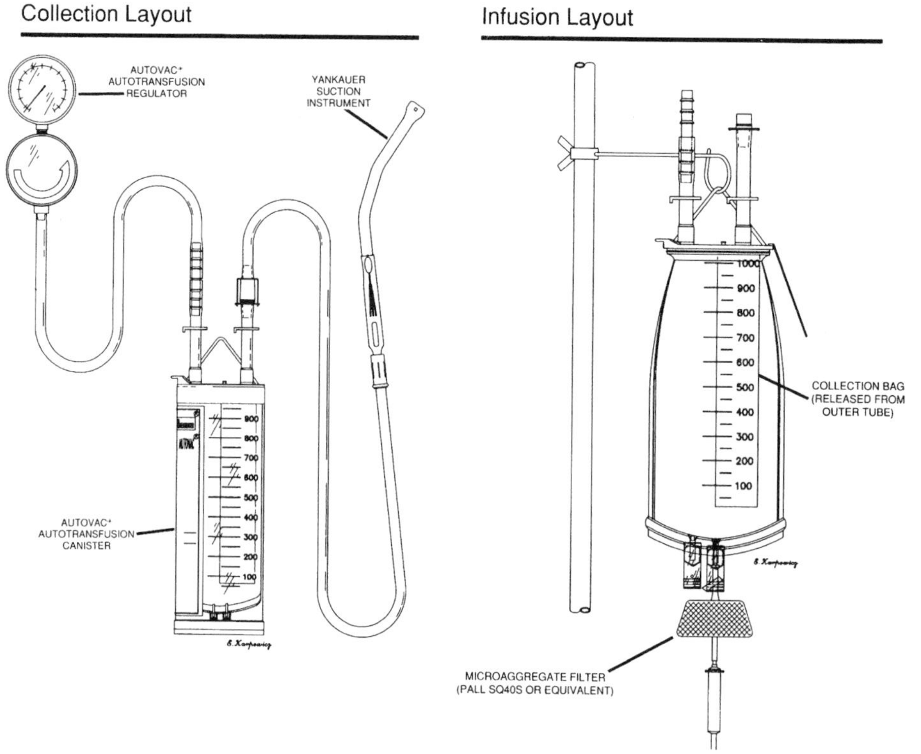

## Collection Layout

## Infusion Layout

**Fig. 9–4.** Schematic diagram of a filtration system. Courtesy of Boehringer Laboratories, Inc., Norristown, PA.

of dual-channeled suction tubing through which shed blood is aspirated and mixed with anticoagulant solution near the tip of a specially designed suction wand.[153,154] Heparinized saline, citrate-phosphate-dextrose (CPD), and acid-citrate-dextrose (ACD) formulas have all been used. Citrate anticoagulants are particularly advantageous in filtration systems because of negligible systemic effects (provided citrated blood is not reinfused too rapidly or in excessive volumes). Anticoagulant requirements may vary depending on the location and extent of bleeding, especially during collection from cavernous sinuses. Intraoperatively, citrated solutions are used in a ratio of one part anticoagulant to seven parts blood. When patients are already heparinized, heparin in a concentration of 20,000–40,000 units/L is usually effective.[155] After collection and course filtration, salvaged blood can be reinfused to the patient. Depending on manufacturer, either part or the entire reservoir can serve as the readministration bag, or blood is transferred to a blood bag before reinfusion.

If blood cannot be immediately reinfused, blood can be stored in a reservoir for up to 6 hours at 20–24°C, according to AABB guidelines.[123] Ideally, the time from initiation of collection of blood to transfusion should not exceed 6 hours. Although these recommendations include replacement of software used for salvaging, this is not always practical in the presence of ongoing blood loss.

The addition of a microaggregate filter (10–50 $\mu$m) is almost universally accepted during reinfusion of salvaged blood, although documentation on the necessity of these filters is not complete. Although Schaff and associates[112] demonstrated that all formed blood elements (RBCs, leukocytes, and platelets) readily pass through 40-$\mu$m filters, others have provided arguments against their routine use. Fine filters are often used as an extra measure to prevent transfusion of microaggregates that may pass through standard 120- to 170-$\mu$m transfusion filters.[156,157] Of particular concern was the effect of platelet and leukocyte microaggregates on the pulmonary microvasculature. Microaggregate embolism of the fine pulmonary vessels has been shown to lead to pulmonary hypertension, resulting in pulmonary insufficiency.[78,107,158–162] Theoretically, these fine-mesh filters, ranging in size between 10 and 50 $\mu$m, should trap platelets.[108,163,164] Because platelet count and function are diminished in banked blood over 48 hours old,[165–167] their use is probably inconsequential and perhaps beneficial. However, their use during transfusion of fresh blood, either banked or autotransfused, or platelet concentrates remains controversial.[108,112,163,168] Furthermore, it has been proposed that the microaggregates in salvaged blood are composed of adhesive platelets that readily dissociate upon reinfusion, as opposed to stored blood aggregates, which do not.[169,170] Because the AABB[123] recommends strict adherence to manufacturer's recommendations, the use of fine filtration during reinfusion is generally accepted.

The principal advantages of blood salvage by filtration are related to the simplicity of their design and ease of operation. Setup and operation of filtration systems do not require specialized training nor is a dedicated operator normally necessary. Other than a vacuum source and an anticoagulant solution, the disposable units are entirely self-contained. Because no blood processing (beyond filtration) is required, shed blood drawn into the collection chamber is immediately available for reinfusion. The cost of blood salvage by filtration is generally lower than that associated with cell processing.

## Cell Processing

Processing (centrifugation and washing) of salvaged blood before reinfusion was first proposed by Wilson and Taswell[60] in the late 1960s for use during transurethral resection of the prostate. Processing provided a means of contaminant removal from salvaged blood, mainly large volumes of irrigation fluid. The heavily diluted blood (with an HCT between 1 and 3%) from the surgical field was aspirated into a continuous-flow centrifuge that separated formed blood elements (RBCs, leukocytes, and platelets) into zones according to their sedimentation rates and buoyant densities. The supernatant fluid consisting of irrigating solution and plasma was passed out of the bowl as waste. After the 240-mL centrifuge bowl filled with RBCs (HCT 60–70%), the RBCs were washed with Ringer's lactate

solution and resuspended to any desired HCT, transferred into plastic blood bags, and reinfused by gravity through a standard blood administration set. No anticoagulants were required because clotting factors in the salvaged blood were highly diluted initially and later almost totally removed with the waste supernatant[60,171,172] (Fig. 9–5).

The first commercially available blood processors for intraoperative use were marketed in the mid-1970s.[68] In basic principle and function, they were similar to the system designed at the Mayo Clinic.[60,171,172] Cell processors are semicontinuous flow devices that filter, wash, and pack shed RBCs collected from the surgical field.[155]

The four manufacturers who now supply the majority of cell-processing devices for perioperative use in the United States are COBE Laboratories (Lakewood, CO), Electromedics (Englewood, CO), Haemonetics (Braintree, MA), and Sorin (Irvine, CA). Each manufacturer provides a variety of instruments with varying degrees of sophistication, functions, and portability. Accordingly, their initial purchase price can vary between $20,000 and $40,000. However, all currently available cell processors do share basic schematic similarities (Fig. 9–6). The use of a cell processor also requires disposable software (collection reservoir, centrifuge bowl, tubing, blood bags, waste container, and suction wand) ($150 to $200), as well as solutions (anticoagulant and washing solutions). Local anticoagulation (in the nonsystemically anticoagulated patient) can be accomplished with either ACD, CPD, or heparin. A metered amount of this anticoagulant is delivered to the suction tip through one lumen of a double-lumened suction wand where it mixes with blood aspirated from the surgical wound. This blood-anticoagulant mixture is drawn into a cardiotomy reservoir with vacuum ($< -100$ mm Hg) usually supplied either from central wall vacuum or an internal vacuum pump. The cardiotomy reservoir contains an integral mesh filter (170 $\mu$m to as low as 20 $\mu$m) whose function is similar to that in filtration salvage systems: removal of gross surgical debris, clots, and microaggregates. Beyond this point, however, any similarity to filtration salvage systems is lost. Although blood salvaged by filtration would be transfused back to the patient after this initial filtration, these previ-

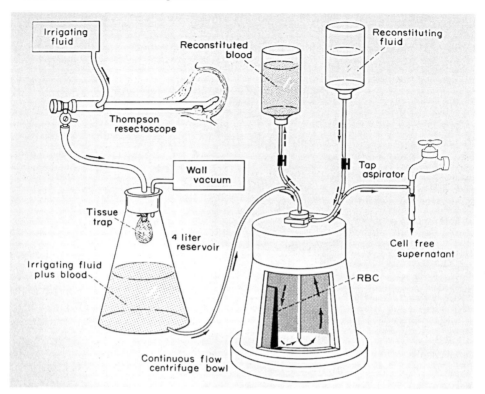

**Fig. 9–5.** Schematic representation of blood processor designed by Wilson and Taswell at the Mayo Clinic for autotransfusion during transurethral resection of the prostrate. From Wilson JD, Taswell HF: Autotransfusion: historical review and preliminary report on a new method. Mayo Clinic Proc 1968; 43:26, with permission.

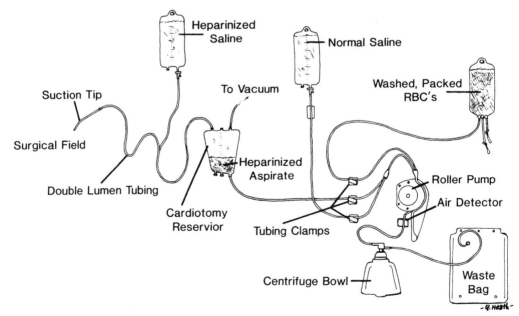

**Fig. 9–6.** Diagram of components of a typical centrifuge-based blood salvage instrument. From Salem MR, Bikhazi GP: Blood conservation. In: Motoyama EK, Davis PJ, eds, Smith's Anesthesia for Infants and Children, 5 ed. St. Louis, 1990, C.V. Mosby, with permission.

ous steps are only preliminary ones for blood that will be further processed.[155]

When sufficient blood has accumulated into the collection reservoir, blood is allowed to flow into a bowl where centrifugation and washing takes place. The processing cycle begins when an electric or pneumatic solenoid valve opens, allowing the collected blood to flow into the spinning centrifuge bowl ($\approx 5000$ rpm). The spinning bowl separates the blood components on the basis of density. The high density of RBCs causes them to line the outer wall of the bowl, whereas components of less density separate at their distinctive levels. As the level of RBCs rises, plasma is continually displaced and eventually spills over into the waste container. An optical scanner or the instrument operator determines when the bowl is full and spill-over of RBCs into the waste is imminent. At this point the solenoid valve closes to prevent further entry of blood. The washing cycle begins immediately after closure of this valve, when a second valve opens to admit the wash solution (usually 0.9% NaCl) into the bowl. While continuously spinning, this wash solution rinses away any remaining low-density constituents. After washing, packed RBCs are pumped from the centrifuge bowl into a transfusion blood bag for reinfusion to the patient. In some center, the washing cycle is sometimes (and even routinely) eliminated, resulting in salvaged blood that is merely packed to a desired HCT.

From the above generic functional description of blood salvaging by cell processing, one is immediately confronted with the major disadvantages of this technique: the procedures of collection, processing, and reinfusion are discontinuous; processing introduces another step into the blood salvage technique; and, finally, the capacity of the system to keep pace with substantial blood loss is limited by the processing time and centrifuge bowl capacity.

The collection, processing, and reinfusion operations are purposely discontinuous, although in certain situations, such as in Jehovah's Witnesses, these functions must necessarily be made continuous[173] (see Chapter 11: Blood Conservation in Jehovah's Witnesses). Significant cost savings are realized by individually packing, collecting, and processing software. In most situations, when the magnitude of blood loss cannot be estimated preoperatively, only the collection apparatus (reservoir,

suction wand and tubing, and anticoagulant) need be set up. If intraoperative blood loss does not warrant processing, the software and personnel costs associated with processing are saved. However, if blood loss does reach a level that makes processing desirable, the processing apparatus can be set up within minutes by an experienced operator. Finally, shed blood suspected of bacterial contamination can be collected and reserved until surgical exploration rules out spillage of enteric contents into the surgical field.

Routine reinfusion of salvaged blood directly to the patient is not recommended because of an increased risk of air embolism.[174] An air detector on the tubing between the centrifuge bowl and transfusion bag is not totally reliable. Thus, either pressure or gravity reinfusion of blood directly from the transfusion bag places the patient at risk. In certain situations—such as Jehovah's Witnesses, who require continuous movement of blood in contact with their own circulation, and during preoperative platelet sequestration in noncardiac surgery—collection, processing, and reinfusion of shed blood can be made continuous. Caution should be exercised by both the salvage system operator and anesthesiologist in these situations to prevent air embolism.[174]

Processing time was once a major concern with the use of cell processors. The limiting factors affecting processor speed are flow rate into the centrifuge (the higher the flow rate, the lower the final HCT), centrifuge speed, and the volume of washing solution. Processing time can take between 2 and 10 minutes depending on the model of cell processor used. Hence, the cell processor can supply approximately 12 units of packed RBCs per hour when functioning at peak efficiency.[175] Efforts by manufacturers have been aimed at increasing processing speed without significantly lessening the quality of final product in terms of HCT or purity.

The rate at which shed blood is pumped into the centrifuge bowl is very important. Slower rates of infusion significantly increase the resultant HCT of the packed RBCs. At an infusion rate of 100 mL/min, the mean HCT can range between 68 and 80% with a mean of 72%. When an infusion rate of 250 mL/min is used, a mean HCT of 61% (range 54–65%) may be obtained.[176,177]

The wash cycle functions to remove any residual contaminants (anticoagulant, plasma free hemoglobin, RBC stroma, and clotting factors) in the packed RBCs. Although Wilson and associates[60,171,172] used lactated Ringer's solution in their initial experience with the cell processor, 0.9% NaCl is now the standard wash solution. The minimum volume of saline wash is between 500 and 700 mL.[178–180] The standard wash solution volume is usually approximately 1000 mL, although 1500–2000 mL may be used in orthopedic procedures where contamination with surgical debris, fat, chemical substances (methylmethacrylate or antibiotic-laden irrigation solutions), and hemostatic agents such as bone wax or absorbable gelatin sponge (Gelfoam®, UpJohn Laboratories, Kalamazoo, MI) may be present. Larger volumes of wash have also been used in cases of suspected or known contamination with enteric contents. Various reports have documented that large wash volumes can significantly reduce but do not completely eliminate bacterial contamination.[181–185] However, most physicians will not reinfuse this salvaged blood, except in extraordinary circumstances (see "Blood Salvage for Trauma Surgery"). When large volumes of blood are lost rapidly and processing cannot keep pace with collection, the washing cycle can be either abbreviated or eliminated.

The minimum volume of salvaged blood required for processing in the standard 225- to 250-mL centrifuge bowl is approximately 500 mL. Because processing should be performed in aliquots of 500 mL, the collection reservoir should have the capacity to store large volumes of blood in case of acute hemorrhage. Some manufacturers offer an oversized (375 mL) bowl for use when substantial blood loss is anticipated. Smaller volume bowls for use in pediatric patients are also now available from all manufacturers. These bowls may range in volume between 125 and 175 mL. When using either oversized or pediatric bowls, minimal salvaged blood requirements are adjusted accordingly. Bowl design has centered around two different types. Most manufacturers offer the Latham-style centrifuge bowl, whereas COBE uses the Baylor-style bowl (Fig. 9–7). The claimed advantage of the Baylor design is faster processing.

When systemic heparinization is not used, local anticoagulation of salvaged blood can be accomplished with either citrate or heparin.

Using a double-lumened suction wand, anticoagulant is mixed with blood at the tip of the wand. By controlling the drip rate of anticoagulant, the salvage operator attempts to introduce anticoagulant in proportion to blood loss. As a rule, citrate should be added to blood in 1:5–1:10 (70 mL of citrate to 500 mL of salvaged blood) proportions. Heparin (30,000 units/L) should be mixed with blood in a 1:7 ratio (10 mL heparin solution to 100 mL of salvaged blood).[155] Because centrifugation and washing removes essentially all anticoagulant, fears of reheparinization or citrate toxicity are virtually eliminated. However, transfusion of large volumes of processed blood may cause dilution of coagulation factors and platelets and increase the requirements of intravenous drugs (heparin, muscle relaxants, narcotics, and anesthetics)[178] (see "Characteristics of Salvaged Blood").

The cell processor has also been used for the collection of platelet-rich plasma, intraoperatively. This practice is similar to plasmapheresis to obtain single-donor platelet packs in the blood bank. Used primarily in cardiac surgery, a quantity of autologous fresh plasma, high in functional platelets and labile coagulation factors, is collected before the initiation of cardiopulmonary bypass (CPB). This plasma is then used after surgery to promote hemostasis. Before instituting CPB, blood is slowly (20–80 mL/min) withdrawn from a side port of the venous line of the extracorporeal circuit and centrifuged but not washed. Blood is infused until spill over of RBCs into the waste bag occurs, by which time a majority of the platelets have been displaced. The waste (platelet-rich plasma) is stored at room temperature for later reinfusion. The packed RBCs can be added to the prime in the extracorporeal circuit or directly (or indirectly) transfused back to the patient.[88,186,187] Although, platelet sequestration is utilized primarily for cardiac surgery involving CPB, its use is not necessarily restricted to this type of surgery.[89,186,188–190]

Finally, the limitations of the cell processor in handling large volumes of blood, such as residual oxygenator blood, have increasingly led to the use of the hemoconcentrator. The hemoconcentrator uses ultrafiltration to effectively and rapidly hemoconcentrate blood by eliminating excessive plasma water. The

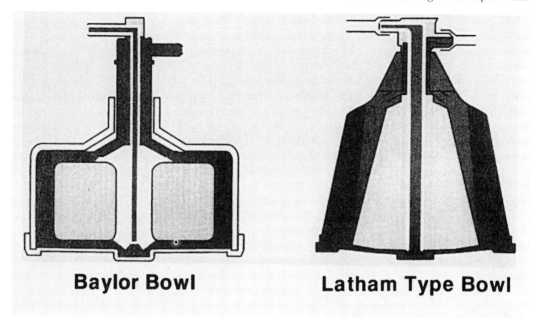

**Baylor Bowl**                    **Latham Type Bowl**

**Fig. 9–7.** Centrifuge bowls. *Left:* Baylor bowl. *Right:* Latham bowl. From Yawn DH: Properties of salvaged blood. In: Taswell HF, Pineda AA, eds, Autologous Transfusion and Hemotherapy. Boston, 1991, Blackwell Scientific Publishers, with permission.

hemoconcentrator is used primarily in association with an extracorporeal circuit and is discussed in Chapter 12: Blood Conservation in Special Situations: Cardiac Surgery.

## CHARACTERISTICS OF SALVAGED BLOOD

Since the first allusion to the salvage of shed blood, there has been constant concern about the quality of salvaged blood and the physiological effects of reinfusion of this extravasated blood. These concerns surround possible physical and biochemical alterations of blood after extravasation, collection and processing, and reinfusion that might render salvaged blood inferior to banked blood or blood products. That salvaged blood differs significantly from allogeneic banked blood or from circulating blood is undisputed (Table 9–5). However, the diverse circumstances under which shed blood can be salvaged and the various techniques used have resulted in salvaged blood products with diverse characteristics.

The earliest practitioners reinfused shed blood after minimal (course filtration) or no processing. The characteristics of the infusate, therefore, closely resembled those of the shed blood. However, many practitioners sus-

pected that blood sometimes containing large concentrations of plasma free hemoglobin, contaminated with cellular and surgical debris and possibly containing procoagulants, microaggregates, and bacteria, was unfit for transfusion. These suspicions, which have only partially been realized, remain today in some circles. Modern technology has evolved systems that can significantly alter the characteristics of salvaged blood by centrifugation, cell washing, and hemofiltration, resulting in an infusate bearing little resemblance to that of the shed blood. Accordingly, when considering the characteristics of salvaged blood and the physiological effects of its reinfusion, it becomes necessary to differentiate the techniques used.

### Filtration

QUANTITATIVE CHARACTERISTICS OF SALVAGED RED BLOOD CELLS

Postoperative anemia is a common occurrence after autotransfusion with filtration devices, particularly when this salvaged blood is the sole or primary source of replacement RBCs. Salvaged blood typically has a low HCT, with hemoglobin values ranging between 6 and 9 g/dL[149,191,192] (Table 9–5).

**Table 9–5.  Hematological Comparison of Bank and Salvaged Blood***

| Index Factor | Processed Salvaged Blood | Unprocessed Salvaged Blood | Bank Blood | Normal Blood |
|---|---|---|---|---|
| Hemoglobin (g/dL) | 17.9 | 6.3 ± 1.1 | 16.0 ± 3.5 | 12–17† |
| HCT (%) | | 17.0 ± 3.3 | 46.5 ± 10.5 | 37–50† |
| RBC (/mm³ × 10⁶) | | 2.0 ± 0.4 | 5.0 ± 1.1 | 4.8–5.8† |
| Leukocytes (/mm³ × 10³) | 1.1 | 3.4 ± 1.3 | 5.3 ± 2.3 | 7.0 |
| Platelets (/mm³ × 10³) | 64 | 384 ± 141 | 149 ± 78 | 250–350 |
| Free hemoglobin (mg/dL) | 123 | 1000 ± 625 | 13.3 ± 10.8 | <2.5 |
| Screen filtration pressure (mm Hg) | | 200 | 170 | N/A |
| pH | | 7.72 ± 0.18 | 6.63 ± 0.06 | 7.33–7.43 |
| $P_{CO_2}$ (mm Hg) | | 8.5 ± 4.0 | 158 ± 68 | 38–50 |
| $P_{O_2}$ (mm Hg) | | 160 ± 17 | 50 ± 25 | 60–108 |
| Sodium (mmol/L) | 147 ± 2.4 | 136 ± 5 | 162 ± 6 | 135–148 |
| Potassium (mmol/L) | 1.6 ± 1.5 | 6.8 ± 1.9 | 12.6 ± 4.6 | 3.5–5.3 |
| Chloride (mmol/L) | 134 ± 3.3 | 123 ± 5 | 76 ± 9 | 98–106 |
| $CO_2$ (mmol/L) | 5.4 ± 1.6 | 6 ± 1 | 11 ± 2 | 19–26 |
| Calcium (ionized) (mmol/L) | 2.3 ± 0.5 | 1.25 ± 0.2 | 2.25 ± 0.1 | 2.1–2.7 |
| SGOT (units) | 9 ± 5 | 128 ± 74 | 14 ± 4 | 6–21 |
| SGPT (units) | 15 ± 9 | 14 ± 6 | 11 ± 5 | 7–14 |
| LDH (units) | 214 ± 103 | 1605 ± 718 | 299 ± 146 | 85–190 |
| CPK (units) | | 1073 ± 983 | 96 ± 27 | 10–65 |
| Direct bilirubin (conjugated) (mg/dL) | | 0.4 ± 0.1 | 0.06 ± 0.02 | 0–0.2 |
| Total bilirubin (mg/dL) | 0.11 ± 0.07 | 0.7 ± 0.2 | 0.41 ± 0.13 | 0.2–1.0 |

* Modified Bentley ATS100 employed for blood salvage
† Range includes both male and female adults
Processed salvage data modified from Yawn DH: Properties of salvaged blood. In: Taswell HF, Pineda AA, eds, Autologous Transfusion and Hemotherapy. Boston, 1991, Blackwell Scientific Publishers, with permission. Filtration data modified from Aaron RK, Beazley RM, Riggle GC: Hematologic integrity after intraoperative allotransfusion. Arch Surg 1974; 108:831, with permission. Normal data from Fiereck EA: Appendix. In: Tietz NW, ed, Fundamentals of Clinical Chemistry, 2 ed. Philadelphia, 1976, W.B. Saunders, pp. 1177–1227, with permission.[490]

The autotransfusion of large volumes of salvaged blood of low HCT without benefit of centrifugation or hemoconcentration can result in unintentional systemic hemodilution. This may be further potentiated with fluid shifts in response to hemorrhage and when large volumes of crystalloid or colloid solutions are concomitantly infused.[119,193]

The low HCT of salvaged blood is related to several factors, including intravascular and extravascular hemolysis and coagulation before collection; dilution with apparatus priming, anticoagulant, and irrigation solutions and serous fluids; hemolysis and coagulation after collection and filtration; and the mass of unrecovered RBCs.[92,93,153,154,194] Thus, the theoretical advantages of salvaging fresh RBCs and avoiding transfusion of stored blood are partially offset by the inevitable loss, hemolysis, and RBC damage before and during the harvesting process.[144]

Although dilution cannot be entirely prevented, it can be lessened by use of modern salvage technology and strict adherence to technique.[195] Dilution occurs when shed blood is allowed to mingle with serous body fluids or wound irrigation solutions and during collection with salvage apparatus priming solutions and anticoagulants. Local anticoagulant volume should be limited to that necessary to prevent coagulation.[108] Unless bleeding is brisk, the addition of anticoagulant is often unnecessary when blood is collected from the cavernous sinuses.[119,123] Dilution with wound irrigation solutions can be limited by thoroughly suctioning shed blood from the surgical field immediately before the use of irrigation solutions and using waste suction after irrigation.

The primary cause of the low HCT of salvaged blood appears to be loss of RBCs to hemolysis, clots, and irretrievable shed blood. Although technique can substantially improve yield, loss of RBCs to these factors cannot be totally eliminated.[191,196] The total amount of RBC hemolysis has been estimated at anywhere between 2.5 and 15%.[197,198] Hemolysis can occur after extravasation but before collection (in situ) or as a result of the collection-reinfusion process.

Blood oozing from traumatically or surgically damaged vessels comes into contact with exposed endothelial tissue, rich in procoagulants, leukoattractants, and lysozymes, leading directly to hemolysis or loss of RBCs sequestered within clots caused by localized activation of the coagulation cascade.[199–201] The degree of damage caused by contact with mesothelial surfaces is probably related to the duration of contact, and thus immediate aspiration of shed blood allows insufficient time for adverse blood-tissue interactions.[202–204] Extravasated blood that remains in contact with the serous lining of cavernous sinuses is not only defibrinogenated but becomes hemolyzed after an extended period. As early as 1928, Filatov[205] demonstrated that blood allowed to remain in the peritoneum began to hemolyze in 16 hours and by 24 hours was grossly hemolyzed. Ricci and DiPalma[206] in 1931 observed that RBC deformation can occur after only 6 hours. Thus, one should be wary of pooled hemothorax or peritoneal blood more than 6 hours old.[65,123,207] Significant hemolysis is an indication that this blood should be discarded.

Damage of RBCs during collection are commonly attributed to trauma of the suction apparatus, filters, reservoir and tubing, the pumping mechanism, and entrapment of RBCs in clots during extravascular coagulation.[80,81,92,93,108,154,194,198,208] The most damaging aspect of collection is probably the aspiration of shed blood. The usual way of suctioning during surgical procedures produces foaming as a result of an intensive blood-air interface. This extensive interface is responsible for a number of complications of massive autotransfusion, that is, hemolysis, coagulation defects, platelet microaggregate formation, and excessive postoperative bleeding. The RBC membrane, subject to high shear stresses by turbulent flow within the suction tubing, can either immediately lyse or deform, thus reducing RBC survival.[209–211] By placing the suction wand tip below the surface of pooled blood to prevent the aspiration of air, this interface can be minimized.[204] For this reason RBC harvest is generally higher in cardiothoracic and abdominal surgeries where blood tends to pool in cavities than in surgical procedures in noncavernous sites, such as spinal fusion or joint arthroplastic procedures.[212] Other techniques, such as limiting the suction-negative pressure generated, the use of the shortest and widest possible suction tubing, and the avoidance of roller pump heads in the autotransfusion system, have been advocated and incorporated into present-day blood salvage technology.[63,83,113,213,214] Although most manufacturers recommend limiting suction below $-150$ mm Hg negative pressure, significantly lower pressures (under $-100$ mm Hg and as low as $-40$ to $-50$ mm Hg) can be used, especially when bleeding is not profuse.[123] Filters can be impregnated with anticoagulant and antifoaming agents to prevent excessive clotting on the filter mesh. As a mesh filter becomes clogged with clots and debris, higher pressures are required for passage of subsequent blood through the filter (screen-filtration pressures). The resultant higher pressures and turbulence increase the likelihood of lysis or deformation of all formed blood elements. The addition of anticoagulant at the suction wand tip is an important factor in reducing the loss and damage to RBCs, platelets, leukocytes, and coagulation factors along apparatus surfaces.

Hemolysis and dilution are not the only factors precipitating postoperative anemia after blood salvaging. All shed blood is not salvageable. Harvest depends on various factors, including the accessibility of the shed blood; the capacity of the salvage apparatus during massive hemorrhage; loss of RBCs to nonanticoagulated surfaces and to filters, sponges, drapes, and disposable suction; the skill and experience of the surgical team; and finally the degree of RBC destruction.[108,159,191,215]

## QUALITATIVE ANALYSIS OF SALVAGED RED BLOOD CELLS

Isotope-labeled RBC studies indicate that those RBCs that are salvaged have a relatively normal half-life,[83,92,93,159,196,216–218] which does not differ from normal RBCs.[191] Concentrations of 2,3-DPG in salvaged RBCs are normal in comparison to nonsalvaged RBCs and significantly higher than banked allogeneic blood.[106,184,191] Autotransfused blood tends to have a higher P50 and a more normal pH than banked blood.[219–221] Salvaged RBCs are more resistant to osmotic lysis. These factors probably represent the survival of the healthiest RBCs, reuptake by the reticuloendothelial system of sublethally damaged RBCs, and hemolysis of the frailest RBCs.[106,149,196,222]

High levels of free plasma hemoglobin and cellular debris resulting from hemolysis have been shown to be nephrotoxic, although the exact mechanism remains in question.[223] This toxicity was demonstrated in one of the first reported deaths specifically identified with autotransfusion, a case of gross hemoglobinuria.[224] Schweitzer[224] reinfused blood that had remained in a body cavity over 24 hours, during which time, although unclotted, had become hemolyzed. Hemolysis can occur in vivo, by mechanical churning and contact with extravascular tissues in blood pooled in a body cavity, and in vitro, with trauma from suction and filtration, compression in roller pump heads, contact with air and tissue, turbulent flow, and foaming.[63,215] Intensive blood-air contact encountered during normally applied suction was found to be the most damaging factor for RBCs and platelets.[204] The degree of hemolysis or, more easily measured, the level of free plasma hemoglobin at which nephrotoxicity should be feared is unknown. Previous observations have confirmed that infusion of plasma free hemoglobin is not detrimental to renal function in the nonacidotic patient with an adequate urine output.[225] Under normal circumstances, the reticuloendothelial system can remove plasma free hemoglobin in concentrations up to 120 mg/dL. Above this level renal excretion occurs. Levels approaching 1600 mg/dL were seen in salvaged blood that was reinfused without consequence.[154,198,226] Whatever the toxic level might be, adequate hydration, avoidance of hypotension and acidosis, and maintenance of urinary output with appropriate use of diuretics or dopamine have been shown to prevent this complication.[107,202]

## PLATELETS, LEUKOCYTES, AND COAGULATION FACTORS

Although platelets, leukocytes, and coagulation factors are reduced in salvaged blood, they may still be substantial.[180,227–231] The concentration of these components in unprocessed salvaged blood is dependant on their concentration in the patient's blood; loss in salvage apparatus; and dilution with anticoagulant, tissue fluids, and irrigation solutions.[149]

Those platelets that are recovered have been shown to have released $\beta$-thromboglobulin, thromboxane $A_2$, serotonin, and lactic dehydrogenase, demonstrating platelet activation.[136,207] Morphological changes in salvaged platelets are difficult to analyze. Platelets have been described under light microscopy as "normal,"[149] shape-changed,[232] and/or degranulated.[233] Neither human[83] nor animal[211,234] aggregation studies have clearly demonstrated that salvaged platelets are functional.

Leukocytes are present in unwashed salvaged blood in varying quantities. Virtually no information is present concerning leukocyte function in salvaged blood or the effects of their depletion during massive autotransfusion.

The concentration of coagulation factors and the clotting competency of salvaged blood are often specifically determined by the location and circumstances of collection. Blood salvaged from the mediastinum, pleural space, and peritoneal cavity has undergone extensive coagulation and clot lysis and is virtually devoid of fibrinogen. Fibrinogen may be significantly higher in blood salvaged from systemically anticoagulated patients. Some investigators ascribe this hypofibrinogenemia to selective fibrinogenolysis; recent work also reveals depleted levels of factor VIII coagulant activity and factor V.[235] Extensive proteolysis is suggested by elevated level of peptides derived from plasmin-lysed fibrin and thrombin-lysed fibrinogen.[230] Antithrombin III and plasminogen concentrations of 40–50% of normal have been found. Fibrin degradation products (FDPs), the result of intravascular and extravascular coagulation and fibrinolysis, are markedly increased in filtered blood.[137,236]

The clotting competency of cavernous sinus blood was examined as early as 1914 by Thies.[4] Rietz[237] believed that defibrination occurred through respiratory movements, and Filatov[205] suggested that it was a selective biochemical reaction between blood and secretions of the serous lining of the cavity. In dogs, Rietz[237] showed that intraperitoneal blood became defibrinated and thus suitable for reinfusion without anticoagulation in as little as 15 minutes. Blood removed from a cavernous space displays increased prothrombin time (PT) and activated partial thromboplastin time (PTT), causing Kongsgaard and associates[231] to believe that most of the fibrinogen is consumed in the cavity, via activation of both the intrinsic and extrinsic, before collection.

## CONSEQUENCES OF REINFUSION OF FILTERED SALVAGED BLOOD

The perioperative autotransfusion of small to moderate volumes of unwashed filtered shed blood has been shown to be safe and effective. Hematological abormalities consequent of the transfusion of this blood product normalize early within the postoperative period and are not usually associated with incrased mortality or hemotological, cardiopulmonary, or renal complications.[236]

Besides the presence of the normal constituents of blood, blood salvaged by filtration may contain various other substances. These substances may have been present in the blood before extravasation or may result from extravasation, collection, and filtration. An inherent property of filtration is that elements smaller than the finest filter (usually 20–50 $\mu m$) or dissolved substances readily pass through and therefore may be present in the infusate. It is the possible presence of these substances, in combination with the dilute nature of salvaged blood, that accounts for much of the concern about reinfusing nonprocessed salvaged blood.

In unknown concentrations, previously administered anesthetic drugs (intact or metabolized), heparin (during systemic anticoagulation), catecholamines (during excision or manipulation of a pheochromocytoma tumor), FDPs and D-dimers (resulting from intravascular fibrinolytic activity), and methylmethacrylate (during cemented joint arthroplasty) may be present in shed blood. After extravasation, blood may become further contaminated by hemolysis, resulting in increased concentrations of free plasma hemoglobin and stoma debris, activated coagulation factors and products released from aggregated platelets (serotonin, histamine, or catecholamines), plasma cardiac enzymes, bacteria from contact with contaminated wound surfaces, topically administered substances (absorbable gelatin sponge, thrombin, oxidized cellulose sponge, microfibrillar collagen hemostat, fibrin glue), and antibiotic and bacteriocidal wash solutions. The vacuum necessary for collection of shed blood and high-screen-filtration pressures can cause excessive stress on cellular membranes of formed blood elements causing deformation or RBC lysis. Stress-induced lysis of RBCs results in further increases in free plasma hemoglobin and RBC stroma; lysis of platelets and leukocytes results in the release of various platelet activators, procoagulants, proteases, and lysozymes. The autotransfusion of blood salvaged after cardiac surgery has resulted in elevated plasma levels of creatine kinase, lactate dehydrogenase, and serum glutamic-oxaloacetic transaminase.[238] Anticoagulation with ACD or CPD solutions alter the composition of shed blood. Although having no systemic anticoagulant effects, citrate anticoagulants bind calcium and if administered in sufficient quantities over a short period of time can lead to citrate toxicity (hypocalcemia).

The reinfusion of blood containing these various contaminants remains controversial. Microaggregates can cause bronchoconstriction, increased pulmonary vascular resistance, and pulmonary hypertension.[16,159,239,240] Thrombocytopenia and coagulation disorder have been reported in patients receiving large quantities of salvaged blood.[84,108,114,116,202,241] The autotransfusion of blood salvaged by filtration has been implicated as a cause of DIC,[170,202] as evidenced by the presence of large quantities of FDPs (D-dimers) in salvaged blood. FDPs interfere with platelet aggregation and the polymerization of fibrin and thus have the potential not only to signal fibrinolysis but also directly to cause or aggravate a coagulopathy.[241] Although there is evidence that systemic anticoagulation can avert considerable loss of RBCs, platelets, and fibrinogen, this is rarely feasible, except when the surgical procedure warrants it.[234]

Salvaged mediastinal blood contains reduced numbers of platelets, either temporarily or permanently dysfunctional; reduced levels of activated coagulation factors; minimal fibrinogen; and fibrin-degradation products. Thus, when larger volumes of shed blood are transfused, signs of clinical bleeding should be monitored and the need for fresh frozen plasma and platelet concentrates considered.[232] However, component replacement is usually unnecessary. The transfusion of even

**Table 9–6.   Changes in Hematological Variables and Proteases During Mediastinal Blood Autotransfusion**

| | Patient Blood Preoperative | Shed Blood Before AT | Shed Blood After AT | Patient Blood After AT |
|---|---|---|---|---|
| Hemoglobin (g/dL) | 12.0 | 9.3 | 7.4 | 9.9 |
| Platelets ($\times 10^9$/L) | 224 | 71 | 119 | 129 |
| Free hemoglobin (mg/dL) | — | 311 | 410 | 430 |
| Total pl protein (g/dL) | — | 5.1 | 5.3 | 5.0 |
| Plasma albumin (g/dL) | — | 2.7 | 2.7 | 3.3 |
| Pthr (%) | 104 | 30 | 23 | 84 |
| AT-III (%) | 95 | 48 | 46 | 79 |
| TT (%) | 98 | 60 | 39 | 79 |
| NT (%) | 100 | 34 | 26 | 88 |
| APTT (sec) | 30 | 166 | 180 | 40 |
| Fibrinogen ($\mu$mol/L) | 7.9 | 0.6 | 0 | 7.1 |
| Pl (units/L) | 24 | 63 | 71 | 24 |
| Plg (%) | 92 | 65 | 68 | 72 |
| API (%) | 87 | 37 | 28 | 72 |
| FDP ($\mu$g/dL) | <100 | >300 | >300 | 100–300 |
| KK (units/L) | 9 | 46 | 58 | 7 |
| PKK (%) | 82 | 56 | 57 | 76 |
| KKI (%) | 92 | 44 | 45 | 87 |

Data compiled in 14 patients after undergoing coronary bypass or valvular replacement surgery. A mean of 482 mL was autotransfused during a mean 6.2-hour period. Note that patient values after 6 hours of autotransfusion are only moderately different from preoperative values, despite significant changes demonstrated in shed blood. pl., plasma; Pthr, prothrombin; AT-III, antithrombin-III; TT, thrombotest; NT, normotest; APTT, activated partial thromboplastin time; Pl, spontaneous plasmin activity; Plg, plasminogen; API, functional anti-plasmin activity; FDP, fibrin degradation products; KK, spontaneous kallikrein activity; PKK, prekallikrein; KKI, functional kallikrein inhibition. Modified from Kongsgaard UE, Tølløfsrud S, Brosstad F, and others: Autotransfusion after open heart surgery: characteristics of shed mediastinal blood and its influence on the plasma proteases in circulating blood. Acta Anaesthesiol Scand 1991; 35:71, with permission.

large volumes of shed blood is usually not accompanied with a low platelet count or increased PT, PTT, or bleeding.[103,112,116,130,242] That only slight decreases in fibrinogen concentration are seen in patients receiving large volumes of defibrinated salvaged blood demonstrates the enormous capacity of the healthy liver to replenish the circulation with fibrinogen within 2 hours.[105] Kongsgaard and associates[231] examined the quality of shed mediastinal blood with special regard to its influences of plasma proteases in the circulating blood (Table 9–6). They concluded that the infusion of moderate volumes shed mediastinal blood and with considerable alterations had minimal influence on the circulating blood.

## Cell Processing

The characteristics of salvaged blood after processing (centrifugation and washing) differ significantly from those of nonprocessed blood (Table 9–5). Centrifugation virtually eliminates all plasma constituents of blood. Washing significantly reduces any residual contaminants, including anticoagulant, free plasma hemoglobin and potassium, FDP and D- dimer fragments, products of platelet activation and lysis ($\beta$- thromboglobulin, thromboxane $A_2$, serotonin, and lactic dehydrogenase), products of complement activation, and tissue debris and microaggregates. The resulting product is similar to packed RBCs but suspended in normal saline rather than plasma. Unlike filtration systems, the HCT of the infusate after cell processing is unrelated to the HCT of the shed blood, dilution with irrigation solutions or serous fluids, and the degree of hemolysis. The HCT of processed RBCs is dependent on the flow rate of salvaged blood into the centrifuge bowl and the rotational speed of the centrifuge and can be further adjusted by varying the volume of saline used for resuspension. The HCT of the packed RBCs usually varies between 45 and 65% and sometimes can be higher.[179,184]

RBC survival assessed by chromium-51 and indium-111 were found to be normal after centrifugation and washing[113,126,216] or slightly reduced[243] and may appear normal or moderately damaged[149,184,243] through electron microscopy. Because isotope- tagged RBCs salvaged by processing appear to have relatively normal survival characteristics upon reinfusion, these RBCs probably represent survival of the most viable RBCs.[216] Older more fragile RBCs most likely are lysed during collection and centrifugation and discarded during washing cycles.[244] Provided that negative pressure in the recovery system is low, hemolysis during harvest and processing is between 2 and 10% of the salvageable RBCs. When processed blood was compared with relatively fresh (mean 4.2 day old) allogeneic banked blood, washed RBCs was found to be more resistant to osmolysis.[245] Salvaged blood has a 2,3-DPG level that is equal to circulating blood as opposed to 1-week-old banked blood, which is 20% of normal.[106,246] This normal 2,3-DPG level translates into a low oxygen affinity that results in increased oxygen unloading to the tissue.

The leukocyte count in salvaged blood has been shown to be high,[184] normal,[179] or low.[106] Leukocytes, generally larger than RBCs, should be lost or significantly reduced during processing. Unfortunately, those remaining are predominantly neutrophils and appear vacuolated, suggesting damage and autolysis. Theoretically, damaged leukocytes would permit leakage of enzymes, including proteases, that have been shown to attack lung interstitium and surfactant apoproteins[247] and lead to respiratory distress syndrome. The clinical significance of the reinfusion of salvaged leukocytes remains unclear. Bull and Bull[248] have advocated a salvaged blood syndrome resulting from the reinfusion of blood that had previously undergone mechanochemical activation of platelets and leukocytes on the walls of the centrifuge bowl. Although the removal of leukocytes through the use of specific leukocyte filters has been advocated, further investigation is required before their use can be recommended.

The platelet count of processed salvaged blood is nominal. As in the case of leukocytes, centrifugation and washing should eliminate platelets. Those platelets remaining may be physically or functionally damaged and may contribute to coagulation defects when reinfused to the patient. Washed RBCs have been found to contain toxic degradation products released from fractured platelets and leukocytes adhering to the centrifuge bowl wall.

The reinfusion of these toxic products can result in DIC and pulmonary occlusive thrombi.[249]

Plasma constituents such as coagulation factors and plasma protein are totally eliminated during processing of salvaged blood. Patients transfused with large volumes of processed RBCs may show a slight reduction of coagulation factors, significant loss of platelets, prolonged PT, PTT, thrombin time (TT), and bleeding time.[179] When compared with patients receiving only allogeneic blood or patients receiving filtered salvaged blood, patients receiving massive autotransfusions of processed blood are more apt to require fresh frozen plasma (FFP).[113] In the past, various formulas for replacement of plasma constituents and platelets have been advanced.[244,250] Sharp and associates[250] suggested the administration of FFP and platelets by formula: three to four units FFP and 12 platelet packs for every 3500 mL salvaged blood transfused. The administration of albumen (50 g)[251] or dextran[179] has been advocated to replace lost proteins and thus increase urinary output. However, the development of a coagulopathy cannot be predicted based on the volume of autotransfusion. Patients receiving in excess of 25,000 mL processed blood have not exhibiting coagulopathy.[106] In most clinical settings, usually several blood volumes are required before the development of a coagulopathy.[86,252] Coagulopathy can be the result of dilution of coagulation factors, fibrinogen, and platelets or due to a consumption process (DIC). Without the benefit of in vitro hemostatic laboratory testing, it is difficult to differentiate dilutional coagulopathy from DIC. Nonetheless, although laboratory analyses of PT, PTT, TT, and platelet count are important, replacement therapy should be based on definite signs of coagulopathy and bleeding or oozing.

Centrifugation and cell washing does not remove all contamination. Smith and associates[239] found very high catecholamine levels in salvaged blood after bilateral adrenalectomy for pheochromocytoma. This was later confirmed by others who detected incredibly high epinephrine and norepinephrine levels in processed salvaged blood during surgery for pheochromocytoma.[240] Evidence of elevated enzyme levels have also been observed in processed blood.[113] Fat globule, bone marrow, and methylmethacrylate contamination during orthopedic procedures has not resulted in adverse reactions, despite the extensive experience with the autotransfusion of processed and unprocessed salvaged blood. During clean procedures, the incidence of positive blood culture or wound infection is not different from patients receiving only allogeneic blood. When blood is positively contaminated with intestinal contents, bile, or urine, prudence dictates that reinfusion should be avoided except under the most dire circumstances.

## Blood Salvage and Hemostatic Drugs

Several blood conservation techniques are often used in a particular procedure. Occasionally, the application of one technique may complicate the use of other techniques. An example may be the use of hemostatic drugs to reduce surgical blood loss, complicating the use of blood salvage techniques. This may be the case with the intraoperative use of microfibrillar collagen hemostats and the use of blood salvage techniques.[253]

Microfibrillar collagen hemostat (Avitene®, FMC Corporation, Princeton, NJ) is a dry, water-insoluble, fibrous hydrochloric acid salt of purified bovine corium collagen. When brought into contact with bleeding tissue, collagen attracts platelets that then adhere to the fibrils, triggering aggregation and thrombi.[253,254] The hemostat has been effectively demonstrated for control of localized and diffuse bleeding in the postperfusion period after cardiac surgery.[255,256] Microfibrillar collagen hemostat remains active despite the presence of heparin.[253] The recycling of blood contaminated with microfibrillar collagen hemostat has become a major concern. During in vitro and in vivo animal studies, Robicsek and coworkers[253] established that the intravenous injection of blood contaminated with hemostat may cause embolization of parenchymal organs and, if administered in sufficient quantity, death. The hemostat can pass unimpeded through both simple filtration and cell-processing salvage apparatus. Although 40-$\mu$m filtration does impede passage of most but not all microfibrillar collagen hemostat, platelet aggregability remains in the filtrate. In the canine kidney-perfusion model, Niebauer and colleagues[254] found similar evidence of microembolization despite 20-$\mu$m filtration. Based on these results, it is recommended that blood contaminated with microfibrillar collagen hemostat not be returned to the circulation.[253,254]

Except for microfibrillar collagen hemostat, the presence of other commonly used hemostatic substances, such as topical thrombin, absorbable gelatin sponge, and oxidized regenerated cellulose, does not contraindicate the use of blood salvaging.

## Massive Autotransfusion

The technical advances in blood salvage apparatus and a greater willingness to use these techniques in emergency situations led to far greater volumes of blood being salvaged than had previously been the case.[80,81,92,93,198,202] Rather than the reinfusion of several hundred milliliters of blood, common during the early experience with blood salvage, as much as 40,000 mL has been reinfused.[195] Most investigators agree that the hematological consequences in the recipient of autotransfused blood depends mainly on the volume of blood reinfused.[80,81,107,195,257] As observed during CPB, blood subjected to repeated passage through extravascular surfaces, suctioning, occlusive pump heads, exhausted filters, and air interfaces will break down.[215,258] The analysis of the hematological effects of massive autotransfusion, in the clinical situation, is often complicated by the concomitant administration of large volumes of allogeneic blood and blood components.[80,81,195,202,220,259,260] Duncan and associates[80,81] examined 53 patients undergoing emergent procedures receiving an average of 3000 mL (range 150–18,000 mL) autotransfused blood. They observed that a grouping of patients receiving between 3500 and 10,000 mL autotransfused blood displayed decreased RBC masses and platelet counts, prolonged PT and PTT, and increased plasma free hemoglobin or hemoglobinuria than those patients receiving between 150 and 3200 mL.[80,81] The autotransfusion of less than 3000–3500 mL of salvaged blood is not usually associated with significant anemia due to hemodilution or RBC damage; from dilution, aggregation or destruction of platelets, and coagulation factors; DIC; reheparinization; or gross hemoglobinuria.[103,107,108,154,158,195,202,213,259] Fear of coagulopathy prompted several investigators to recommend that coagulation factors be replenished by administering FFP, platelet concentrates, and/or cryoprecipitates routinely after infusion of 3500 mL salvaged blood.[108,261] Although it is justifiable to obtain a coagulation profile as autotransfusion approaches this volume, coagulation factor and platelet replacement should be based on some indication of coagulopathy resulting in increased bleeding or oozing rather than by formulas based on a preconceived volume of autotransfusion or laboratory analyses.

## BLOOD SALVAGE FOR SPECIAL SITUATIONS
### Blood Salvage for Cardiac Surgery

In 1973, an average of eight units of allogeneic blood were transfused in adult patients undergoing cardiac surgery. Following a prediction in 1973 by Roche and Stengle[262] that without significant efforts toward blood conservation the national blood supply could easily be consumed by patients undergoing cardiac surgery, cardiac surgeons began to institute measures to reduce blood consumption, the most significant being the switch to crystalloid priming solutions and thus the acceptance of a lower perioperative HCT.[131,177,263–265] Other measures included autologous blood predonation,[266–270] isovolemic hemodilution by preoperative blood withdrawal,[271–275] return of shed blood to the oxygenator,[270,273,275–278] intraoperative blood salvaging,[275,279,280,282] reinfusion of residual oxygenator blood,[178,275,276,278] and postoperative autotransfusion of shed mediastinal blood.[112,275,280,281] Using multiple techniques to minimize blood loss and allogeneic blood transfusion have been effective, especially during reoperation when dissection of adhesions in the chest may increase blood loss.[270,275] Typically, a protocol calling for the use of multiple measures to limit and recycle blood loss results in a 50% or greater reduction, even complete elimination in some instances of allogeneic blood usage for cardiac surgery.[180,189,251,280,282–287] Dietrich and colleagues[288] showed that allogeneic blood bank usage progressively decreased from a mean of 2132 mL per procedure to 408 mL per procedure with increasing use of multiple

blood conservation techniques during myocardial revascularization.

Currently, the most widespread use of blood salvaging is in cardiac surgery. The volume of anticipated blood loss (and the potential for massive blood loss) during and after cardiac surgery generally meets indication criteria for the use of a blood salvage technique. Many patients arriving for cardiac surgery are at particular risk of increased blood loss because of preoperative fibrinolytic intervention (e.g., aspirin, dipyridamole, sodium warfarin, or heparin therapy).[289] The technology and techniques used during extracorporeal circulation lend themselves itself to the intraoperative collection of shed blood. Systemic heparinization, as a necessary part of extracorporeal circulation, avoided many of the problems associated with anticoagulating salvaged blood. When blood salvaging is used, the most common technique is cell processing.[113]

Blood salvage has also been shown to be especially effective during open heart surgery in children. The autotransfusion of small quantities of perioperatively salvaged blood can sometimes eliminate the need for allogeneic blood transfusion.[259,290]

### INTRAOPERATIVE BLOOD SALVAGE

The cardiac surgical field is ideal for blood salvage because it is usually aseptic, free of neoplastic cells, systemically anticoagulated, and the chest cavity provides a site for blood pooling and thus easy accessibility for aspiration.[64,291] Cardiotomy suction is an integral part of the CPB circuit, functioning to return shed blood to the oxygenator for reinfusion. Although familiarity with such devices enhanced the cardiac surgeon's acceptance of blood salvage technology, early filtration salvage systems did not offer major benefits over the use of cardiotomy suction. The use of the cardiotomy suction as the intraoperative salvage device has several drawbacks because it is generally intended for aspiration of blood from the surface of the heart or from the interior of the heart and thus blood aspirated for return directly into the oxygenator is essentially free of contamination (i.e., debris, cardioplegia, or irrigating solutions). However, blood found pooled in the chest cavity may be extremely hemodiluted with cardioplegia and irrigation solutions and may contain tissue and bone debris and high levels of potassium.[292] Early cardiotomy reservoirs were not particularly effective in removing particulate microaggregates.[293] Furthermore, cardiotomy suction is not available before or after the discontinuation of extracorporeal circulation.[278,294] Finally, at the conclusion of extracorporeal circulation, excess blood remaining in the oxygenator that cannot be immediately transfused is wasted. The residual oxygenator blood may be heparinized, hemodiluted, and somewhat hemolyzed.[292] The intraoperative use of filtration salvage devices is not generally advantageous under most of these circumstances. Reports have described the use of filtration apparatus for procedures performed without extracorporeal circulation[295] or in the event of hemorrhage after discontinuation of CPB.[64]

The introduction of commercial cell-processing devices significantly increased the utility of intraoperative blood salvage. Cell centrifugation and washing provided fresh autologous RBCs to maintain oxygen-carrying capacity after, or if necessary during, extracorporeal circulation without fear of further hemodilution, hyperkalemia, reheparinization, or transfusion reaction.[278] When using a blood processor, shed blood is collected to the cell processor before CPB and after protamine reversal of heparin. During CPB, aspirated blood is generally returned to the oxygenator by cardiotomy suction. The cell processor is especially useful during dissection of adhesions in reoperations or in patients previously treated by radiation therapy for thoracic tumors.[246,275,292,296]

Intraoperative blood salvage is now a routine part of cardiac surgery and has been shown to decrease both intraoperative and postoperative blood usage. Although it can usually be predicted which patients are at particular risk of excessive blood loss,[297] unexpected bleeding occurs often enough to warrant the routine use of blood salvage technology for cardiac surgery.[298]

Cell washing and centrifugation have been shown to alter the concentration of intravenously administered drugs (heparin, fentanyl, d-tubocurarine, and so on). This is especially true for fentanyl, which firmly binds to plasma proteins that are effectively reduced by as much as 74% during processing. Thus, in a procedure with 1000 mL blood loss in a 70-kg patient, the elimination of approximately 15% of the intravascular concentration can be anticipated. During procedures with abnormally high blood loss (several blood volumes), this removal of fentanyl may become clinically significant.[299] Shanks and coworkers[300] found a 7.2% increase in clearance of d-tubocurarine during cell processing. Cell washing also removes heparin from salvaged blood, increasing the heparin requirement.[178,301]

By combining several methods of blood conservation, Cosgrove and coworkers[302] were able to completely eliminate allogeneic blood transfusion in 94% of patients undergoing elective coronary artery surgery. Meticulous surgical hemostasis, acceptance of postoperative isovolemic anemia, and autologous blood provided by preoperative blood withdrawal (0.5–1.5 units) and relatively minor intraoperative (mean 260 mL) and postoperative (mean 195 mL) salvage volumes combined to limit the use of allogeneic blood to only 3 of 50 patients. Similar results using multiple blood conservation measures have been obtained by other investigators.[264,283,303–307]

The cost-effectiveness of the routine use of intraoperative blood salvage is difficult to calculate during cardiac surgery, because multiple techniques to reduce homologus blood requirement are usually used.[265] Breyer and associates[308] acknowledged that the intraoperative use of the cell processor during coronary artery surgery significantly decreases transfusion requirements and that the combined use of intraoperative salvage of shed mediastinal blood resulted in further savings. The costs incurred in blood salvage were completely offset by savings resulting from decreased allogeneic blood usage. However, there have been reports of disappointingly low RBC yield, increased costs, and excessive postoperative bleeding during intraoperative and postoperative salvage for cardiac surgery.[131,132,147,294,309] Typically, dissatisfaction with RBC yield or cost-effectiveness results from either poor methodology or failure to use multiple blood conservation techniques and account for savings from these methods in calculating cost-effectiveness. Even well-controlled cost analyses have difficulty figuring the costs related to the complications of allogeneic blood transfusion that may be avoided or reduced by reduction in allogeneic blood product usage.[147]

## POSTOPERATIVE SALVAGE OF MEDIASTINAL BLOOD

Schaff and colleagues[112] first described collection and reinfusion of postoperatively shed mediastinal blood after cardiac surgery. It has since become a routine part of the postoperative care in patients after cardiac surgery in some practices.[130,133,230,235,281,302,306,310,311]

Although mediastinal chest drainage has been carried out with both filtration and cell-processing salvage devices, filtration devices predominate in the postoperative period. They are simple to set up and operate and easily fit within the limited space at the bedside. Mediastinal chest drains are connected to a regulated vacuum source at a negative pressure of $-20$ cm $H_2O$. The addition of an underwater seal to a mediastinal filtration system increases patient safety because there is potential communication between the pleural cavity, mediastinum, and the ambient environment.[312]

When more than 250–400 mL shed blood accumulates, the salvaged blood is reinfused through a standard transfusion set. Blood is not allowed to stand in the collection canister for more than 6 hours. Because mediastinal blood has been shown to be defibrinogenated and will not clot, anticoagulation was unnecessary. Normal mediastinal drainage can range between 500 and 1000 mL/m² body surface area during the first 24 hours and most filtration systems seem to function well under these conditions.[313,314] However, these systems are not designed for massive hemorrhage, and consequently reexploration is indicated if chest tube drainage exceeds 500 mL for 1 hour or greater than 300 mL for 3 consecutive hours.[278,315]

The quality of pleural cavity blood has always been a major concern. These concerns centered upon four issues: the effect of infusing defibrinogenated blood on the patient's coagulation mechanism, risk of contamination and subsequent infection, risk of reinfusing hemolyzed blood, and risk of microembolism.[112,310]

The foremost consideration of recycling mediastinal blood is the effects on coagulation after reinfusion. Brawley and Schaff[310] found that although hemoglobin, HCT, and fibrinogen were low compared with banked blood, platelets, factor VIII, and factor IX levels in shed mediastinal blood were near normal. However, the quality of the platelets salvaged was not examined. Despite the autotransfusion of a mean of 900 mL salvaged blood with an average HCT of 25% and a platelet count of 60,800/mm³, Schaff and coworkers[112] found no difference in postoperative PT and PTT, factors VIII and IX levels, and free plasma hemoglobin levels. Although the reinfusion of shed mediastinal blood (in excess of 2000 mL in some patients) did not result in DIC,[112,130,281,310] others have found that without washing some evidence of coagulation is present.[137,316] These findings have motivated some to recommend that the routine infusion of unwashed shed mediastinal blood should be no longer used.[137,317,318] The introduction of fully automated and smaller cell-processing devices designed for bedside use offer an option. The use of a hemoconcentrator to concentrate shed mediastinal blood has also been suggested.[319]

The savings in allogeneic blood usage usually depends on the amount of postoperative drainage and the HCT of shed blood.[320,321] When compared with patients receiving only allogeneic blood, patients in whom postoperative blood salvage is used do not differ in postoperative blood loss and total blood transfusion (allogeneic + autologous) requirements.[112,310,322] According to various investigators, postoperative allogeneic blood requirements were reduced by 50% in patients receiving salvaged blood.[112,132,322,323] Reductions in allogeneic blood use may be difficult to attain when postoperative mediastinal blood salvage is used in the excessively hemodiluted patients. Thurer and associates[130] found the HCT of mediastinal blood to be 19% in hemodiluted patients as compared with 25% in nonhemodiluted patients.[281,310]

Cost savings have been effected by use of the cardiotomy reservoir used intraoperatively as the reservoir for postoperative mediastinal drainage.[324] In such cases, an infusion pump (with air detector) can reinfuse shed blood. This results in relatively inexpensive postoperative salvage because the cardiotomy was previously used and the infusion pump is reusable.[320]

Another major concern is the possibility of

bacterial contamination of salvaged blood. Cultures of salvaged blood have yielded some positive cultures. Most are considered common skin and operating room contaminants (diptheriods).[325] However, most authors have not noted an increased incidence of systemic infection among patients receiving either intraoperative or postoperative autotransfusion as compared with those receiving banked blood.[112,130,143,281,310] Standard procedures dictate that blood more than 6 hours old not be reinfused on the theoretical basis of possible bacterial growth.[123]

Levels of free plasma hemoglobin and other cellular debris, products of fibrin and fibrinogen degradation, and D-dimers can be signficantly elevated in shed mediastinal blood.[316] However, reinfusion of small to moderate volumes of such blood after filtration does not appear to be clinically significant.

Bennett and coworkers[159] compared the effects of autotransfused blood and allogeneic blood on the pulmonary microvasculature in a lung perfusion animal model. They selectively perfused dog lungs with either fresh blood salvaged from the pleural cavity or with 24-hour and 21-day-old banked blood. Upon examining the biopsy, a near 100% incidence of interstitial edema, perivascular and intraalveolar hemorrhage, and intraalveolar fluid and congestion was noted in tissue perfused by 21-day-old blood, despite filtration with the standard 170-$\mu$m transfusion filter. These morphological changes were significantly less in specimens perfused by autotransfused blood and fresh banked blood (24 hours) (Table 9–7). Their conclusion was that filtered autotransfused blood was significantly less injurious to the lung than filtered blood stored 3 weeks.

## BLOOD SALVAGE IN THE PEDIATRIC CARDIAC PATIENT

Surgery without donor blood transfusion is possible in children (over 10 kg body weight) with simple congenital heart disease (atrial or ventricular septal defects or pulmonary stenosis) but only if intraoperative blood loss is under 20 mL/kg. When surgical blood loss exceeds this limit, some transfusion therapy becomes necessary. Even small volumes of salvaged blood can significantly reduce the need for allogeneic blood transfusion.[290] In infants and children below 10 kg body weight, the low total blood volume (<860 mL) severely restricts allowable blood loss or generally precludes strict reliance on salvage techniques for blood replacement.[326] Blood loss in children must be carefully and completely computed. Blood soaked sponges (if used) should be weighed and then placed in saline-filled basins and agitated. The saline-blood solution can be aspirated into a cell processor or hemoconcentrator for processing. Ronai and colleagues[327] were able to increase RBC harvest from 50% to approximately 90% by salvaging blood in soaked sponges. Cell processors are now available with pediatric-sized bowls that reduce the minimum salvaged blood requirement for these instruments.

## Blood Salvage for Vascular Surgery

Blood salvage techniques are particularly appropriate during vascular surgery.[113,217,221,228,328,329] The volume of blood loss is usually predictable depending on the size and location of the aneurysm[236,330] and occurs principally during dissection of large blood vessels and during preclotting and flushing of porous grafts.[198,228,236] Blood loss may be substantial and is typically easily salvaged from within an aneurysm cavity or periaortic space.[331] Finally, most elective procedures and many emergency procedures are performed in an uncontaminated surgical field. Age and total blood loss have been identified as the primary deter-

**Table 9–7.   Morphological Alterations\* in Lungs Perfused with Autotransfused, Fresh, and Stored Blood**

| Finding | Autotransfused Blood | 24-Hour Blood | 21-Day Blood |
|---|---|---|---|
| Interstitial edema | 3/10 | 2/7 | 7/7 |
| Perivascular hemorrhage | 2/10 | 2/7 | 6/7 |
| Intraalveolar hemorrhage | 1/10 | 1/7 | 6/7 |
| Intraalveolar fluid | 1/10 | 1/7 | 5/7 |
| Alveolar congestion | 2/10 | 3/7 | 6/7 |

\* Expressed as the number of lungs exhibiting the specified histological changes.
Modified from Bennett SH, Geelhoed GW, Terrill RE, and others: Pulmonary effects of autotransfused blood. A comparison of fresh autologous and stored blood with blood retrieved from the pleural cavity in an *in situ* lung perfusion model. Am J Surg 1973; 125:696, with permission.

minants of survival during ruptured aortic aneurysm surgery.[332] The patients who die tend to be older and have a twofold greater blood loss than survivors.[228]

In 1973, Brener and coworkers[198] reported the first series of patients that had intraoperative blood salvage technology during elective abdominal aortic aneurysm repair. Salvaging between 200 and 15,000 mL of blood, there was evidence of extravascular coagulation and only moderate hemolysis. Autotransfusion in excess of 60,000 mL has been reported without significant complications, other than dilution of platelets and coagulation factors remedied by allogeneic platelets and FFP.[333] It has been concluded that intraoperative blood salvage is applicable during elective vascular surgery where moderate blood loss (>1000 mL) is anticipated.[198,213,217,220,236,309,334,336]

The indications for emergency vascular surgery are acute vascular occlusion or threatening hemorrhage (aortic aneurysm, aortoiliac resection, aortocaval fistula, and so on). Although only moderate blood loss may be anticipated, blood salvage techniques may be essential in maintaining adequate circulating volume if bleeding becomes excessive.[217,227,309,337-339] Aortic repair, whether for ruptured aneurysm or trauma, is nearly always complicated with massive blood loss.[340] Rapid exsanguination after rupture of an aortic aneurysm is almost invariably fatal without immediate surgical intervention,[341] precluding the normal preoperative preparation of the patient, including prior notification to the blood bank or discontinuation of antifibrinolytic therapy.

Blood salvage can provide a significant portion (40–100%) of the total transfusion requirement.[114,191,233,251,330,342-347] Cali and coworkers[348] examined the influence of autotransfusion on allogeneic blood requirements during aortic reconstruction. In 557 patients undergoing aortic reconstruction without the benefit of blood salvage, a mean volume of 5.9 units of allogeneic blood was administered perioperatively. In 150 patients who underwent similar surgery but with blood salvage, total allogeneic blood usage was reduced to 3.0 units. Furthermore, they found a reduction in the incidence of postoperative complications (19.7 versus 11.4%) and mortality (5.6 versus 2.7%). Stanton and associates[349] found that patients receiving salvaged blood not only

had lower incidences of morbidity and mortality, they tended to have more complete replacement of their lost blood volume.

The cost-effectiveness of the routine use of blood salvage has been an issue. Although Winton and colleagues[294] determined that blood salvage was not necessarily cost-effective when used routinely for cardiac surgery, Salerno[350] later found that its use is probably more justified for vascular surgery where blood loss is predictable. The typical savings is not enormous in the routine vascular procedure ($30.00 per patient) but may be significantly larger when large volumes of blood are lost.[147,331,334,335,343,351]

Excessive use of discard suction to maintain a relatively dry surgical field is wasteful. However, maintaining a dry surgical field enables more expedient surgical repairs, which translates into significantly less blood loss. Galbut and Bolooki[352] believed that the use of blood salvage apparatus not only preserved blood volume but enabled the reanastomoses of more intercostal arteries during descending aortic aneurysm repair, the ligation of which is a risk factor in postoperative paraplegia.

The early cell processors were seriously limited in capacity to recycle blood when massive rapid blood loss occurred.[229,347,353,354] This was usually due to inadequate suction at the operative field, limited capacity of the cardiotomy reservoir, and excessive time lapse recycling the collected blood for reinfusion.[229] Warnock and associates[353] modified a cell processor to allow bypass of the centrifuge and thus directly reinfused filtered but unprocessed blood from the cardiotomy reservoir. This modification transformed the cell processor to a system resembling the Bentley ATS100. Processing time can also be reduced by eliminating the washing cycle. Elimination of the wash spares some coagulation factors and is possible during many vascular procedures because the surgical field is rarely contaminated. Later enhancements made in blood processors have significantly reduced processing time, thus reducing the need to reinfuse unprocessed or partially processed blood.[221,236] Cardiotomy capacity can be increased by the simple addition of a second reservoir for collection of overflow volume during those few procedures when blood loss is excessive.[229]

Blood salvage techniques are often combined with other blood conservation techniques during vascular surgery. These may include the use of surgical techniques designed to minimize dissection and unnecessary blood loss, preoperative autologous donation (in elective procedures), normovolemic hemodilution, induced hypotension or control of hypertension (during aortic crossclamp), and hemoconcentration using a hemofilter (during partial or full CPB).[191,343,355,356]

## Blood Salvage for Trauma Surgery

Trauma surgery is often accompanied by massive hemorrhage. Along with orthotopic liver transplantation and aortic reconstruction, trauma surgery is a major consumer of blood and blood products. Although not all trauma surgery is emergent in nature, those procedures that do require immediate surgery are usually rushed directly from the emergency room to the operating room without the benefit of the usual presurgical preparation. The bleeding patient may arrive in the operating room with or without blood, and available blood may either be typed and compatible (if time allowed) or more probably emergency release blood (type-specific, uncross matched, or universal-donor untyped) and nearly always in inadequate amounts.[102,117,167,357]

Massive autotransfusion in the trauma patient, up to 30,000 mL of estimated autotransfusion volume in addition to allogeneic blood and blood products, has been described.[202] Although massive autotransfusion shares few of the potentially deleterious effects of the massive transfusion of stored blood (Table 9–8), this does not minimize the deleterious effects of autotransfusion that do occur. The major problem encountered is in the maintenance of intraoperative hemostasis. The intraoperative dilution of coagulation factors and platelets, postoperative thrombocytopenia, hypofibrinogenemia, and elevated plasma levels of FDPs characterize massive autotransfusion.[80,81,202] Glover and associates[201] found that those patients receiving in excess of 5000 mL salvaged blood displayed generalized oozing in the operative field, although postoperative course may not be affected. Most authors agree that autotransfusion of 2000–3000 mL can be accomplished without major coagulopathy or clinical sequelae.[93,107,111,358,359]

**Table 9–8. Potentially Deleterious Effects of Massive Autotransfusion and Stored Blood Transfusion**

| | Allogeneic Blood | Salvaged Blood |
|---|---|---|
| Volume-related factors | | |
| Transmission of disease | + | − |
| Immunological mismatch | + | − |
| Immunization of the patient | + | − |
| Rate and volume related factors | | |
| Altered P50 | + | − |
| Coagulation abnormalities | + | + |
| Acid-base imbalance | + | − |
| Citrate toxicity | + | −* |
| Hypothermia | + | − |
| Microembolization | + | +† |
| Impaired RBC deformability | + | − |
| Infusion of plasticizers | + | − |
| Infusion of denatured proteins | + | + |
| Infusion of vasoactive substances | + | +† |
| Elevated potassium, phosphate, ammonia levels | + | +† |
| Impaired antibacterial defenses | + | +† |
| Graft-vs.-host reactions | + | − |
| Toxicity of additives | + | − |

* Except when citrate local anticoagulation is used in a filtration salvage system.
† When filtration salvage devices are used.
Modified from Collins JA: Problems associated with the massive transfusion of stored blood. Surgery 1974; 75:274, with permission.

Blood aspirated from body cavities usually does not require anticoagulation. The mechanical churning action of the heart, lungs, and diaphragm causes defibrinogenation of extravasated blood.[63,92,93,208] However, during massive bleeding, blood may be aspirated before having sufficient contact with serous linings and may clot.[111,117] Thus, local citrate[105,107,110,111,360] or heparin[65,134,358] anticoagulation has been advocated. Systemic heparinization is usually contraindicated in trauma patients.[257,360] When massive volumes of allogeneic and autotransfused blood and blood products are transfused, micropore filtration (20–40 μm) is recommended.[146]

Duncan and associates[81] noted that several patient deaths from exsanguinating hemorrhage was averted when over 3000 mL shed blood was autotransfused before allogeneic blood could be obtained from the blood bank. Autotransfusion is especially important when used to support circulation during evacuation of tamponade, both thoracic and abdominal. When the cavity is opened and tamponade released, sudden collapse from fresh hemorrhage is a common event. Slow decompression of the chest or abdomen while suctioning accumulated and fresh blood into a salvage device for rapid reinfusion can often sustain arterial blood pressure for a time, allowing the surgeon to apply clamps or sutures.[361]

Hemorrhagic shock or an anticipated blood loss in excess of 1000–1500 mL is an indication for the use of an autotransfusion system.[80,81,195,257] The autotransfusion of salvaged blood can have an impact on allogeneic blood use in the treatment of trauma. Salvaged blood is not necessarily a replacement for allogeneic blood or blood products, especially in cases of massive blood loss when large amounts of allogeneic and salvaged blood may be transfused. Furthermore, the use of massive autotransfusion by either filtration or cell processing can result in dilution of coagulation factors, anemia (especially in filtration systems), and thrombocytopenia. Careful monitoring of the hemostatic mechanism and early treatment of coagulation abnormalities is of utmost importance. FFP, platelet concentrate, cryoprecipitates, and individual factor administration may be necessary to provide hemostasis during massive transfusion of blood (salvaged or allogeneic).[86]

The discontinuous collection-transfusion nature of filtration and cell-processing salvage systems is a major disadvantage of autotransfusion systems.[84] One of the prime objectives in the management of shock in the severely traumatized patient is prompt and vigorous restoration of the circulating blood volume. Trauma victims often require administration of unusually large volumes of fluid over a brief period of time. Various manufacturers now market rapid infusion systems specifically designed to warm and infuse multiple units of blood[362] (see Chapter 1: Principles of Blood Transfusion).

All experience with blood salvage in trauma surgery has not been positive. Inadequate scavenging techniques, extensive contamination, and delayed reinfusion because of processing limited autotransfusion to only 26% of patients in one series of trauma patients.[139] Air, fat, microaggregate, and macroaggregate embolism during infusion of salvaged blood

have been reported.[82,363] Oozing as a result of dilution of coagulation factors and thrombocytopenia can complicate fluid resuscitation in the hemorrhaging patient.

Blood salvaging in trauma patients has not been limited to the operating room or even to surgical candidates. Hemothorax blood drained through chest tubes can be collected, filtered, and autotransfused in almost any location.[86,107,111,117,152,360,364,365] Autotransfusion systems with a larger capacity (up to 2500 mL) have been designed specifically for use in the emergency department.[111,117] Blood salvage volumes from the chest drainage in the emergency room have ranged as high as 14,000 mL.[65] Blood salvaged preoperatively can be used for fluid resuscitation and hemodynamic stabilization before surgery.[134,366,367]

## ENTERIC CONTAMINATION OF SALVAGED BLOOD

The presence of contaminants in salvaged blood is a major concern in traumatized patients.[136,364] Frequently, injury to the bowel concurrent with injuries to the liver, spleen, and major blood vessels, particular in penetrating trauma, limits the usage of blood salvage in trauma surgery.[368,369] Contaminants may include gross fecal material, urine, stomach and intestinal contents, fat, tissue, and bile, among others. Contamination may also arise from the skin immediately adjacent to the wound and from airborne operating room contaminants.[364] The autotransfusion of blood contaminated or suspected of contamination remains controversial. In 100 patients reported by Griswold and Ortner,[50] many patients received blood contaminated with "toxins" from necrotic tissue, bile, macerated liver tissue, and bacterial contamination from penetration of the hollow viscus. They noted that although a temporary bacteriemia did occur, bacterial infection did not complicate postoperative recovery. They credited this to the fact that if adequate circulating volume was maintained and anemia avoided, the body's own defense mechanisms were adequate.[50]

During the initial testing of the prototypes of the Bentley ATS100 in a small series of dogs, autotransfusion with contaminated blood showed positive postoperative blood cultures but no resultant sepsis with and without short-term antibiotic therapy.[79] Yaw and coworkers[368] studied exaggerated levels of colon contamination in dogs. They found that the safety of autotransfusion of 20–30% of the blood volume was as much related to the severity of hemorrhage as it was to the presence or absence of contamination. Thus, survival was unaffected when small volumes of contaminated blood were autotransfused. However, when large volumes (40% of blood volume) were autotransfused, survival was only 30% compared with 90% in dogs receiving uncontaminated blood. The administration of small doses of antibiotics in another group of dogs reversed this high mortality (to 90% survival). Data from many sources have not proven that the reinfusion of blood contaminated with enteric contents is associated with significantly higher morbidity or mortality.[50,79,81,82,183,185,201,257,369,370] Duncan and associates[80,81] did not hesitate to salvage blood in patients with wounds of the stomach, liver, kidney, or small intestine when blood loss was large. Many have argued that when autotransfusion is a life-saving measure, the presence of contamination should not automatically preclude its use.[201,257,370] Despite these results, there is reluctance among most physicians to reinfuse blood salvaged under contaminated conditions, especially when banked blood is available. Purulent infection or colon injury is considered as absolute contraindications by some[80,81] but not by others.[201,257]

Neither filtration nor cell processing can reliably eliminate bacterial contamination from blood.[181–183,185] Cell processing results in logarithmic reduction (up to 80%) but not elimination of bacterial contamination.[183] The addition of antibiotics (Keflin 1 g/L, Garamycin 80 mg/L, or Cleocin 600 mg/L) to the saline wash solution eliminated culture growth of coliforms and bacteroides species and reduced fecal strep counts.[182] Bacteria may remain attached to RBCs despite several washing cycles even when antibiotics are added.[183,369] An antibacterial membrane (a charged cellulose membrane coated with an analog of polymyxin B) has been shown to be significantly more effective in removing fecal contamination than cell processing.[371] Ozman and associates[369] found no significant increase in site-specific infection risk associated with the autotransfusion of potentially

culture-positive shed blood in abdominal trauma.

Bacterial contamination of shed blood is also seen in nontraumatic surgery.[112,115,143,372] Very often, blood aspirated from the open chest is contaminated with microorganisms, usually due to airbourne contamination or skin commensals.[143,373] Despite high incidences of contamination, the reinfusion of this salvaged blood is rarely associated with any sign of even transient bacteremia.

## Blood Salvage for Urological Surgery

Blood salvage during urological surgery poses a particular problem for surgeons. Shed blood from the urethra during transurethral resection of the prostate is necessarily highly diluted with irrigation fluid (HCT 1–3%) as well as contaminated with tissue and urine. Blood filtration devices, although able to remove particulate matter such as tissue with use of appropriate filters, were unable to concentrate RBCs and remove urine contamination. Toward this end, Wilson and Taswell[60] developed the first blood salvage processing device for intraoperative use (Figure 9–5). During controlled clinical trials with a prototype cell processor, Wilson and coworkers[60,171,172] established the effectiveness and safety of this type of blood salvage for urological surgery. Klimberg and associates[374–376] demonstrated the safety and efficacy of cell processing in large groups of patients undergoing resection of urological neoplasms. The contamination of shed blood with urine did not increase the incidence of postoperative sequelae.[172] The composition of the irrigating fluid should be altered to prevent hemolysis and agglutination and development of a positive direct Coombs' reaction.[172]

### MALIGNANT CELL CONTAMINATION IN SALVAGED BLOOD

Concerns about the dissemination of cancer cells contaminating salvaged blood has led to the general contraindication of blood salvaging during cancer surgery.[61,377] That blood filtration or cell centrifugation and washing will not remove cancer cell contamination from blood has been established.[368,378] The concept that autotransfusion leads to disseminated disease and widespread metastases has not yet been unsubstantiated and thus is purely a theoretical concern.[374,375] Furthermore, studies and case reports support the contention that autotransfusion is safe in patients with malignant disease.[180,376,378–383] A correlation between circulating tumor cells and the subsequent development of metastases in patients undergoing surgery has not been established.[384–386] Klimberg and colleagues[374] attempted to dispel fears that prevented the use of blood salvaging techniques during surgical oncology. In a series of 49 patients undergoing surgery for surgical extirpation of urological malignant neoplasms, they salvaged a median of 1300 mL. After 1 year, 45 (91.8%) of 49 patients were alive, 43 (89.6%) of whom were free of disease. There were only five (10.4%) documented cases of recurrences, and one patient was lost to follow-up as to cause of death. These figures compare favorably with statistics on bladder cancer survival after treatment.[387] Klimberg[375] and Hart and associates,[376] in 54 and 49 patients, respectively, reported that despite recurrence in some patients, no patient developed diffuse metastatic disease compatible with intravascular dissemination of tumors. Similar work by Zulim and associates[383] and Fujimoto and coworkers[388] in patients undergoing hepatic resection for malignancy concur with these[374,375] findings.

Despite the fact that the above findings tend to dispel the myth that salvage and reinfusion of blood contaminated with cancer cells can cause metastases, they do not offer proof. Until such proof is forthcoming, autotransfusion continues to be considered absolutely or relatively contraindicated during cancer surgery. Other blood conservation measures, such as intraoperative hemodilution or use of predeposit blood donation programs, have proved successful[375] and thus should be considered whenever possible.

## Blood Salvage for Orthopedic Surgery

Blood salvaging techniques are used extensively for major orthopedic procedures in which moderate blood loss is anticipated. Autologous transfusion, by predeposit of blood or by intraoperative salvage or both, should be considered by orthopedic surgeons for all patients who have an elective procedure.[389]

The modern experience with intraoperative blood salvage in orthopedic surgery is mainly during hip arthroplasty in adult patients and spinal fusion in both adults and children.[121,125,126,138,180,212,244,251,390–402] These studies demonstrated that intraoperative blood salvage alone (or used in conjunction with predonated autologous blood) can significantly reduce or in some cases eliminate the need for allogeneic blood transfusion during the intraoperative and postoperative periods (Table 9–9).

A reduction in allogeneic blood usage as a result of blood salvage may not translate into a decrease in total transfusion volume when both autotransfused and allogeneic units are totaled.[397] This may indicate an increase in bleeding, especially when salvaged blood is processed by washing and centrifugation. Although severe coagulopathy, characterized by thrombocytopenia, hypofibrinogenemia, and platelet dysfunction, has occurred during massive autologous transfusion with autotransfusion of blood salvaged by both filtration and processing, moderate amounts (<3000 mL) have not been associated with such events.[234,401] To some extent, this increased number may reflect an increased likelihood that a physician will transfuse an available autologous unit of blood over a allogeneic unit.[403] This is further evidenced by a similar increase in the volume of blood transfused when predeposited autologous blood is available.[404] The practice of transfusing autologous blood simply because it is available is not recommended.[103]

The combined use of intraoperative blood salvage and predeposited autologous blood has been advocated as a means of further reduction and in many cases elimination of the need for allogeneic blood.[393,397,398] The combination of these two techniques should intuitively decrease the allogeneic blood requirement, although no convincing evidence of an additive affect is available. Certainly, measures such as iron or erythropoietin therapy should be considered during autologous blood donation to prevent a low presurgical HCT.[405–407] However, the patient's age, size, and medical condition may limit the use of preoperative autologous blood donation.[402,408] A low preoperative HCT combined with the relatively

**Table 9–9.   Erythrocyte Harvest During Blood Salvage for Orthopedic Surgery**

| Author, Year | Number of Cases | Type of Surgery | Estimated Blood Loss (mL) | Preoperative HCT (%) | RBC Yield (mL) | RBC Harvest (%) | Salvage HCT (%) |
|---|---|---|---|---|---|---|---|
| Lehner et al., 1981[391] | 16 | S | 1496 | — | 367 | 20 | 45 |
| Turner and Steady, 1981[390] | 99 | S | 1000 | 39 | 225 | 52 | — |
| Flynn et al., 1982[244] | 99 | S | 1082 | 36 | 217 | 54 | 60 |
| Young et al., 1982[251] | 93 | H | 2000 | — | 662 | — | — |
| Keeling et al., 1983[180] | 34 | S & H | — | — | 500 | — | 50 |
| Kruger and Calbert, 1985[125] | 28 | S | 1350 | 39 | 400 | 52 | 52 |
| Ray et al., 1986[126] | 239 | S & H | 976 | 31 | 354 | 60 | 60 |
| Bovill et al., 1986[121] | 24 | SH | 960 | 43 | 518 | — | — |
| Bovill et al., 1986[121] | 12 | H | 870 | — | 518 | — | — |
| Goulet et al., 1989[397] | 175 | S & H | 746 | — | 448 | 60 | 55 |
| Wilson, 1989[396] | 50 | H | 1455 | 40 | 685 | 47 | — |
| Behrman and Keim, 1982[489] | 25 | S | 1055 | 39 | 447 | 74 | — |
| Endresen et al., 1991[399] | 17 | H | 880 | 36 | 670 | 76 | — |

low RBC harvests common in orthopedic surgery (30–50%) may increase the intraoperative demand for allogeneic blood. Low harvest during orthopedic surgery results from technical difficulties in recovering shed blood and RBC damage during collection.[244,400] During most orthopedic operations, blood tends to ooze from bony surfaces with no cavity to pool. Suctioning blood in this manner causes excessive amount of air-blood interface, resulting in foaming and RBC damage.[406] Henn and associates[409] demonstrated that cell processing does not completely remove plasma free hemoglobin. Ray and associates,[126] in 239 spinal fusion patients, found that RBC survival was unaffected by blood salvaging and processing over a 30-day period.

Blood salvage can also be combined with other blood conservation techniques, such as normovolemic hemodilution and deliberate hypotension. The combined use of blood salvaging and normovolemic hemodilution during orthopedic surgery has not been adequately studied. However, a wealth of knowledge is available in the cardiovascular surgery literature, where intraoperative and postoperative blood salvage and hemodilution are routinely used during cardiovascular surgery. Haberkern and Dangel[410] recently reported the use in children of intraoperative blood salvage, normovolemic hemodilution, induced hypotension, and mild hypothermia in orthopedic surgery. Compared with an earlier series wherein all patients received banked blood, allogeneic blood transfusion was re-

duced by approximately 75%. Such results were achieved by combining these various techniques with painstaking surgical hemostasis and restrictive indications for allogeneic transfusion.

Intraoperative blood salvage may also be combined with deliberate hypotension. The effectiveness of deliberate hypotension as a blood conservation technique in orthopedic surgery for both adults and children has been well demonstrated.[411–417] As yet, there is no data on the effectiveness of the combined use of blood salvage and deliberate hypotension in orthopedic surgery. Lennon and associates[394] studied both blood conservation techniques for spinal surgery but in separate groups of patients. Blood loss and transfusion requirements were similar when comparing the blood salvage group to the deliberate hypotensive group or a group of patients in which neither method was used, but allogeneic blood use was reduced by 50% in the blood salvage group.[394]

Intraoperative blood salvage has been used in the pediatric orthopedic surgery, with most experience in spinal fusion patients for scoliosis correction.[212,418] Originally there was difficulty with commercially available blood salvage devices, both filtration and processing devices, when used in pediatric surgery. These devices were originally designed for use in adults and thus required correspondingly large volumes of shed blood. These early difficulties have been overcome with devices designed specifically for use in pediatrics.[244] In

26 elective spinal fusions for scoliosis and kyphosis, Csencsitz and Flynn[212] were able to achieve results comparable with adults in a program where intraoperative blood salvage is combined with predeposit of autologous blood.[212,244]

Finally, both filtration and processed methods of blood transfusion are effective in decreasing or eliminating particulate debris such as bone fragments, marrow, and fat that are of concern to orthopedic surgeons.[197,390] Furthermore, potentially toxic antibiotics (clindamycin, tobramycin, bacitracin, and polymyxin) not ordinarily administered systemically or in the doses used in topical washes are effectively removed during processing.[390] This may be of special importance when intraoperative blood salvage is used in nonelective surgical procedures.[392] Drug removal by washing of salvaged blood has also been studied during orthopedic surgery. Cell processing removed significant quantities of fentanyl, probably the result of binding to plasma proteins or adsorption to the components of the cell-saving device.[299] Shanks and associates[300] found a relatively small reduction (7%) in d-tubocurarine levels. Thus, blood salvage may radically alter blood concentrations of intravenous drugs.

Semkiw and associates[138] extended the use of blood salvage to the postoperative period after total hip and knee replacement operations. Considerable experience in postoperative blood salvage techniques after cardiac and thoracic surgery has demonstrated the effectiveness and safety of drainage blood collection for autotransfusion. Using either cell-processing[138,402] or filtration[402,419,420] systems, a 300- to 400-mL wound drainage was reinfused. They found that postoperative blood salvage was most effective in procedures such as revision and bilateral arthroplasty and in patients where noncemented components were used. These cases usually resulted in larger blood loss and longer stays in the recovery room, thereby increasing the effectiveness of blood salvaging. Healy and colleagues[421] demonstrated that methylmethacrylate levels as high as 496 $\mu g/mL$ and minute (<9 $\mu m$) fat globules are present in unwashed shed blood. The significance of these findings are unknown because in those cases where filtration apparatus has been used, no evidence of increased bleeding, renal failure, cardiopulmonary compromise, or infection has been found.

## Blood Salvage for Organ Transplantation

Transfusion requirements for organ transplantation surgery are among the largest for any surgical procedure. However, these requirements vary depending on the organ affected. Uncomplicated heart and kidney transplantation may require minimal blood, one to two units of packed RBCs,[76,422,423] although combination heart and lung transplants and repeat heart transplants can require considerably more blood components.[424] In contrast, Butler and associates[425] described an orthotopic liver transplant requiring 251 units of packed RBCs, 107 platelet concentrates, and 206 units of FFP. Although such excessive usage of blood and blood products is exceptional, even the routine blood requirement for orthotopic liver transplantation is large.

Since the first orthotopic liver transplantation in 1963,[426] the requirements for blood and blood products have gradually decreased. This decrease is the result of improved surgical and anesthetic techniques, particularly venovenous bypass to decrease venous congestion; intraoperative coagulation monitoring; and treatment of fibrinolysis.[427-429] Despite these advances, the blood requirements remain significant and tax the abilities of blood banks.

Motschman and associates,[428] reviewing the literature on blood usage for orthotopic liver transplantation, found the mean intraoperative use of blood and blood products in adult patients ranged from 12.5 to 56.3 RBC units (packed RBCs and whole blood), from 6.0 to 40.4 units FFP, from 3.9 to 25.4 units cryoprecipitate, and from 13.6 to 25.4 units platelet concentrates. These were based on reports appearing in the literature between 1985 and 1987. Excessive blood loss during orthotopic liver transplantation has been traced to various causes. Decreased production of coagulation factors produced in the hepatocyte is a major consideration. The coagulation factors produced in the hepatocyte include fibrinogen, prothrombin (factor II), labile factor proaccelerin (factor V), stabile factor proconvertin (factor VII), Christmas factor (factor IX), Stuart Prower factor (factor X), plasma thromboplastin antecedent (factor

XI), Hageman factor (factor XII), and fibrin stabilizing factor (factor XIII). The deficits of vitamin K-dependant factors (factors II, VII, IX, and X) and fibrinogen have the greatest effect on coagulation dysfunction. Although normal coagulation function is maintained at concentrations as low as 30% below normal in other coagulation factors, decreases of only 20–25% in fibrinogen levels (150–200 mg/dL) can result in coagulation abnormalities. Other considerations may include long-standing portal hypertension and thrombocytopenia-related to gastrointestinal bleeding, splenomegaly, and malnutrition.[428] These chronic abnormalities related to end-stage liver disease are frequently accompanied by perihepatic scarring from previous surgeries, bleeding at the time of large vessel anastomoses, bleeding secondary to coagulopathy resulting from inactivation of procoagulants and fibrinolytic activators, and FDPs generated during surgery.[430,431]

Intraoperative blood salvage is uniquely suited for procedures such as orthotopic liver transplantation where massive blood loss is anticipated, some patients are systemically anticoagulated, and blood tends to pools in an accessible body cavity where it can be readily aspirated. Furthermore, the usual poor health of the patient before transplantation would ordinarily prohibit preoperative donation of autologous blood. The use of blood salvage during orthotopic liver transplantation is widely accepted, and although not eliminating the need for allogeneic banked blood, it has reduced the blood requirement.[122,429,431–433] The use of blood salvaging techniques has been shown to decrease the allogeneic blood requirements from anywhere between 20 and 50%.[122,428,429,432,434]

Theoretically, patients undergoing massive transfusion are at particular risk of dilutional coagulopathy. Banked blood (unless fresh) is devoid of platelets and labile coagulation factors (V and VIII), and cells salvaged by processing yield packed RBCs, without platelets or coagulation factors. Any coagulation abnormality resulting from blood transfusion should be particularly evident during orthotopic liver transplantation. In practice, however, dilutional coagulopathy is uncommon as demonstrated by Mendel and associates,[435] who failed to show any untoward postoperative biochemical or hematological

findings in patients receiving an average of 1.65 L processed blood and 6.23 L allogeneic blood during orthotopic liver transplantation.

The rate of blood loss varies during the different phases of orthotopic liver transplantation.[120,175,428] Motschman and colleagues[428] showed that the rate of transfusion, blood salvage, and autotransfusion is highest immediately after reperfusion of the transplanted liver. During periods of excessive blood loss requiring immediate transfusion of large quantities of blood, concentrated but unwashed salvaged blood has been shown to be safe.[136,431] At the Mayo Clinic, a specially manufactured cell-washing system has reduced the processing time to as little as 4 minutes, thus eliminating the necessity of infusing unwashed packed RBCs.[120,175]

## Blood Salvage for Obstetrical and Gynecological Surgery

The earliest experiences with blood salvage were largely in connection with obstetrical and gynecological emergencies. Despite the fact that the early experience with blood salvage for obstetrical and gynecological procedures was remarkably free of complications, today blood salvage techniques are not routinely used in obstetrical and gynecological surgery.[436] The reasons for the abandonment of blood salvage as a clinical tool during obstetrical and gynecological surgery are varied.

First, the need for blood transfusion in obstetrical and gynecological surgery has declined over the years. Historically, acute hemorrhage from ruptured ectopic pregnancies was the major impetus to salvage shed blood. Although the incidence of ectopic pregnancies remains high, the death-to-case ratio has declined.[437–440] Major advances in the early detection and treatment of ectopic pregnancy, improved prenatal care, and heightened patient awareness of possible complications of pregnancy have decreased the incidence of hemorrhagic emergencies from ectopic pregnancies in developed nations. Similarly, blood transfusion (and maternal mortality from hemorrhage) during cesarean section has declined.[441–444]

Second, the fear of transfusion-transmitted disease has resulted in a reassessment of the need for transfusion, particularly when the patient expresses a wish to avoid allogeneic blood transfusion. This can often be accomplished by acceptance of a lower postpartum hemoglobin concentration (8 gm/dL rather than 10 gm/dL) in the nonbleeding patient.[443] An increased maternal blood volume (1000–2000 mL by the second trimester) that accompanies pregnancy is usually sufficient to cover blood lost during the antepartum period and delivery, which has been estimated at between 200 and 500 mL during normal spontaneous vaginal delivery and as much as a liter or more during cesarean section.[441,445]

Finally, the quality of salvaged blood has remained suspect. Filtration techniques for salvaging blood in nonsystemically anticoagulated patients have been implicated as a cause of DIC[63] and may thus initiate or aggravate coagulation defects in the parturient. Hypofibrinogenemia and FDPs and prolongation of the thrombin, prothrombin, and activated partial thromboplastin times are frequently associated with intraoperative blood salvage.[80,202] Findings consistent with DIC induced by autotransfusion have been reported by others.[80,81,107,158] Beller and associates[446] and Carty and associates[447] showed that peritoneal blood recovered during ruptured ectopic pregnancies (blood that may be salvaged and reinfused) has pronounced depletion of coagulation factors and grossly elevated levels of FDPs. Pregnancy can be associated with a variety of hematological complications, including aplastic anemia,[448] factor deficiency,[449] DIC,[441,450] sickle cell disease and other hemoglobinopathies,[451,452] and thrombocytopenia (hemolysis, elevated liver enzymes, and low platelet count [HELLP] syndrome).[453–455] DIC has been associated with amniotic fluid, fat or tissue embolism, septic abortion and uterine infection, retained (dead) fetal tissue, hydatidiform mole, preeclampsia and eclampsia, and placental rupture or abruptio.[441,456] The initiation of the coagulation cascade by any of these processes leads to the formation of fibrin. If this process is a widely disseminated one, a consumption of coagulation factors may occur. Particularly affected will be the labile factors (V and VIII), as well as the fibrinogen level. Finally, clot lysis activity results in the abnormal appearance of FDPs in the blood.[456] Furthermore, DIC results in platelet consumption and dysfunction (see Chapter 2: Coagulation and Hemostasis). These coagulation defects can be exacerbated by the infusion of blood salvaged by filtration. All of these factors can contribute to increased surgical blood loss. Preoperative or intraoperative laboratory testing that reveals an abnormally low platelet count and bleeding time and extended partial thromboplastin, prothrombin, and thrombin times should increase suspicion of DIC.

Although cell-processing equipment is rarely immediately available in the obstetrical unit, when used, care must be taken to monitor the coagulation profile of obstetrical and gynecological patients during and after intraoperative autotransfusion. Blood component therapy (FFP, platelets, or cryoprecipitate) may be required to promote hemostasis when large volumes of processed blood are autotransfused.

Nevertheless, obstetrical hemorrhage (defined as blood loss of 500 mL or more in excess of normal) can occur. Antepartum hemorrhage is usually confined to those patients with placental abruption, placenta previa, and uterine rupture, either spontaneous or traumatic.[445] Most obstetrical hemorrhages occur in the postpartum period. Placental atony, vaginal or cervical lacerations, uterine inversions, and coagulopathies occur from various causes.[441,457] Although in the presence of risk factors the likelihood of obstetrical hemorrhage can often be predicted, hemorrhage can also occur on rare occasions in the patient in whom hemorrhage would ordinarily be deemed unlikely. Today's conservative blood policy usually prohibits type- and cross-matching allogeneic blood (or predonation of autologous blood) unless some risk factors are present.[458,459] Thus, unanticipated hemorrhage in these patients must be initially treated without the benefits of readily available typed-compatible blood. In such situations, blood salvage may represent the only source of RBC until banked blood becomes available. In Third World countries, hemorrhage from ruptured ectopic pregnancy is significantly more common and is the most frequently encountered gynecological emergency.[98,99,101,102,460] Lichtiger and associates[380] obtained consent to use blood salvaging from two Jehovah's Witness patients undergoing laparotomy for cancerous tumors of the uterus and ovary. Consent for salvaging was contingent upon the blood being in continual movement and never separated from the body.

In the only large series (39 gynecological patients), Merrill and associates[261] were able to retrieve and autotransfuse 59% of their transfusion requirements during surgery for ruptured ectopic pregnancy. There were no deaths or bacterial-positive blood cultures in this series of patients. Morbidity connected to blood transfusion was limited to six patients and included coagulopathy, thrombocytopenia, transient transfusion rashes related to the concomitant administration of allogeneic blood, and pulmonary edema from excessive fluid therapy. Other investigators showed similar reductions in allogeneic blood use for ruptured ectopic pregnancies and a bleeding corpus luteum cyst.[80,436,461,462]

Autotransfusion has been safely used in patients with ruptured ectopic pregnancies complicated with pelvic inflammatory disease,[261] in surgery for excision of ovarian and uterine tumor, and in the presence of amniotic fluid during cesarean section.[380,436,463]

## DOES POSSIBLE AMNIOTIC FLUID CONTAMINATION CONTRAINDICATE BLOOD SALVAGE?

The procoagulant activity of amniotic fluid is well recognized, as are the resulting risks of mixing amniotic fluid with blood. Thus, it has been suggested that blood salvage techniques are contraindicated during cesarean section because of possible contamination of salvaged blood with amniotic fluid.[436] This contraindication remains theoretical because there have been no reported cases of amniotic fluid embolism secondary to the autotransfusion of salvaged blood. There have been numerous reports of the use of blood salvaging procedures during massive hemorrhage from ruptured ectopic pregnancy, placenta previa, and placental rupture and from cesarean section without incident.[226,261,380,462-464] Furthermore, the exact mechanism of amniotic fluid embolism is not fully understood. Although insoluble fetal debris has traditionally been considered the causative agent, it has been shown that such debris is found in women not affected by amniotic fluid embolism.[465] It is known that the introduction of fetal material into the maternal circulation can precipitate a massive conversion of fibrinogen to fibrin that effectively blocks the pulmonary circulation whereas fibrinogen depletion causes uncon-

trollable hemorrhage due to coagulation failure.[466-469] Whether occurrence of amniotic fluid embolism is affected by the degree of insoluble fetal debris contamination or caused in part or totally by some soluble substance is not known.[465,470]

Autotransfusion systems rely on either filtration or cell processing (cell washing and centrifugation) to remove contaminants before reinfusion. Filtration (40–120 $\mu$m) can be expected to remove many insoluble contaminants but not the soluble elements. Cell-processing systems should reduce or eliminate both soluble and insoluble elements of amniotic fluid. Thornhill and associates[463] demonstrated that when $\alpha$-fetal protein concentration and fetal debris are used as markers, the cell processor appears to completely remove the $\alpha$-fetal proteins and significantly reduce but not eliminate fetal debris contamination. Zichella and Gramolini[464] safely autotransfused eight women undergoing elective cesarean section after demonstrating a lack of coagulant activity and the virtual elimination of phosphatidylglycerol in processed blood salvaged.

Based on the limited recent experience with and research in blood salvage in obstetrical patients, their appears to be a logical possibility of adverse reaction to the reinfusion of blood contaminated with amniotic fluid. Without further research or demonstrated incidence of amniotic fluid embolism resulting from autotransfusion, this remains theoretical. Until such information is available, it seems wise to avoid reinfusing shed blood suspected of amniotic fluid contamination.

## Blood Salvage for Jehovah's Witness Patients

Although the Jehovah's Witness religious doctrine demands strict abstinence from blood transfusion, there is some variation in acceptance of this conviction. Some are willing to accept autologous blood in some form (preoperative donation, very rarely), blood salvage techniques (occasionally for cardiac surgery but rarely for other procedures), and intraoperative acute normovolemic hemodilution; some are willing to accept synthetic blood (perfluorocarbons usually acceptable, hemoglobin solutions rarely acceptable);

whereas others refuse all blood, blood products, and substitutes.[471–474]

The acceptance of the CPB circuit, cardiotomy suction, and recirculators involved in cardiac surgery as temporary appendages of the body has somewhat increased the acceptance of blood salvage technology among Jehovah's Witness patients undergoing a wide variety of noncardiac surgical procedures. Strictly speaking, removal of blood from the body for reinfusion is usually only acceptable if it does not lose contact with the patient's circulation. The technological and functional similarity between blood salvage apparatus and the CPB circuit facilitated acceptance of blood salvage technology among Jehovah's Witnesses.[475–477] The cell processor has also been used for both intraoperative blood salvage[179,244,474,478–480] and as a component of a continuous-flow blood storage reservoir during normovolemic hemodilution.[179,380,481] After CPB, the hemoconcentrator has been used to reverse severe hemodilution[480] resulting from use of totally nonsanguinous priming solutions. After cardiovascular procedures, shed mediastinal blood can be captured and continuously reinfused.[480]

The use of blood salvage techniques should be carefully explained to the Jehovah's Witness patient and family. That the salvage circuit provides for continuous flow between the collection and reinfusion sites should be emphasized.[473] This may require modification of the usual blood salvaging techniques because some systems use discontinuous collection-reinfusion processes.[482]

## Blood Salvage for Sickle Cell Patients

Blood salvage in patients with sickle cell trait or disease is somewhat controversial.[483–485] In a 1986 report on the efficacy of blood conservation methods during vascular surgery, Tawes and colleagues[334] stated that the use of the cell processor was "ill-advised" in patients with sickle cell anemia. This statement was made without further explanation nor was this statement referenced. It can only be assumed they believed that mechanical damage to fragile RBCs may cause undue hemolysis or that these conditions might promote sickling.

Traditional therapy for the anemic sickle cell patient about to undergo surgery has been partial exchange transfusion to improve oxygen-carrying capacity and to reduce the proportion of hemoglobin-S and improve microvascular perfusion. This partial exchange transfusion is aimed at reducing the hemoglobin-S level below 30% without increasing HCT over 36%. However, exchange transfusion has become a complicated issue and its efficacy is currently being investigated.[486] Alloimmunization to RBC antigens is a common problem in sickle cell patients and presents significant limitations to transfusion therapy, including difficult compatability testing because of multiple RBC alloantibodies[487] and an increased risk of severe delayed hemolytic reactions. The sickle cell patient's concerns about transfusion-transmitted infection, particular the acquired immunodeficiency virus, must be considered. More likely to require blood transfusion than the average patient, these patients are at particular risk.[488] These risks must be weighed against proceeding with surgery with high levels of hemoglobin-S. Sickle cell crisis related to unintentional hypothermia, acidosis, and hypoxemia can ensue during the perioperative period. Anemia can be worsened by intraoperative blood loss and hemolysis. Preoperative autologous blood donation and frozen storage has been suggested[489] but has not gained popularity.[485,488] Intraoperative autotransfusion of salvaged blood offers several advantages over banked blood for patients requiring transfusion in the sickle cell patient: the risk of alloimmunization to donor cells and HLA antigens is reduced and autotransfused blood is warm, has higher 2,3-DPG levels, and has a more normal pH.

The safety of blood salvage in patients with sickle cell disease or trait has not been adequately studied, as literature is limited to occasional case reports.[483–485] In a patient with sickle cell disease, Castro and associates[488] positively demonstrated that sickled RBCs tended to clump in the centrifuge bowl and that this could be avoided by dilution with saline. Brajtbord and associates[483] noted significant sickling of RBCs after cell processing in a sickle cell trait (heterozygous) patient. However, Black and Dearing[482] used the cell processor in a sickle cell trait patient for total exchange transfusion before CPB without incident. In this case, only platelet-rich plasma

**Table 9–10.   Characteristics of Blood from Various Sites During Autotransfusion in a Sickle Cell Patient**

|  | Preoperative Venous | Reservoir Sample | Reinfused Blood | Discard Solution | Postoperative Arterial |
|---|---|---|---|---|---|
| pH | — | 7.78 | 7.81 | 7.77 | 7.34 |
| $PO_2$ (mm Hg) | — | 173 | 217 | 191 | 108 |
| $SaO_2$ (%) | — | 100 | 100 | 100 | 96 |
| WBC ($10^3$/mL) | 9.0 | 6.3 | 12.7 | — | 28.8 |
| Hemoglobin (g/dL) | 11.6 | 6.8 | 15.5 | 1.5 | 9.1 |
| HCT (%) | 34.7 | 16.4 | 46.2 | — | 26.9 |
| Platelets ($10^3$/mL) | 282 | — | — | — | 182 |
| $K^+$ (mmol/L) | 3.8 | 10.2 | 2.1 | 5.7 | 4.1 |
| Sickling | Marked | Occasional | Slight | — | Slight/moderate |

Modified from Cook A, Hanowell LH: Intraoperative autotransfusion for a patient with homozygous sickle cell disease. Anesthesiology 1990; 73:177, with permission.

was reinfused and the concentrated sickle cell RBCs discarded.

Cook and Hanowell[484] demonstrated the safety of blood salvage by cell processing in a sickle cell disease (homozygous) patient undergoing hip replacement surgery. After preoperative exchange transfusion (2 months being required to obtain sufficient bank blood for anticipated perioperative transfusion due to acquired RBC antibodies), electrophoresis showed hemoglobin-S 25% and hemoglobin-A 71%; preoperative hemoglobin was 11.5 g/dL. Using a cell-processing device, 2200 mL blood loss resulted in an RBC harvest of 675 mL. There was only slight sickling in reinfused blood and no adverse sequelae from blood sal-

vaging occurred (Table 9–10). This appears in contrast to the report by Brajtbord and colleagues[483] in a patient with sickle cell trait. The reason for this discrepancy is unclear. Nevertheless, autotransfusion in sickle cell trait and disease appears to be possible, provided that the quality of the salvaged blood is carefully monitored. Suggested perioperative considerations are listed in Table 9–11.[485]

## SUMMARY

Today, blood salvage is an integral component of a comprehensive approach to blood conservation. Although in some situations the use of blood salvage has resulted in the elimination of allogeneic blood transfusion, it cannot necessarily be viewed as a substitute for allogeneic blood. In an effort to conserve the allogeneic blood supply and reduce the risks of allogeneic blood transfusion, blood salvage should be considered a complement to allogeneic blood. Whenever possible, blood salvage techniques should be combined with any number of other blood conservation techniques appropriate for the situation. These include surgical and anesthetic techniques aimed at reducing blood loss or increasing salvage harvest, preoperative autologous blood donation, acute normovolemic hemodilution, deliberate hypotension, induced hypothermia, and, finally, a rational basis for the decision to transfuse a unit of blood or blood product perioperatively (allogeneic or autologous).

**Table 9–11.   Suggested Guidelines for Intraoperative Autotransfusion in Patients with Sickle Cell Disease**

Preoperative considerations
  Exchange transfuse to attain 60–70% hemoglobin-A and HCT 30–36%
  Bank autologous blood if feasible
Intraoperative considerations
  Solutions with physiologic pH for wound lavage and cell washing
  Limit negative pressure at tip of suction cannulae to <100 mm Hg
  Compare smears of venous and processed blood before reinfusion to assess sickling
  Monitor pH, $PO_2$, and HCT of processed blood
  Anticoagulate harvested blood (heparin) until processing
  Wash RBC with 1–2 L 0.9% NaCl to remove waste products and filter before reinfusion

HBGB = hemoglobin; HCT = hematocrit. From Cook A and Hanowell LH: Intraoperative autotransfusion for a patient with homozygous sickle cell disease. Anesthesiology 73:177, 1990, with permission.

### REFERENCES

1. Highmore W: Practical remarks on an overlooked source of blood-supply for transfusion in post-partum haemorrhage. Lancet 1874; 1:89.

2. Duncan J: On re-infusion of blood in primary and other amputations. Br Med J 1886; 1:192.
3. Miller AG: Case of amputation at hip-joint, in which reinjection of blood was performed, and rapid recovery took place. Edinburgh Med J 1986; 31:721.
4. Thies HJ: Zür behandlung der extrautering gravidi tat. Zentralbl Gynakol 1914; 38:1191.
5. Elmendorf: Über wiederinfusion nach punktion eines frischen hämatothorax. Münchener Med Woch 1917; 64:36.
6. Farrar LKP: Auto blood transfusion in gynecology. Surg Gynecol Obstet 1923; 36:454.
7. Coley BL: Traumatic rupture of spleen splenectomy: autotransfusion. Am J Surg 1928; 6:334.
8. Watson CM, Watson JR: Autotransfusion in the treatment of wounds of the heart. JAMA 1936; 106:520.
9. Rossi EC, Simon TL, Moss GS: Transfusion in transition. In: Rossi EC, Simon TL, Moss GS, eds, Principles of Transfusion Medicine. Baltimore, 1991, Williams & Wilkins, pp. 1–11.
10. Blundell J: Experiments on the transfusion of blood by the syringe. Med Chir Trans 1818; 9:57.
11. Blundell J: Some account of a case of obstinate vomiting in which an attempt was made to prolong life by the injection of blood into the veins. Med Chir Trans 1819; 10:296.
12. Blundell J: Observations on transfusion of blood. 1928; Lancet 2:321.
13. Jones HW, Mackmull G: The influence of James Blundell on the development of blood transfusion. Ann Hist Med 1928; 20:242.
14. Burch LE: Autotransfusion. Surg Gynecol Obstet 1922; 811.
15. Burch LE: Autotransfusion. Trans South Surg Assoc 1922; 35:25.
16. Lichtenstein F: Eigenbluttransfusion bei extrauteringraviditaet und uterusruptur. München Med Woch 1915; 42:1597.
17. Schaefer A: Ruecktransfusion des koerpereigenen blutenach masssenblutungen in die grossen koerpers hoehlen. Zentralbl Chir 1916; 43:417.
18. Lichtenstein F: Ohne Eigenbluttransfusion sollte keine wegen tubenusur operierte frau mehr an verblutung sterben. Arch Gynakol 1918; 109:599.
19. Ostwald E: Über wiederinfusion abdominaler massenblutungen. München Med Woch 1918; 65:678.
20. Roedelius E: Zur technik der direkten blut- und eigenbluttransfusion. Zentralbl Chir 1918; 45:599.
21. Schaefer A: Intravenoese intramuskulaere und rektale infusion koerpereigenen blutes nach schweren blutungen. München Med Woch 1918; 65:908.
22. Blechschmidt: Über eigenblutinfusion, dissertation. Leipzig, 1919, Lehmann.
23. Lichtenstein F: Technisches sur eigenbluttransfusion bei extrauteringraviditaet. Zentralbl Gynakol 1919; 43:433.
24. Roedelius E: Eigenbluttransfusion bei geplatzter tubargraviditaet. Berl Klin Woch 1919; 56:820.
25. Schaefer A: Die autoinfusion in der geburtshuelfe. Monatsschr Geburtsh Gynakol 1919; 49:162.
26. Von Arnim E: Über reinfusion von eigenblut bei extrauteringraviditaet. Zentralbl Gynakol 1919; 43: 971.
27. Zapelloni LG: La reinfusione del sangue stravasato nelleg gravdisierose. Riforma Med 1919; 32:932.
28. Bumm E: Zur frage de bluttransfusion. Zentralbl Gynakol 40:286, 1920.
29. Doederlein A: Über eigenblutinfusion. Deutsche Med Wchnschr 1920; 56:449.
30. Kulenkampff D: Die technik der laparatomie bei der eigenblutinfusion. Sentralbl Gynakol 1920; 44: 396.
31. Opitz: Gefahren der bluttransfusion in der geburtshilfe. Zentralbl Gynakol 1920; 44:6.
32. Toepler B: Über blutreinfusion bei 24 faellen von graviditas extrauterine rupta. Deutsche Med Woch 1922; 64:92.
33. Kreuter E: Zur wiederinfusion abdomineller blutungen. München Med Woch 1916; 43:1498.
34. Kreuter E: Ein weiterer fall von wiederinfusion einer intra-abdominellen massenblutung bei leberruptur. Zentralbl Chir 1917; 44:765.
35. Peiser: Über eigenbluttransfusion bei milzzerreissung. Zentralbl Chir 1917; 44:71.
36. Ranft G: Autotransfusion nach milzruptur. Zentralbl Chir 1917; 44:1019.
37. Feiber EL: Eigenbluttransfusion bei milzzerreissung. Zentralbl Chir 1918; 45:413.
38. Laewen A: Die schussverletzungen des bauches und der nieren. Ergeb Chir Orthop 1918; 10:611.
39. Davis MB: Autotransfusion. J Tenn Med Asso 1922; 15:292.
40. Burchhardt F, Landois: Die brustverletzungen im kriege. Ergeb Chir Orthop 1918; 10:467.
41. Burchhardt F: Zur urheberschaft der eigenblutinfusion. Zentralbl Gynakol 1920; 44:724.
42. Eberle D: Aus der praxis der eigenblut und der indirekten fremblut transfusion bei akuten bluverlusten. Schweiz Med Wochenschr 1920; 1:961.
43. Loehnberg E: Zur kinik der tubargraviditaet insbesondere über die reinfusion bei rupturen. Z Geburtsh Gynakol 1921; 84:404.
44. Lockwood CD: Surgical treatment of Banti's disease: report of three cases. Surg Gynecol Obstet 1916; 25:188.
45. White CS: Rupture of the liver: with report of a case in which autotransfusion was employed. Surg Gynecol Obstet 1923; 36:343.
46. Brown AL, Debenham MW: Autotransfusion: use of blood from hemothorax. JAMA 1931; 96:1223.
47. Davis LE, Cushing H: Experiences with blood replacement during or after major intracranial operations. Surg Gynecol Obstet 1925; 40:310.
48. May GE: Auto blood transfusion. N Engl J Med 1930; 203:1197.
49. Rumbaugh MC: Ruptured tubal pregnancy: report of a case in which life was saved by autotransfusion of blood. Penn Med J 1931; 34:7100.
50. Griswold RA, Ortner AB: The use of autotransfusion in surgery of the serous cavities. Surg Gynecol Obstet 1943; 77:167.
51. Rous P, Turner JR: The preservation of living red blood cells in vitro. J Exp Med 1916; 23:219.
52. Grant FC: Autotransfusion. Ann Surg 1921; 74: 253.
53. Brown AL: A closed method for the transfusion of citrated blood. Calif West Med 1929; 31:205.
54. Loutit JF, Mollison PL: Advantages of a disodium-citrate-glucose mixture as a blood preservative. Br Med J 1943; 2:744.
55. Weil R: Sodium citrate in the transfusion of blood. JAMA 1915; 64:425.
56. Robertson OH: Transfusion with preserved red blood cells. Br Med J 1918; 1:691.
57. Duran-Jorda F: The Barcelona blood transfusion service. Lancet 1939; 1:773.

58. Fantus B: Therapeutics: the therapy of Cook County Hospital. JAMA 1937; 109:128.

59. Fantus B, Schirmer EH: Blood preservation technic. JAMA 1938; 111:317.

60. Wilson JD, Taswell HF: Autotransfusion: historical review and preliminary report on a new method. Mayo Clin Proc 1968; 43:26.

61. Thurer RL, Hauer JM: Autotransfusion and blood conservation. Curr Probl Surg 1982; 19:97.

62. Ferrara BE: Autotransfusion: its use in acute hemothorax. South Med J 1957; 50:516.

63. Brzica SM Jr, Pineda AA, Taswell HF: Autologous blood transfusion. Mayo Clin Proc 1976; 51:723.

64. Ellison N, Wurzel HA: The blood shortage: is autotransfusion an answer? Anesthesiology 1975; 43: 288.

65. O'Riordan WD: Autotransfusion in the emergency department of a community hospital. J Am Coll Emerg Phys 1977; 6:233.

66. Dyer RH Jr: Intraoperative autotransfusion: a preliminary report and new method. Am J Surg 1966; 112:874.

67. Saarela E: Autotransfusion: review. Ann Clin Res 1981; 13(suppl 13):48.

68. Solem JO, Vagianos C: Perioperative blood salvage. Acta Anaesth Scand 1988; 89:71.

69. Rumisek JD: Autotransfusion of shed blood: an untapped battlefield resource. Milit Med 1982; 147: 193.

70. Langston HT, Milles G, Dalessandro W: Further experiences with autogenous blood transfusions. Ann Surg 1963; 158:333.

71. Tarasov MM: Cadaveric blood transfusion. Ann N Y Acad Sci 1960; 87:512.

72. Yudin SS: Transfusion of cadaver blood. JAMA 1936; 106:997.

73. Vaughn J: Blood transfusion in the U.S.S.R. Transfusion 1967; 7:212.

74. Kevorkian J, Bylsma GW: Transfusion of postmortem human blood. Am J Clin Pathol 1961; 35:413.

75. Kevorkian J, Marra JJ: Transfusion of human corpse blood without additives. Transfusion 1964; 4:112.

76. Valbonesi M, Ferrari M, Zia S, et al: New application of the autotrans: autologous support of the organ donor and salvage of the donor's red blood cells for the transfusion support of organ recipients. J Clin Apheresis 1988; 4:166.

77. Klebanoff G, Watkins D: A disposable auto-transfusion unit. Am J Surg 1968; 116:475.

78. Klebanoff G: Early clinical experience with a disposable unit for the intraoperative salvage and reinfusion of blood loss (intraoperative autotransfusion). Am J Surg 1970; 120:718.

79. Klebanoff G, Phillps J, Evans W: Use of a disposable autotransfusion unit under varying conditions of contamination. Am J Surg 1970; 120:351.

80. Duncan SE, Edwards WH, Dale WA: Caution regarding autotransfusion. Surgery 1974; 76:1024.

81. Duncan SE, Klebanoff G, Rogers W: A clinical experience with intraoperative autotransfusion. Ann Surg 1974; 180:296.

82. Deysine M: Intraoperative autotransfusion and air embolism. Surgery 1977; 81:729.

83. Noon GP, Solis RT, Natelson EA: A simple method of intraoperative autotransfusion. Surg Gynecol Obstet 1976; 143:65.

84. Noon GP: Intraoperative autotransfusion. Surgery 1978; 84:719.

85. Tullis JL, Tinch RJ, Gibson JG II, et al: A simplified centrifuge for the separation and processing of blood cells. Transfusion 1967; 7:232.

86. Hauer JM: Autotransfusion in trauma surgery. In: Hauer JM, Thurer RL, Dawson RB, eds, Autotransfusion. New York, 1981, Elsevier-North Holland, pp. 93–103.

87. Mohr R, Golan M, Martinowitz U, et al: Effect of cardiac operation on platelets. J Thorac Cardiovasc Surg 1986; 92:434.

88. Giordano GF, Rivers SL, Chung GKT, et al: Autologous platelet-rich plasma in cardiac surgery: effect on intraoperative and postoperative transfusion requirements. Ann Thorac Surg 1988; 46:416.

89. Tawes RL Jr, Sydorak GR, Duvall TB, et al: The plasma collection system: a new concept in autotransfusion. Ann Vasc Surg 1989; 3:304.

90. Breyer RH, Engelman RM, Rousou JA, et al: A comparison of cell saver versus ultrafilter during coronary artery bypass operations. J Thorac Cardiovasc Surg 1985; 90:736.

91. Solem JO, Steen S, Olin C: A new method for autotransfusion of shed blood. Acta Chir Scand 1986; 152:421.

92. Symbas PN, Levin JM, Ferrier FL, et al: A study on autotransfusion from hemothorax. South Med J 1969a; 62:671.

93. Symbas PN, Levin JM, Ferrier FL: Autotransfusion and its effects upon the blood components and the recipient. Curr Top Surg Res 1969b; 1:387.

94. Symbas PN: Autotransfusion from hemothorax: experimental and clinical studies. J Trauma 1972; 12: 689.

95. Bunn HF: The use of hemoglobin as a blood substitute. Am J Hematol 1993; 42:112.

96. Crosby ET: Perioperative haemotherapy. I. Indications for blood component transfusion. Can J Anaesth 1992; 39:695.

97. Beal R: Transfusion science and practice in developing countries: " . . . a high frequency of empty shelves . . . ." Transfusion 1993; 33:276.

98. Lawson JB, Stewart DB: Obstetrics and Gynaecology in the Tropics and Developing Countries. London, 1967, Edward Arnold LTD.

99. Pathak UN, Stewart DB: Autotransfusion in ruptured ectopic pregnancy. Lancet 1970; 1:961.

100. Whitehead SM: Using blood bags for autotransfusion. Trop Doct 1982; 12:189.

101. Price ME, Kembey TY: Collecting blood: autotransfusion in ectopic pregnancy. Trop Doct 1985; 15: 67.

102. Paika RL: Autotransfusion in splenic rupture. P N G Med J 1993; 36:56.

103. Bell WR: The hematology of autotransfusion. Surgery 1978; 84:695.

104. Mattox KL, Espada R, Beall AC, et al: Performing thoracotomy in the emergency center. JACEP 1974; 3:13.

105. Young GP, Purcell TB: Emergency autotransfusion. Ann Emerg Med 1983; 12:180.

106. Orr MD: Autotransfusion: the use of washed red cells as an adjunct to component therapy. Surgery 1978; 84:728.

107. Reul GJ Jr, Solis RT, Greenberg SD, et al: Experience with autotransfusion in the surgical management of trauma. Surgery 1974; 76:546.

108. Raines J, Buth J, Brewster DC, et al: Intraoperative autotransfusion: equipment, protocols, and guidelines. J Trauma 1976; 16:616.

109. Nightingale CH, Robotti J, Deckers PJ, et al: Qual-

ity care and cost-effectiveness: an organized approach to problem solving. Arch Surg 1987; 122: 451.

110. Von Koch L, Defore WW, Mattox KL: A practical method of autotransfusion in the emergency center. Am J Surg 1977; 133:770.

111. Davidson SJ: Emergency unit autotransfusion. Surgery 1978; 84:703.

112. Schaff HV, Hauer JM, Bell WR, et al: Autotransfusion of shed mediastinal blood after cardiac surgery: a prospective study. J Thorac Cardiovasc Surg 1978; 75:632.

113. Cordell AR, Lavender SW: An appraisal of blood salvage techniques in vascular and cardiac operations. Ann Thorac Surg 1981; 31:421.

114. Adhoute BG, Bleyn JA: Autotransfusion in vascular surgical practice. In: Hauer JM, Thurer RL, Dawson RB, eds, Autotransfusion. New York, 1981, Elsevier-North Holland, pp. 29–41.

115. Bennett JG: Autotransfusion of drained mediastinal blood. Thorac Cardiovasc Surg 1982; 30:28.

116. Brawley RK: Autotransfusion in postoperative cardiac surgical patients. In: Hauer JM, Thurer RL, Dawson RB, eds, Autotransfusion. New York, 1981, Elsevier-North Holland, pp. 51–62.

117. Sinclair A, Jacobs LM Jr: Emergency department autotransfusion for trauma victims. Med Instrum 1982; 16:283.

118. Williamson KR, Taswell HF: Intraoperative Blood Salvage. In: Taswell HF, Pineda AA, eds, Autologous Transfusion and Hemotherapy. Boston, 1991, Blackwell Scientific Publications, pp. 122–154.

119. Stehling LC: Trends in transfusion therapy. Anesthesiol Clin North Am 1990; 8:519.

120. Popovsky MA, Devine PA, Taswell HF: Intraoperative autologous transfusion. Mayo Clin Proc 1985; 60:125.

121. Bovill DF, Moulton CW, Jackson WST, et al: The efficacy of intraoperative autologous transfusion in major orthopedic surgery: a regression analysis. Orthopedics 1986; 9:1403.

122. Dale RF, Lindop MJ, Farman JV, et al: Autotransfusion: an experience of seventy six cases. Ann R Coll Surg 1986; 68:295.

123. American Association of Blood Banks: Guidelines for blood salvage and reinfusion in surgery and trauma. Arlington, VA, 1990, American Association of Blood Banks.

124. Honek T, Horvath P, Kucera V, et al: Minimization of priming volume and blood saving in paediatric cardiac surgery. Eur J Cardiothorac Surg 1992; 6: 308.

125. Kruger LM, Colbert JM: Intraoperative autologous transfusion in children undergoing spinal surgery. J Pediatr Orthop 1985; 5:330.

126. Ray JM, Flynn JC, Bierman AH: Erythrocyte survival following intraoperative autotransfusion in spinal surgery. An *in vivo* comparative study and 5-year update. Spine 1986; 11:879.

127. Salem MR, Bikhazi G: Blood Conservation. In: Motoyama EK, Davis PJ, eds, Smith's Anesthesia for Infants and Children. St. Louis, 1990, C.V. Mosby.

128. Brecher ME, Moore SB, Taswell HF: Minimal-exposure transfusion: a new approach to homologous blood transfusion. Mayo Clin Proc 1988; 63:903.

129. Salem MR, Podraza AG: Blood conservation and massive transfusion. Semin Anesth 1992; 11:339.

130. Thurer RL, Lytle BW, Cosgrove DM, et al: Auto-transfusion following cardiac operations: a randomized, prospective study. Ann Thorac Surg 1979; 27: 500.

131. Thurer RL, Loop FD, Lytle BW, et al: The conservation of blood during cardiac surgery. Clin Cardiol 1979; 2:155.

132. Johnson RG, Rosenkrantz KR, Preston RA, et al: The efficacy of postoperative autotransfusion in patients undergoing cardiac operations. Ann Thorac Surg 1983; 36:173.

133. Solem JO, Olin C, Tengborn L, et al: Postoperative autotransfusion of concentrated drainage blood in cardiac surgery. Experience with a new autotransfusion system. Scand J Thorac Cardiovasc Surg 1987; 21:153.

134. Von Hippel A: Autotransfusion of major hemothorax in a simple country hospital. Alaska Med 1975; 17:62.

135. Solot JA: Autotransfusion: an update. J Am Osteopath Assoc 1982; 81:618.

136. Hauer JM, Thurer RL: Controversies in autotransfusion. Vox Sang 1984; 46:8.

137. Griffith LD, Billman GF, Daily PO, et al: Apparent coagulopathy caused by infusion of shed mediastinal blood and its prevention by washing of the infusate. Ann Thorac Surg 1989; 47:400.

138. Semkiw LB, Schurman DJ, Goodman SB, et al: Postoperative blood salvage using the cell saver after total joint arthroplasty. J Bone Joint Surg [Am] 1989; 71A:823.

139. Jurkovich GJ, Moore EE, Medina G: Autotransfusion in trauma. A pragmatic analysis. Am J Surg 1984; 148:782.

140. Wodo R, Tetzlaff JE: Upper airway oedema following autologous blood transfusion form a wound drainage system. Can J Anaesth 1992; 39:290.

141. Bengston J-P, Backman L, Stenqvist O, et al: Complement activation and reinfusion of wound drainage blood. Anesthesiology 1990; 73:376.

142. Jacob HS, Craddock PR, Hammerschmidt DE, et al: Complement-induced granulocyte aggregation. N Engl J Med 1980; 302:789.

143. Bland LA, Villarino ME, Arduino MJ, et al: Bacteriologic and endotoxin analysis of salvaged blood used in autologous transfusions during cardiac operations. J Thorac Cardiovasc Surg 1992; 103:582.

144. Eisenstaedt RS: Operative red cell salvage and autotransfusion. Transfus Sci 1989; 10:185.

145. Koehler LC, Williamson KR, Taswell HF: A comprehensive program to ensure quality in intraoperative blood salvage. J Intraven Nursing 1991; 14: 193.

146. Jacobs LM, Hsieh JW: A clinical review of autotransfusion and its role in trauma. JAMA 1984; 251: 3283.

147. Solomon MD, Rutledge ML, Kane LE, et al: Cost comparison of intraoperative autologous versus homologous transfusion. Transfusion 1988; 28:379.

148. Giordano GF: Intraoperative salvage: administrative aspects. In: Maffei LM, Thurer RL, eds, Autologous Blood Transfusion: Current Issues. Arlington, TX, 1988, American Association of Blood Banks, pp. 21–32.

149. Yawn DH: Properties of salvaged blood. In: Taswell HF, Pineda AA, eds, Autologous Transfusion and Hemotherapy. Boston, 1991, Blackwell Scientific, pp. 194–206.

150. Popovsky MA, Taswell HF: Role of i.v. and transfusion nurses in autologous transfusion. NITA 1984; 7:385.

151. DeCrosta T: Autotransfusion: risks and rewards in emergency care. Nurs Life 1983; 3:52.

152. Madden K, Adams L: Autotransfusion: now it's saving lives in the ED. RN 1983; 46:50.

153. Bennett SH, Hoye RC, Riggle GC: Intraoperative autotransfusion: preliminary report of a new blood suction device for anticoagulation of autologous blood. Am J Surg 1972; 123:257.

154. Aaron RK, Beazley RM, Riggle GC: Hematologic integrity after intraoperative allotransfusion. Arch Surg 1974; 108:831.

155. Zauder HL: Intraoperative and postoperative blood salvage devices. In: Stehling LC, ed, Perioperative Autologous Transfusion. Arlington, VA, 1991, American Association of Blood Banks, pp. 25–36.

156. Moseley RV, Doty DB: Changes in the filtration characteristics of stored blood. Ann Surg 1970; 171:329.

157. McNamara JJ Burran EL, Larson E, et al: Effect of debris in stored blood on pulmonary microvasculature. Ann Thorac Surg 1972; 14:133.

158. Klebanoff G, Dorang LA, Kemmerer WT, et al: Repair of suprahepatic caval laceration employing autotransfusion: an experimental model to demonstrate the effectiveness of intraoperative blood salvage under conditions of massive hemorrhage. J Trauma 1972; 12:422.

159. Bennett SH, Geelhoed GW, Terrill RE, et al: Pulmonary effects of autotransfused blood: a comparison of fresh autologous and stored blood with blood retrieved from the pleural cavity in an *in situ* lung perfusion model. Am J Surg 1973; 125:696.

160. Connell RS, Swank RL: Pulmonary microembolism after blood transfusions: an electron microscopic study. Ann Surg 1973; 177:40.

161. Davies GG, Wells DG, Mabee TM, et al: Platelet-leukocyte plasmapheresis attenuates the deleterious effects of cardiopulmonary bypass. Ann Thorac Surg 1992; 53:274.

162. Wells DG, Davies GG: Platelet salvage in cardiac surgery. J Cardiothorac Vasc Anesth 1993; 7:448.

163. Gervin AS, Limbird TJ, Puckett CL, et al: Ultrapore hemofiltration: the effects on the coagulation and fibrinolytic mechanisms in fresh and stored blood. Arch Surg 1973; 106:333.

164. Dunbar RW, Price KA, Cannarella CF: Microaggregate blood filters: effect on filtration time plasma hemoglobin and fresh blood platelets. Anesth Analg 1974; 53:577.

165. Levine RH, Freireich EJ, Chappel W: Effect of storage up to 48 hours on response to transfusion of platelet-rich plasma. Transfusion 1964; 4:251.

166. McNamara JJ, Anderson BS, Hayashi T: Stored blood, platelets and microaggregate formation. Surg Gynecol Obstet 1978; 147:507.

167. Moore SB: Management of transfusion in the massively bleeding patient. Hum Pathol 1983; 14:267.

168. Welch J, Weintraub H, Gutterman BJ, et al: Laboratory experience with a new autotransfusion device. Arch Surg 1976; 111:1374.

169. Geelhoed GW, Bennett SH, McCune WS: Pulmonary effects of autotransfusion with and without dacron wool filtration. Bull Soc Int Chir 1975; 6:549.

170. Stillman RM, Wrezlewicz WW, Stanczewski B, et al: The haematological hazards of autotransfusion. Br J Surg 1976; 63:651.

171. Wilson JD, Utz DC, Taswell HF: Autotransfusion during transurethral resection of the prostate: technique and preliminary clinical evaluation. Mayo Clin Proc 1969; 44:374.

172. Wilson JD, Taswell HF, Utz DC: Autotransfusion: urologic applications and the development of a modified irrigating fluid. J Urol 1971; 105:873.

173. Dixon JL, Smalley G: Jehovah's Witnesses: the surgical/ethical challenge. JAMA 1981; 246:2471.

174. Sade RM, Dearing JP, Wilds SL: Massive air embolus due to Pall filter malfunction. J Thorac Cardiovasc Surg 1983; 86:156.

175. Williamson KR, Taswell HF, Rettke SR, et al: Intraoperative transfusion: its role in orthotopic liver transplantation. Mayo Clin Proc 1989; 28:546.

176. Moran JM, Babka R, Silberman S, et al: Role of the Haemonetics cell saver following cardiopulmonary bypass. Proc Adv Comp Sem, Chicago, Illinois, 1977.

177. Moran JM, Babka R, Silberman S, et al: Immediate centrifugation of oxygenator contents after cardiopulmonary bypass: role in maximum blood conservation. J Thorac Cardiovasc Surg 1978; 76:510.

178. Umlas J, O'Neill TP: Heparin removal in an autotransfusor device. Transfusion 1981; 21:70.

179. Ottesen S, Frøysaker T: Use of Haemonetics cell saver for autotransfusion in cardiovascular surgery. Scand J Thorac Cardiovasc Surg 1982; 16:263.

180. Keeling MM, Gray LA Jr, Brink MA, et al: Intraoperative autotransfusion: experience in 725 consecutive cases. Ann Surg 1983; 197:536.

181. Mattox KL, Allen MK, Lockhart C, et al: Improved techniques for intraoperative autotransfusion in the trauma patient. Proc Blood Conserv Inst, Chicago, Illinois, 1978.

182. Rumisek JD, Weddle RL: Autotransfusion in penetrating abdominal trauma. In: Hauer JM, Thurer RL, Dawson RB, eds, Autotransfusion. New York, 1981, Elsevier-North Holland, pp. 105–113.

183. Boudreaux JP, Bornside GH, Cohn I Jr: Emergency autotransfusion: partial cleansing of bacteria-laden blood by cell washing. J Trauma 1983; 23:31.

184. McShane AJ, Power C, Jackson JF, et al: Autotransfusion: quality of blood prepared with a red cell processing device. Br J Anaesth 1987; 59:1035.

185. Timberlake GA, McSwain NE Jr: Autotransfusion of blood contaminated by enteric contents: a potentially life-saving measure in the massively hemorrhaging trauma patient? J Trauma 1988; 28:855.

186. Cohn LH, Solomon S, Lee-Son S, et al: Sequestration of platelet-rich plasma for patients undergoing coronary bypass operations. Proc Blood Conserv Inst, 1978.

187. Giordano GF Sr, Giordano GF Jr, Rivers SL, et al: Determinants of homologous blood usage utilizing autologous platelet-rich plasma in cardiac operations. Ann Thorac Surg 1989; 47:897.

188. Ferrari M, Zia S, Valbonesi M, et al: A new technique for hemodilution, preparation of autologous platelet-rich plasma and intraoperative blood salvage in cardiac surgery. Int J Artif Organs 1987; 10:47.

189. Boldt J, von Bormann B, Kling D, et al: Preoperative plasmapheresis in patients undergoing cardiac procedures. Anesthesiology 1990; 72:282.

190. Jones JW, McCoy TA, Rawitscher RE, et al: Effects

of intraoperative plasmapheresis on blood loss in cardiac surgery. Ann Thorac Surg 1990; 49:585.

191. Davies MJ, Cronin KD, Moran P, et al: Autologous blood transfusion for major vascular surgery using the Sorenson Receptal device. Anaesth Intens Care 1987; 15:282.

192. Pineda AA, Valbonesi M: Intraoperative blood salvage. Clin Haematol 1990; 3:385.

193. Nelson CL, Nelson RL, Cone J: Blood conservation techniques in orthopaedic surgery. Instruct Course Lec 1990, 53:425.

194. Dyer RH Jr, Alexander JT, Brighton CT: Atraumatic aspiration of whole blood for intraoperative autotransfusion. Am J Surg 1972; 123:510.

195. Stehling LC, Zauder HL, Rogers W: Intraoperative autotransfusion. Anesthesiology 1975; 43:337.

196. Buth J, Raines JK, Kolodny GM, et al: Effect of intraoperative autotransfusion on red cell mass and red cell survival. Surg Forum 1975; 26:276.

197. Dorang LA, Klebanoff G, Kemmerer WT: Autotransfusion in long-segment spinal fusion: an experimental model to demonstrate the efficacy of salvaging blood contaminated with bone fragments and marrow. Am J Surg 1972; 123:686.

198. Brener BJ, Raines JK, Darling RC: Intraoperative autotransfusion in abdominal aortic resections. Arch Surg 1973; 107:78.

199. Murray DJ, Gress K, Weinstein SL: Coagulopathy after reinfusion of autologous scavenged red blood cells. Anesth Analg 1992; 75:125.

200. Tyras DH, DiOrio DA, Stone HH, et al: Autotransfusion of intraperitoneal blood: an experimental study. Am Surg 1973; 39:652.

201. Glover JL, Smith R, Yaw PB, et al: Intraoperative autotransfusion: an underutilized technique. Surgery 1976; 80:474.

202. Rakower SR, Worth MH Jr, Lackner H: Massive intraoperative autotransfusion of blood. Surg Gynecol Obstet 1973; 137:633.

203. Rakower SR, Worth MH Jr: Autotransfusion: perspective and critical problems. J Trauma 1973; 13:573.

204. Ten Duis HJ, Harder MP, Webeke E, et al: An automatic autotransfusion system with a centrifugal pump: a hematologic evaluation in dogs. Surgery 1988; 103:74.

205. Filatov A: Klinische und expperimentelle beiträge zur reinfusion des in die körperhöhlen ergossenen blutes. Arch Klin Chir 1928; 151:184.

206. Ricci JV, DiPalma S: Analysis of 100 cases of ruptured ectopic gestation: technic and evaluation of autohemofusion. Am J Obstet Gynecol 1931; 22:857.

207. Faris PM, Ritter MA, Keating EM, et al: Unwashed filtered shed blood collected after knee and hip arthroplasties. J Bone Joint Surg [Am] 1991; 73A:1169.

208. Broadie TA, Glover JL, Bang N, et al: Clotting competence of intracavitary blood in trauma victims. Ann Emerg Med 1981; 10:127.

209. Wright G: Haematological effects of cardiotomy suction. In: Longmore DB, ed, Towards Safer Cardiac Surgery. Lancaster, England, 1979, MTP Press Ltd., pp. 313–323.

210. Wright G, Anderson JM: Cellular aggregation and trauma in cardiotomy suction systems. Thorax 1979; 34:621.

211. Ten Duis HJ, Binnendijk B, Wildevuur CR: Intra-

operative autotransfusion. Acta Anaesthesiol Belg 1984; 35(suppl):27.

212. Csencsitz TA, Flynn JC: Intraoperative blood salvage in spinal deformity surgery in children. J Fla Med Assoc 1979; 66:31.

213. Wall W, Heimbecker RO, McKenzie FN, et al: Intraoperative autotransfusion in major elective vascular operations: a clinical assessment. Surgery 1976; 79:82.

214. Andrews NJ, Bloor K: Autologous blood collection in abdominal vascular surgery: assessment of a low pressure blood salvage system with particular reference to the preservation of cellular elements, triglyceride, complement and bacterial content in the collected blood. Clin Lab Haematol 1983; 5:361.

215. Glover JL, Broadie TA: Intraoperative autotransfusion. In: Collins JA, Murawski K, Shafer AW, eds, Massive Transfusion in Surgery and Trauma. New York, 1982, Alan R. Liss, Inc., pp. 151–170.

216. Ansell J, Parrilla N, King M, et al: Survival of autotransfused red blood cells recovered from the surgical field during cardiovascular operations. J Thorac Cardiovasc Surg 1982; 84:387.

217. O'Hara PJ, Hertzer NR, Santilli PH, et al: Intraoperative autotransfusion during abdominal aortic reconstruction. Am J Surg 1983; 145:215.

218. Gray A, Valeri CR: Survival and function of washed and non-washed red blood cells in dog shed blood. Transfusion 1989; 29:24S.

219. Weisel RD, Denis RC, Manny J, et al: Adverse effects of transfusion therapy during abdominal aortic aneurysmectomy. Surgery 1978; 83:682.

220. Bjerre-Jepsen K, Kristensen P, Horn A, et al: Intraoperative autotransfusion. Acta Chir Scand 1982; 148:557.

221. Hallett JW Jr, Popovsky M, Ilstrup D: Minimizing blood transfusions during abdominal aortic surgery: recent advances in rapid autotransfusion. J Vasc Surg 1987; 5:601-606.

222. Bernstein EF, Indeglia Ra, Shea MA, et al: Sublethal damage to the red blood cell from pumping. Circulation 1969; 35 (suppl 1):226.

223. Peskin GW, O'Brien K, Rabiner SF: Stroma-free hemoglobin solution: the "ideal" blood substitute? Surgery 1969; 66:135.

224. Schweitzer B: Erfahrungen mit der eigenblutretransfusion bei extrauteringraviditaet. München Med Woch 1921; 68:699.

225. Relihan M, Olsen RE, Litwin MS: Clearance rate and effect on renal function of stroma-free hemoglobin following renal ischemia. Ann Surg 1972; 176:700.

226. Bonfils-Roberts EA, Stutman L, Nealon TF Jr: Autologous blood in the treatment of intraoperative hemorrhage. Ann Surg 1977; 185:321.

227. McKenzie FN, Heimbecker RO, Wall W, et al: Intraoperative autotransfusion in elective and emergency vascular surgery. Surgery 1978; 83:470.

228. Thomas GI, Jones TW, Stavney LS, et al: Experiences with autotransfusion during abdominal aortic aneurysm resection. Am J Surg 1980; 139:628.

229. Gillott A, Thomas JM: Clinical investigation involving the use of the haemonetics cell saver in elective and emergency vascular operations. Am Surg 1984; 50:609.

230. Hartz RS, Smith JA, Green D: Autotransfusion after cardiac operation. Assessment of hemostatic factors. J Thorac Cardiovasc Surg 1988; 96:178.

231. Kongsgaard UE, Tølløfsrud S, Brosstad F, et al: Autotransfusion after open heart surgery: characteristics of shed mediastinal blood and its influence on the plasma proteases in circulating blood. Acta Anaesthesiol Scand 1991; 35:71.

232. Kongsgaard UE, Hovig T, Brosstad F, et al: Platelets in shed mediastinal blood used for postoperative autotransfusion. Acta Anaesthesiol Scand 1993; 37:265.

233. Wilson AJ Cuddigan BJ, Wyatt AP: Early experience of intraoperative autotransfusion. J Roy Soc Med 1988; 81:389.

234. Moore EE, Dunn EL, Breslich DJ, et al: Platelet abnormalities associated with massive autotransfusion. J Trauma 1980; 20:1052.

235. Solem JO, Steen S, Tengborn L, et al: Mediastinal drainage blood potentialities for autotransfusion after cardiac surgery. Scand J Thorac Cardiovasc Surg 1987; 21:149.

236. Long GW, Glover JL, Bendick PJ, et al: Cell washing versus immediate reinfusion of intraoperatively shed blood during abdominal aortic aneurysm repair. Am J Surg 1993; 166:97.

237. Rietz T: Reinfusion of extravasated blood. Lyon Chir 1922; 19:358.

238. Wahl GW, Feins RH, Alfieres G, et al: Reinfusion of shed blood after coronary operation causes elevation of cardiac enzymes. Ann Thorac Surg 1992; 53:625.

239. Smith DF, Mihm FG, Mefford I: Hypertension after intraoperative autotransfusion in bilateral adrenalectomy for pheochromocytoma. Anesthesiology 1983; 58:182.

240. Rice MJ, Violante EV, Kreul JF: The effect of autotransfusion on catecholamine levels during pheochromocytoma. Anesthesiology 1987; 67:1017.

241. Lawrence-Brown MM, Couch C, Halliday M, et al: D-dimer levels in blood salvage for autotransfusion. Aust N Z J Surg 1989; 59:67.

242. Thompson JF, Clifford PC, Webster JHH, et al: Acquired platelet dysfunction and sequestration during autotransfusion: clinical and *in vivo* studies. Eur Surg Res 1989; 21:13.

243. Paravicini D, Wasylewski AH, Rassat J, et al: Red blood cell survival and morphology during and after intraoperative autotransfusion. Acta Anaesthesiol Belg 1984; 35(suppl):43.

244. Flynn JC, Metzger CR, Csencsitz TA: Intraoperative autotransfusion (IAT) in spinal surgery. Spine 1982; 7:432.

245. Von Finck M, Schmidt R, Schneider W, et al: The quality of washed autotransfused erythrocytes. The elimination of plasma hemoglobin, osmotic fragility and survival rate of transfused erythrocytes. Der Anaesthetist 1986; 35:686.

246. Orr MD, Blenko JW: Autotransfusion of concentrated, selected washed red cells from the surgical field: a biochemical and physiological comparison with homologous cell transfusion. Proc Blood Conserv Inst, 1978.

247. Janoff A, White R, Carp, H, et al: Lung injury induced by leukocytic proteases. Am J Pathol 1979; 97:111.

248. Bull BS, Bull MH: The salvaged blood syndrome: a sequel to mechanochemical activation of platelets and leukocytes. Blood Cells 1990; 16:5.

249. Bull MH, Bull BS, Van Arsdell GS, et al: Clinical implications of procoagulant and leukoattractant

250. Sharp WV, Stark M, Donovan DL: Modern autotransfusion. Experience with a washed red cell processing technique. Am J Surg 1981; 142:522.

251. Young JN, Ecker RR, Moretti RL, et al: Autologous blood retrieval in thoracic, cardiovascular, and orthopedic surgery. Am J Surg 1982; 144:48.

252. Bell WR: Hematologic aspects of autotransfusion. In: Hauer JM, Thurer RL, Dawson RB, eds, Autotransfusion. New York, 1981, Elsevier-North Holland, pp. 1–9.

253. Robicsek F, Duncan GD, Born GVR, et al: Inherent dangers of simultaneous application of microfibrillar collagen hemostat and blood-saving devices. J Thorac Cardiovasc Surg 1986; 92:766.

254. Niebauer GW, Oz MC, Goldschmidt M, et al: Simultaneous use of microfibrillar collagen hemostat and blood saving devices in a canine kidney perfusion model. Ann Thorac Surg 1989; 48:523.

255. Harjola PT, Kyosola K: Collagen hemostatic felt in coronary bypass surgery. Thorac Cardiovasc Surg 1981; 29:127.

256. Robicsek F, Born GVR: The control of bleeding after cardiopulmonary bypass by intrapericardial instillation of fresh frozen plasma and platelets with microfibrillar collagen. Thorac Cardiovasc Surg 1984; 32:127.

257. Due TL, Johnson JM, Wood M, et al: Intraoperative autotransfusion in the management of massive hemorrhage. Am J Surg 1975; 130:652.

258. Bachmann F, McKenna R, Cole ER, et al: The hemostatic mechanism after open-heart surgery: studies on plasma coagulation factors and fibrinolysis in 512 patients after extracorporeal circulation. J Thorac Cardiovasc Surg 1975; 70:76.

259. Bregman D, Parodi EN, Hutchinson JE III, et al: Intraoperative autotransfusion during emergency thoracic and elective open-heart surgery. Ann Thorac Surg 1974; 18:590.

260. Collins JA: Problems associated with the massive transfusion of stored blood. Surgery 1974; 75:274.

261. Merrill BS, Mitts DL, Rogers W, et al: Autotransfusion: intraoperative use in ruptured ectopic pregnancy. J Reprod Med 1980; 24:14.

262. Roche JK, Stengle JM: Open-heart surgery and the demand for blood. JAMA 1973; 225:1516.

263. Rajan RS, Barratt-Boyes BG, Woodfield DG: Blood utilisation in open heart surgery at Green Lane Hospital. N Z Med J 1983; 96:575.

264. Vertrees RA, Engelman RM, Johnson JW III, et al: Blood Conservation during open heart surgery: a literature review. J Extra-Corp Technol 1986; 18:200.

265. Scott WJ, Rode R, Castlemain B, et al: Efficacy, complications, and cost of a comprehensive blood conservation program for cardiac operations. J Thorac Cardiovasc Surg 1992; 103:1001.

266. Cuello L, Vazquez E, Rios R, et al: Autologous blood transfusion in thoracic and cardiovascular surgery. Surgery 1967; 62:814.

267. Newman MM, Hamstra R, Block M: Use of banked autologous blood in elective surgery. JAMA 1971; 218:861.

268. Lubin JJ Jr, Greenberg WZ, Yahr JL, et al: The use of autologous blood in open heart surgery. Transfusion 1974; 14:602.

269. Cove H, Matloff J, Sacks HJ, et al: Autologous

blood transfusion in coronary artery bypass surgery. Transfusion 1976; 16:245.

270. Tector AJ, Gabriel RP, Mateicka WE, et al: Reduction of blood usage in open heart surgery. Chest 1976; 70:454.

271. Hardesty RL, Bayer WL, Bahnson HT: A technique for the use of autologous fresh blood during open-heart surgery. J Thorac Cardiovasc Surg 1968; 56: 683.

272. Hallowell P, Bland JHL, Buckley MJ: Transfusion of fresh autologous blood in open-heart surgery. A method for reducing bank blood requirements. J Thorac Cardiovasc Surg 1972; 64:941.

273. Zubiate P, Kay JH, Mendez AM, et al: Coronary artery surgery: a new technique with the use of little blood, if any. J Thorac Cardiovasc Surg 1974; 68: 263.

274. Kaplan JA, Cannarella C, Jones EL, et al: Autologous blood transfusion during cardiac surgery: a re-evaluation of three methods. J Thorac Cardiovasc Surg 1977; 74:4.

275. Loop FD, Cosgrove DM, Sheldon WC: Reoperations in coronary artery surgery. Cardiovasc Clin 1981; 12:23.

276. Newland PE, Pastoriza-Pinol J, McMillan J, et al: Maximal conservation and minimal usage of blood products in open heart surgery. Anaesth Intens Care 1980; 8:178.

277. Cosgrove DM, Loop FD, Lytle BW: Blood conservation in cardiac surgery. Cardiovasc Clin 1981; 12: 165.

278. Utley JR, Moores WY, Stephens DB: Blood conservation techniques. Ann Thorac Surg 1981; 31:482.

279. Messick KD, Gibbons GA, Fosburg RG, et al: Intraoperative use of the Haemonetics Cellsaver. Proc Blood Conserv Inst, Chicago, Illinois, 1978.

280. Weniger J, Shanahan R: Reduction of blood bank requirements in cardiac surgery. Thorac Cardiovasc Surg 1982; 30:142.

281. Schaff HV, Hauer JM, Gardner TJ, et al: Routine use of autotransfusion following cardiac surgery: experience in 700 patients. Ann Thorac Surg 1979; 27:493.

282. Davies MJ, Picken J, Buxton BF, et al: Blood-conservation techniques for coronary-artery bypass surgery at a private hospital. Med J Aust 1988; 149: 517.

283. Hiratzka LF, Richardson JV, Brandt B II, et al: The effect of autologous blood salvage techniques upon blood bank usage and the cost of routine coronary revascularization. Perfusion 1986; 1:239.

284. McCarthy PM, Popovsky MA, Schaff HV, et al: Effect of blood conservation efforts in cardiac operations at the Mayo Clinic. Mayo Clin Proc 1988; 63:225.

285. Szécsi J, Batonyi E, Liptay P, et al: Early clinical experience with a simple method for autotransfusion in cardiac surgery. Scand J Thorac Cardiovasc Surg 1989; 23:51.

286. Scott WJ, Kessler R, Wernley JA: Blood conservation in cardiac surgery. Ann Thorac Surg 1990; 50: 843.

287. Laub GW, Dharan M, Riebman JB, et al: The impact of intraoperative autotransfusion on cardiac surgery: a prospective randomized double-blind study. Chest 1993; 104:686.

288. Dietrich W, Barankay A, Dilthey G, et al: Reduction

of blood utilization during myocardial revascularization. J Thorac Cardiovasc Surg 1989; 97:213.

289. Barner HB: Coronary artery bypass surgery with minimal use of homologous blood. Effect of a simple and inexpensive blood conservation programme (Letter). Eur J Cardiothorac Surg 1991; 5:111.

290. Matsumoto K, Tomita M, Koga Y, et al: Intra- and postoperative autotransfusion in open heart surgery under simple hypothermia in children. Jpn J Surg 1980; 10:39.

291. Couch NP, Laks H, Pilon RN: Autotransfusion in three variations. Arch Surg 1974; 108:121.

292. Thurer RL: Blood conservation in cardiac surgery: the role of intraoperative autotransfusion. In: Hauer JM, Thurer RL, Dawson RB, eds, Autotransfusion. New York, 1981, Elsevier- North Holland, pp. 63–69.

293. Solis RT, Scott MA, Kennedy PS, et al: Filtration of cardiotomy reservoir blood. J Extra-Corp Technol 1976; 8:1.

294. Winton TL, Charrette EJ, Salerno TA: The cell saver during cardiac surgery. Does it save? Ann Thorac Surg 1982; 33:379.

295. Khan RA, Bassett HFM: Intraoperative autologous blood transfusion: report of a technique. Thorax 1975; 30:447.

296. Cosgrove DM, Loop FD, Lytle BW, et al: Determinants of blood utilization during myocardial revascularization. Ann Thorac Surg 1985; 40:380.

297. Ferraris VA, Gildengorin V: Predictors of excessive blood use after coronary artery bypass grafting: a multivariate analysis. J Thorac Cardiovasc Surg 1989; 98:492.

298. Giordano GF, Goldman DS, Mammana RB, et al: Intraoperative autotransfusion in cardiac operations effect on intraoperative and postoperative transfusion requirements. J Thorac Cardiovasc Surg 1988; 96:382.

299. Hanowell LH, Eisele JH, Erskine EV: Autotransfusor removal of fentanyl from blood. Anesth Analg 1989; 69:239.

300. Shanks CA, Avram MJ, Ronai AK, et al: The pharmacokinetics of d-tubocurarine with surgery involving salvaged autologous blood. Anesthesiology 1985; 62:161.

301. Mummaneni N, Istanbouli M, Pifarre R, et al: Increased heparin requirements with autotransfusion. Thorac Cardiovasc Surg 1983; 86:446.

302. Cosgrove DM, Thurer RL, Lytle BW, et al: Blood conservation during myocardial revascularization. Ann Thorac Surg 1979; 28:184.

303. Richardson JV, Cyrus RJ: Blood conservation in cardiac surgery. J Med Assoc Ala 1982; 52:45.

304. Finegan BA, Calthorpe DA, Moriarty DC: Autotransfusion—a brief review. Irish Med J 1983; 76: 503.

305. Davies MJ, Cronin KD: Blood conservation in elective surgery. Anaesth Intens Care 1984; 12:229.

306. Øvrum E, Åm Holen E, Lindstein-Ringdal M-A: Coronary artery bypass surgery with minimal use of homologous blood: effects of a simple and inexpensive blood conservation programme. Eur J Cardiothorac Surg 1990; 4:644.

307. Ikeda S, Johnston MFM, Yagi K, et al: Intraoperative autologous blood salvage with cardiac surgery: an analysis of five years' experience in more than 3,000 patients. J Clin Anesth 1992; 4:359.

308. Breyer RH, Engelman RM, Rousou JA, et al: Blood conservation for myocardial revascularization: is it cost effective? J Thorac Cardiovasc Surg 1987; 93: 512.

309. Hall RI, Schweiger IA, Finlayson DC: The benefit of the Haemonetics cell saver apparatus during cardiac surgery. Can J Anaesth 1990; 37:618.

310. Brawley RK, Schaff HV: Autotransfusion following cardiac surgery. Surg Rounds 1980; 3:58.

311. Eng J, Kay PH, Murday AJ, et al: Postoperative autologous transfusion in cardiac surgery: a prospective, randomized study. Eur J Cardiothorac Surg 1990; 4:595.

312. Voegele LD, Causby G, Utley T, et al: An improved method for collection of shed mediastinal blood for autotransfusion. Ann Thorac Surg 1982; 34:471.

313. Tector AJ, Dressler DK, Glassner-Davis RM: A new method of autotransfusing blood drained after cardiac surgery. Ann Thorac Surg 1985; 40:305.

314. Zollinger RW II, Andrews DS, Taylor FH, et al: Autotransfusion in bilateral internal mammary artery bypass: cost effectiveness in the 1980s. N C Med J 1986; 47:523.

315. Thurer RL, Popovsky MA, Johnson RG: Shed mediastinal blood transfusion in open heart surgery. Lancet 1991; 338:1078.

316. Fuller JA, Buxton BF, Picken J, et al: Haematological effects of reinfused mediastinal blood after cardiac surgery. Med J Aust 1991; 154:737.

317. Parrot D, Lançon JP, Merle JP, et al: Blood salvage in cardiac surgery. J Cardiothorac Vasc Anesth 1991; 5:454.

318. Ward HB, Smith RRA, Landis KP, et al: Prospective, randomized trial of autotransfusion after routine cardiac operations. Ann Thorac Surg 1993; 56: 137.

319. Solem JO, Tengborn L, Steen S, et al: Cell saver versus hemofilter for concentration of oxygenator blood after cardiopulmonary bypass. Thorac Cardiovasc Surg 1987; 35:42.

320. Stephens DB, Stephens E: Continuous autotransfusion after coronary bypass surgery. J Miss Med Assoc 1988; 29:343.

321. Roberts SR, Early GL, Brown B, et al: Autotransfusion of unwashed mediastinal shed blood fails to decrease banked blood requirements in patients undergoing aortocoronary bypass surgery. Am J Surg 1991; 162:47.

322. Adan A, de la Riviere A, Haas F, et al: Autotransfusion of drained mediastinal blood after cardiac surgery: a reappraisal. Thorac Cardiovasc Surg 1988; 36:10.

323. Johnson RG: Postoperative salvage: autologous blood transfusion. Current issues. Arlington, VA, American Asociation of Blood Banks, 1988, pp. 57–65.

324. Øvrum E, Åm Holen E, Lindstein-Ringdal M-A: Elective coronary artery bypass surgery without homologous blood transfusion. Scand J Thorac Cardiovasc Surg 1991; 25:13.

325. Blakemore WS, McGarrity CJ, Thurer RJ, et al: Infection by air-borne bacteria with cardiopulmonary bypass. Surgery 1971; 70:830.

326. Levine AH, Imai PK: Hypothermia and hemodilution with autologous transfusion. AORN J 1983; 37:1060.

327. Ronai AK, Glass JJ, Shapiro AS: Improving autologous blood harvest recovery of red cells from sponges and suction. Anaesth Intens Care 1987; 15:421.

328. Allums JA, Gordon FT, Moore CH, et al: Intraoperative autotransfusion for abdominal aortic aneurysm repair. Texas Med 1978; 74:55.

329. Adhoute BG, Nahaboo K, Reymondon L, et al: Autotransfusion applied in elective vascular surgery. J Cardiovasc Surg 1979; 20:177.

330. Pittman RD, Inahara T: Eliminating homologous blood transfusions during abdominal aortic aneurysm repair. Am J Surg 1990; 159:522.

331. Ouriel K, Shortell CK, Green RM, et al: Intraoperative autotransfusion in aortic surgery. J Vasc Surg 1993; 18:16- 22.

332. Lawrie GM, Morris GC, Crawford ES, et al: Improved results of operation for ruptured abdominal aortic aneurysm. Surgery 1989; 85:483.

333. Strom JA, Towne JB, Quebbeman EJ, et al: Autotransfusion in complex abdominal aneurysms. Surg Gynecol Obstet 1984; 159:59.

334. Tawes RL Jr, Scribner RG, Duval TB, et al: The cell saver and autologous transfusion and underutilized resource in vascular surgery. Am J Surg 1986; 152: 105.

335. Kelley-Patteson C, Ammar AD, Kelley H: Should the cell-saver autotransfusion device be used routinely in all infrarenal abdominal aortic bypass operations. J Vasc Surg 1993; 18:26.

336. Doty DB, Wright CB, Lamberth WC, et al: Aortocaval fistula associated with aneurysm of the abdominal aorta: current management using autotransfusion techniques. Surgery 1978; 84:250.

337. Brewster DC, Ambrosino JJ, Darling RC, et al: Intraoperative autotransfusion in major vascular surgery. Am J Surg 1979; 137:507.

338. Odagiri S, Tokunaga H, Ishikura Y, et al: An isolated aneurysm of the common iliac artery associated with an arterio-venous fistula: autotransfusion technique and postoperative hemodynamic monitoring. A case report. Jpn J Surg 1988; 18:601.

339. Cunningham AJ: Anesthesia for abdominal aortic surgery—a review (Part II). Can J Anaesth 1989; 36:568.

340. Cunningham AJ: Anaesthesia for abdominal aortic surgery—a review (Part I). Can J Anaesth 1989; 36:426.

341. Wakefield TW, Whitehouse WM, Wu SC, et al: Abdominal aortic aneurysm rupture: statistical analysis of factors affecting outcome of surgical treatment. Surgery 1982; 91:586.

342. Shehata S: Autotransfusion in vascular surgery. Int Surg 1983; 68:33.

343. Cutler BS: Avoidance of homologous transfusion in aortic operations: the role of autotransfusion, hemodilution, and surgical technique. Surgery 1984; 95:717.

344. Clifford PC, Kruger AR, Smith A, et al: Salvage autotransfusion in aortic surgery: initial studies using a disposable reservoir. Br J Surg 1987; 74: 755.

345. Freeman JM, Roberts MH, Donnan AS: Surgical treatment of abdominal aortic aneurysms using cell saver. J Med Assoc Ga 1989; 78:33.

346. Reddy DJ, Ryan CJ, Shepard AD, et al: Intraoperative autotransfusion in vascular surgery. Arch Surg 1990; 125:1012.

347. Thompson JF, Webster JHH, Chant ADB: Prospective randomised evaluation of a new cell saving

device in elective aortic reconstruction. Eur J Vasc Surg 1990; 4:507.

348. Cali RF, O'Hara PJ, Hertzer NR, et al: The influence of autotransfusion on homologous blood requirements during aortic reconstruction. Cleve Clinic Quart 51:143, 1984.

349. Stanton PE Jr, Shannon J, Rosenthal D, et al: Intraoperative autologous transfusion during major aortic reconstructive procedures. South Med J 1987; 80:315.

350. Salerno TA: Cell saver in noncardiac surgery. Ann Thorac Surg 1983; 35:575.

351. Reid CBA, Graham AR, Lord RSA: Initial experience of intra-operative red cell salvage. Aust N Z J Surg 1990; 60:959.

352. Galbut DL, Bolooki H: Surgery of descending aorta. A method of autotransfusion and intercostal artery preservation. Chest 1982; 82:590.

353. Warnock DF, Davison JK, Brewster DC, et al: Modification of the haemonetics cell saver for optional high flow rate autotransfusion. Am J Surg 1982; 143:765.

354. Allen P, O'Rourke JS, Swan P, et al: The use of autologous blood recovery in major aortic surgery: experience of cases with Haemonetics Cell-Saver III system. Irish J Med Sci 1985; 154:14.

355. Urbanyi B, Spillner G, Breymann T, et al: Autotransfusion with hemodilution in vascular surgery. Int Surg 1983; 68:37.

356. Tulloh BR, Brakespear CP, Bates SC, et al: Autologous predonation, haemodilution and intraoperative blood salvage in elective abdominal aortic aneurysm repair. Br J Surg 1993; 80:313.

357. Kruskall MS, Mintz PD, Bergin JJ, et al: Transfusion therapy in emergency medicine. Ann Emerg Med 1988; 17:327.

358. Mattox KL, Walker LE, Beall AC, et al: Blood availability for the trauma patient—autotransfusion. J Trauma 1975; 15:663.

359. Solem JO, Tengborn L, Olin C, et al: Autotransfusion of whole blood in massive bleeding. An experimental study in the pig. Acta Chir Scand 1986; 152:427.

360. Mattox KL: Autotransfusion in the emergency department. JACEP 1975; 4:218.

361. Wesson DE, Ein SH, Villamater J: Intraoperative autotransfusion in blunt abdominal trauma. J Pediatr Surg 1980; 15:735.

362. Nicholls BJ, Cullen BF: Anesthesia for trauma. J Clin Anesth 1988; 1:115.

363. Bretton P, Reines HD, Sade RM: Air embolization during autotransfusion for abdominal trauma. J Trauma 1985; 25:165.

364. Emminizer S, Klopp EH, Hauer JM: Autotransfusion: current status. Heart Lung 1981; 10:83.

365. Wood L: Autotransfusion in the postanesthesia care unit. J Post Anesth Nurs 1991; 6:98.

366. Anderson CB: Autotransfusion in traumatic hemothorax. Missouri Med 1975; 72:541.

367. Mattox KL, Beall AC: Autotransfusion: use in penetrating trauma. Texas Med 1975; 71:69.

368. Yaw PB, Sentany M, Link WJ, et al: Tumor cells carried through autotransfusion: contraindication to intraoperative blood recovery? JAMA 1975; 231:490.

369. Ozman V, McSwain NE Jr, Nichols RL, et al: Autotransfusion of potentially culture-positive blood (CPB) in abdominal trauma: preliminary data from a prospective study. J Trauma 1992; 32:36.

370. Glover JL, Smith R, Yaw PB, et al: Autotransfusion of blood contaminated by intestinal contents. J Am Coll Emerg Phys 1978; 7:142.

371. Marks DH, Medina F, Hou KC, et al: Efficacy of antibacterial membrane and effect on blood components. Milit Med 1988; 153:337.

372. Schweiger IM, Gallagher CJ, Finlayson DC, et al: Incidence of cell-saver contamination during cardiopulmonary bypass. Ann Thorac Surg 1989; 48:51.

373. Kluge RM, Calia FM, McLaughlin JS: Sources of contamination in open heart surgery. JAMA 1974; 230:1415.

374. Klimberg IW, Sirois R, Wajsman Z, et al: Intraoperative autotransfusion in urologic oncology. Arch Surg 1986; 121:1326.

375. Klimberg IW: Autotransfusion and blood conservation in urologic oncology. Semin Surg Oncol 1989; 5:286.

376. Hart OJ, Klimberg IW, Wajsman Z, et al: Intraoperative autotransfusion in radical cystectomy for carcinoma of the bladder. Surg Obstet Gyecol 1989; 168:302.

377. Miller GV, Ramsden CW, Primrose JN: Autologous transfusion: an alternative to transfusion with banked blood during surgery for cancer. Br J Surg 1991; 78:713.

378. Dale RF, Kipling RM, Smith MF, et al: Separation of malignant cells during autotransfusion. Br J Surg 1988; 75:581.

379. McCullough DL, Gittes RF: Vena cava resection for renal cell carcinomas. J Urol 1974; 112:162.

380. Lichtiger B, Dupuis JF, Seski J: Hemotherapy during surgery for Jehovah's Witnesses: a new method. Anesth Analg 1982; 61:618.

381. Glover JL, Broadie TA: Intraoperative autotransfusion. Surg Ann 1984; 16:39.

382. Krane RJ, deVere White R, Davis Z, et al: Removal of renal cell carcinoma extending into the right atrium using cardiopulmonary bypass, profound hypothermia and circulatory arrest. J Urol 1984; 131:945.

383. Zulim RA, Rocco M, Goodnight JE Jr, et al: Intraoperative autotransfusion in hepatic resection for malignancy: is it safe? Arch Surg 1993; 128:206.

384. Cole WH: The mechanisms of the spread of cancer. Surg Gynecol Obstet 1973; 137:853.

385. Griffiths JD, McKinna JA, Rowththam HD, et al, Carcinoma of the colon and rectum: circulating malignant cells and five year survival. Cancer 1973; 31:226.

386. Salsbury AJ: The significance of the circulating cancer cell. Cancer Treat Rev 1975; 2:55.

387. Marshall VF, McCarron LP: The curability of vesical cancer: greater now or then? Cancer 1977; 37:2753.

388. Fujimoto J, Okamoto E, Yamanaka N, et al: Efficacy of autotransfusion in hepatectomy for hepatocellular carcinoma. Arch Surg 1993; 128:1065.

389. Cowell HR: Perioperative red blood-cell transfusion. J Bone Joint Surg [Am] 1989; 71A:1.

390. Turner RH, Steady HM: Cell washing in orthopedic surgery. In Hauer JM, Thurer RL, Dawson RB, eds, Autotransfusion. New York, 1981, Elsevier-North Holland, pp. 43–50.

391. Lehner JT, Van Peteghem PK, Leatherman KD, et al: Experience with an intraoperative autogenous blood recovery system in scoliosis and spinal surgery. Spine 1981; 6:131.

392. Huth JF, Maier RV, Pavlin E, et al: Utilization of blood recycling in nonelective surgery. Arch Surg 1983; 118:626.

393. Bunch WH: Posterior fusion for idiopathic scoliosis. In: Stauffer ES, ed, Instructional Course Lectures. St. Louis, 1985, C.V. Mosby, pp. 140–152.

394. Lennon RL, Hosking MP, Gray JR, et al: The effects of intraoperative blood salvage and induced hypotension on transfusion requirements during spinal surgical procedures. Mayo Clin Proc 1987; 62:1090.

395. Phillips WA, Hensinger RN: Control of blood loss during scoliosis surgery. Clin Orthop Rel Res 1988; 229:88.

396. Wilson WJ: Intraoperative autologous transfusion in revision total hip arthroplasty. J Bone Joint Surg [Am] 1989; 71A:8.

397. Goulet JA, Bray TJ, Timmerman LA: et al: Intraoperative autologous transfusion in orthopaedic patients. J Bone Joint Surg [Am] 1989; 71A:3.

398. Brown MD, Seltzer DG: Perioperative care in lumbar spine surgery. Orthop Clin North Am 1991; 22:353.

399. Endresen GKM, Spiechowicz J, Pahle JA, et al: Intraoperative autotransfusion in reconstructive hip joint surgery of patients with rheumatoid arthritis and alkylosing spondylitis. Scand J Rheumatol 1991; 20:28.

400. Tate DE, Friedman RJ: Blood conservation in spinal surgery. Review of current techniques. Spine 1992; 17:1450.

401. Blevins FT, Shaw B, Valeri CR, et al: Reinfusion of shed blood after orthopedic procedures in children and adolescents. J Bone Joint Surg [Am] 1993; 75A:363.

402. Keeling MM, Schmidt-Clay P, Kotcamp WW, et al: Autotransfusion in the postoperative orthopedic patient. Clin Orthop Rel Res 1993; 291:251.

403. Giordano GF, Giordano DM, Wallace BA, et al: An analysis of 9,918 consecutive perioperative autotransfusions. Surg Gyecol Obset 1993; 176:103.

404. MacFarlane BJ, Marx L, Anquist K, et al: Analysis of a protocol for an autologous blood transfusion program for total joint replacement surgery. Can J Surg 1988; 31:126.

405. Finch S, Haskins D, Finch CA: Iron metabolism: hematopoiesis following phlebotomy; iron as a limiting factor. J Clin Invest 1950; 29:1078.

406. Goodnough LT, Rudnick S, Price TH, et al: Increased preoperative collection of autologous blood with recombinant human erythropoietin therapy. N Engl J Med 1989; 321:1163.

407. Goodnough LT, Wasman J, Corlucci K, et al: Limitations to donating adequate autologous blood prior to elective orthopedic surgery. Arch Surg 1989; 124:494.

408. Goodnough LT, Vizmeg K, Marcus RE: Blood lost and transfused in patients undergoing elective orthopedic operation. Surg Obstet Gynecol 1993; 176:235.

409. Henn A, Hoffmann R, Müller HAG: Haptoglobinbestimmung im patientenserum nach intraoperativer autotransfusion mit dem Hämonetics Cell-Saver III. Der Anaesthesist 1988; 37:741.

410. Haberkern M, Dangel P: Normovolaemic haemodilution and intraoperative autotransfusion in children: experience with 30 cases of spinal fusion. Eur J Pediatr Surg 1991; 1:30.

411. McNeill TW, Dewald RL, Kuo KN, et al: Controlled hypotensive anesthesia in scoliosis surgery. J Bone Joint Surg [Am] 1974; 56A:1167.

412. Bennett EJ, Salem MR, Sakul P, et al: Induced hypotension for spinal corrective procedures. Middle East J Anaesth 1974; 4:177.

413. Salem MR, Wong AY, Bennett EJ, et al: Deliberate hypotension in infants and children. Anesth Analg 1974; 53:975.

414. Mallory TH, Kennedy M: The use of banked autologous blood in total hip replacement surgery. Clin Orthop Rel Res 1976; 117:254.

415. Mandel RJ, Brown MD, McCollough NC, et al: Hypotensive anesthesia and autotransfusion in spinal surgery. Clin Orthop Rel Res 1981; 154:27.

416. Malcolm-Smith NA, McMaster MJ: The uses of induced hypotension to control bleeding during posterior spinal fusion for scoliosis. J Bone Joint Surg [Br] 1983; 65B:255.

417. Nelson CL, Bowen WS: Total hip arthroplasty in Jehovah's witnesses without blood transfusion. J Bone Joint Surg [Am] 1986; 68A:350.

418. Salem MR, Klowden, AJ: Anesthesia for orthopedic surgery. In: Gregory GA, ed, Pediatric Anesthesia. New York, 1994, Churchill Livingstone.

419. Groh GI, Buchert PK, Allen WC: A comparison of transfusion requirements after total knee arthroplasty using the solcotrans autotransfusion system. J Arthroplast 1990; 3:291.

420. Gannon DM, Lombardi AV, Mallory TH, et al: An evaluation of the efficacy of postoperative blood salvage after total joint arthroplasty. J Arthroplasty 1991; 1:109.

421. Healy WL, Wasilewski SA, Pfeifer BA, et al: Methylmethacrylate monomer and fat content in shed blood after total joint arthroplasty. Clin Orthop Rel Res 1993; 286:15.

422. Corno AF, Laks H, Stevenson LW, et al: Heart transplantation in a Jehovah's Witness. J Heart Transplant 1986; 5:175.

423. Kaufman DB, Sutherland DER, Fryd DS, et al: A single- center experience of renal transplantation in thirteen Jehovah's Witnesses. Transplantation 1988; 45:1045.

424. Hunt BJ, Sack D, Amin S, et al: The perioperative use of blood components during heart and heart-lung transplantation. Transfusion 1992; 32:57.

425. Butler P, Israel L, Nusbacher J, et al: Blood transfusion in liver transplantation. Transfusion 1985; 25: 120.

426. Starzl TE, Marchioro TL, von Kaulla KN, et al: Homotransplantation of the liver in humans. Surg Gynecol Obstet 1963; 117:659.

427. Lewis JH, Bontempo FA, Cornell F, et al: Blood use in liver transplantation. Transfusion 1987; 27: 222.

428. Motschman TL, Taswell HF, Brecher M, et al: Blood bank support of a liver transplantation program. Mayo Clin Proc 1989; 64:103.

429. Kang YG, Aggarwal S, Virji M, et al: Clinical evaluation of autotransfusion during liver transplantation. Anesth Analg 1991; 72:94.

430. Bohmig HJ: The coagulation disorder of rthotopic hepatic transplantation. Semin Thromb Hemost 1977; 4:57.

431. Dzik WH, Jenkins R: Use of intraoperative blood

salvage during orthotopic liver transplantation. Arch Surg 1985; 120:946.

432. Van Voorst SJ, Peters TG, Williams JW, et al: Autotransfusion in hepatic transplantation. Am Surg 1985; 51:623.

433. Brown MR, Ramsay MA, Swygert TH: Exchange autotransfusion using the cell saver during liver transplantation. Anesthesiology 1989; 70:168.

434. Lindop MJ, Farman JV, Smith MF: Anesthesia: assessment and intraoperative management. In: Calne RY, ed, Liver Transplantation. London, 1983, Grune & Stratton, pp. 128–129.

435. Mendel L, Smith MF, Park GR: Lack of haematological and biochemical consequences following autologous blood transfusion. Anaesthesia 1986; 41:1259.

436. Grimes DA: A simplified device for intraoperative autotransfusion. Obstet Gynecol 1988; 72:947.

437. Weinstein L, Morris MB, Dotters D, et al: Ectopic pregnancy—a new surgical epidemic. Obstet Gynecol 1983; 61:698.

438. Dorfman SF: Deaths from ectopic pregnancy, United States, 1979 to 1980. Obstet Gynecol 1983; 62:334.

439. MacKay HT, Hughes JM, Hogue CR: Ectopic pregnancy in the United States, 1979–1980. MMWR 1984; 33:1SS.

440. Strathy JH, Coulam CB, Marchbanks P, et al: Incidence of ectopic pregnancy in Rochester, Minnesota, 1950–1981. Obstet Gynecol 1984; 64:37.

441. Boulton FE, Letsky E: Obstetric haemorrhage: causes and management. Clin Haematol 1985; 14:683.

442. Bukovsky I, Schneider DF, Langer R, et al: Elective caesarean hysterectomy. Indications and outcome: a 17-year experience of 140 cases. Aust N Z J Obstet Gynaecol 1989; 29:287.

443. Maxwell CN: Blood transfusion and caesarean section. Aust N Z J Obstet Gynaecol 1989; 29:121.

444. Imberti R, Preseglio I, Trotta V, et al: Blood transfusion during cesarean section. A 12 year retrospective analysis. Acta Anaesthesiol Belg 1990; 41:139.

445. Hayashi RH: Hemorrhagic shock in obstetrics. Clin Perinatal 1986; 13:755.

446. Beller FK, Maki M, Epstein MD: Incoagulability of intraperitoneal blood. Am J Obstet Gynecol 1968; 102:1121.

447. Carty MJ, Barr RD, Ouna N: The coagulation and fibrinolytic properties of peritoneal and venous blood in patients with rupture ectopic pregnancies. J Obstet Gyaecol Br Commonw 1973; 80:701.

448. Majer RV, Green PJ: Recurrent reversible pure red cell aplasia in pregnancy. Clin Lab Haematol 1988; 10:101.

449. Rodeghiero F, Castaman GC, Di Bona E, et al: Successful pregnancy in a woman with congenital factor XIII deficiency treated with substitutive therapy. Blut 1987; 55:45.

450. Weiner CP: The obstetric patient and disseminated intravascular coagulation. Clin Pernatol 1986; 13:705.

451. Davies S: Obstetric implications of sickle cell disease. Midwife Health Visit Commun Nurs 1988; 24:361.

452. Ogedengbe OK, Akinyanju OO: The hemoglobinopathies and pregnancy in Lagos. Int J Gynecol Obstet 1988; 26:229.

453. Erkkola R, Eklad U, Kero P, et al: HELLP syndrome. Ann Chir Gynaecol 1987; 202:26.

454. Duffy BL: HELLP syndrome and the anaesthetist. Anaesthesia 1988; 43:223.

455. Martin JN Jr, Blake PG, Perry KG Jr, et al: The natural history of HELLP syndrome: patterns of disease progression and regression. Am J Obstet Gynecol 1991; 164:1500.

456. Nolan TE, Smith RP, Devoe LD: Maternal plasma d-dimer levels in normal and complicated pregnancies. Obstet Gynecol 1993; 81:235.

457. Dorman KF: Hemorrhagic emergencies in obstetrics. J Perinat Neonatal Nurs 1989; 3:23

458. Kruskall MS, Leonard S, Klapholz H: Autologous blood donation during pregnancy: analysis of safety and blood use. Obstet Gynecol 1987; 70:938.

459. Herbert WNP, Owen HG, Collins ML: Autologous blood storage in obstetrics. Obstet Gynecol 1988; 72:166.

460. Malik LR: Autotransfusion in ruptured tubal pregnancy. J Pakist Med Assoc 1987; 37:78.

461. Silva PD, Geguin EA Jr: Intraoperative rapid autologous blood transfusion. Am J Obstet Gynecol 1989; 160:1226.

462. Curtis CH: Autotransfusion in gynecologic hemoperitoneum. Am J Obstet Gynecol 1983; 146:501.

463. Thornhill ML, O'Leary AJ, Lussos SA, et al: An in-vitro assessment of amniotic fluid removal from human blood through cell saver processing. Anesthesiology 1991; 75:A830.

464. Zichella L, Gramolini R: Autotransfusion during cesarean section (Letter). Am J Obstet Gynecol 1990; 162:295.

465. Kuhlman K, Hidvegi D, Tamura RK, et al: Is amniotic fluid material in the central circulation of peripartum patients pathologic? Am J Perinatol 1985; 2:295.

466. Price TM, Baker VV, Cefalo RC: Amniotic fluid embolism. Three cases with a review of the literature. Obstet Gynecol 1985; 40:462.

467. Giampaolo C, Schneider V, Kowalski BH, et al: The cytologic diagnosis of amniotic fluid embolism: a critical reappraisal. Diagn Cytopathol 1987; 3:126.

468. Attwood HD, Delprado WJ: Amniotic fluid embolism: fatal case confirmed at autopsy five weeks after delivery. Pathology 1988; 20:381.

469. Shapiro SH, Wessley Z: Rhodamine B fluorescence as a stain for amniotic fluid squames in maternal pulmonary embolism and fetal lungs. Ann Clin Lab Sci 1988; 18:451.

470. Clark SL: New concepts of amniotic fluid embolism: a review. Obstet Gynecol Surv 1990; 45:360.

471. Fatteh MM: Jehovah's Witnesses. How can we help them. J Med Assoc Ga 1980; 69:977

472. Popovsky MA, Moore SB: Autologous transfusion in Jehovah's Witnesses. Transfusion 1985; 25:444.

473. Rothenberg DM: The approach to the Jehovah's witness patient. Anesth Clin North Am 1990; 8:589.

474. Cooley DA, Lewis CTP: Blood Saving in Jehovah's Witnesses (Letter). Ann Thorac Surg 1991; 52:900.

475. Annexion M: Autotransfusion for surgery: a comeback? JAMA 1978; 240:2710.

476. Cundy JM: Jehovah's Witnesses and haemorrhage. Anaesthesia 1980; 35:1013.

477. Clarke JMF: Surgery in Jehovah's Witnesses. Br J Hosp Med 1992; 27:497.

478. Lindop MJ, Farman JV, Smith MF, et al: Haemo-

netics cell saver. Anaesthesia 1987; 42: 85.

479. Olsen JB, Alstrup P, Madsen T: Open-heart surgery in Jehovah's Witnesses. Scand J Thorac Cardiovasc Surg 1990; 24:165.

480. Vanelli P, Castelli P, Condemi AM, et al: Blood Saving in Jehovah's Witnesses (Letter). Ann Thorac Surg 1991; 52:899.

481. Cooper JR Jr: Perioperative considerations in Jehovah's Witnesses. Int Anesthesiol Clin 1990; 28: 210.

482. Black HA, Dearing JP: Exchange transfusion prior to cardiopulmonary bypass in sickle cell anemia. J Extra-Corp Technol 1980; 12:82.

483. Brajtbord D, Johnson D, Ramsay M: Use of the cell saver in patients with sickle cell trait. Anesthesiology 1989; 70:878.

484. Cook A, Hanowell LH: Intraoperative autotransfu-sion for a patient with homozygous sickle cell disease. Anesthesiology 1990; 73:177.

485. Wayne AS, Levy SV, Nathan DG: Transfusion management of sickle cell diseases. Blood 1993; 81: 1109.

486. Castro O: Autotransfusion: a management option for alloimmunized sickle cell patients? Prog Clin Biol Res 1982; 98:117.

487. Charache S: Problems in transfusion therapy. N Engl J Med 1990; 322:1666.

488. Castro O, Finke-Castro H, Coats D: Improved method for automated red cell exchange in sickle cell disease. J Clin Apheresis 1986; 3:93.

489. Behrman MJ, Keim HA: Perioperative red blood cell salvage in spine surgery: a prospective analysis. Clin Orthop Rel Res 1982; 278:51.

490. Fiereck EA: Appendix. In: Tietz NW, ed, Fundamentals of Clinical Chemistry, 2 ed. Philadelphia, 1976, W.B. Saunders, pp. 1177–1227.

# 10

# BLOOD SUBSTITUTES

*Steven A. Gould, Lakshman R. Sehgal,*
*Hansa L. Sehgal, and Gerald S. Moss*

## INTRODUCTION

The development of a safe and effective red blood cell substitute for use in resuscitation is an exciting prospect. Such a product has been sought over the past century for several reasons. The most important functions of a red blood cell (RBC) substitute are to transport oxygen and carbon dioxide effectively and to support circulatory dynamics. From a logisti-

cal point of view, a suitable product should be readily available, nontoxic, temperature stable, and universally compatible. In addition, it should have a long shelf storage time and satisfactory intravascular persistence and should be effective during room-air breathing. Clinically, the risk-to-benefit ratio would be improved by the availability of such a product because serious transfusion hazards such as hepatitis and acquired immunodeficiency syndrome (AIDS) would not be a consideration. Hemoglobin solutions and perfluorochemical (FC) emulsions are the two products that have been most extensively evaluated and are discussed below.

Aside from these solutions, there are no other oxygen-carrying blood substitutes that are currently being evaluated. There is great interest in the use of asanguinous fluids for use in intravascular volume expansion after blood loss. A brief discussion follows of the currently available choices for intravenous fluid infusion in acute hypovolemia.

## INTRAVASCULAR VOLUME EXPANSION

The infusion of fluid is the fundamental treatment of acute hypovolemia. All commercially available intravenous fluids (Table 10–1) share the ability to replenish the circulation once appropriate intravenous access is established. The challenge inherent with the use of these solutions is to promote the prompt and adequate restoration of cardiac filling pressures to optimum values without compromising ventilation secondary to fluid overload. Regardless of the fluid used for re-

**Table 10–1. Characteristics of fluids used for resuscitation**

| | Sodium chloride (0.9%) | Ringer's lactate | Hypertonic saline solution (3%) | Albumin (5%) | Hetastarch (6%) | Dextran 70 (6%) | Fresh-frozen plasma |
|---|---|---|---|---|---|---|---|
| Na (mmol/L) | 154 | 130 | 513 | 130–160 | 154 | 154 | 170 |
| Cl (mmol/L) | 154 | 109 | 513 | 130–160 | 154 | 154 | 100 |
| Osmolarity (mOsm/L) | 310 | 275 | 1025 | 310 | 310 | 310 | 300 |
| Oncotic pressure (mm Hg) | 0 | 0 | 0 | 20 | 30 | 60 | 20 |
| Lactate (mmol/L) | 0 | 28 | 0 | 0 | 0 | 0 | 4 |
| pH | 5.0 | 6.5 | 6.0 | 6.9 | 5.5 | 3.8–7.0 | Variable |
| Cost* (L) | $0.60 | $0.75 | $0.84 | $80.00 | $76.00 | $25.00 | $120.00 |

* Prices reflect costs charged to our hospital, as of 1990. Patient charges will vary from institution to institution.
From Rosen B, Rosen AL, Schegal H, et al.: In: Rippe JM, Irwin RS, Alpert JS, and others, eds., *Intensive Care Medicine*, 2nd ed. Boston, MA, 1991, Little, Brown, and Company, pp. 1435–1443, with permission.

suscitation, it is therefore imperative to use physiological endpoints to gauge the initial response to treatment and to adjust the therapy to meet the individual needs of the patient.

## Normal Fluid Dynamics

On examination of the fluid distribution in adults, approximately two-thirds of the total body water is intracellular; the remaining one-third present in the extracellular compartment is distributed between the interstitial and intravascular spaces at a ratio of 3:1. The movement of fluids between the major compartments of the body is governed by the number of particles, or osmoles, in solution. Under steady-state conditions, the osmolality of the intracellular and extracellular compartments is maintained between 280 and 300 mOsm by the Na-K adenosine triphosphatase pump. In contrast, the distribution of fluid between the intravascular and extravascular spaces, as defined by the Starling equation, is dependent on the transcapillary hydrostatic and oncotic pressures and the relative permeability of the capillary membranes that separate these spaces. Although controversy exists regarding the absolute values of these forces, the net effect is a small efflux of fluid into the interstitium, which is returned to the circulation via the lymphatics.

## Crystalloid Solutions

The osmolality of a solution is dependent on the number of particles in solution. The functional osmolality, or tonicity, of a solution is defined by the ability of the particles in solution to permeate cell membranes. Accordingly, isotonic solutions such as 0.9% sodium chloride and Ringer's lactate freely equilibrate between the intravascular and interstitial spaces but do not promote intracellular fluid shifts. In contrast, the osmotic pressure exerted at the cell membrane by the infusion of hypertonic saline solutions leads to the redistribution of intracellular fluid into the extracellular compartment.

Isotonic crystalloid solutions are universally recognized as the primary fluid for acute intravascular volume expansion. When care is taken to titrate total infusion volume to physiological endpoints, resuscitation is usually successful without the development of pulmonary edema. A concern with isotonic fluids is the large volume often required for resuscitation. This usually results in peripheral edema, which clears within several days. The large volume requirements may also represent a logistical problem in some settings. For these reasons, hypertonic saline solutions have been studied.

The theoretical advantage of hypertonic saline solution relates to the reduced total infusion volume required for adequate resuscitation. The greater the sodium concentration, the less total volume is necessary for satisfactory resuscitation when compared with isotonic saline solution. In addition to the osmotic effects, hypertonic solutions are believed to exert a positive inotropic effect on the myocardium and a direct effect on the peripheral vasculature leading to vasodilation.[1-3] The principal disadvantage of hypertonic saline is the danger of hypernatremia. Serum sodium levels above 170 mmol/L produce extreme brain dehydration and can be fatal.[4]

The primary mechanism for the maintenance of relatively constant serum sodium levels in the face of hypertonic infusions involves the movement of intracellular water into the extracellular compartment. Thus, the infusion of exogenous hypertonic saline solution is always accompanied by an endogenous infusion of free water into the extracellular space. A simple method of calculating the expected endogenous infusion is to examine the ratio of the infused fluid to the normal serum sodium concentration. For example, a solution containing 300 mmol/L of sodium would produce a 2:1 endogenous infusion, whereas a solution containing 1200 mmol/L of sodium would produce a 7:1 infusion volume. The safety of hypertonic solutions depends on how much of the intracellular volume can be safely transferred to the extracellular compartment without injuring cell function or leading to hypernatremia in a given clinical situation.

## Colloid Solutions

Intravenous colloid solutions share the presence of large molecules that are relatively impermeable to the capillary membranes. These oncotically active particles produce an effective volume expansion with little loss into the interstitial space, as occurs with the simple salt solutions. In addition, the intravascular persistence of these molecules increases their duration of action. The net effect of colloid administration is a marked reduction in the volume of infusate necessary to expand the intravascular space, as compared with isotonic saline solutions.

One of the most commonly used colloid preparations is 5% albumin (Table 10–1). It is prepared from normal donor plasma that is heat treated to eliminate the potential for disease transmission. Once administered, it leads to an effective intravascular volume expansion of approximately one-half of the volume infused, with a duration of action of 24 hours. Side effects include the rare occurrence of anaphylactic reactions (0.5%) and inhibition of hemostasis.[5]

The high cost and limited availability of albumin solutions led to the development of synthetic colloid preparations such as 6% hetastarch and 6% dextran solutions (Table 10–1). Hetastarch is an amylopectin-derived polymer with an average molecular weight of 450,000 d. Dextran 70 is a polysaccharide formed by bacterial growth and digestion in sucrose media. Administration of these solutions leads to a plasma volume expansion and duration of action approximately 50% greater than 5% albumin. Side effects of these solutions are similar to albumin, with the exception of the documented inhibition of platelet aggregation and interference with RBC cross matching with dextran 70. In addition, concern has been raised over the long-term effects that these synthetic macromolecules might have on immune function secondary to their incomplete elimination by the reticuloendothelial system.

Theoretically, fresh frozen plasma also can be used as a volume expander. It is similar to 5% albumin in electrolyte concentration and oncotic pressure. In addition, it contains all the naturally occurring immunoglobulins and all the clotting factors except platelets. At first glance, it appears to be an ideal volume expander. Unfortunately, as is the case with all currently used blood components, the risk of hepatitis and AIDS is real, and neither risk can be totally eliminated by current screening techniques. Accordingly, its use after acute blood loss should be limited to the treatment of clinically significant coagulopathies after large volume resuscitation, as discussed later in this chapter.

## Experimental Comparisons of Intravenous Solutions

### LABORATORY STUDIES

There has been considerable controversy over the role of resuscitation with crystalloid or colloid solutions in the subsequent development of deranged pulmonary function after major nonthoracic trauma. Proponents of colloid therapy cite the following points derived from laboratory studies.

1. Resuscitation with colloid leads to a more rapid and effective correction of the intravascular volume deficits that follow acute hemorrhage.[6]
2. Colloid resuscitation prevents pulmonary edema formation through maintenance of the intravascular colloid osmotic pressure (COP).[7]

3. Crystalloid resuscitation dilutes the plasma protein pool, thereby reducing plasma oncotic pressure and setting the stage for the development of pulmonary edema.[8,9]
4. The peripheral edema that follows large-volume crystalloid infusions may impair wound healing and nutrient transport.[10]

Crystalloid proponents cite the following:

5. Crystalloid administration most effectively replaces the interstitial fluid deficits that follow hemorrhagic shock.[11]
6. The rapid intravascular-extravascular fluid equilibrium that follows crystalloid resuscitation may reduce the incidence of pulmonary edema by promoting a less rapid rise in the pulmonary artery occlusion pressure.[12]
7. Albumin normally enters the pulmonary interstitium relatively freely and is returned to the circulation via the lymphatic system. The exogenous administration of colloid solutions increases the albumin pool in the pulmonary interstitium, promoting the accumulation of interstitial fluid.[13,14]

It is evident from this discussion that the arguments supporting either treatment regiment are in direct conflict with respect to the physiological changes that are believed to follow resuscitation with either crystalloid or colloid solutions. Much of this conflict stems from the divergent study conditions used to answer these questions in the laboratory setting. Nevertheless, numerous clinical studies designed to compare the efficacy and safety of these resuscitation regiments after acute blood loss have failed to demonstrate a clear advantage of colloid administration to justify its cost. The following section reviews these clinical trials, with particular emphasis on the resuscitation from hemorrhagic shock.

## RANDOMIZED TRIALS IN HUMAN SUBJECTS

### Crystalloid versus Colloid

One of the first trials comparing crystalloid and colloid resuscitation was reported by Skillman et al.,[7] in which 16 patients undergoing elective abdominal aortic operations received either colloid or crystalloid in the perioperative period. They noted a significant difference during the immediate postoperative period in plasma colloid oncotic pressure

between the Ringer's lactate-treated group and the colloid-treated group (22 and 27 mm Hg, respectively) but no alveolar-arterial oxygen tension difference. They also reported a significant correlation between the amount of infused sodium and the alveolar-arterial oxygen difference in the Ringer's lactate-treated group but not in the albumin-treated group. It was concluded that albumin-rich fluid was preferable because it reduced the amount of sodium-containing fluid required for adequate resuscitation. This study does not represent a strong argument for albumin-rich fluids, because both groups received albumin in the form of whole blood administered intraoperatively. Furthermore, the test fluid was given by formula rather than by titration to physiological endpoints. The positive correlation between infused sodium and pulmonary function was not confirmed in several subsequent studies by other investigators.

Another study involving patients undergoing elective vascular operations was published in 1979 by Virgilio et al.[12] During the operation, patients received either Ringer's lactate (14 patients) or 5% albumin in Ringer's lactate (15 patients) to maintain preoperative filling pressures, cardiac output, and urine output. Blood loss was replaced by packed cells. Patients assigned to the Ringer's lactate-treated group received approximately 11 L test fluid on the day of operation, whereas those in the albumin-treated group received 6 L. Both groups required approximately 6.5 units of packed RBCs. Patients receiving Ringer's lactate gained 10% of their original body weight and had a 40% reduction in plasma colloid oncotic pressure.

During the study, no deaths occurred in either group. No difference was noted between groups in regard to the intrapulmonary shunt on any day of the study. Furthermore, no correlation was found between the intrapulmonary shunt and the plasma colloid oncotic pressure-hydrostatic pressure gradient. Mean postoperative ventilator time was 23 hours in both groups. Pulmonary edema developed in two patients receiving albumin. No patients treated with Ringer's lactate manifested evidence of pulmonary edema despite reduced colloid oncotic pressures. It was concluded that safe resuscitation without albumin could be achieved in patients undergoing elective vascular operations.

Numerous clinical trials have compared the effects of crystalloid or colloid administration in the resuscitation of trauma patients. In 1977, Lowe et al.[15] reported a clinical trial in 141 trauma victims from Cook County Hospital in Chicago. Thirty-six of these patients were in shock on admission. Patients received, in random sequence, either Ringer's lactate (84 patients) or 4% albumin solution (55 patients) in volumes sufficient to restore normal vital signs and urine output. This was the first report in the literature of a group of human subjects resuscitated without any albumin. RBC losses were replaced with washed RBCs. These patients received an average of 5.5 L test fluid and 2 units RBCs before operation.

Three deaths occurred in each group. Eight patients (14%) in the albumin-treated group required ventilatory support after operation, whereas three (3.6%) assigned to the Ringer's lactate-treated group required ventilatory support. There were no changes in the results of a battery of pulmonary function tests, including intrapulmonary shunt fraction and alveolar-arterial oxygen tension difference. In addition, no correlation was found between the amount of sodium infused and any pulmonary function test result in either group. Lowe et al.[15] concluded that the addition of albumin in Ringer's lactate was unnecessary to achieve successful resuscitation in this group of patients. A criticism of this study was that too few patients were in shock on admission so the failure to find differences in mortality or pulmonary function with either test fluid was not surprising.[16]

In 1981, further findings in the 36 patients at Cook County Hospital who were in shock on admission were published by Moss et al.[17] Twenty patients were assigned to the Ringer's lactate-treated group and 16 received albumin. These patients received an average of 8 units packed RBCs and 9 L test fluid, indicating severe injury and blood loss. Only one death occurred. Two patients in each group required ventilatory support, and no differences were noted in the pulmonary function test results. Once again, no evidence could be found that albumin added to Ringer's lactate was necessary to prevent adult respiratory distress syndrome.

In an effort to determine the relative mortality after resuscitation with either crystalloid or colloid solutions, Velanovich[18] pooled the results of these and other clinical trials and compared the mortality rates by metaanalysis. On examination of results from clinical trials derived from trauma patients, the mortality rate was 12% lower for those that received crystalloid. In contrast, the relative difference in mortality from studied performed on nontrauma patients was 8% in favor of colloid treatment. Based on these results, it was concluded that crystalloid administration may be more efficacious than colloids in the trauma setting.

Hypertonic Saline Solutions

Hypertonic saline solution is an attractive fluid in the treatment of burn resuscitation because peripheral edema is frequently seen after conventional resuscitation and may complicate local burn tissue management. If resuscitation with hypertonic saline solution resulted in a smaller infusion volume and less peripheral edema, then this would constitute an argument in favor of its use in burns. The effect of varying the concentration of sodium in resuscitative fluids for burn victims has been reported.[19] Three groups of patients were studied. One group was given saline solution with sodium concentrations of 116–140 mmol/L, the second group was given saline solutions with sodium concentrations between 150 and 199 mmol/L, and the third group was given saline solutions with sodium concentration of 200–250 mmol/L. The total volume infused decreased as the sodium concentration in the infusate increased. No increase was seen in sodium loading. However, in two instances, the serum sodium concentration increased to greater than 170 mmol/L. Similar results with hypertonic saline solution have been reported in young and aged burn victims.[20,21] Weight gain was noted to be minimal in children treated with hypertonic saline solution, and the problem of hypernatremia was avoided by serial monitoring of serum sodium levels. Hypertonic saline solution has become an acceptable form of therapy in burn resuscitation.

Clinical studies of hypertonic saline solutions for resuscitation of hemorrhage have been reported. In a study of 58 patients undergoing vascular operations, Shackford et al.[22] showed that the hypertonic saline solution group required less fluid during operation than did the isotonic saline solution group (4.5 and 9.5 L, respectively) and gained less weight. They concluded that the use of hypertonic saline solution during operation resulted in a reduction in infusion volume but demanded careful monitoring of serum osmolarity to avoid hypernatremia. In a clinical study in trauma victims, one group of 10 patients received 3% saline solution at a volume of 4 mL/kg for no more than 3 hours, whereas the control group received isotonic saline solution.[23] The hypertonic saline solution group required less fluid and produced more urine than the isotonic saline solution group.

### Summary of Clinical Studies

1. Isotonic solutions are effective plasma expanders. There is no good evidence that resuscitation with these fluids in the treatment of hemorrhagic shock produces increased pulmonary interstitial water.
2. There is some evidence that albumin resuscitation may result in albumin accumulation in the lung interstitium. The clinical significance of this observation is not clear.
3. A major increase in pulmonary microvascular pressure is the most important determinant of transvascular movement of water into the pulmonary interstitium. The clinical implication of this observation is that careful monitoring of pulmonary hydrostatic pressure is crucial during resuscitation.
4. Most clinical studies suggest there is no advantage to the administration of colloid solution rather than crystalloid in the treatment of hemorrhagic shock.
5. Preliminary studies with hypertonic saline solutions suggest effective resuscitation can be achieved using relatively small volumes of fluid. Further clinical studies are necessary to verify the safety and efficacy of this therapy after hemorrhagic shock.

## ACELLULAR OXYGEN CARRIERS
### Perfluorochemical Emulsions
#### PHYSIOLOGICAL CONSIDERATIONS

The FCs are potential oxygen carriers because of their relatively high oxygen solubility compared with blood or plasma.[24] However, this high solubility exists only for pure FCs. Because they are not miscible with water (i.e., plasma), current FC products are prepared as an emulsion, which lowers their concentration. Their properties can best be understood

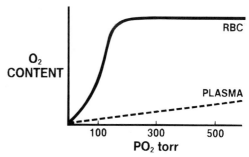

**Fig. 10–1.** [$O_2$] curves for RBCs and plasma. From Gould SA, Moss GS, Rosen AL, et al.: Red cell substitutes. In: Civetta JM, Taylor RW, Kirby RR, eds, Critical Care. Philadelphia, 1988, J.B. Lippincott, pp. 1495–1502, with permission.

by looking at several oxygen content curves. The oxygen content [$O_2$] curve for whole blood is actually the composite of the [$O_2$] curves for RBC hemoglobin and plasma (Figure 10–1).[25] The majority of oxygen is chemically bound to the hemoglobin molecule, which becomes fully saturated at a $PO_2$ of 150 mm Hg. Above this level, a further increase in whole blood oxygen reflects the dissolved oxygen in the aqueous phase of plasma. Because this amount is only 0.3 mL/dL at the alveolar $PO_2$ of 100 mm Hg, it is generally ignored when discussing [$O_2$].

The potential value of FCs as oxygen carriers is illustrated in Figure 10–2.[26] Pure FCs have a solubility coefficient that is approximately 10–20 times that of plasma. In a sense, they function as a "super water." Unfortunately, however, they cannot be administered

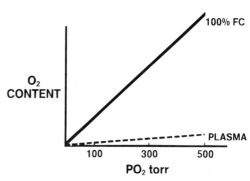

**Fig. 10–2.** [$O_2$] curves for 100% FCs and plasma. From Gould SA, Moss GS, Rosen AL, et al.: Red cell substitutes. In: Civetta JM, Taylor RW, Kirby RR, eds, Critical Care. Philadelphia, 1988, J.B. Lippincott, pp. 1495–1502, with permission.

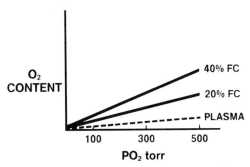

**Fig. 10–3.** [$O_2$] curves for plasma and 20% and 40% FCs. From Gould SA, Moss GS, Rosen AL, et al.: Red cell substitutes. In: Civetta JM, Taylor RW, Kirby RR, eds, Critical Care. Philadelphia, 1988, J.B. Lippincott, pp. 1495–1502, with permission.

in this form. A major development in FC research was the ability to make a stable emulsion using pluronic F-68 as the emulsifying agent. With this emulsion, the concentration of FC is lowered dramatically, as is the [$O_2$] (Figure 10–3). The [$O_2$] depends on both the $PO_2$ and the volume concentration of FC (fluorocrit). For any given fluorocrit, the higher the $PO_2$, the higher the concentration of dissolved oxygen. Similarly, for any given $PO_2$, the higher the amount of fluorocarbon, the higher the [$O_2$].

The commercially prepared FC emulsion is Fluosol-DA 20% (FL-DA 20%). This product has been evaluated extensively in animals and humans in Japan and in several series in the United States. A comparison of whole blood with a hemoglobin of 15 g/dL and FL-DA 20% is shown in Figure 10–4.[26] Although FL-

DA 20% offers some value as an oxygen carrier, several limiting factors are present. First, the patient must breathe a high concentration of inspired oxygen to maximize FL-DA [$O_2$]. Second, even at a $PO_2$ of 500 mm Hg [fraction of inspired oxygen (FIO$_2$) = 1.0], with the maximum achievable fluorocrit, the [$O_2$] is still less than 5 mL/dL compared with the normal 20 mL/dL of whole blood. The infusion of FL-DA 20%, therefore, adds very little to the total [$O_2$] unless the hemoglobin is considerably reduced from normal. Finally, the amount of FL-DA 20% that can be administered to any patient (40 mL/kg) limits the achievable fluorocrit, further decreasing the amount of oxygen that can be carried.

## LABORATORY STUDIES

Our initial effort was to answer the question, How good are FC emulsions as oxygen carriers? Because the principal requirement of any oxygen carrier is the ability to load and unload oxygen, these functions must be assessed accurately. We have shown that adult baboons can survive a total exchange transfusion to zero hematocrit with FL-DA if they are ventilated with pure oxygen.[27] The animals maintain normal hemodynamic and oxygen transport functions in the virtual absence of RBCs. Although these data suggest that FL-DA is an effective oxygen carrier, we also demonstrated that control animals survive at zero hematocrit and an FIO$_2$ of 1.0 without FL-DA. This remarkable observation leads to the conclusion that FL-DA is not necessary, at least in this acute setting.

These results can be explained by an understanding of the way in which the fluorocarbons carry oxygen. In the presence of RBCs and FC, the total oxygen content in the blood can be considered the sum of three separate oxygen carriers.

$$[O_2] \text{ Total} = [O_2] \text{ RBC} + [O_2] \text{ Plasma} + [O_2] \text{ FC}$$

Survival depends on total [$O_2$], but the body does not distinguish among the oxygen carriers.[28] At a $PO_2$ of 500 mm Hg, the plasma becomes a significant carrier of oxygen that is capable of supporting oxygen consumption ($\dot{V}O_2$) even in the complete absence of both RBC and FC. Because the [$O_2$] plasma will

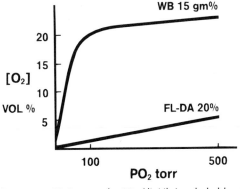

**Fig. 10–4.** [$O_2$] curves for 15 g/dL Hb in whole blood (WB) and for 20% FL-DA. From Gould SA, Moss GS, Rosen AL, and others: Red cell substitutes. In: Civetta JM, Taylor RW, Kirby RR, eds, Critical Care. Philadelphia, 1988, J.B. Lippincott, pp. 1495–1502, with permission.

always be increased at an $FIO_2$ of 1.0, the actual need for FL-DA is unclear.

Although this study documents the efficacy of plasma as an oxygen carrier, we are concerned about the potential risk of pulmonary oxygen toxicity in the clinical setting. The safe level of supplemental oxygen is thought to be an $FIO_2$ less than 0.6. Although our data suggest that FL-DA is unnecessary at an $FIO_2$ of 1.0, we cannot assume the same is true at lower levels of supplemental oxygen.

## CLINICAL TRIAL

The results of our animal study[27] led us to design a clinical trial.[29] We sought to distinguish between the contributions of the $[O_2]$ plasma and $[O_2]$ FL-DA. Further, we wanted to minimize the risk of toxicity associated with breathing 100% oxygen. The objective, therefore, was to provide sufficient oxygen delivery with FL-DA at an $FIO_2$ less than 0.6. Unlike most clinical trials, the protocol for FL-DA was nonblinded and had a crossover design, with each patient serving as his or her own control for each oxygen carrier. This design allowed us to define the physiological need for, and evaluate the efficacy of, FL-DA in acute anemia.

Physiological criteria of need derived from our control studies in baboons included [Hb] < 3.5 g/dL, partial pressure of oxygen in mixed venous blood oxygen pressure ($P\bar{v}O_2$) < 25 mm Hg, and oxygen extraction ratio > 50%. We evaluated 23 surgical patients with blood loss and religious objections to receiving blood transfusions. Of these 23, 15 moderately anemic patients with a mean [Hb] ($\pm$ SE) of 7.2 $\pm$ 0.5 g/dL had no evidence of a physiological need for increased arterial oxygen content and did not receive FL-DA. Eight severely anemic patients with a mean [Hb] of 3.0 $\pm$ 0.4 g/dL met one or more of our criteria and received FL-DA until the physiological need disappeared or a maximal dose of 40 mL/kg of body weight was reached. All patients breathed supplemental oxygen. We observed no adverse reactions. The volume of FL-DA infused ranged from 2 to 10 units. Six of the eight patients received the maximal allowable dose; one patient survived after receiving only 2 units and another died before the total dosage had been infused.

The maximal FL-DA $[O_2]$ ranged from 0.3

**Table 10–2. Arterial oxygen content at peak effect of FL-DA**

| Measure | Mean $\pm$ SE |
|---|---|
| Partial pressure of arterial $O_2$ (mm Hg) | 430 $\pm$ 19 |
| Fluorocrit (%) | 5 $\pm$ 1 |
| $FIO_2$ | 1.0 $\pm$ 0.0 |
| Arterial $[O_2]$ | |
| FL-DA phase (mL/dL) | 0.7 $\pm$ 0.1 |
| Plasma phase (mL/dL) | 1.3 $\pm$ 0.1 |
| Red cells (mL/dL) | 2.8 $\pm$ 0.6 |

From Gould SA, Moss GS, Rosen AL, et al.: Red cell substitutes. In: Civetta JM, Taylor RW, Kirby RR, eds, Critical Care. Philadelphia, 1988, JB Lippincott, pp. 1495–1502, with permission.

to 1.2 mL/dL, with a mean increment of 0.7 $\pm$ 0.1 mL/dL. The simultaneous level of arterial oxygen carried by the plasma was 1.3 $\pm$ 0.1 mL/dL and the level of oxygen carried by the RBCs was 2.8 $\pm$ 0.6 mL/dL (Table 10–2).

Eighty-two percent of the plasma and FL-DA oxygen phases was unloaded. In contrast, only 19% was unloaded from the RBC phase (Table 10–3). The relative contribution to total oxygen consumption for each of the three phases is also shown in Table 10–3. The plasma contributed 50%, whereas FL-DA contributed 28% and the RBCs only 22%.

The only statistically significant differences in hemodynamic and oxygen transport values before and after FL-DA were a minor reduction in heart rate and an increase in $PaO_2$ (which followed an increased fractional inspired oxygen concentration in one patient) (Table 10–4). Intravascular persistence of FL-DA was determined in five patients. The mean half-life was 24.3 $\pm$ 4.3 hours, with a range of 12–37 hours.

Of the eight patients who received FL-DA, six died. The minimal hemoglobin level observed in these eight patients was 1.8 $\pm$ 0.4 g/dL. Fourteen of 15 patients who did not receive FL-DA survived.

These data illustrate that FL-DA is a poor oxygen loader and that the fluorocrit that can be achieved clinically with the currently available product is only approximately 5%. A 5% concentration of FL-DA at an oxygen partial pressure of 430 mm Hg carries 0.7 mL/dL of oxygen, or approximately half the oxygen carried by plasma (1.3 mL/dL). This value is

**Table 10–3.   Oxygen dynamics of three phases at peak effect of FL-DA (mean ± SE)**

| Measure | FL-DA | Plasma | Red cells |
|---|---|---|---|
| Arterial [O$_2$] (mL/dL) | 0.7 ± 0.1 | 1.3 ± 0.1 | 2.8 ± 0.6 |
| Venous [O$_2$] (mL/dL) | 0.2 ± 0.1 | 0.2 ± 0.1 | 2.2 ± 0.4 |
| Oxygen unloaded (%) | 82 ± 5 | 82 ± 5 | 19 ± 5 |
| Contribution to V$_{O_2}$ (%) | 28 ± 5 | 50 ± 5 | 22 ± 7 |

From Gould SA, Moss GS, Rosen AL, et al.: Red cell substitutes. In: Civetta JM, Taylor RW, Kirby RR, eds, Critical Care. Philadelphia, 1988, JB Lippincott, pp. 1495–1502, with permission.

equivalent to an increase in [Hb] of only 0.5 g/dL. The relationship between FL-DA [O$_2$] at this fluorocrit and the amount carried by plasma holds regardless of the partial pressure of oxygen, because the oxygen content curves for both carriers are linear (Figure 10–5). The potential benefit of FL-DA is that even this small amount of oxygen is additive to the amount carried by plasma. However, the observed increase in total [O$_2$] of 0.7 mL/dL was not clinically important, as evidenced by the absence of any discernible physiological benefit after the FL-DA infusion.

In contrast, FL-DA unloads oxygen very effectively. The difference between the arterial and venous FL-DA [O$_2$] is 0.5 mL/dL (Table 10–3). Most of the oxygen carried by FL-DA is thus unloaded. However, the lack of any apparent physiological benefit despite this effi-

cient unloading again suggests that this contribution is inadequate.

The intravascular persistence of FL-DA is also insufficient, at least when RBCs cannot be used subsequently. The half-life of 24 hours and the maximal allowable dose of 40 mL/kg led to a loss of FL-DA from the circulation before the patients were able to regenerate an adequate RBC mass to recover from their severe anemia. The mean hemoglobin level in the eight patients fell from an initial value of 3.0 g/dL to a low of 1.8 g/dL. This level usually is not compatible with survival. The combination of an insufficient increase in arterial oxygen content and an inadequate duration of FL-DA probably contributed to this unsatisfactory outcome. One of the two survivors eventually received RBCs against his wishes after the total FL-DA dose had been infused. An evaluation of FL-DA during short-term unavailability of RBCs might result in a better outcome.

In earlier reports, representing a total of 200 patients, only 3 had a [Hb] less than 3

**Table 10–4.   Hemodynamics and oxygen transport before and after FL-DA administration (mean ± SE)**

| Measure | Before FL-DA | After FL-DA* |
|---|---|---|
| Heart rate (bpm) | 117 ± 5 | 106 ± 4† |
| Mean arterial (mm Hg) pressure | 74 ± 6 | 78 ± 5 |
| Cardiac index (L/min/ m$^2$) | 4.5 ± 0.7 | 4.2 ± 0.7 |
| Hemoglobin (g/dL) | 3.0 ± 0.4 | 2.0 ± 0.4 |
| Arterial [O$_2$] (mL/dL) | 5.3 ± 0.5 | 4.8 ± 0.6 |
| Oxygen delivery (mL/ min/m$^2$) | 235 ± 27 | 197 ± 32 |
| V$_{O_2}$ (mL/min/m$^2$) | 109 ± 13 | 88 ± 11 |
| Pa$_{O_2}$ (mm Hg) | 356 ± 24 | 430 ± 19† |
| P$\bar{v}_{O_2}$ (mm Hg) | 40.0 ± 3.9 | 78.2 ± 23.3 |
| Oxygen extraction ratio (%) | 46.0 ± 2.5 | 47.6 ± 3.8 |

* Data were obtained at peak arterial oxygen content after FL-DA.
† The difference between values before and after FL-DA is significant (P < .05).
From Gould SA, Moss GS, Rosen AL, et al.: Red cell substitutes. In: Civetta JM, Taylor RW, Kirby RR, eds, Critical Care. Philadelphia, 1988, JB Lippincott, pp. 1495–1502, with permission.

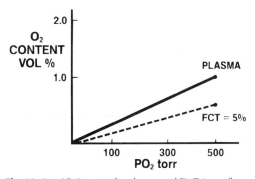

**Fig. 10–5.** [O$_2$] curves for plasma and FL-DA at a fluorocrit of 5%. From Gould SA, Moss GS, Rosen AL, et al.: Red cell substitutes. In: Civetta JM, Taylor RW, Kirby RR, eds, Critical Care. Philadelphia, 1988, J.B. Lippincott, pp. 1495–1502, with permission.

g/dL. Two of these three patients died. The less severely anemic patients receiving FL-DA had satisfactory outcomes. Fifteen of our 23 patients had no physiological evidence of a need for increased arterial oxygen content despite their minimal hemoglobin level of 7.2 g/dL. Fourteen of these 15 moderately anemic patients survived without FL-DA. This good outcome raises some questions about the manner in which decisions about transfusions are made. The mortality rate is high among severely anemic patients who refuse RBCs, despite FL-DA therapy. Patients with less extreme blood loss who refuse RBCs do well, with or without FL-DA.

The results illustrate that FL-DA is unnecessary when anemia is moderate and ineffective when it is severe. It is, therefore, an inadequate RBC substitute. New formulations of FCs that correct the observed shortcomings of FL-DA may be more effective by providing higher FC concentrations and longer intravascular persistence.[30,31]

There are two clinical trials underway with higher FC concentrations. The requirement for supplemental $O_2$ and the small increase in $[O_2]$ will remain and are likely to limit the clinical utility. The results of these clinical trials will determine the potential role of FC in transfusion practice.

## HEMOGLOBIN SOLUTIONS

For many years, we have pursued the concept that a hemoglobin solution prepared from outdated blood could serve as a temporary substitute for RBCs.[32-34] This interest is based on several characteristics of the hemoglobin molecule. For example, 1 g hemoglobin binds 1.39 mL oxygen and is almost fully saturated with oxygen at ambient pressure. Few, if any, biologically acceptable substances have a greater oxygen-binding capacity. Oxygen is normally unloaded from hemoglobin in the capillaries at a partial pressure of approximately 40 mm Hg, allowing oxygen molecules to diffuse from hemoglobin to the intracellular mitochondria without producing interstitial hypoxia. Despite these features, an acceptable hemoglobin solution has not yet been used in the clinical setting.

Efforts to produce a clinically acceptable hemoglobin solution that functions as a temporary oxygen carrier have evolved through several stages. Starting with the simple tetramer, we have normalized the affinity of hemoglobin for oxygen by pyridoxylation and then polymerized the modified tetramer. This new substance, polyhemoglobin, has a normal oxygen-carrying capacity and a half-life of 38 hours. The following sections review the evolution of polymerized pyridoxylated hemoglobin solution.

## Hemoglobin Solution: An Effective Oxygen Carrier?

In 1934, Mulder et al.[35] published a classic study that was, unfortunately, ignored for more than 30 years. In this research, oxygen consumption was measured in dogs and cats breathing room air before and after total exchange transfusion with hemoglobin solution. The results are shown in Figure 10–6. Mulder and associates were the first to report no change in oxygen consumption at zero hematocrit with hemoglobin solution. In addition, they reported that after total exchange transfusion, cats were capable of landing on their feet when dropped in an upside-down position from a modest height.

In 1976, this study was repeated using baboons as the experimental animals.[33] Hemoglobin was prepared from outdated blood. The constituents are shown in Table 10–5. The hemoglobin solution was anemic and the hemoglobin oxygen affinity state was increased, as reflected by the reduced oxygen half-saturation pressure ($P_{50}$) value (12–14 mm Hg, compared with a normal of 26–28 mm Hg for fresh blood). Of the 18 animals in the study, 9 underwent total exchange transfusion with hemoglobin solution and 9 control animals underwent exchange transfusion with dextran 70. All nine animals given hemoglobin solution survived to zero hematocrit. In contrast, all nine control animals died at hematocrit levels of approximately 5%.

The dextran-treated animals responded to isovolemic anemia with an increase in cardiac output, an increase in oxygen extraction, and a decrease in $P\bar{v}O_2$. The hemoglobin-treated animals developed no changes in oxygen consumption at zero hematocrit when compared with baseline levels, thereby confirming the observations made by Mulder et al.[35] The maintenance of normal oxygen consumption at zero hematocrit was achieved solely

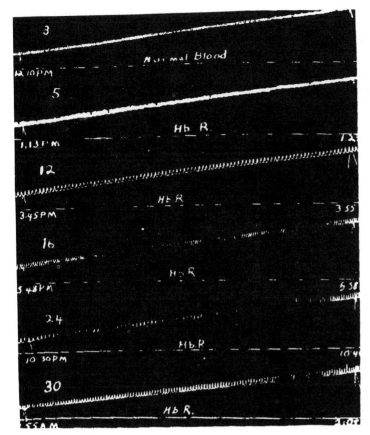

**Fig. 10–6.** Original smoked drum recording of respiratory excursion of a cat during exchange transfusion with hemoglobin solution. Slope of the line represents oxygen consumption. Panel 3 is the control. All subsequent panels represent measurements made after total exchange transfusion. There is no change in oxygen consumption at zero hematocrit. From Moss GS, Sehgal LR, Gould SA: Hemoglobin solution as an acellular oxygen carrier. In: Rossi EC, Simon TL, Moss GS, eds, Principles of Transfusion Medicine. Baltimore, 1991, Williams and Wilkins, pp. 443–451, with permission.

through the mechanism of increased oxygen extraction leading to low $P\bar{v}O_2$ levels. That oxygen consumption was unchanged at zero hematocrit was remarkable, especially because a radical change in the circulation had occurred. Blood containing hemoglobin of 12 g/dL with a $P_{50}$ of 32 mm Hg was replaced acutely with anemic blood of 7 g/dL with a $P_{50}$ of 12 mm Hg. Also remarkable was the maintenance of normal oxygen consumption at zero hematocrit. In view of the profound

**Table 10–5. Properties of hemoglobin-saline solution**

| | |
|---|---|
| Hemoglobin concentration | 6–9 g/dL |
| Methemoglobin | 2–4% |
| Total phospholipids | <1 mg/dL |
| pH | 7.35–7.45 |
| $P_{50}$ | 14.0 mm Hg |

From Moss GS, Sehgal LR, Gould SA: Hemoglobin solution as an accelular oxygen carrier. In: Rossi EC, Simon TL, Moss GS, eds, Principles of Transfusion Medicine. Baltimore, 1991, Williams and Wilkins, pp. 443–451, with permission.

shift in the affinity state, an increase in cardiac output rather than an elevation in oxygen extraction would have been the expected response.

That baboons could temporarily survive such a massive assault on their circulation was surprising and encouraging. A number of questions surfaced from this study. One question concerned the dramatic reduction in $P\bar{v}O_2$ to 20 mm Hg in the hemoglobin-treated animals at zero hematocrit. The $P\bar{v}O_2$ is the tension at which oxygen unloads from the hemoglobin and is in equilibrium with the tissue arterial oxygen pressure ($PO_2$). Such a low $P\bar{v}O_2$ was alarming and led to an attempt at correction.

## Normalization of Mixed Venous Oxygen Tension

Factors that affect $P\bar{v}O_2$ include an increase in oxygen consumption and a decrease in cardiac output, arterial saturation, hemoglobin mass, and affinity state. In reviewing the ba-

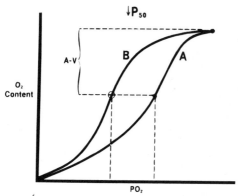

**Fig. 10–7.** Effect of a leftward shift in the oxygen content curve. *Curve A:* normal position. *Curve B:* shifted leftward. Assuming no change in AVDO$_2$, the result must be a decline in the P$\bar{v}$O$_2$. From Moss GS, Sehgal LR, Gould SA: Hemoglobin solution as an acellular oxygen carrier. In: Rossi EC, Simon TL, Moss GS, eds, Principles of Transfusion Medicine. Baltimore, 1991, Williams and Wilkins, pp. 443–451, with permission.

boon data, changes in oxygen consumption, arterial saturation, and cardiac output could be eliminated as possible explanations for the decline in P$\bar{v}$O$_2$, because they remained at baseline values. That left changes in hemoglobin mass and affinity state remaining for further consideration. Affinity state changes were examined first. Figure 10–7 demonstrates how a leftward shift in the content curve produces a decrease in the tension at which oxygen unloading occurs—the P$\bar{v}$O$_2$. This possibility was confirmed by Riggs et al.,[36] who exchanged transfused blood in monkeys with high-affinity banked monkey blood. No changes in cardiac output or arteriovenous oxygen content difference (AVDO$_2$) were noted, but there was a significant decrease in P$\bar{v}$O$_2$. No data exist concerning the consequences of normalizing a leftward-shifted curve.

The increase in affinity state in the hemoglobin solution is related to the loss of the organic ligand 2,3-diphosphoglycerate (2,3-DPG), normally found within the RBC. Attempts to normalize P$_{50}$ by the addition of 2,3-DPG to the hemoglobin solution were unsuccessful, because the DPG rapidly disappears from the circulation after infusion.[37] Benesch et al.,[38] Greenberg et al.,[39] and Sehgal et al.[40] described a modification of the hemoglobin molecule by the addition of pyridoxal-phosphate. The resulting compound,

pyridoxylated hemoglobin, exhibits a P$_{50}$ considerably higher than the P$_{50}$ of unmodified hemoglobin. This modification allowed for an examination of the P$\bar{v}$O$_2$ in animal exchange transfusion with pyridoxylated hemoglobin.[41]

Eight baboons were the test animals. Four received unmodified hemoglobin (P$_{50}$ = 12 mm Hg), and four received pyridoxylated hemoglobin (P$_{50}$ = 22 mm Hg). The exchange transfusion was carried out until zero hematocrit was achieved. The hemoglobin concentration of both solutions was approximately 7 g/dL. No important changes were noted after exchange transfusion in either group in terms of oxygen consumption, cardiac output, or AVDO$_2$. Figure 10–8 demonstrates that animals undergoing exchange transfusion with pyridoxylated hemoglobin developed significantly higher whole blood P$_{50}$ levels than animals given unmodified hemoglobin when the hematocrit levels decline to 10%. From this point, P$\bar{v}$O$_2$ levels were substantially higher in the animals given pyridoxylated hemoglobin (Fig. 10–9).

These data illustrate two points. First, they confirm the concept that rightward shifts in the dissociation curve result in an increased P$\bar{v}$O$_2$, as long as cardiac output and AVDO$_2$ remain constant. This is important because it allows for unloading to occur at a higher tissue PO$_2$. Second, the P$\bar{v}$O$_2$ level in the animals treated with pyridoxylated hemoglobin was still substantially lower than the 40–50 mm Hg found in control animals. Thus, other means for normalizing the P$\bar{v}$O$_2$ in animals

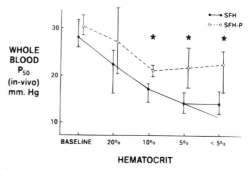

**Fig. 10–8.** Whole blood in vivo P$_{50}$ versus hematocrit (mean value and range). Significant difference ($P < .05$). From Moss GS, Sehgal LR, Gould SA: Hemoglobin solution as an acellular oxygen carrier. In: Rossi EC, Simon TL, Moss GS, eds, Principles of Transfusion Medicine. Baltimore, 1991, Williams and Wilkins, pp. 443–451, with permission.

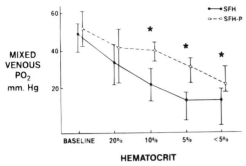

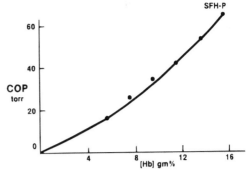

**Fig. 10–9.** Mixed venous oxygen tension versus hematocrit (mean value and range). Significant difference ($P <$ .05). From Moss GS, Sehgal LR, Gould SA: Hemoglobin solution as an acellular oxygen carrier. In: Rossi EC, Simon TL, Moss GS, eds, Principles of Transfusion Medicine. Baltimore, 1991, Williams and Wilkins, pp. 443–451, with permission.

**Fig. 10–10.** Relationship between COP and hemoglobin concentration ([Hb]) for polymerized stroma-free hemoglobin (SFH-P). From Moss GS, Sehgal LR, Gould SA: Hemoglobin solution as an acellular oxygen carrier. In: Rossi EC, Simon TL, Moss GS, eds, Principles of Transfusion Medicine. Baltimore, 1991, Williams and Wilkins, pp. 443–451, with permission.

undergoing total exchange transfusion with hemoglobin solution had to be found. This led to an examination of the quantitative relationships among changes in hemoglobin concentration, $P_{50}$ levels, and $P\bar{v}O_2$.

## Hemoglobin Concentration, Oxygen Half-Saturation Pressure, and Mixed Venous Oxygen Tension

Little information exists concerning the relationship among changes in hemoglobin concentration, the oxygen half-saturation pressure of hemoglobin ($P_{50}$), and the resultant $P\bar{v}O_2$ in animals receiving hemoglobin solution. Such information might provide a clue concerning whether or not further efforts should be made to increase the $P_{50}$ of the hemoglobin solution or whether attempts to increase the hemoglobin concentration should be continued.

In this study, 15 baboons underwent total exchange transfusion with pyridoxylated hemoglobin with a $P_{50}$ of 21 mm Hg and a hemoglobin concentration of 7 g/dL (Fig. 10–10). The result involved simultaneous changes in the recipient hemoglobin concentration and $P_{50}$. To assess the effect of each variable on $P\bar{v}O_2$, a multiple linear regression model was used. The equation was as follows:

$$P\bar{v}O_2 = a \times [Hb] + b \times P_{50}$$

where a is the coefficient for hemoglobin concentration and b is the coefficient for $P_{50}$. The results are shown in Table 10–6. The important results include a decrease in hemoglobin concentration of 6.5 g/dL and a decrease in $P_{50}$ of 21.5 mm Hg. These changes were associated with a decline in $P\bar{v}O_2$ of 29 mm Hg.

The coefficients of each variable (calculated

**Table 10–6.** Preexchange and postexchange oxygen transport variables (mean ± SE)

| Variable | Baseline | After exchange |
|---|---|---|
| $P\bar{v}O_2$ (mm Hg) | 51.4 ± 1.5 | 22.4 ± 2.6* |
| Hemoglobin concentration (g/dL) | 11.6 ± 0.3 | 5.1 ± 0.4* |
| $P_{50}$ (mm Hg) | 31.0 ± 0.9 | 19.5 ± 1.6* |
| Oxygen consumption (mL/min/kg) | 4.5 ± 0.3 | 3.2 ± 0.3* |
| Cardiac output (L/min) | 3.3 ± 0.2 | 2.8 ± 0.2 |
| Oxygen saturation | 0.96 ± 0.003 | 0.96 ± 0.007 |

* Significantly different from baseline ($P <$ .001).
From Moss GS, Sehgal LR, Gould SA: Hemoglobin solution as an acellular oxygen carrier. In: Rossi EC, Simon TL, Moss GS, eds, Principles of Transfusion Medicine. Baltimore, 1991, Williams and Wilkins, pp. 443–451, with permission.

**Table 10–7.** Calculated changes in mixed venous oxygen tension

| Variable | Average total change | Multiple regression coefficient | Contribution to P$\bar{v}O_2$ (mm Hg) |
|---|---|---|---|
| Hemoglobin concentration | −6.5 | 4.0 | −26.0 |
| P$_{50}$ | −11.5 | 0.33 | −3.8 |
| Total calculated | | | −29.8 |
| P$\bar{v}O_2$ vs. | | | −29.0 |
| observed | | | |
| P$\bar{v}O_2$ | | | |

From Gould SA, Sehgal LR, Rosen AL, et al.: Hemoglobin solution: is a normal [Hb] or P$_{50}$ more important? J Surg Res 1982; 33:189–193; and Moss GS, Sehgal LR, Gould SA: Hemoglobin solution as an acellular oxygen carrier. In: Rossi EC, Simon TL, Moss GS, eds, Principles of Transfusion Medicine. Baltimore, 1991, Williams and Wilkins, pp. 443–451, with permission.

# POLYMERIZATION

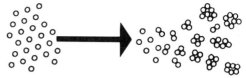

[Hb]−15 gm/dl   [Hb]−15 gm/dl
COP > 70 torr  →  COP = 25 torr

**Fig. 10–11.** Polymerization results in a reduction in COP, whereas a constant hemoglobin concentration ([Hb]) is maintained. From Moss GS, Sehgal LR, Gould SA: Hemoglobin solution as an acellular oxygen carrier. In: Rossi EC, Simon TL, Moss GS, eds, Principles of Transfusion Medicine. Baltimore, 1991, Williams and Wilkins, pp. 443–451, with permission.

from the equation) and contribution of each variable to the change in P$\bar{v}O_2$ are shown in Table 10–7. The results show that the 6.5-g/dL decrease in hemoglobin concentration produced a 26-mm Hg decline in P$\bar{v}O_2$, whereas an 11.5-mm Hg decline in P$_{50}$ produced only a 3.8-mm Hg decrease in P$\bar{v}O_2$. These changes clearly indicate that further efforts should be directed toward normalizing the hemoglobin concentration.

## Nonanemic Isooncotic Hemoglobin Solution?

The advantages of a nonanemic hemoglobin solution are self-evident. Such a solution would have the same oxygen-carrying capacity as whole blood. In addition, according to established data, the infusion of a nonanemic solution should be associated with normal P$\bar{v}O_2$[42] levels, even at zero hematocrit. The principal obstacle to normalization of hemoglobin concentration is the effect of an elevation in protein concentration on oncotic pressure.

The relationship between hemoglobin concentration and oncotic pressure is shown in Figure 10–10.[43] At hemoglobin concentrations of 7 g/dL, the oncotic pressure is similar to that of plasma—20 mm Hg. In contrast, at hemoglobin levels of 15 g/dL, oncotic pressure increases by more than 300%. The infusion of such a solution would theoretically produce large shifts of fluid from the extravascular space into the intravascular space. These changes are likely to be exceedingly harmful.

One approach to producing a nonanemic hemoglobin solution with normal COP values is polymerization of the hemoglobin. The COP of any solution is proportional to the number of colloidal particles. If a 15-g/dL solution of hemoglobin could be polymerized, the result would be reduction in COP, whereas no change would occur in hemoglobin concentration (Figure 10– 11).

This idea was tested in the research laboratory.[44] Approximately 14 L of the hemoglobin solution obtained in the manner already discussed was pyridoxylated by modification of previously described techniques.[38,39] Briefly, pyridoxal-5′-phosphate is added to the solution on a 4:1 molar ratio. The solu-

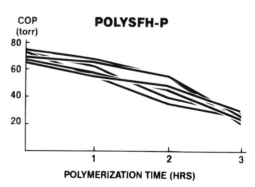

**Fig. 10–12.** Decrease in COP measured during the course of polymerization for five different batches. From Moss GS, Sehgal LR, Gould SA: Hemoglobin solution as an acellular oxygen carrier. In: Rossi EC, Simon TL, Moss GS, eds, Principles of Transfusion Medicine. Baltimore, 1991, Williams and Wilkins, pp. 443–451, with permission.

tion is transferred to a 20-L sealed reservoir (Millipore Corporation, Bedford, MA) and deoxygenated with nitrogen ($N_2$) using a gas exchanger (William Harvey Company, Santa Ana, CA). Deoxygenation of the solution is continued until the $PO_2$ is below 10 mm Hg and the oxygen content is below 1 vol%.[44] Sodium borohydride is then added to the solution, and the reaction is continued for 2–4 hours. The goal of the polymerization is to normalize the $O_2$ capacity while still maintaining the COP within normal limits (20–25 mm Hg). There are several parameters that can be manipulated to obtain, in a reproducible way, the polymerized solution of choice.[45] These parameters include the hemoglobin concentration, the concentration of the polymerizing agent, the rate of addition of the latter, and the rate of mixing. Finally, the duration in which the above parameters are controlled determines the reaction yield, the molecular weight distribution of the polymeric species, the oxygen affinity ($P_{50}$), and the viscosity of the solution.

The details of polymerization have been described previously.[46] Polymerization is conducted to a physiological endpoint with respect to COP. The reaction is monitored by the decrease in COP. Figure 10–12 shows the changes in COP monitored during the polymerization process conducted over a 3-hour period. As seen from the figure, the reproducibility of the process over five batches is quite acceptable.

The polymerization and the evolution of the polymeric species are also followed by sodium dodecyl sulfate-polyacrylamide gel electrophoresis (SDS-PAGE) technique. Figure 10–13 shows the formation of new polypeptide bands over the duration of the process. Typically, four to six bands are seen, ranging in molecular weights from 16 to 96 kd. The first four bands (16–64 kd) represent more than 90% of all species.

With the formation of polymers, changes in the viscosity of the solution should be anticipated. Figure 10–14 shows changes in viscosity observed over five different batches. The

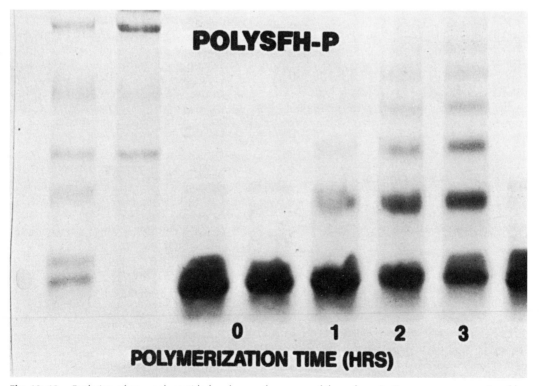

**Fig. 10–13.** Evolution of new polypeptide bands over the course of the polymerization process, as monitored by SDS-PAGE. From Moss GS, Sehgal LR, Gould SA: Hemoglobin solution as an acellular oxygen carrier. In: Rossi EC, Simon TL, Moss GS, eds, Principles of Transfusion Medicine. Baltimore, 1991, Williams and Wilkins, pp. 443–451, with permission.

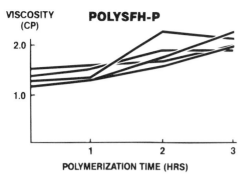

**Fig. 10–14.** Changes in viscosity of five batches of hemoglobin solution during polymerization. From Moss GS, Sehgal LR, Gould SA: Hemoglobin solution as an acellular oxygen carrier. In: Rossi EC, Simon TL, Moss GS, eds, Principles of Transfusion Medicine. Baltimore, 1991, Williams and Wilkins, pp. 443–451, with permission.

**Table 10–8.   Characteristics of polymerized pyridoxylated hemoglobin**

| | |
|---|---|
| Hemoglobin concentration | 12–14 g/dL |
| Methemoglobin concentration | <5% |
| Molecular weight range | 64–400 × kd |
| Number average molecular weight | 150 kd |
| $P_{50}$ | 18–22 mm Hg |
| Binding coefficient | 1.30 mL $O_2$/g Hb |
| Hill coefficient | 1.5–2.0 |
| Bohr coefficient | −0.12 to −0.25 |
| Colloid osmotic pressure | 15–20 mm Hg |
| Viscosity | 2–3 cp |
| Phospholipids | <0.4 mg/dL |
| Limulus-amebocyte lysate assay | <0.625 ESU/mL |
| Rabbit pyrogen test | Pass |

From Moss GS, Sehgal LR, Gould SA: Hemoglobin solution as an acellular oxygen carrier. In: Rossi EC, Simon TL, Moss GS, eds, Principles of Transfusion Medicine. Baltimore, 1991, Williams and Wilkins, pp. 443–451, with permission.

viscosity at the start of polymerization ranges from 1.0 to 1.5 cp and increases to a range of 1.9–2.1 cp at the end. This represents a relatively modest increase, but it is consistent with the absence of large molecular weight species in the solution, as demonstrated by SDS-PAGE.

The changes in $P_{50}$ during the polymerization were tracked and are shown in Figure 10–15. There was a modest increase in $P_{50}$ in all five batches, which reflects a decrease in the buffering capacity of the solution with polymerization. It is consistent with the observation that a drop in pH is observed during poly-

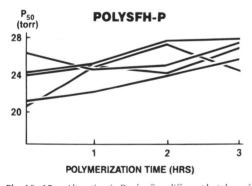

**Fig. 10–15.** Alteration in $P_{50}$ for five different batches of hemoglobin solution during polymerization. From Moss GS, Sehgal LR, Gould SA: Hemoglobin solution as an acellular oxygen carrier. In: Rossi EC, Simon TL, Moss GS, eds, Principles of Transfusion Medicine. Baltimore, 1991, Williams and Wilkins, pp. 443–451, with permission.

merization, which is not surprising because some of the same amino groups involved in the buffering are involved in the cross-linking as well.

The characteristics of the final product are listed in Table 10–8. The solution at 12–15 g/dL has a COP between 15 and 20 mm Hg. The molecular weight range based on SDS-PAGE and high-pressure liquid chromatography (HPLC) is between 16 and 96 kd. The number average molecular weight calculated from the COP is 150 kd. The weight average molecular weight, obtained by ultracentrifugation, is 120 kd. The $P_{50}$ of the solution under standard conditions (pH 7.40, $PCO_2$ 35 mm Hg, temperature 35°C) ranges from 18 to 22 mm Hg. The viscosity of the solution ([Hb] = 8.0 g/dL) ranges from 2 to 3 cp. The phospholipid content is below the detection limits of the thin-layer chromatography technique (<0.4 mg/dL).

The stability of the polymerized solution when stored at 4–8°C as a sterile pyrogen-free product has been traced, and this stability, with respect to rate of conversion to methemoglobin, is shown in Figure 10–16. The methemoglobin remains below 2% for a 150-day period.

The stability of the polymeric species was followed by monitoring the solution over time by HPLC, SDS-PAGE, and viscosity. No changes were observed for at least a 1-year period. Thus, the polymerized pyridoxylated

## STABILITY OF POLYSFH-P

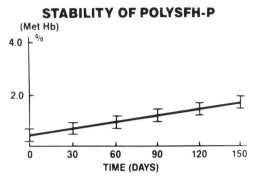

**Fig. 10-16.** Changes in methemoglobin concentration upon storage at 4–8°C as a sterile pyrogen-free solution. Each point represents mean ± SE for five different batches. From Moss GS, Sehgal LR, Gould SA: Hemoglobin solution as an acellular oxygen carrier. In: Rossi EC, Simon TL, Moss GS, eds, Principles of Transfusion Medicine. Baltimore, 1991, Williams and Wilkins, pp. 443–451, with permission.

## STABILITY OF POLYSFH-P

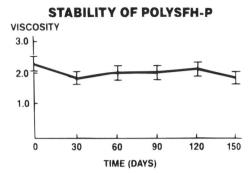

**Fig. 10-18.** Changes in viscosity of five batches, observed over a 150-day period. Each point represents the mean ± SE. No changes in viscosity are observed. From Moss GS, Sehgal LR, Gould SA: Hemoglobin solution as an acellular oxygen carrier. In: Rossi EC, Simon TL, Moss GS, eds, Principles of Transfusion Medicine. Baltimore, 1991, Williams and Wilkins, pp. 443–451, with permission.

stroma-free hemoglobin (poly-SFH-P), when stored at 4–8°C, appears to be very stable. Figure 10–17 shows the HPLC scans for three different batches at the time of manufacture and at 150 days later. No visible changes occurred. Finally, Figure 10–18 shows the changes in viscosity over a 150-day storage period. Once again, no change in viscosity is seen.

### Efficacy of Polymerized Pyridoxylated Stroma-Free Hemoglobin

Seven adult baboons were anesthetized, paralyzed, intubated, and mechanically venti-lated on room air. The respiratory rate and tidal volume were adjusted to maintain an arterial carbon dioxide pressure ($PaCO_2$) between 35 and 45 mm Hg before the start of the study; these values were not changed during the study. The animals were prepared surgically with arterial and central venous catheters for infusion, blood sampling, and monitoring. A thermal dilution balloon-tipped catheter was floated into the pulmonary artery. A Foley catheter was inserted into the urinary bladder. Standard hemodynamic monitoring was performed for electrocardiogram, arterial pressures, pulmonary capillary wedge pressure (PCWP), and central venous

## STABILITY OF POLYSFH-P

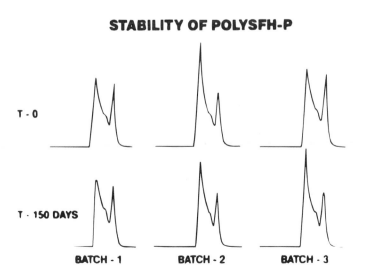

**Fig. 10-17.** HPLC scans for three batches at the time of manufacture and 150 days later. No changes are noted. From Moss GS, Sehgal LR, Gould SA: Hemoglobin solution as an acellular oxygen carrier. In: Rossi EC, Simon TL, Moss GS, eds, Principles of Transfusion Medicine. Baltimore, 1991, Williams and Wilkins, pp. 443–451, with permission.

pressures. Cardiac output was determined by the thermal dilution method.

The study was conducted under ketamine anesthesia. After stabilization of the animals, a set of baseline measurements was obtained. An isovolemic exchange transfusion with the poly-SFH-P was then performed. Historical control animals, exchange transfused with SFH-P, were used for comparison. Whole blood was removed in 50-mL aliquots and was replaced with approximately equal volumes of the infusate. Additional volume adjustments were made, as required, to maintain the PCWP at baseline values. The exchange was stopped at hematocrits of 20, 10, and 5% to obtain additional sets of measurements. The exchange transfusion was then carried out to obtain a complete washout of the RBCs. A hematocrit of less than 1% was achieved.

These animals, at zero hematocrit, had a poly-SFH-P concentration of approximately 10 g/dL. An exchange transfusion with dextran 70 to a hemoglobin concentration of 1 g/dL was then performed. The data from the second half of the study were compared with that of a control group ($n = 6$) that underwent an exchange transfusion with dextran 70 to a hemoglobin concentration of 1 g/dL.

Arterial and mixed venous blood gases were measured by standard electrodes [IL-813]. Whole blood and plasma hemoglobin levels were determined on the IL-282 Co-oximeter.[47] Oxygen carried by whole blood hemoglobin also was measured by the IL-282 Co-oximeter. The physically dissolved oxygen in the aqueous phase was calculated from the $PO_2$ of the plasma separated by centrifugation. The poly-SFH-P $O_2$ content was measured by the IL-282 Co-oximeter. Hematocrits were determined by the microhematocrit method, and $P_{50}$ values of whole blood and plasma hemoglobin were determined with the hemoglobin $O_2$ dissociation curve analyzer (Hem-O-Scan).[48]

The efficacy of the poly-SFH-P was calculated as previously described.[49] At each hematocrit level, the $O_2$ content was determined for each compartment by direct measurement or calculation. Total $O_2$ delivery was calculated as the product of the cardiac output and the total arteriovenous $O_2$ content difference [$AVDO_2$]. The contribution of poly-SFH-P to $O_2$ delivery was calculated as the ratio of the poly-SFH-P to total arterial $O_2$ content:[42]

*Poly-SFH-P $O_2$ delivery*

$$= \frac{[O_2]_a, \, poly\text{-}SFH\text{-}P}{[O_2], \, total}$$

The contribution of poly-SFH-P to $O_2$ consumption was calculated as the ratio of poly-SFH-P to total $AVDO_2$:

$$Poly\text{-}SFH\text{-}P \; VO_2 = \frac{[AVDO_2] \, poly\text{-}SFH\text{-}P}{[AVDO_2] \, total}$$

All contributions were expressed as percent values.

All animals receiving poly-SFH-P survived the exchange transfusion, as did the previous animals receiving SFH-P.[41] The final hematocrit was $0.8 \pm 0.4\%$ (mean $\pm$ SE). The difference in the initial bag $P_{50}$ values of the two infusates was statistically significant ($P < .05$). The mean in vivo plasma $P_{50}$ for the poly-SFH-P, however, was $17.0 \pm 0.5$ mm Hg, which was not significantly different from the mean value of $17.6 \pm 0.8$ mm Hg for the SFH-P. Both of these plasma $P_{50}$ values are significantly below the mean baboon RBC $P_{50}$ of $31.3 \pm 0.8$ mm Hg. The poly-SFH-P $[O_2]_a$ is significantly greater than the SFH-P value at all hematocrits ($P < .001$). At a hematocrit of 5%, the $(O_2)_a$ was $9.5 \pm 0.2$ vol% for poly-SFH-P and $5.0 \pm 0.4$ vol% for SFH-P. Poly-SFH-P makes a greater ($P < .02$) contribution to total $O_2$ delivery than SFH-P at all hematocrits. The contribution to total $O_2$ consumption is greater by poly-SFH-P at all hematocrits, with the difference becoming significant ($P < .005$) at a hematocrit of 20%.

The in vivo $P_{50}$ in the poly-SFH-P animals undergoing the second exchange transfusion with dextran 70 ranged from 18 to 11 mm Hg.[50] In contrast, the in vivo $P_{50}$ of the control group ranged from 31.5 to 25.5 mm Hg. The $P\bar{v}O_2$ was significantly lower in the poly-SFH-P group than in the control group. Both groups of animals raised their cardiac output in an identical manner in response to their anemia. The critical $O_2$ delivery in the control group was 6.6 mL/min/kg compared with 5.7 mL/min/kg in the noncontrol group.

## SAFETY OF POLYMERIZED PYRIDOXYLATED STROMA-FREE HEMOGLOBIN

So far, the efficacy of hemoglobin solution has been discussed with regard to oxygen dynamic properties. The next issue is safety, with concern focused in two areas: nephrotoxicity and immunocompetence.

Nephrotoxicity after the infusion of hemoglobin solution was reported in early studies.[51] Further investigation suggested that the stroma was the toxic factor, probably because of thrombosis of the small renal vasculature.[52] In 1967, Rabiner et al.[53] reported that hemoglobin solution (relatively free of stroma) produced no deterioration in renal function after infusion in dogs. These findings were subsequently confirmed in monkeys under such stressful circumstances as dehydration and shock.[54]

In 1978, Savitsky et al.[55] reported the results of a clinical safety trial in humans using SFH. Eight healthy male volunteers received a 250 mL infusion of SFH at a rate of 2–4 mL/min. The hemoglobin concentration of this solution was 6.4 g/dL. The $P_{50}$ was not reported. Two control patients received similar infusions of 5% albumin.

The most striking finding of this study was a decline in creatinine clearance in the hemoglobin solution recipients, from a baseline value of 148 mL/min to one of 73 mL/min 1 hour after infusion. This value returned to normal in the second hour after infusion. The alteration in kidney function was accompanied by a sharp decline in urine volume. In the albumin control patients, no changes were seen in urine volume or creatinine clearance. The authors stressed that this deterioration in kidney function was transient and not associated with permanent renal damage. Nevertheless, these results had a chilling effect on further clinical research.

As Savitsky et al.[55] pointed out, there are three possible explanations for the observed nephrotoxicity. The first is stromal toxicity. They did report a stroma lipid level of 1.6 mg/dL. Because this represents only 1% of the original level of phospholipid and because the infusion of hemoglobin solution did not produce detectable disseminated intravascular coagulation in the recipients, stromal toxicity is an unlikely explanation.

A second possibility is the presence of a vasoactive substance in the hemoglobin solution that affects renal blood flow. This is supported by the observation that recipients developed transient bradycardia and mild hypertension during the infusion. Similar findings discovered in earlier hemoglobin solution studies in baboons[56] led to the belief that prospective hemoglobin solutions should be tested for the presence of vasoactive substances by bioassay techniques before clinical testing.

A third possibility is that the changes in renal function were simply related to the filtration of free hemoglobin through kidneys. Perhaps hemoglobin filtration interferes in some way with normal kidney function. Once the hemoglobinemia disappears, renal function returns to normal. This is an interesting argument, because the highest level of plasma hemoglobin in the human volunteers was only 57 mg/dL. In actual clinical practice, plasma hemoglobin levels can be expected to rise as high as 6–8 g/dL, a 1000-fold increase over the levels in the clinical safety trials. It is likely that elevations of plasma hemoglobin of that magnitude would produce even greater changes in renal function, especially in a setting of hemorrhagic shock.

In this regard, polyhemoglobin has theoretical appeal. The large molecular size of a polymer should rule out renal excretion. The principal route of excretion is presumably the reticuloendothelial system. Nephrotoxicity is, therefore, less likely to occur with a polymer than it is with the hemoglobin tetramer.

Our second major concern is postinfusion immunosuppression. Because sepsis is one of the most serious complications that can develop in circumstances in which hemoglobin solution is used, it is important to establish whether or not the infusion of hemoglobin solution impairs the host defense mechanism.

The effect of hemoglobin solution on granulocyte function was studied by Hau and Simmons.[37] They showed that hemoglobin acted as an adjuvant in experimental peritonitis in rats by interfering with granulocyte phagocytosis and bacterial killing capability. The significance of this finding is not clear, because the hemoglobin acted only as an adjuvant when it was injected intravenously or intramuscularly. In another report, Hoyt et al.[57] studied the ability of rats to withstand peritonitis after exposure to hemoglobin solution used as a volume expander in the treatment of hemorrhagic shock. They found no evidence that hemoglobin solution depressed host defense mechanisms.

Whether polyhemoglobin alters immunocompetence is not known. What is known, however, is that the infusion of colloid particles produces blockage of the reticuloendothelial system and thereby enhances susceptibility to bacterial toxins.[58] Stein and Saba[59] showed that the infusion of colloid particles not only blocks the reticuloendothelial system but also acutely depletes plasma fibronectin levels. Thus, studies designed to investigate the effects of polyhemoglobin on immunocompetence must be done before clinical trials.

The polyhemoglobin solution passes the rabbit pyrogen test and, from batch to batch, remained at levels between 0.3125 and 0.625 ESU/mL as determined by the limulus-amebocyte lysate assay. In addition, the solution passes the United States Pharmacopeia (USP) safety test as well as the USP systemic toxicity test and shows no pressor effects (as measured by the USP pressor test).

In addition to the above standard tests, baboons receiving from 1 to 8 g/kg body weight of the solution (followed for a period of 3–6 months) showed no alteration in renal function, blood chemistry, or coagulation profile. On the basis of all the data on safety and efficacy, a further modification of the polyhemoglobin product was made, leading to the approval of clinical trials in humans. Preliminary results from the trials confirm the preclinical data.[33]

## Clinical Trials

Based on these preclinical observations, we began clinical trials in both healthy volunteers and patients to assess the safety and efficacy of poly-SFH-P. For these trials a decision was made to prepare the poly-SFH-P in a fashion that would allow 1 unit of poly-SFH-P to deliver the equivalent amount of hemoglobin contained in a 1-unit blood transfusion. Therefore, each unit contains 500 mL at a 10-g/dL concentration, thereby delivering 50 g of hemoglobin. In addition, continued improvement in the process enabled the $P_{50}$ to be increased to 30 mm Hg. The characteristics of 1 unit of poly-SFH-P used for clinical trials

**Table 10–9.  Characteristics of poly-SFH-P for clinical trials**

- Hb = 10 g/dL
- $P_{50}$ = 30 mm Hg
- Met Hb < 3%
- Tetramer < 1%
- 1 unit = 500 mL (50 g)

From Anderson KC, ed, Transfusion Science. Exeter, UK, 1994, Elsevier Science Ltd., with permission.

are shown in Table 10–9. To date, the phase I clinical trials have included both healthy volunteers, stable patients, and patients being resuscitated from hemorrhagic shock after major trauma. The poly-SFH-P was successfully infused in doses up to the equivalent of a 1-unit transfusion of blood (50 g) in these recipients without the undesirable effects historically associated with hemoglobin solutions, including vasoconstriction, kidney dysfunction, or gastrointestinal distress. We have recently been approved to begin phase II trials in patients. The protocol will involve increasing the dose to 3 units (150 g) in patients suffering acute blood loss after major trauma and during major surgery. Although the work is still in progress, the preliminary results appear to confirm the safety and efficacy observations from the preclinical studies. The lack of observed toxicity to date suggests the proposed mechanisms of toxicity discussed earlier in this paper, as well as the attempts to prevent these by polymerization, appear to be accurate. Further clinical testing will be required to fully assess the ultimate clinical utility of poly-SFH-P.

## SUMMARY

Attempts to develop a hemoglobin-based RBC substitute have spanned many decades,[33,35] but no clinically useful product has been produced to date. The issues preventing clinical application primarily are ones of safety and not efficacy.[52] Numerous animal studies have documented the efficacy of SFH.[33,50] Although effective, the solution has limitations that have caused concern. Oncotic considerations limit the concentration of the infusate SFH to 6–8 g/dL, or half-normal. Owing to the loss of organic phosphate modulators of $P_{50}$, such as 2,3-DPG, the $P_{50}$ of SFH is typically between 12 and 14 mm Hg, which is also half the normal value. And finally, the intravascular half-life of SFH is too short, ranging only from 2 to 6 hours.[60]

Polymerization provides a means of correcting these limitations. The high $O_2$ affinity can be greatly diminished by covalent binding of pyridoxal-5′-phosphate to the N-terminal of the chains. COP exerted by a protein solution is proportional to the number of discrete colloid particles. Through polymerization, the number of colloid particles are reduced, leading to a decrease in COP. Data show this can be achieved in a reproducible fashion. The rate at which COP diminishes determines the yield of polymeric species, as well as their molecular weight distribution. Polymerization can be controlled to result in a yield of 75–85% polymers, with a molecular weight distribution of 128–400 kd.[44] The number average and the weight average molecular weights indicate that the large proportion of polymers represent the cross-linking of two tetramers.

The data that reflect the interaction of $O_2$ with poly-SFH-P indicate that the $O_2$-carrying function of hemoglobin has not been significantly altered by the chemical modifications. The binding coefficient of $O_2$ is unchanged. As anticipated, there is a loss of cooperativity (diminished Hill coefficient) between the hemoglobin chains, suggesting structural restrictions in the polymeric species because of cross-linking. A reduced alkaline Bohr effect is the expected result, and data confirm this.[44] Finally, some increase in $O_2$ affinity is to be expected with polymerization. This is indeed the case, although the $P_{50}$ of poly-SFH-P is comparable with banked blood (18–22 mm Hg).

To be clinically useful, a modified hemoglobin solution requires a reasonable shelf-life. Data demonstrate that polymerized hemoglobin can be stored in the cold (4–8°C) for several months with minimum change in the methemoglobin concentration. Furthermore, HPLC and viscosity data clearly indicate that no significant alterations in the polymeric species occur during storage.

## REFERENCES

1. Marshall RJ, Shepherd JT: Effect of injections of hypertonic solutions on blood flow through the femoral artery of the dog. Am J Physiol 1959; 97:951.
2. Templeton GH, Mitchell JH, Wildenthal K: Influence of hyperosmolarity on left ventricular stiffness. Am J Physiol 1972; 222:1406.
3. Wildenthal K, Mierzwiak DS, Mitchell JH: Acute effects of increased serum osmolality on left ventricular performance. Am J Physiol 1969; 216:898.
4. Kleeman CR: The kidney in health and disease. X. CNS manifestations of disordered salt and water balance. Hosp Pract 1979; 14:59.
5. Lucas CE, Ledgerwood AM, Mammen EF: Altered coagulation protein content after albumin resuscitation. Ann Surg 1982; 196:198.
6. Shoemaker MC, Schluchter M, Hopkins JA, et al.: Fluid therapy in emergency resuscitation: clinical evaluation of colloid and crystalloid regimens. Crit Care Med 1981; 9:367.
7. Skillman JJ, Restall DS, Salzman EW: Randomized trial of albumin vs. electrolyte solutions during abdominal aortic operations. Surgery 1975; 78:291.
8. Moore FD, Lyons JH, Pierce EC: Posttraumatic Pulmonary Insufficiency. Philadelphia, 1969, W.B. Saunders.
9. Rackow EC, Falk JL, Fein IA, et al.: Fluid resuscitation in circulatory shock: a comparison of the cardiorespiratory effects of albumin, hetastarch, and saline solutions in patients with hypovolemic and septic shock. Crit Care Med 1983; 11:839.
10. Hauser CJ, Shoemaker WC, Turpin I, et al.: Oxygen transport responses to colloids and crystalloids in critically ill surgical patients. Surg Gynecol Obstet 1980; 150:811.
11. Shires GT, Braun FT, Canizaro PC, et al.: Distributional changes in extracellular fluid during acute hemorrhagic shock. Surg Forum 1960; 11:115.
12. Virgilio RW, Rice CL, Smith DE, et al.: Crystalloid vs. colloid resuscitation: is one better? A Randomized clinical study. Surgery 1979; 85:129.
13. Lucas CE, Denis R, Ledgerwood AM, et al.: The effect of hespan on serum and lymphatic albumin, globulin and coagulant protein. Ann Surg 1988; 207:416.
14. Siegel DC, Moss GS, Cochin A: Pulmonary changes following treatment for hemorrhagic shock: saline versus colloid infusion. Surg Forum 1970; 21:17.
15. Lowe RJ, Moss GS, Jilek J, et al.: Crystalloid vs. colloid in the etiology of pulmonary failure after trauma: a randomized trial in man. Surgery 1977; 81:676.
16. Shoemaker WC, Hauser CJ: Critique of crystalloid vs. colloid therapy in shock and shock lung. Crit Care Med 1979; 7:117.
17. Moss GS, Lowe RJ, Jilek J, et al.: Colloid or crystalloid in the resuscitation of hemorrhagic shock: a controlled clinical trial. Surgery 1981; 89:434.
18. Velanovich V: Crystalloid versus colloid fluid resuscitation: a meta-analysis of mortality. Surgery 1989; 105:65.
19. Monafo WW, Halverson JD, Schechtman K: The role of concentrated sodium solutions in the resuscitation of patients with severe burns. Surgery 1984; 95:129.
20. Bowser-Wallace BH, Caldwell FT Jr: A prospective analysis of hypertonic lactated saline vs. Ringer's lactate-colloid for the resuscitation of severely burned children. Burns 1986; 12:402.
21. Bowser-Wallace BH, Cone JB, Caldwell FT Jr: Hypertonic lactated saline resuscitation of severely burned patients over 60 years of age. J Trauma 1985; 25:22.
22. Shackford SR, Sise MJ, Fridlund PH, et al.: Hypertonic sodium lactate versus lactated Ringer's solution

for intravenous fluid therapy in operations on the abdominal aorta. Surgery 1983; 94:41.

23. Holcroft JW, Vassar MJ, Blaisdell FW: 3% NaCl and 7.5% NaCl/dextran 70 in the resuscitation of severely injured patients. Ann Surg 1987; 206:279.

24. Biro GP, Blais P: Perfluorocarbon blood substitutes. Crit Rev Oncol Hematol 1987; 6:311.

25. Gould SA, Rosen AL, Sehgal LR, et al.: Clinical experience with Fluosol-DA. In: Bolin RB, Geyer RP, Nemo GJ, eds, Advances in Blood Substitute Research. New York, 1983, Alan R. Liss, p. 331.

26. Gould SA, Sehgal LR, Rosen AL, et al.: Red cell substitutes: an update. Ann Emerg Med 1985; 14:798.

27. Gould SA, Rosen AL, Sehgal LR, et al.: How good are fluorocarbon emulsions as $O_2$ carriers? Surg Forum 1981; 32:299.

28. Gould SA, Rosen AL, Sehgal LR, et al.: Red cell substitutes: hemoglobin solution or fluorocarbon? J Trauma 1982; 22:736.

29. Gould SA, Rosen AL, Sehgal, LR, et al.: Fluosol-DA as a red cell substitute in acute anemia. N Engl J Med 1986; 314:1653.

30. Clark LC Jr, Clark EW, Moore RE, et al.: Room temperature-stable biocompatible fluorocarbon emulsions. In: Bolin RB, Geyer RP, Nemo GJ, eds, Advances in Blood Substitute Research. New York, 1983, Alan R. Liss, p. 169.

31. Sloviter HA, Mukherji B: Prolonged retention in the circulation of emulsified lipid-coated perfluorochemicals. In: Bolin RB, Geyer RP, Nemo GJ, eds, Advances in Blood Substitute Research. New York, 1983, Alan R. Liss, p. 181.

32. Gould SA, Sehgal LR, Rosen AL, et al.: The development of polymerized pyridoxylated hemoglobin solution as a red cell substitute. Ann Emerg Med 1986; 15:1416.

33. Moss GS, DeWoskin R, Rosen AL, et al.: Transport of oxygen and carbon dioxide by hemoglobin-saline solution in the red cell-free primate. Surg Gynecol Obstet 1976; 142:357.

34. Moss GS, Gould SA, Sehgal LR, et al.: Hemoglobin solution from tetramer to polymer. Surgery 1984; 95:249.

35. Mulder AG, Amberson WR, Steggerda FR, et al.: Oxygen consumption with hemoglobin-ringer. J Cell Comp Physiol 1934; 5:383.

36. Riggs TE, Shafer AW, Guenter CA: Acute changes in oxyhemoglobin affinity. Effects on oxygen transport and utilization. J Clin Invest 1973; 52:2660.

37. Hau T, Simmons RL: Mechanisms of the adjuvant effect of hemoglobin in experimental peritonitis. III. The influence of hemoglobin on phagocytosis and intracellular killing by human granulocytes. Surgery 1980; 87:588.

38. Benesch RE, Benesch R, Renthal RD, et al.: Affinity labeling of the polyphosphate binding site of hemoglobin. Biochemistry 1972; 11:3576.

39. Greenberg AG, Hayashi R, Siefert I, et al.: Intravascular persistence and oxygen delivery of pyridoxylated, stroma-free hemoglobin during gradations of hypotension. Surgery 1979; 86:13.

40. Sehgal LR, Rosen AL, Noud G, et al.: Large volume preparation of pyridoxylated hemoglobin with high $P_{50}$. J Surg Res 1981; 30:14.

41. Gould SA, Rosen AL, Sehgal LR, et al.: The effect of altered hemoglobin-oxygen affinity on oxygen transport by hemoglobin solution. J Surg Res 1980; 28:246.

42. Gould SA, Sehgal LR, Rosen AL, et al.: Hemoglobin solution: is a normal [Hb] or $P_{50}$ more important? J Surg Res 1982; 33:189.

43. Sehgal LR, Rosen AL, Gould SA, et al.: An appraisal of polymerized pyridoxylated hemoglobin as an acellular oxygen carrier. In: Bolin RB, Geyer RP, eds, Blood Substitutes. New York, 1983, Alan R. Liss, pp. 19–28.

44. Sehgal LR, Rosen AL, Gould SA, et al.: Preparation of *in vitro* characteristics of polymerized pyridoxylated hemoglobin. Transfusion 1983; 23:148.

45. Sehgal LR, Rosen AL, Gould SA, et al.: Characteristics of polymerized pyridoxylated hemoglobin. Biomater Artif Cells Artif Organs 1988; 16:173.

46. Sehgal LR, et al.: *In vitro* and *in vivo* characteristics of polymerized pyridoxylated hemoglobin solutions. Fed Proc 1980; 38:718.

47. Sehgal HL, Sehgal LR, Rosen AL, et al.: Sensitivity of the IL-282 Co-oximeter to low hemoglobin concentrations and high proportions of methemoglobin. Clin Chem 1980; 26:362.

48. Sehgal HL, Sehgal LR, Rosen AL, et al.: Performance of the oxygen-hemoglobin dissociation analyzer (Hem-O-Scan) compared with the IL-282 Co-oximeter (Letter). Clin Chem 1980; 26:784.

49. Rosen AL, Gould SA, Sehgal LR, et al.: Evaluation of efficacy of stroma-free hemoglobin solutions. In: Bolin RB, Geyer RP, eds, Blood Substitutes. New York, 1983, Alan R. Liss, pp. 79–88.

50. Rosen AL, Gould SA, Sehgal LR, et al.: Effect of hemoglobin solution on compensation to anemia in the erythrocyte free primate. J Appl Physiol 1990; 68:938.

51. Hamilton PB, Hiller A, Van Slyke DD: Renal effects of hemoglobin infusions in dogs in hemorrhagic shock. J Exp Med 1948; 85:477.

52. Rabiner SF, Friedman LH: The role of intravascular hemolysis and the reticuloendothelial system in the production of a hypercoagulable state. Br J Haematol 1968; 14:105.

53. Rabiner SF, Helbert JR, Lopas H, et al.: Evaluation of a stroma-free hemoglobin solution for use as a plasma expander. J Exp Med 1967; 126:1127.

54. Birndorf NI, Lopas H: Effects of red cell stroma-free hemoglobin solution on renal function in monkeys. J Appl Physiol 1970; 29:573.

55. Savitsky JP, Doczi J, Black J, et al.: A clinical safety trial of stroma-free hemoglobin. Clin Pharmacol Ther 1978; 23:73.

56. Moss GS, Gould SA, Rosen AL, et al.: Animal model for nephrotoxicity of haemoglobin tetramer (Letter). Lancet 1986; 1:1219.

57. Hoyt DB, Greenberg AG, Peskin CW, et al.: Resuscitation with pyridoxylated stroma free hemoglobin: tolerance to sepsis. J Trauma 1981; 21:938.

58. Litwin MD, Walter CW, Ejarque P, et al.: Synergistic toxicity of Gram-negative bacteria and free colloidal hemoglobin. Ann Surg 1963; 157:485.

59. Stein PM, Saba TM: Cardiovascular response to hemorrhage in the dog as modified by colloid induced opsonic deficiency and reticuloendothelial blockade. Fed Proc 1979; 38:1115.

60. DeVenuto F, Friedman H, Neville JR, et al.: Appraisal of hemoglobin solution as a blood substitute. Surg Gynecol Obstet 1979; 149:417.

# 11

# BLOOD CONSERVATION IN JEHOVAH'S WITNESSES

## David J. Lang and M. Ramez Salem

## INTRODUCTION

The Jehovah's Witness (JW) surgical patient presents the surgeon and anesthesiologist with special ethical, legal, and medical considerations that arise from the Witnesses' refusal of blood transfusion.

The JWs are a fundamentalist Christian sect that believes in the literal interpretation of the Bible. They are descendants of a Bible study group led by Charles Taze Russell in Pennsylvania in the late 1870s. Originally known as "Russellism" or "Millenial Darwinism," by 1931 the group became known as the JWs. The name is adopted from a verse in Isaiah (43:10) "Ye are my witnesses saith the Lord [Jehovah], and my servant whom I have chosen." Although this verse does not make a distinction between Jew and non-Jew, the JWs accept Jesus as the ultimate JW of their faith:

Wherefore, seeing we also are compassed about with so great a cloud of witnesses, let us lay aside every weight, and the sin which do so easily beset us, and let us run with patience the race that is set before us, looking unto Jesus the author and finisher of our faith. (Hebrews 12:1,2)

The JWs' refusal of blood transfusions is based on strict interpretation of several verses of the Old and New Testaments and was formalized in July 1945 after discussion in the group's journal *Watch Tower*. The first referral to this "blood guilt" appeared in the *Watch Tower* on December 15, 1927, but the point was made clear in 1945 that taking blood into the body would result in the loss of eternal life.

Although eating blood and receiving a transfusion of blood or blood products might seem to be totally different, the JW will point out that it is not the route that is the issue, but the blood itself.[1,2]

A later publication, *Jehovah's Witnesses and the Question of Blood*, published in 1977 before the acquired immunodeficiency syndrome epidemic, highlighted transmission of disease as a risk of blood transfusion but stressed that the JW objection to transfusion is rooted in the Bible, that is, the objection is religious and not medical.

Everything that lives and moves will be food for you . . . . But you must not eat meat that has its lifeblood still in it. (Genesis 9:3,4)

If anyone of the House of Israel or of the strangers who reside among them partake of any blood, I will set my face against the person who partakes of the blood, and I will cut him off from among his kin. For the life of the flesh is in the blood. (Leviticus 17:10,11)

. . . for it seemed to the Holy Ghost, and to us, to lay upon you no greater burden than these necessary things; that ye abstain from meats offered to idols, and from blood, and from things strangled, and from fornication; from which if ye keep yourselves ye shall do well. (Acts 15:19–21)

Unlike members of the Christian Scientist faith, JWs actively seek medical help but refuse transfusion of blood or blood products, believing these will jeopardize their soul on earth and their obtaining eternal life after death.

In general, JWs believe the use of blood

327

components, for example, white blood cells, albumin, platelets, or plasma, is the same as the use of blood. However, in a study of a JW congregation in Colorado, 12% of the members would consider accepting plasma as an alternative to blood transfusion.[3] Most JWs also consider autologous transfusion to be unacceptable because, even though it is their own blood, it has not been kept in continuity with the circulation and hence should be "poured out on the ground as water" to show that it was for God and not humans to sustain the life of some earthly creature.[1]

Individual JWs make their own decisions based on their interpretation of biblical teachings (in consultation with family and church elders) that leave them with a clear conscience before God.[3,4]

Extracorporeal circulation and hemodialysis are readily accepted by JWs provided the machines are not primed with blood. Blood salvage and normovolemic hemodilution devices are viewed as extensions of the circulatory system and are acceptable provided there is continuity between the collection site and the reinfusion port.[5–7]

Bearb and Pennant[8] reported on a JW accepting an epidural blood patch for a postlumbar puncture headache. They used extension tubes and a series of stopcocks to inject 20 mL of the patient's blood into the epidural space without interrupting continuity between the intravenous line and the epidural needle.

Vaccines that are made with the use of recombinant DNA are acceptable to JWs. The choice of accepting a serum-derived vaccine is left to the individual.[1] Decisions regarding human tissue donation and transplantation (other than bone marrow) have also been left to individual members.[9] JWs believe the cells of a transplanted organ are replaced by the patient's own cells; therefore, organ transplantation is acceptable.[2]

## ETHICAL CONSIDERATIONS

There are varying degrees of strictness among JWs in adhering to the proscription against blood and blood products. Some may accept transfusion in a last-ditch attempt to save their lives; many others would rather die than receive a transfusion. Many JWs will accept biological tissues, including transplanted organs and homograft heart valves.

In the past, patients whose religious beliefs preclude blood transfusion have been denied major surgery. Many physicians believe that undertaking major surgical procedures without the option of transfusion poses an unacceptable risk to the patient, unreasonably circumscribes the quality of care that can be given by the surgical team, and poses an ethical dilemma.[10] From the physician's viewpoint, being obliged to let a patient die for want of transfusion is against the Hippocratic Oath and is considered by many to be substandard and/or unethical care. This conflict (respecting the patient's wishes even if it means letting the patient die) is even greater when the patient is a minor and the directive comes from the parents.

There have been numerous situations in which physicians and hospitals have turned to the courts in an attempt to force a JW patient to receive a transfusion. The central issues of this ethical conflict are the patient's right of religious freedom and the physician's right to practice medicine according to accepted standards.[11] In cases involving a competent adult JW without minor dependents, the courts have generally upheld their right to refuse blood or blood product transfusions. In contrast, incompetent adults, adults with dependent minors, and pregnant patients have often been given blood by court order when the courts were petitioned by hospitals and physicians. Similarly, critically ill children have been transfused by court order. There is presently no statutory law to provide guidance in these situations, and case law is continuing to evolve.

When caring for a JW, it is imperative to discuss beforehand with the patient, if at all possible, the planned management of the case [i.e., measures to increase preoperative red blood cell (RBC) mass and decrease intraoperative blood loss, e.g., hypothermia, deliberate hypotension, vasoconstrictors, hemodilution, hemostatic drugs, and blood salvage techniques] as well as potential complications and whether the patient will accept blood or blood products in a life-threatening situation. The fact that the discussion took place, what was discussed, and the patient's expressed wishes as to how to proceed in a life-threatening situation need to be documented fully in the chart and signed by the patient (in the case of a competent adult) and the patient's family. A special consent form releasing the hospital and physician from liability for withholding blood and blood products should also be signed by the physician, the patient, and the patient's family and placed in the chart. The plan regarding transfusion must be made clear before surgery to the surgeons, anesthesiologists, and nurses. If any doubt exists, the hospital's legal counsel (and perhaps ethicist or ethics committee) should be consulted preoperatively.

## LEGAL CONSIDERATIONS

Despite their attempts to understand the religious convictions of the JW patient, the physician's and hospital's concerns to save a life (and for their liability in the event of a death) have caused those involved to seek guidance from the courts. Many middle-of-the-night petitions for conservatorship have been filed in an attempt to force a nonconsenting patient to receive a transfusion.[2]

Because it relates to the First Amendment right of freedom of religion, the courts have not been wholly consistent in their rulings. The patient's right to refuse blood is not absolute; this must be balanced against the state's interests. These interests have been cited in a number of court decisions and include preserving life; protecting the interest of third parties, for example, minors and/or other dependents; preventing suicide; and maintaining the ethical integrity of the medical profession. A court decision overruling a JW patient's refusal of blood or blood products based on the state's interest has been cited only in emergency cases or when the patient is incompetent, pregnant, or a minor. Case law regarding transfusion for the JW patient has been reviewed by Rothenberg in 1990[2]; the reader who desires a greater discussion of case law is referred to this article.

## PREOPERATIVE PREPARATION

Patients whose religious beliefs preclude acceptance of blood transfusion should not be denied the potential benefits of major surgical procedures. Management of these patients has contributed to our knowledge of the physiology of isovolemic hemodilution. Furthermore, the old dictum that a hemoglobin (HGB) level of 10 g/dL is necessary for optimal perioperative management of surgical patients cannot be justified (see Chapter 5: Perioperative Hemoglobin Requirements). Despite the contribution of severe anemia to the mortality of JW patients undergoing major surgical procedure, it must be emphasized that the vast majority of patients survive. With proper preoperative planning, adequate preparation, and skilled anesthesia and surgical management as well as vigilant postoperative care, major surgical procedures can be successfully undertaken in JW patients.

Preoperative assessment and preparation do not differ markedly from other patients; however, extra attention is paid to HGB levels, coagulation profile, and the anticipated blood loss. Any treatable conditions resulting in decreased HGB or altered hemostasis must be identified and treated. The use of blood conservation measures to minimize perioperative blood loss must be discussed with the patient and documented in the chart. Whenever possible, these measures must be thought of and implemented weeks or even months before surgery. A hematology consultation may be indicated if there is a history suggestive of coagulopathy or anemia of unknown etiology. When these patients who refuse blood transfusion do undergo major surgery, they can be expected to have a prolonged convalescence after major blood loss.

A normal to high preoperative HGB to compensate for operative blood loss and enhance recovery is desirable in these patients.[12] Hemograms may be repeated to ensure accuracy. If a substantial blood loss is anticipated, a low preoperative HGB level is an indication to postpone nonurgent surgery until it can be increased.

Iron therapy (oral or intravenous) alone or in combination with recombinant human erythropoietin has been used to raise preoperative HGB. If the patient does not have a chronic disease that blunts the response to iron therapy, iron therapy alone can be expected to raise HGB levels by 50% toward normal in 3 weeks.[13] A recent study[14] that compared iron alone to iron plus erythropoietin in postpartum anemia showed that the addition of erythropoietin resulted in a more rapid and steeper increase in HGB. Case histories[12] showed that within a relatively short time the combination of iron and erythropoietin raises the HGB level high enough to compensate for perioperative blood loss. The dosage for erythropoietin is 150 units/kg subcutaneously three times a week, and for ferrous sulfate 300 mg, orally three times daily for up to 10 weeks (but should be started at least 4 weeks before the planned surgery). If the patient is unable to tolerate oral iron, iron dextran injection can be used. The total iron required equals[15]

$$Fe = 0.66 \times BW \times \left(100 - \frac{HGB \times 100}{14.8}\right)$$

where Fe is the iron required in mg, BW is the body weight in kg, and HGB is the patient hemoglobin.

Recombinant human erythropoietin is supplied in buffered saline containing human albumin,[16] which falls into a grey zone of acceptability; some JW patients will accept albumin, whereas others will not. Only transfusions of whole blood, RBCs, white cells, platelets, and plasma are specifically prohibited.[17] Until a new formulation of recombinant human erythropoietin without albumin is available, this issue must be discussed with the patient before starting this course of action.

Medications that affect platelet function (see Chapter 2: Coagulation and Hemostasis) should be discontinued at least 1 week before elective surgery. Anticoagulants should also be discontinued unless their continued use is essential, as in patients with a history of emboli from prosthetic heart valves or deep venous thrombosis. If continued anticoagulation is necessary, long-acting anticoagulants may be replaced by intravenous heparin that can be stopped before surgery and then restarted 12 hours after surgery.

Diagnostic procedures requiring frequent blood sampling, such as cardiac catheterization, may be performed during a separate admission to allow time for restoration of normal to high HGB levels before surgery.[10] The amount of blood drawn for laboratory tests should be minimized; microchemistry instruments can be used with minimal effects on accuracy.[18]

Perioperative blood conservation measures (Table 11–1) must be discussed with the patient and explained in detail. The Watchtower Bible and Tract Society of New York, Inc. publishes and distributes to its membership a document entitled *Strategies for Avoiding and*

*Controlling Hemorrhage and Anemia Without Blood Transfusion.* Patients may bring this document with them when meeting with their anesthesiologist or surgeon. The physician must be prepared to discuss the various strategies outlined in this tract with the patient and which ones will be applicable to the planned surgery. Measures such as tourniquets, infiltration with vasoconstrictors, and deliberate hypotension aiming at reducing blood loss are readily acceptable to JW patients. It has been the authors' experience, as well as others, that deliberate hypotension as the sole blood conservation measure in certain procedures, such as hip replacement, has been effective in reducing blood loss to a minimum in JW patients.[19,20] Obviously, preoperative blood donation is not acceptable to JW patients because the blood is removed from the body[17] (see Chapter 6: Preoperative Autologous Blood Donation). However, they may accept acute normovolemic or hypervolemic hemodilution if the blood that is removed from the patient remains in uninterrupted contact with the patient's circulation (Fig. 11–1). In patients undergoing procedures where substantial blood loss is anticipated, hemodilution to a hematocrit (HCT) less than 20% may be acceptable. Additionally, hemodilution can be combined with hypotension or with hypotension and hypothermia to further reduce blood loss (see Chapter 7: Acute Normovolemic Hemodilution). Coagulopathy usually does not occur during acute normovolemic hemodilution if the HCT is kept above 20%; if coagulopathy does occur with extreme hemodilution, which may be necessary in some patients, the administration of a diuretic will usually cause a rise in the HCT and improved hemostasis.

Blood salvage techniques are acceptable to the JW patient undergoing cardiopulmonary bypass (CPB) as long as the blood in the extracorporeal circuit remains in constant contact with the patient's own circulation. It has been the authors' experience that most JW patients do not accept blood salvage techniques in noncardiac procedures such as orthopedic surgery. Diagrams need to be drawn to explain in detail the use of blood salvage techniques to JW patients to assure them that these techniques conform to their religious beliefs (Fig. 11–2) (see Chapter 9: Blood Salvage Techniques).

**Table 11–1.  Alternative strategies for avoiding and controlling hemorrhage and anemia without blood transfusion**

I. SURGICAL DEVICES AND TECHNIQUES TO LOCATE AND ARREST INTERNAL BLEEDING:
   A. Electrocautery
   B. Laser surgery
   C. Argon beam coagulator
   D. Gamma knife radiosurgery
   E. Microwave coagulating scalpel
   F. Shaw hemostatic scalpel
   G. Endoscope
   H. Arterial embolization
   I. Tissue adhesives
II. TECHNIQUES AND DEVICES TO CONTROL EXTERNAL BLEEDING AND SHOCK:
   A. For bleeding:
      1. Direct pressure
      2. Ice packs
      3. Elevate body part above level of heart
      4. Hemostatic agents (see Section VI)
      5. Prompt surgery
      6. Tourniquet
   B. For shock:
      1. Trendelenburg/shock position (patient supine with head lower than legs)
      2. Medical Antishock Trousers (M.A.S.T.)
      3. Appropriate volume replacement after bleeding controlled
III. OPERATIVE AND ANESTHETIC TECHNIQUES TO LIMIT BLOOD LOSS DURING SURGERY:
   A. Hypotensive anesthesia
   B. Induced hypothermia
   C. Intraoperative hemodilution
   D. Hypervolemic hemodilution
   E. Intraoperative blood salvage
   F. Mechanical occlusion of bleeding vessels
   G. Reduce blood flow to skin
   H. Meticulous hemostasis
   I. Preoperative planning
      1. Enlarged surgical team/Minimal time
      2. Surgical positioning
      3. Staging of complex procedures
IV. BLOOD-OXYGEN MONITORING DEVICES AND TECHNIQUES THAT LIMIT BLOOD SAMPLING:
   A. Transcutaneous pulse oximeter
   B. Pulse oximeter
   C. Pediatric microsampling equipment
   D. Multiple tests per sample
V. VOLUME EXPANDERS:
   A. Crystalloids:
      1. Ringer's lactate
      2. Normal saline
      3. Hypertonic saline
   B. Colloids:
      1. Dextran
      2. Gelatin
      3. Hetastarch
   C. Perfluorochemical:
      1. Fluosol-DA-20

**Table 11–1.**   *(continued)*

VI. HEMOSTATIC AGENTS FOR BLEEDING/CLOTTING PROBLEMS:
   A. Topical:
      1. Avitene
      2. Gelfoam
      3. Oxycel
      4. Surgicel
      5. Many others
   B. Injectable:
      1. Desmopressin
      2. $\epsilon$-Aminocaproic acid
      3. Tranexamic acid
      4. Vitamin K
   C. Other drugs:
      1. Vasopressin
      2. Conjugated estrogens
      3. Aprotinin
      4. Vincristine
VII. THERAPEUTIC AGENTS AND TECHNIQUES FOR MANAGING ANEMIA:
   A. Stop any bleeding
   B. Oxygen support
   C. Maintain intravascular volume
   D. Iron Dextran (Imferon)
   E. Folic acid
   F. Vitamin $B_{12}$
   G. Erythropoietin
   H. Nutritional support
   I. Immunosuppressive agents if indicated
   J. Perfluorocarbon solutions (FL-DL)
   K. Granulocyte-colony stimulating factor
   L. Hyperbaric oxygen therapy
   M. 10/30 rule for minimum RBC level has no scientific basis

This table appears in the publication Family Care and Medical Management for Jehovah's Witnesses, published by Watchtower Bible and Tract Society[37] and is distributed to their members. Patients may show this document to their physician who must be prepared to discuss the applicability of various measures to the planned surgery. Printed with permission.

In certain operations, a transient state of hypervolemia may be needed such as before the removal of the aortic cross-clamp during aortic procedures. This is easily accomplished using crystalloids or colloids. This transient hypervolemic hemodilution may help to reduce the amount of RBC mass lost in shed blood. Use of certain colloids, such as hydroxyethyl starch and low molecular weight dextrans, must be limited because large volumes (>1.5 mL/kg for hydroxyethyl starch) may result in a coagulopathy[21] (see Chapter 2: Coagulation and Hemostasis).

In small children undergoing CPB, the minimum volume of crystalloid needed to prime the oxygenator may exceed the child's blood volume and result in severe hemodilution (HCT < 20%). The risk is less in polycythemic and older children. Definitive procedures requiring CPB in small JW children are better postponed if possible and a palliative procedure performed instead. When the definitive procedure cannot be postponed, the risk that the minimum safe priming volume in the oxygenator might produce anemia severe enough to cause insufficient oxygen delivery must be accepted.[10,22] Henling and associates[22] reported on 110 JW children undergoing a variety of open heart procedures. In children weighing less than 10 kg, HGB levels during CPB averaged 4.5 g/dL. None of these patients developed lactic acidosis or inadequate cerebral perfusion as evidenced by electroencephalographic monitoring. Although two of these children died postoperatively, these deaths were attributed to myocardial failure and not to anemia.[10,22] After the termination of CPB in JW children, the volume remaining in the bypass circuit is slowly reinfused through the aortic cannula. If the

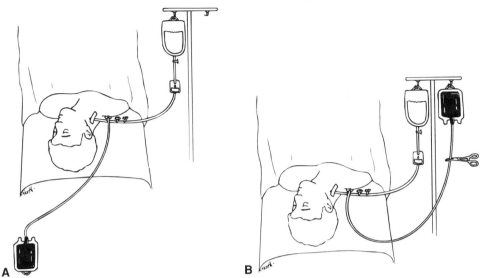

**Fig. 11–1.** *A:* Arrangement used to harvest blood from a Jehovah's Witness before cardiopulmonary bypass. A 3-stopcock manifold is placed on the sidearm of the percutaneous introducer for the pulmonary artery catheter. A blood collection bag containing CPD solution is connected to one of the stopcocks, lowered below the level of the heart, and allowed to fill. *B:* Once the bag is filled, it is hung on an intravenous pole and the tubing from the bag to the patient partially occluded with a surgical clamp so the blood is reinfused extremely slowly. This way the blood in the bag is kept in continuity with the circulatory system, and the patient's concerns about removing the blood from the body are satisfactorily addressed.

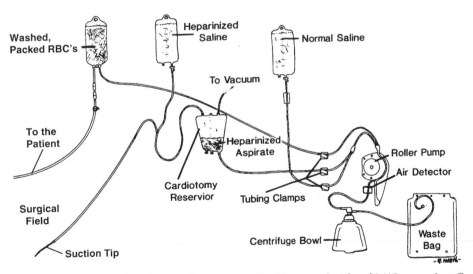

**Fig. 11–2.**   Schematic diagram of a cell-processing system modified for use in the Jehovah's Witness patient. Continuous reinfusion of blood from the blood collection bag ensures that salvaged blood remains in an unbroken circuit with the patient's own circulation. Modified from Salem MR, Bikhazi G: Blood Conservation. In: Motoyama EK: Davis PJ, eds, Smith's Anesthesia for Infants and Children. St. Louis, 1990, C. V. Mosby.[38]

heart cannot tolerate this volume without overdistension, then diuresis, which is usually brisk because of the glucose load in the prime, is increased with furosemide.[10]

The surgeon's role in minimizing perioperative blood loss cannot be underestimated. The surgeon should use the approach most comfortable for him or her, incorporating Halstedian principles of meticulous dissection and gentle handling of tissues.[23] Prolonged bypass time must be avoided as much as possible to avoid post-CPB coagulopathies. Alterations in platelet function worsen as bypass time lengthens.[24]

## POSTOPERATIVE MANAGEMENT

Infusion of crystalloids is continued postoperatively to maintain adequate circulatory volume, filling pressures, and urine output. Scavenging of shed mediastinal blood and re-infusion are accepted by some JW patients if given in a closed circuit. However, this method has the disadvantage of infusing activated procoagulant factors that may lead to disseminated intravascular coagulation.[25]

Persistent hemodilution in the postoperative period may be associated with lower arterial pressure due to decreased systemic vascular resistance. Lower blood pressure postoperatively may not require treatment as long as cardiac output is adequate, as evidenced by warm dry skin, adequate urine output, absence of metabolic acidosis, and normal mentation.

Sometimes, despite intraoperative blood conservation measures, the patient will still end up with a low postoperative HGB. Levels as low as 1.4 g/dL have been reported, with the patient surviving intact, although with a prolonged recovery.[26] Perfusion and oxygenation must be evaluated and steps taken, as needed, to optimize each one. A pulmonary artery catheter can be used to evaluate left ventricular end-diastolic pressures, with volume resuscitation guided by these readings. A pulmonary artery catheter capable of monitoring mixed venous oxygen saturations ($S\bar{v}O_2$) can be used to follow the adequacy of oxygen transport and delivery. If the $S\bar{v}O_2$ is low, steps to maximize oxygen delivery and minimize consumption can be initiated. There is, in actuality, little that can be done to increase oxygen delivery without a blood transfusion. On a theoretical basis, hyperbaric oxygen, by increasing dissolved oxygen, will improve oxygen delivery, but there are no reported cases of hyperbaric oxygen being used for this indication. Additional measures to minimize oxygen consumption include keeping the patient intubated, sedated, pharmacologically paralyzed, and mechanically ventilated.[27] Simultaneously, supportive treatment to aid the patient in restoring their RBC mass, for example, iron supplementation, erythropoietin, and enteral or parenteral nutrition, is started.

Although controversial, the prophylactic use of desmopressin acetate 0.3 $\mu$g/kg intravenously has been accepted as a current standard for postoperative care of JW patients.[10] The drug is given slowly either in the operating room or immediately after arrival in the intensive care unit. It has been reported by some to reduce postoperative bleeding after cardiac surgery[28] and by others to be of no benefit[29] (see Chapter 2: Coagulation and Hemostasis).

Also controversial is the prophylactic use of antifibrinolytic agents such as $\epsilon$-aminocaproic acid, tranexamic acid, and aprotinin in JW patients undergoing open heart surgery where fibrinolytic substances are released during sternotomy, pericardiotomy, and while on CPB. $\epsilon$-Aminocaproic acid and tranexamic acid have each been reported to have either beneficial effects[30,31] or no effects[24] on hemostasis after cardiac surgery as evidenced by chest tube drainage and by postoperative requirement for transfusion. Aprotinin, in addition to preventing hyperfibrinolysis during cardiac surgery,[32] also appears to have a protective effect on platelets,[33] preserving both numbers and function.

Dipyridamole is another drug that has been reported to preserve platelet numbers and function after cardiopulmonary bypass. Given intravenously or orally in the perioperative period, dipyridamole preserves platelet adhesion while inhibiting activation, aggregation, and degranulation; thus, it does not interfere with the platelet's hemostatic function.[34]

Mediastinal drainage in excess of 400 mL during the first postoperative hour in a JW patient is an indication for reexploration. If reexploration is delayed, severe life-threatening anemia or excessive bleeding due to coagulopathy may ensue. The seriousness of the situation should be discussed with the family, and a decision that represents the patient's wishes regarding transfusion of blood and/or blood products should be made and documented in the patient's chart. In the case of minor children, even if both parents are participating in the decision to transfuse or not, only one parent needs to consent to transfusion for it to be carried out.[10] Some centers have gained wide experience in the management of JW patients. Two reports from the Texas Heart Institute described their results in adult and pediatric cardiovascular and noncardiovascular procedures.[22,35] Procedures performed on 1105 JW patients between 1963 and 1989 included coronary artery bypass grafting (31.7%), valve repair (32.6%), repair of congenital heart disease (18.8%), vascular operations (4.4%), and noncardiovascular procedures (9.4%).[10] They reported an overall mortality rate of approximately 2.9%. Factors that were associated with mortality included reoperation, use of the internal mammary artery (or arteries) for coronary artery bypass grafting, left ventricular dysfunction (ejection fraction < 35%), and anemia. These results suggest that cardiac operations associated with increased blood loss, for example, reoperation procedures and use of the internal mammary artery, carry a higher mortality for JW patients.[10] The average HGB for nonsurvivors was 5.6 g/dL at the time of death, compared with 9.2 g/dL in survivors at the time they left the hospital. Carson and associates[36] found a higher mortality rate in 125 JWs undergoing surgery when their HGB was less than 8 g/dL before operation or when blood loss exceeded 2000 mL.

## SUMMARY

The JW patient should not be denied the potential benefits of major surgery because of refusal to accept transfusions of blood and blood products. With proper planning, beginning as early as possible and involving the patient and the surgical and anesthesia teams, the patient's RBC mass can be maximized preoperatively and perioperative blood loss minimized while simultaneously observing the patient's religious beliefs.

### REFERENCES

1. Watch Tower Bible and Tract Society: Appreciating the sacredness of life and blood. The Watchtower 1978; June 15:16.
2. Rothenberg DM: The approach to the Jehovah's Witness patient. Anesthesiol Clin North Am 1990; 8:589.
3. Findley LJ, Redstone PM: Blood transfusion in adult Jehovah's Witnesses: a case study of one congregation. Arch Intern Med 1982; 142:606.
4. Schechter DC: Problems relevant to major surgical operations in Jehovah's Witnesses. Am J Surg 1968; 116:73.
5. Laver MB, Bland JHL: Anesthetic management of the pediatric patient during open-heart surgery. Int Anesthesiol Clin 1975; 13:179.
6. Lichtiger B, Dupuis JF, Secki J: Hemotherapy during surgery for Jehovah's Witnesses: a new method. Anesth Analg 1982; 61:618.
7. Schaller RT, Schaller J, Morgan A, et al: Hemodilution anesthesia: a valuable aid to major cancer surgery in children. Am J Surg 1983; 146:79.
8. Bearb ME, Pennant JH: Epidural blood patch in Jehovah's Witness. Anesth Analg 1987; 66:1052.
9. Cleveland SE: Jehovah's Witnesses and human tissue donation. J Clin Psychol 1976; 32:453.
10. Cooper JR: Perioperative considerations in Jehovah's Witnesses. Int Anesthesiol Clin 1990: 28:210.
11. Tierney WM, Weinberger M, Greene JY, et al: Jehovah's Witnesses and blood transfusion: physicians attitudes and legal precedents. South Med J 1984; 77:473.
12. Green D, Handley E: Erythropoietin for anemia in Jehovah's Witnesses. Ann Intern Med 1990; 113:720.
13. Wintrobe MM, Lee GR, Boggs DR, et al: Clinical Hematology. Philadelphia, 1981, Lea & Febiger.
14. Danko J, Huch R, Huch A: Epoietin alfa for treatment of postpartum anaemia (Letter). Lancet 1990; 1:737.
15. American Medical Association: Hematinic agents and hematopoietic growth factors. In: Drug Evaluation Annual. Milwaukee, 1991, American Medical Association.
16. Hillman RS: Hematopoietic agents: growth factors, minerals, and vitamins. In: Gilman AG, ed, Goodman and Gilman's The Pharmacological Basis for Therapeutics, 8 ed. New York, 1990, Pergamon Press.
17. Watch Tower Bible and Tract Society of Pennsylvania: How can blood save your life? New York, 1990, Watch Tower Bible and Tract Society of New York.
18. Salem M, Chernow B, Burke R, et al: Bedside diagnostic blood testing. JAMA 1991; 266:382.
19. Fahmy NR: Techniques for deliberate hypotension: haemodilution and hypotension. In: Enderby GEH, ed, Hypotensive Anaesthesia. London, 1985, Churchill-Livingstone.
20. Nelson CL, Bowen WJ: Total hip arthroplasty in Jehovah's Witnesses without blood transfusions. J Bone Joint Surg [Am] 1986; 68A:350.
21. Lockwood DNJ, Bullen C, Machin SJ: A severe coagulopathy following volume replacement with hydroxyethyl starch in a Jehovah's Witness. Anaesthesia 1988; 43:391.
22. Henling CE, Carmichael MJ, Keats AS, et al: Cardiac operations for congenital heart disease in children of Jehovah's Witnesses. J Thorac Cardiovasc Surg 1985; 89:914.
23. Spence RK, Alexander JB, DelRossi AJ, et al: Transfusion guidelines for cardiovascular surgery: lessons

learned from operations in Jehovah's Witnesses. J Vasc Surg 1992; 16:825.

24. Woodman RC, Harker LA: Bleeding complications associated with cardiopulmonary bypass. Blood 1990; 76:1680.

25. Marrowitz MJ, Mannen EF, Brown M: Autotransfusion of mediastinal shed blood: hematologic effects (Abstract). Anesth Analg 1990: 70:S257.

26. Brimacomb J, Skippen P, Talbutt, T: Acute anaemia to a haemoglobin of 14 gl$^{-1}$. Anaesthesia Intensive Care 1991; 19:581.

27. Nussbaum W, deCastro N: Perioperative challenges in the care of the Jehovah's Witness: a case report. JAANA 1994; 62:160.

28. Salzman EW, Weinstein MJ, Weintraub RM, et al: Treatment with desmopressin acetate to reduce blood loss after cardiac surgery. N Engl J Med 1986; 314:1402

29. Hackmann T, Gascoyne RD, Naiman SC, et al: A trial of desmopressin (1-deamino-8-D-arginine vasopressin) to reduce blood loss in uncomplicated cardiac surgery. N Engl J Med 1989; 321:1437.

30. Lambert CJ, Marengo-Rowe AJ, Leveson JE, et al: The treatment of postperfusion bleeding using $\epsilon$-aminocaproic acid, cryoprecipitate, fresh-frozen plasma, and protamine sulfate. Ann Thorac Surg 1979; 28:440.

31. DelRossi AJ, Cernaianu AC, Botros S, et al: Prophylactic treatment of postperfusion bleeding using EACA. Chest 1989; 96:27.

32. Havel M, Teufelsbauer H, Knöbl P, et al: Effect of intraoperative aprotinin administration on postoperative bleeding in patients undergoing cardiopulmonary bypass operation. J Thorac Cardiovasc Surg 1991; 101:968.

33. Blauhut B, Gross C, Necek S, et al: Effects of high-dose aprotinin on blood loss, platelet function, fibrinolysis, complement, and renal function after cardiopulmonary bypass. J Thorac Cardiovasc Surg 1991; 101:958.

34. Teoh KH, Christakis GT, Weisel RD, et al: Dipyridamole preserved platelets and reduced blood loss after cardiopulmonary bypass. J Thorac Cardiovasc Surg 1988; 96:332.

35. Ott DA, Cooley DA: Cardiovascular surgery in Jehovah's Witnesses. JAMA 1977; 238:1256.

36. Carson JL, Posea RM, Spence RK, et al: Severity of anaemia and operative mortality and morbidity. Lancet 1988; 1:727.

37. Hospital Liaison Committee for Jehovah's Witnesses: Strategies for avoiding and controlling hemorrhage and anemia without blood transfusion. In: Family Care and Medical Management for Jehovah's Witnesses. New York, 1992, Watchtower Bible and Tract Society.

38. Salem MR, Bikhazi G: Blood Conservation. In: Motoyama EK, Davis PJ, eds, Smith's Anesthesia for Infants and Children. St. Louis, 1990, C. V. Mosby.

# 12

# BLOOD CONSERVATION IN SPECIAL SITUATIONS—ANESTHESIOLOGISTS' VIEWPOINTS

## OBSTETRICS AND GYNECOLOGY

### *Harold J. Heyman*

Blood conservation techniques in obstetrics include preoperative autologous blood donation and the recently introduced experimental technique of blood salvage with a cell processor device during cases of major obstetrical hemorrhage. The number of parturients requiring allogeneic transfusion is low, and the type and screen has replaced the routine type and cross-match order for the usual cesarean section. Because of the low transfusion rate, acute normovolemic hemodilution is not performed at cesarean section.

Preoperative autologous blood donation is the only blood conservation technique in obstetrics that has undergone extensive clinical trials. However, it is still a controversial technique, because the number of parturients requiring allogeneic transfusion remains low and difficult to predict in advance.

Although several studies have demonstrated that autologous blood donation is safe for both the parturient and fetus,[1] the Committee on Obstetrics: Maternal and Fetal Medicine of the American College of Obstetricians and Gynecologists stated in May 1987 that data in pregnant patients were insufficient to allow endorsement of autologous blood storage. Concern exists that a phlebotomy may be blamed for any adverse outcome, such as spontaneous abortion, premature labor, or birth defects.[2]

When fetal monitoring of pregnant women donating blood (100 women donating 139 units) was studied,[3-6] all adverse effects (uterine contractions, fetal bradycardia, and hypotension) occurred during the third trimester. Other studies of small series have shown uneventful donations by patients during all trimesters of pregnancy.[7-10]

Herbert and associates[6] performed preoperative autologous blood donation in obstetrics by performing a total of 55 phlebotomies in 30 pregnant patients at a significant risk for transfusion. Average gestational age was 32.4 weeks. Ultimately, 15 patients from this group received 29 units of packed red blood cells (RBCs); this consisted of 23 autologous and 6 allogeneic units. The authors concluded that allogeneic transfusion was avoided in 86.7% of patients receiving blood and that preoperative autologous blood donation was safe and useful in pregnancy. The authors did not state the total number of deliveries in their series, what percentage of all deliveries constituted patients at significant risk for transfusion, or the percentage of patients who required transfusion.

McVay and associates[11] retrospectively identified 268 third-trimester patients who participated in a preoperative autologous blood program and donated 341 units. Most predelivery donations were for anticipated repeat cesarean section. Only 3% had significant blood loss at delivery. The major cause of large blood loss in parturients was placenta previa. The percentage of patients with significant hemorrhage and need for transfusion was not stated. They required a minimum hemoglobin and hematocrit of 11 g/dL and 34%, respectively, with donations every 5–7 days. Donations were begun 4 weeks before the estimated date of confinement and ended 2 weeks before. This would make the average donation 1–2 units before surgery (see Chapter 6: Preoperative Autologous Blood Donation).

Andres and coworkers[12] prospectively studied 2265 deliveries over a 6-month period. Of these, 13 (0.57%) required transfusion. Traditionally accepted risk factors were identified in 251 patients, with only 4 out of this group requiring transfusion. Of 150 repeat cesarean sections, only 1 (0.7%) required transfusion. They concluded that preoperative autologous blood donation is not needed because of the low frequency of blood transfusion in a high-risk population and the difficulty of predicting those individuals likely to receive blood transfusions. However, it should be noted that two of eight patients with placenta previa received a blood transfusion. Therefore, according to this study, one could make a case for a limited role for preoperative autologous blood storage for the patient with placenta previa. However, at our own institution, the author obtained the retrospective data on peripartum blood transfusion from 1988 to 1990.[13] Of 31 parturients who entered the hospital with the diagnosis of placenta previa, only 5 received allogeneic blood transfusion. Fifteen of the last 16 patients with this diagnosis did not receive any blood transfusion. This latter fact may reflect patient concerns about the risk of transmission of infectious diseases, as well as increasing physician tolerance for lower hemoglobin levels perioperatively and at the time of discharge from the hospital.

Kruskall[14] determined that although preoperative blood storage was safe for the mother and fetus, only 1.7% of all parturients received blood transfusion and only 1.2% of parturients who donated blood preoperatively received blood transfusion. She concluded that, at present, preoperative blood donation and storage is an extremely expensive investment of medical technology in obstetrics.

Goldfinger,[15] however, noted that although only 1.7% of obstetrical patients usually received blood transfusion, additional patients had sufficient peripartum blood loss to become significantly anemic but were not transfused. Had autologous blood been available, transfusion would have been appropriate for some of these patients.

In summary, although preoperative blood donation and storage may be helpful in some cases of anticipated placenta previa who develop low perioperative hemoglobin levels, the overall low perioperative transfusion rate and the cost of such a blood donation service would require more supportive data before such a service could be recommended.

The use of a cell-processing device during cases of major obstetrical hemorrhage has always seemed like an attractive idea. The major disadvantage of this technique is that scavenged maternal blood could be contaminated with amniotic fluid, which contains fetal cells and other debris. These could cause amniotic fluid embolism, leading to coagulopathy and maternal death. Thornhill and coworkers[16] performed a study suggesting that the cell saver can remove amniotic fluid and reduce the quantity of fetal debris in salvaged blood. Whole blood was mixed with large quantities of amniotic fluid previously obtained from women undergoing cesarean section. Samples were passed through a 40-$\mu$m cardiotomy filter and washed with normal saline in a cell processor. This process reduced a marker for the presence of amniotic fluid, $\alpha$-fetoprotein, from a range of 36–83 units before washing to zero after the wash. The cell processor eliminated most, but not all, fetal debris. Much further work remains to be done before use of the cell processor is proved safe for cases of obstetrical hemorrhage; however, it is still not known which substances in amniotic fluid are responsible for the signs and symptoms of amniotic fluid embolism. If the use of such a device was perfected, this technique could greatly reduce the incidence of maternal morbidity-mortality in cases of major obstetrical hemorrhage (see Chapter 9: Blood Salvage Techniques).

Several investigations, reporting in obstetrical literature, have contended that general anesthesia for cesarean section and second-trimester abortion results in significantly more blood loss than regional anesthesia for the former or local anesthesia for the latter procedure. Gilstrap and coworkers,[17] comparing preoperative versus postoperative hematocrit to assess blood loss during cesarean section, reported that the addition of 0.3–1% halothane to nitrous oxide was associated with much more bleeding than with nitrous oxide alone or with regional anesthesia. Also, they reported that 18% of 114 patients receiving halothane were given blood transfusions, whereas only 1 of the 150 patients in the regional anesthesia group received blood. Approximately 60% of the patients administered halothane received it both before and after delivery. However, Thirion and coworkers[18] studied 60 patients undergoing cesarean section. Those receiving general anesthesia, either with halothane 0.3–0.8% before delivery or before and after delivery, had no greater decrease in hematocrit or greater need for blood transfusion than did a similar group receiving epidural anesthesia.

MacKay and associates[19] studied complications of second-trimester abortions and attributed a greater incidence of hemorrhage requiring transfusion if general anesthesia, as opposed to local anesthesia, was used. Although it is true that a potent inhalation agent like halothane will produce dose-dependent uterine relaxation, and therefore increased uterine bleeding, clinical experience has shown that nitrous oxide has little effect on uterine contractibility.[20] The reason for the increased hemorrhage in the general anesthesia group in the MacKay study may have been the longer duration and increased vigor of curettage that is likely to occur when that procedure is performed under general anesthesia.

Preoperative autologous blood donation has not been reported for gynecological patients at risk for major hemorrhage. Curtis[21] described intraoperative blood salvage in two patients with "gynecologic hemoperitoneum" with the use of a cell-processor unit. One case was a ruptured ectopic pregnancy and the other, a ruptured corpus luteum cyst. These cases resulted in the intraoperative transfusion of 600–1200 mL packed RBCs, respectively. The authors concluded that intraoperative blood salvage could be useful in these situations; however, because of the expense of the supplies and the cost of the technicians to operate the cell processor, an intraperitoneal blood loss of at least 1000 mL should be anticipated to justify this expense. Intraoperative blood salvage would be contraindicated for the gynecology oncology patient because of the risk of dissemination of

tumor cells (see Chapter 9: Blood Salvage Techniques).

In the performance of vaginal hysterectomy, some surgeons infiltrate the junction of the vagina and cervix with a dilute solution of epinephrine[22] to cause local vasoconstriction, minimizing blood loss during incision of the cervix. Depending on the dose injected and the vascularity of the cervix, a transient tachycardia and widened pulse pressure could occur from systemic absorption of this drug. Other surgeons use dilute solutions of vasopressin or phenylephrine, which upon systemic uptake could be expected to produce transient episodes of hypertension and bradycardia. Normal saline without vasoactive substances (30–40 mL) has also been infiltrated at this junction to reduce blood loss.

## REFERENCES

1. Reisner L: Type and screen for elective cesarean section. Anesthesiology 1983; 58:476.
2. Sandler SG, Naiman JL, Fletcher JL: Alternative approaches to transfusion: autologous blood and directed blood donation. Prog Hematol 1987; 15: 183.
3. Davis R: Banked autologous blood for caesarean section. Anaesth Intens Care 1979; 7:358.
4. Kruskall MS, Leonard S, Klapholz H: Autologous blood donation during pregnancy: analysis of safety and blood uses. Obstet Gynecol 1987; 70:938.
5. Druzin ML, Wold CF, Edersheim TG, et al.: Donation of blood by the pregnant patient for autologous transfusion. Am J Obstet Gynecol 1988; 159:1023.
6. Herbert WNP, Owen NG, Collins ML: Autologous blood storage in obstetrics. Obstet Gynecol 1988; 72:166.
7. Katz AR, Walker WA, Ross PJ, et al.: Autologous transfusion in obstetrics and gynecology. Int J Gynaecol Obstet 1978–1979; 16:345.
8. Sandler SG, Beyth Y, Laufer N, et al.: Autologous blood transfusion and pregnancy. Obstet Gynecol Suppl 1979; 53:62.
9. Mann M, Sacks HJ, Goldfinger D: Safety of autologous blood donation prior to elective surgery for a variety of potentially "high risk" patients. Transfusion 1986; 26:355.
10. Lindenbaum CR, Schwartz IR, Chhibber G, et al.: Safety of predeposit autologous blood donation in the third trimester of pregnancy. J Reprod Med 1990; 35:537.
11. McVay PA, Hoag RW, Hoag MS, et al.: Safety and use of autologous blood donation during the third trimester of pregnancy. Am J Obstet Gynecol 1989; 160:1479.
12. Andres RL, Piacquaido KM, Resnik R: A reappraisal of the need for autologous blood donation in the obstetric patient. Am J Obstet Gynecol 1990; 163: 1551.
13. Heyman HF, Barton JJ: Safety of local versus gener anesthesia for second-trimester dilatation and evacu

ation abortion [Reply]. Obstet Gynecol 1986; 68: 877.

14. Kruskall MS: Are autologous transfusions necessary for pregnant women? In: Maffei LM, Thurer RL, eds, Autologous Blood Transfusion: Current Issues. Baltimore, MD, 1988, American Association of Blood Banks, p. 83.

15. Goldfinger D: Strategies for reducing risk of transfusion in pregnancy: unanswered questions regarding safety and effectiveness. In: Maffei LM, Thurer RL, eds, Autologous Blood Transfusion: Current Issues. Baltimore, MD, 1988, American Association of Blood Banks, p. 89.

16. Thornhill ML, O'Leary AJ, Lussos SA, et al.: An *in vitro* assessment of amniotic fluid removal through cell saver processing (Abstract). Anesthesiology 1991; 75:A830.

17. Gilstrap LC, Hauth UC, Hankins GD, et al.: Effect of type anesthesia on blood loss at cesarean section. Obstet Gynecol 1987; 69:328.

18. Thirion AV, Wright RG, Messer CP, et al.: Maternal blood loss associated with low dose halothane administration for cesarean section (Abstract). Anesthesiology 1988; 69:A693.

19. MacKay HT, Schulz KF, Grimes DA: Safety of local versus general anesthesia for second-trimester dilatation and evacuation abortion. Obstet Gynecol 1985; 66:661.

20. Cullen BF, Margolis AJ, Eger EI: The effects of anesthesia and pulmonary ventilation on blood loss during elective therapeutic abortion. Anesthesiology 1970; 32:108.

21. Curtis CH: Autotransfusion in gynecologic hemoperitoneum. Am J Obstet Gynecol 1983; 146:501.

22. Summers P: Medical and surgical consideration in gynecology. In: Pernoll ML, Benson RC, eds, Current Obstetric and Gynecologic Diagnosis and Treatment. Norwalk, CT, 1987, Appleton and Lange, p. 838.

# ORTHOTOPIC LIVER TRANSPLANTATION

## *Victor Scott and Peter J. Davis*

Since 1980 orthotopic liver transplantation (OLT) has become the preferred surgical procedure for end-stage liver disease of varied etiologies. The number of procedures being performed has increased exponentially, and presently 2500–3000 procedures are performed annually; of these, 350 are in the pediatric population. With the introduction of cyclosporine in the past decade, and more recently of FK-506, graft and patient survival have improved dramatically. Current survival rates are reported of 80–90% at 1 year and 70% at 5 years.[1]

Indications for OLT are varied.[1–4] The range of diseases contraindicating transplantation has also changed in the past year. Most notable are patients with hepatitis B who are known to be hepatitis B e antigen positive and appear to have a 100% recurrence rate of disease in the grafted organ. Transplantation in this subpopulation of patients is now being abandoned.[2]

## STAGES OF LIVER TRANSPLANTATION

OLT is classically divided into three separate stages. Stage I, the preanhepatic stage, begins with a wide bilateral subcostal incision and ends when the liver is freed up to its vascular pedicle. Stage II, the anhepatic phase, begins with the interruption of the liver's vascular supply and ends with the revascularization of the donor organ. During this stage the patient's suprahepatic and infrahepatic vena cava, portal vein, and hepatic artery are cross-clamped. Stage III, the neohepatic stage, begins with reperfusion of the grafted liver and ends with the completion of surgery. During this stage blood flow is restored via the inferior vena cava and the portal vein. Because of the liver's blood supply, it is not essential that the hepatic arterial blood supply be restored before unclamping the vena cava and portal vein.[3] The exact timing of the reanastomosis of the hepatic artery is determined by technical considerations. The biliary anastomosis, the last phase of the surgical procedure, is performed after the revascularization of the donor organ is complete and adequate hemostasis has been achieved.

The major intraoperative problems occurring during these stages of OLT include cardiovascular instability, coagulation disorders, metabolic derangements, and hypothermia. In this discussion, only the first two issues are addressed. However, it must be remembered that all of these problems are somewhat interrelated. Consequently, the persistence of hypothermia or metabolic derangements (e.g., acidosis) can significantly affect the patient's underlying hemodynamic stability and coagulation profile.

# HEMODYNAMIC CONSIDERATIONS
## Preanhepatic Stage

The hemodynamic alterations and the coagulopathy seen during OLT are best viewed in relation to the three stages of the surgical procedure. During stage I, the recipient's liver is freed from the diaphragm and vena cava. Although this maneuver seems easy, technically it is difficult and accounts for most of the blood lost during the surgical procedure.[3] Other factors that may contribute to blood loss during stage I are extensive vascular collaterals and recently treated peritonitis. In patients with a history of abdominal surgery or preexisting thrombosis in the portal vein, additional blood loss occurs because of the dense adhesions and collateral vessel formation. Massive blood loss during stage I, thus, partly accounts for hemodynamic instability.

Massive transfusion of packed red blood cells (RBCs) and fresh frozen plasma (FFP) will eventually lead to the accumulation of citrate toward the end of stage I and a subsequent decrease in the level of serum ionized calcium.[4,5] This low level of serum ionized calcium is the second greatest contributor of hemodynamic instability in stage I. Because of the technique used to fractionate blood into its components, FFP contains the greatest amount of citrate per unit volume of any blood product. Consequently, its effect on cardiovascular stability may be more pronounced than infusions of equal volumes of packed RBCs. Coté[6] demonstrated that infusion of FFP at rates of 1–2.5 mL/kg/min is associated with transient decreases in serum ionized calcium levels and significant decreases in arterial blood pressure. Inhalation anesthetics accentuate the hemodynamic effects of citrate intoxication. Marquez and associates[7] reported profound myocardial dysfunction at a serum ionized calcium level of less than 0.56 mg/L.

## Anhepatic Stage

Although the vascular supply to the liver is interrupted and controlled during stage II, blood loss continues. In addition to the causes previously noted, the absence of the liver further exacerbates the continued bleeding and hemodynamic instability. During the anhepatic phase, citrate accumulates and hypocalcemia worsens. Acidemia and hyperkalemia also occur and may worsen myocardial function. Cross-clamping of the inferior vena cava and the portal vein results in a 50% loss of venous return, which results in hypotension, decreased cardiac output, increased systemic vascular resistance, and compensatory tachycardia.[4,8]

The hemodynamic changes observed in stage II can be attenuated by the use of venoveno bypass or "piggybacking" the donor liver to support the recipient's circulation.[9] With venoveno bypass the femoral and portal veins are cannulated, and venous return from splanchnic bed, kidneys, and lower extremities to the axillary vein is aided by a centrifugal pump. Flow rates on venoveno bypass are usually maintained between 20 and 40% of the cardiac output.[9] The augmented venous return is usually sufficient to maintain adequate blood pressure without the use of vasoactive agents. In adults without the use of venoveno bypass, the addition of dopamine or phenylephrine hydrochloride to increase the blood pressure may be essential. Children, however, appear to have a lower incidence of hemodynamic instability during vena cava cross-clamping in the absence of venoveno bypass. Whether this is a result of a more extensive collateral circulation or a better functioning myocardium is unclear. In the piggyback technique the donor's liver suprahepatic vena cava is anastomosed to the recipient's hepatic veins rather than vena cava. Thus, venous return to the heart from the femoral area is maintained. A temporary portacaval shunt occasionally is used during the procedure to augment venous return from the splanchnic bed.

## Neohepatic Stage

The beginning of the neohepatic stage is the time of greatest hemodynamic consequence. Graft reperfusion initially restores the preload to the level seen in stage I.[10] Hypotension is often seen at the beginning of this stage. Initially, this effect may be due to the release of cold, acidotic, hyperkalemic effluent from the grafted liver. The postreperfusion syndrome (hypotension, bradycardia, conduction defects, decreased systemic vascular resistance index [SVRI], and increased atrial filling pressures) occurs in 30% of patients upon graft reperfusion.[11] In adults, vasoactive agents (primarily epinephrine, 5–10 $\mu$g) are usually required to restore the decrease in mean arterial pressure. Continued hypotension in stage III is usually a result of a low SVRI. The etiology of this low SVRI is thought to be related to mediators released from the grafted liver. In children, postreperfusion syndrome does not appear to be as significant as it is in adults, and the use of vasoactive agents is not uncommon.

## COAGULATION CONSIDERATIONS
### Preanhepatic Stage

The sequence of changes in coagulation during OLT is unique to this surgical procedure.[12–18] Although changes in the coagulation profile as assessed by the thromboelastogram (Figure 12–1 in adults and children undergoing OLT are similar (e.g., poor preoperative coagulation and severe coagulopathy on reperfusion), the coagulatory changes in children appeared to be less severe than those in adults.[13]

In both adults and children, alterations of the coagulation cascade are frequent before surgery (Fig. 12–2). With the exception of factor VIII, all other coagulation factors are synthesized in the liver. Defective synthesis of essential factors and inadequate clearance of

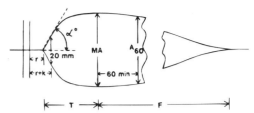

**Fig. 12–1.** The reaction time (r) as measured by the thromboelastograph (TEG) denotes the time to onset of the start of coagulation and should be approximately 6–8 minutes. It represents the rate of thromboplastin formation. Prolongation of this portion of the TEG usually represents factor deficiency and is treated with the administration of FFP. The coagulation time (r + k) is the period between the start of the TEG recording and the time to the operation of an amplitude of 20 mm. It is a measurement of the speed of solid clot formation. The clot formation rate is measured by the $\alpha$ angle and normally is greater than 50°. Abnormalities of the $\alpha$ angle represent platelet function, fibrinogen, and the intrinsic pathway. $\alpha$ angle abnormalities are usually corrected by cryoprecipitate administration. The maximum amplitude (MA) is most indicative of platelet function and normally measures between 50 and 70 mm.

activated factors by the recipient's diseased liver account for a significant portion of abnormal bleeding. Factor VIII and fibrinogen levels are usually normal or increased, although an abnormal fibrinogen is often synthesized.[14] Thrombocytopenia, which occurs in over 50% of the patients, is often a consequence of hypersplenism and bone marrow suppression. In addition, platelet function is abnormal. A low-grade fibrinolysis, a consequence of low antiplasmin levels and diminished clearance of tissue plasminogen activator (tPA), often is present before OLT.[15] An increase in fibrinolytic split products indicates this process.

## Anhepatic Stage

During the anhepatic stage, a dilutional coagulopathy resulting from the massive administration of blood exacerbates the existing coagulopathy. However, continued replacement factors with FFP abates this process. Factor VIII and fibrinogen are usually not replaced during this stage because their levels are elevated before surgery. Fibrinolysis occurring during this stage is usually mild; however, the presence of severe fibrinolysis may require therapy with $\epsilon$-aminocaproic acid (EACA). Early treatment of fibrinolysis may help prevent severe blood loss and its consequences. Coagulation defects seen during the anhepatic stage are a direct consequence of the liver's inability to metabolize tPA.[15] The underlying coagulopathy may be exacerbated by continued blood replacement as well as the

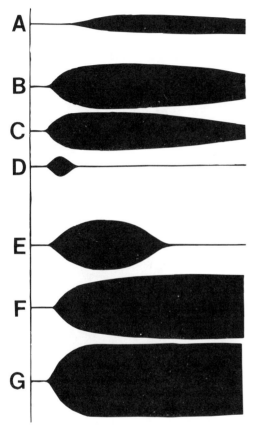

**Fig. 12–2.** *A:* This is a representation of the abnormalities of coagulation noted before surgery. There is a prolongation of the r time and a diminution of the α angle as well as the maximum amplitude (MA). *B:* Improved coagulation during stage I is noted as there is administration of FFP and platelets as the surgery progresses. Note the improved MA and r time. There is also an improved α angle. *C:* This TEG is representative of the continued coagulopathy seen during stage II of the surgery. Note the progressive diminution of the MA and the progressive tapering of the MA that suggest possible fibrinolysis. *D:* This is a classic representation of fibrinolysis occasionally seen late in stage I. Note there is clot formation that is dissolved as represented by the straight line seen on the right of this picture. *E:* Again fibrinolysis is seen immediately on graft reperfusion. Note in this case the clot formed takes somewhat longer before dissolution occurs. *F:* EACA-treated TEG is represented that demonstrates dramatic improvement of the fibrinolytic state. Note the improved MA, R time, and α angle. *G:* The end of TEG shows a normal coagulation profile that is representative of normal liver function from the graft as well as continued administration of coagulation factors.

use of heparin flush during insertion of the femoral, portal, and axillary vein cannulas for venoveno bypass. This heparin effect, however, is mild, dissipates within 30–60 minutes, and generally does not require treatment.[4] Primary fibrinolysis occurs in approximately 30% of patients by the end of stage II. Judicious use of EACA is recommended for the treatment of fibrinolysis during this stage because of the potential for thromboembolism with the use of venoveno bypass.

## Neohepatic Stage

Changes in coagulation at the onset of the neohepatic stage are common and multifactorial. Continued blood loss and massive transfusion requirements result in diminution in platelets and in levels of factors V and VII. By the beginning of stage III, with the onset of graft reperfusion, primary fibrinolysis, thought to be secondary to the release of tPA from the grafted liver, occurs in 80% of patients but does not appear to be the main factor contributing to ongoing blood loss.[16] Although primary fibrinolysis is common, specific treatment is required in only 20% of patients, probably because a functional hepatic graft can metabolize tPA, thereby making primary fibrinolysis a self-limiting process. In the few patients who do require treatment for primary fibrinolysis, Kang and coworkers[17] demonstrated that small doses of EACA (250 mg/kg) effectively reversed this problem.

Endogenous release of heparin from the previously ischemic hepatocytes also occurs at this time and can contribute to the underlying coagulopathy.[20] However, by 30 minutes after graft reperfusion, the heparin effect resolves and treatment is seldom necessary. If the heparin effect persists, then protamine (25–50 mg) is administered.

## AUTOLOGOUS TRANSFUSION

As previously stated, liver disease and liver transplant surgery are associated with underlying coagulopathies, massive blood loss, massive blood transfusion, hemodynamic instability, and metabolic derangement. The use of autologous transfusion decreases the blood requirement during surgery, increases blood bank resources, assures blood supply safety, and decreases the risk of autoimmunization, providing significant benefits in the overall anesthetic and surgical treatment of patients undergoing OLT.

Autologous transfusion is the collection and reinfusion of the patient's own blood, and it appears to have a positive role in liver transplantation.[19–24] There are three methods of autologous transfusion: preoperative autologous blood donation, perioperative blood salvage, and acute normovolemic hemodilution. Preoperative autologous blood donation and acute normovolemic hemodilution are usually not feasible options for patients undergoing OLT, because the average amount of blood required during surgery for adults is approximately 10 units each of packed RBCs and FFP. Acute normovolemic hemodilution, although not fully explored as an option, carries some risks, as these patients are usually anemic and thrombocytopenic before surgery. Thus, further hemodilution would significantly compromise oxygen transport. Recently, acute normovolemic hemodilution and preoperative erythropoietin therapy have been used in Jehovah's Witnesses undergoing OLT. However, this form of autologous transfusion in patients receiving transfusions of four to five times their total blood volume appears less practicable than cell salvage techniques.

The use of blood salvage has been reported in patients undergoing OLT. In 1989, Williamson and associates[22] reported their experience of 89 patients undergoing OLT with autologous transfusion. Of the 89 patients, intraoperative blood salvage with sodium citrate resulted in the collection of 586 units of salvaged RBCs (mean 6.6 units/patient). These 586 units of salvaged blood accounted for one-third of the RBC units needed intraoperatively. Dzik and Jenkins[20] reported that intraoperative blood salvage during OLT supplied roughly 45% of the patient's packed RBC requirements. The clinical evaluation of autotransfusion during OLT has also been reported by Kang and associates.[24] In this series of 25 patients, blood salvage was with acid-citrate-dextrose solution, and autotransfusion did not alter coagulation, electrolyte balance, or hematological findings. Although one-third of the patients had bacterial contamination of their salvaged blood, it was not sufficient to cause infections in these immunocompromised patients who were receiving antimicrobial prophylaxis.

At present, existing abdominal infection, viral hepatitis, or malignancy are the only absolute contraindications to the use of autologous transfusion. However, the rapidity with which blood can be collected, processed, and returned to the patient by the cell processor may also be a limiting factor in its usage. Blood loss during OLT may exceed this rate of return, thus requiring the use of the rapid infusion system with banked blood to maintain hemoglobin at a safe level for adequate oxygen transport and delivery (see Chapter 9: Blood Salvage Techniques).

## REFERENCES

1. Gordon RD, Bismuth H: Liver transplant registry for the Pittsburgh UNOS liver transplant registry and the European liver transplant registry. Transplant Proc 1991; 23:58.
2. Todo S, Demetris AJ, Van Thiel D, et al.: Orthotopic liver transplantation for patients with hepatitis B virus-related liver disease. Hepatology 1991; 13:619.
3. Starzl TE, Iwatsuki S, Van Thiel D, et al.: Evaluation of liver transplantation. Hepatology 1982; 2:614.
4. Kang Y: Anesthesia for liver transplantation. Int Anesthesiol Clin 1991; 29:59.
5. Martin TJ, Kang Y, Marquez JM, et al.: Ionization and hemodynamic effects of calcium chloride and calcium gluconate in the absence of hepatic function. Anesthesiology 1990; 73:62.
6. Coté CJ: Depth of halothane anesthesia potentiates citrate-induced ionized hypocalcemia and adverse cardiovascular events in dogs. Anesthesiology 1987; 67:676.
7. Marquez JM, Martin DJ, Virji M, et al.: Cardiovascular depression secondary to citrate intoxication during orthotopic liver transplantation in man. Anesthesiology 1986; 65:457.
8. Pappas G, Palmer WM, Martineau GI, et al.: Hemodynamic alterations caused during orthotopic liver transplantation in humans. Surgery 1971; 70:872.
9. Shaw BW, Martin DJ, Marquez JM, et al.: Advantages of venous bypass during orthotopic transplantation of the liver. Semin Liver Dis 1985; 5:344.
10. DeWolf A, Gasior T, Begliomini B, et al.: Right ventricular function during orthotopic liver transplantation (Abstract). Anesthesiology 1990; 73:A97.
11. Aggarwal S, Kang Y, Freeman JA, et al.: Postreperfusion syndrome: cardiovascular collapse following hepatic reperfusion during liver transplantation. Transplant Proc 1987; 19:54.
12. Lewis JH, Bontempo FA, Awad SA, et al.: Liver transplantation: intraoperative changes in coagulation factors in the 100 first transplants. Hepatology 1989; 9:710.
13. Kang Y, Borland LM, Picone J, et al.: Intraoperative coagulation changes in children undergoing liver transplantation. Anesthesiology 1989; 71:44.
14. Martinez J, Plalsacak JE, Kwasniak D: Abnormal sialic acid content of the dysfibrinogenemia associated with liver disease. J Clin Invest 1978; 61:535.
15. Lewis JA, Bontempo FA, Kang Y, et al.: Intraoperative coagulation changes in liver transplantation. In: Winter PM, Kang Y, eds, Anesthetic and Peri-

operative Management. New York, 1986, Prager Publishers, p. 142.

16. Kang Y, Martin DJ, Marquez JM, et al.: Intraoperative changes in coagulation and thromboelastographic monitoring in liver transplantation. Anesth Analg 1985; 64:888.

17. Kang Y, Lewis JH, Navalgund A, et al.: Epsilon-aminocaproic acid for treatment of fibrinolysis during liver transplantation. Anesthesiology 1987; 66:766.

18. Groth GC, Pechet L, Starzl TE: Coagulation during and after orthotopic transplantation of the human liver. Arch Surg 1969; 98:31.

19. AMA Council on Scientific Affairs: Autologous blood transfusions. JAMA 1986; 256:2378.

20. Dzik WH, Jenkins R: Use of intraoperative blood salvage during orthotopic liver transplantation. Arch Surg 1985; 120:946.

21. Popovsky MA, Devine PA, Taswell HF: Intraoperative autologous transfusion. Mayo Clin Proc 1985; 60:125.

22. Williamson KR, Taswell HF, Retke SR, et al.: Intraoperative autologous transfusion: its role in orthotopic liver transplantation. Mayo Clin Proc 1989; 64:340.

23. Toy PTCY: Autologous transfusion. Anesthesiol Clin North Am 1990; 8:533.

24. Kang Y, Aggarwal S, Virji M, et al.: Clinical evaluation of autotransfusion during liver transplantation. Anesth Analg 1991; 72:94.

# NEUROSURGERY

## Usharani Nimmagadda

The neurosurgical procedures commonly associated with significant blood loss include head trauma, correction of craniosynostosis, resection of vascular tumors, ligation of arteriovenous malformations (AVMs), clipping of aneurysms, and major spinal fusion procedures. At this time, preoperative autologous blood donation, and if necessary intraoperative transfusion of that blood, is used frequently for major spine surgery and is occasionally extended to other neurosurgical procedures such as craniotomies. Acute normovolemic hemodilution is not currently used in neurosurgery. Blood salvage procedures have been used in many institutions for major spine surgery and occasionally during surgery for head trauma or craniotomy.

Other blood conservation measures in neurosurgery include a well-planned and conducted anesthetic; appropriate positioning of the patient; control of blood pressure; addition of vasoconstrictor to the local anesthetic; and the use of various electrical, mechanical, and chemical hemostatic methods.

A well-planned and conducted anesthetic technique is vital in neuroanesthesia (see Chapter 4: Blood Conservation Techniques). Although the choice of an anesthetic agent may not play an important role in decreasing the blood loss during neurosurgery, meticulous control of the airway and the avoidance of coughing, bucking, and obstruction to venous drainage are essential. Because ventilation is controlled and end tidal or arterial $CO_2$ is monitored during neurosurgery, bleeding secondary to hypercapnia is uncommon.

Positioning the patient properly is important to decrease the blood loss. If the operative field is kept at a higher level than the rest of the body, venous drainage from the surgical site is more effective and venous bleeding is reduced. When the prone position is used for surgery of the spine and for posterior fossa surgery, proper padding of the anterior chest wall and abdomen prevents interference with respiration and compression of the inferior vena cava. Special frames, such as Relton Hall operative frame,[1] Andrews spinal surgery frame (Orthopedic Systems Inc., Hayward, CA), and Cloward surgical saddle (Surgical Equipment International Inc., Honolulu, HI), can be effectively used to reduce the pressure on the chest and abdomen during spinal surgery. Legs should always be wrapped with ace bandages to improve the venous return (see Chapter 4: Blood Conservation Techniques).

A few neurosurgeons prefer the lateral position for spine surgery to avoid problems with the prone position. But in this position, the spine may not be aligned properly, making the surgical orientation more difficult. The lateral sitting position provides maximal flexion instead of lateral position of the thoracolumbar spine and better drainage of the blood and cerebrospinal fluid.[2]

The sitting position provides several advantages when used for posterior fossa craniotomy and cervical spine surgery. It allows access to the face, airway, and extremities; does not interfere with respirations; provides better surgical exposure by draining cerebrospinal fluid and blood; and allows maximal flexion of the cervical spine. In addition, it has been shown that the use of blood transfusions is less in the sitting position than in various horizontal positions (supine, prone, lateral, park bench). A retrospective study involving 579 patients who underwent posterior fossa craniotomy showed that only 3% of patients in the sitting position received more than 2 units of blood compared with 13% of patients in the horizontal position.[3] Despite the above advantages, in recent years, the sitting position is less frequently used because of major complications, such as hemodynamic instability,[4] venous or arterial air emboli,[5] and cervical spinal cord compression with resulting quadriplegia.[6,7]

Avoiding sudden changes in mean arterial blood pressure and maintaining it close to the preoperative values can play an important role in the outcome of patients after neurosurgical procedures. In patients with cerebrovascular disease, decreases in blood pressure can lead to cerebral ischemia, whereas increases in blood pressure can lead to disruption of the blood-brain barrier and increases in cerebral blood flow and edema formation. Although unintentional decreases in blood pressure can be detrimental to patients with cerebrovascular disease, deliberate hypotension can be used to facilitate intracranial vessel surgery. Carefully controlled decreases in blood pressure allow easier clipping of the aneurysm by reducing the pressure across the aneurysm wall and by softening the neck and sac of the aneurysm. The decreased blood pressure also decreases the risk of rupture.[8] Intraoperative rupture of aneurysm has been shown not only to increase blood loss but also to increase postoperative neurological dysfunction.[9] In the event of a rupture during surgery, decreasing the blood pressure further reduces blood loss and allows

the surgeon to locate the bleeding site and apply the clip properly.

In recent years, improved surgical techniques and fear of cerebral vasospasm have resulted in avoidance of excessive hypotension during cerebrovascular surgery. Cerebral vasospasm leading to ischemia is a major concern after bleeding from cerebral aneurysms because it leads to permanent neurological deficits or death in 10–20% of patients.[10] Increasing the systemic arterial pressure by volume loading and by the use of vasopressors has been used with encouraging results either to prevent the occurrence of delayed neurological deficits or to reverse the deficits that have already developed. In recent years several investigators have shown that hypervolemic hemodilution with or without induced hypertension is useful in the treatment of vasospasm.[11–13]

When deliberate hypotension is used, careful selection of the hypotensive drug is essential. Sodium nitroprusside,[14] nitroglycerin,[15] trimethaphan,[16] and deep inhalation anesthesia have all been used (see Chapter 8: Deliberate Hypotension). Sodium nitroprusside is a direct arteriolar vasodilator and can increase cerebral blood flow and intracranial pressure in patients with decreased intracranial compliance.[17] Nitroglycerin is primarily a venodilator and can also increase cerebral blood flow and intracranial pressure.[18] Trimethaphan is a ganglionic blocking agent and causes smaller increases in cerebral blood flow than sodium nitroprusside or nitroglycerin. However, if mean arterial pressure is decreased below 50 mm Hg, it may precipitate cerebral ischemia.[16] Furthermore, cycloplegia resulting from ganglionic blockade may interfere with the neurological assessment of the patient. Deep inhalation anesthesia with either halothane[19,20] or isoflurane[21] can be used to provide hypotension. The advantage of isoflurane over halothane is twofold. Isoflurane progressively decreases the cerebral metabolic rate for oxygen ($CMRO_2$) only until cortical electrical activity ceases, and further increases in isoflurane concentration do not decrease $CMRO_2$ any lower. Also, isoflurane does not alter oxidative phosphorylation and maintains cerebral energy stores,[22] thus providing some cerebral protection. On the other hand, increasing concentrations of halothane decreases $CMRO_2$ even after the cessation of cortical electrical activity and decreases cerebral tissue concentrations of adenosine triphosphate and phosphocreatinine and causes large increases in cerebral lactate levels. In addition, concentrations of halothane above 2% alter mitochondrial electron transport and respiratory control.[23]

Since 1961, antifibrinolytic therapy has been used to prevent the recurrence of bleeding after subarachnoid hemorrhage, but the benefits obtained from the antifibrinolytic agents remain controversial. Many recent studies have shown that tranexamic acid[24] or ε-aminocaproic acid,[25] despite decreasing the rebleeding rate, do not improve the overall mortality rate. This is because of the higher incidence of cerebral infarction with these agents. A review article in 1981 suggested that antifibrinolytic therapy has no favorable influence on the natural history of aneurysmal subarachnoid hemorrhage.[26]

Some AVMs are not accessible for surgery because of either their size or their location. Furthermore, some patients may not tolerate these extensive microsurgical procedures that may take many hours and may be associated with large amounts of blood loss. Thus, some carefully selected AVMs can be embolized with neuroradiological procedures to reduce their size before the surgical procedure. Recently, isobutyl-2-cyanoacrylate[27] (Bucrylate, Ethicon Inc., Somerville, NJ) and conjugated estrogen[28] have been used for this purpose. Once the embolization is done, the neurosurgeon can then extirpate the lesion with much less blood loss or the lesion can be obliterated by using various stereotactic procedures, such as Bragg peak proton beam radiosurgery[29,30] or 201-source cobalt-60 γ knife.[30]

When neurosurgical procedures such as burr holes or insertion of intracranial pressure monitor are performed under local anesthesia, epinephrine may be added as a vasoconstrictor. Catecholamines have little effect on cerebral blood flow and cerebral metabolic rate when blood-brain barrier and autoregulation are intact. But with disruption of these, both epinephrine and norepinephrine can raise cerebral blood flow and cerebral metabolic rate. In this respect, epinephrine causes more increases than norepinephrine.[31,32]

A small amount of bleeding into the brain can cause serious consequences as compared with the same amount of blood left in other areas, such as the abdominal cavity. Thus, meticulous and complete hemostasis is critical in neurosurgery. The bony confinement, depth of surgery, and the indispensability of the brain tissue make hemostasis more difficult (hemostasis is usually accomplished without the use of ligature)[33] (see Chapter 13: Surgical Hemostasis and Blood Conservation).

## REFERENCES

1. Relton JES, Hall JE: An operation frame for spinal fusion: a new apparatus designed to reduce hemorrhage during operation. J Bone Joint Surg [Br] 1967; 49B:327.
2. Garcia-Bengochia F, Munson EJ, Freeman JV: The lateral sitting position for neurosurgery. Anesth Analg 1976; 55:326.
3. Black S, Ockert DB, Oliver WC, et al.: Comparison of outcome following posterior fossa craniotomy done either in a sitting or horizontal position. Anesthesiology 1988; 69:49.
4. Marshall WK, Bedford RF, Miller ED: Hemodynamics in the seated position. Anesth Analg 1982; 61:201.
5. Cucchiara RF, Nugent M, Seward JB, et al.: Air embolism in upright neurosurgical patients: detection and localization by 2-D transesophageal echocardiography. Anesthesiology 1984; 60:353.
6. Hitselberger WE, House WF: A warning regarding the sitting position for acoustic tumor surgery. Arch Otolaryngol 1980; 106:69.
7. Wilder BL: Hypotheses: etiology of midcervical quadriplegia after operation with the patient in sitting position. Neurosurgery 1982; 6:530.
8. Yasargil MG, Smith RD: Management of aneurysms of anterior circulation by intracranial procedures. In: Youmans JR, ed, Neurological Surgery, 2 ed. Philadelphia, 1982, W.B. Saunders, vol. 3, p. 1668.
9. Batyer H, Samson D: Intraoperative aneurysmal rupture: incidence, outcome and suggestions for surgical management. Neurosurgery 1986; 18:701.
10. Kassell NF, Sasaki T, Colchan ART, et al.: Cerebral vasospasm following aneurysmal subarachnoid hemorrhage. Stroke 1985; 16:562.
11. Kassell NF, Peerless ST, Durward QJ, et al.: Treatment of ischemic deficits from vasospasm with intravascular volume expansion and induced arterial hypertension. Neurosurgery 1982; 11:377.
12. Finn SS, Stephenson SS, Miller CA, et al.: Observations on the perioperative management of aneurysmal subarachnoid hemorrhage. J Neurosurg 1986; 65:48.
13. Awad IA, Carter LP, Spetzler RF, et al.: Clinical vasospasm after subarachnoid hemorrhage: response to hypervolemic hemodilution and arterial hypertension. Stroke 1987; 18:365.
14. Henriksen L, Thorshauge C, Harmsen A, et al.: Controlled hypotension with sodium nitroprusside: effects of cerebral blood flow and cerebral venous blood gases in patients operated for cerebral aneurysms. Acta Anaesthesiol Scand 1983; 27:62.
15. Maktabi M, Warner D, Sokoll M, et al.: Comparison of nitroprusside, nitroglycerin and deep isoflurane anesthesia for induced hypotension. Neurosurgery 1986; 19:350.

16. Michenfelder JD, Theye RA: Canine systemic and cerebral effects of hypotension induced by hemorrhage, trimethaphan, halothane or nitroprusside. Anesthesiology 1977; 46:188.
17. Larson R, Teichmann J, Hilfiker O, et al.: Nitroprusside—hypotension, cerebral blood flow and cerebral oxygen consumption in neurosurgical patients. Acta Anaesthesiol Scand 1982; 26:327.
18. Essen CV, Kistler JP, Lees RS, et al.: Cerebral blood flow and intracranial pressure in the dog during intravenous infusion of nitroglycerin alone and in combination with dopamine. Stroke 1981; 12:331.
19. Murtagh GP: Controlled hypotension with halothane. Anaesthesia 1960; 15:235.
20. Prys-Roberts C, Lloyd JW, Fisher A, et al.: Deliberate profound hypotension induced with halothane: studies of hemodynamics and pulmonary gas exchange. Br J Anaesth 1974; 46:105.
21. Lam AM, Gelb AW: Cardiovascular effects of isoflurane-induced hypotension for cerebral aneurysm surgery. Anesth Analg 1983; 62:742.
22. Newberg LA, Milde JH, Michenfelder JD: The cerebral metabolic effects of isoflurane at and above concentrations that suppress cortical electrical activity. Anesthesiology 1983; 59:23.
23. Cohen PJ: Effects of anesthetics on mitochondrial function. Anesthesiology 1973; 39:153.
24. Fodstad H, Forssell A, Liliequist B, et al.: Antifibrinolysis with tranexamic acid in aneurysmal subarachnoid hemorrhage: a consecutive controlled clinical trial. Neurosurgery 1981; 8:158.
25. Shucart WA, Hussain SK, Cooper PR: Epsilon aminocaproic acid and recurrent subarachnoid hemorrhage. A clinical trial. J Neurosurg 1980; 53:28.
26. Ramirez-Lassepas M: Antifibrinolytic therapy in subarachnoid hemorrhage caused by ruptured intracranial aneurysm. Neurology 1981; 31:316.
27. Cromwell LD, Freeny PC, Kerber CW, et al.: Histologic analysis of tissue response to bucrylate-pantopaque mixture. AJR Am J Roentgenol 1986; 147:627.
28. Negamine Y, Komatsu S, Sujuki J: New embolization method using estrogen: effect of estrogen on microcirculation. Surg Neurol 1983; 20:269.
29. Kjellberg RN: Stereotactic Bragg peak proton beam surgery for cerebral arteriovenous malformations. Ann Clin Res 1986; 47:17.
30. Lunsford LD, Kondziolka D, Flickenger JC, et al.: Stereotactic radiosurgery for arteriovenous malformations of the brain. J Neurosurg 1991; 175:512.
31. Berntman L, Dahlgren N, Siesjo BK: Influence of intravenously administered catecholamines on cerebral oxygen consumption and blood flow in the rat. Acta Physiol Scand 1978; 104:101.
32. Abdul-Rahman A, Dahlgren N, Johansson BB, et al.: Increase in local cerebral blood flow induced by circulating adrenaline: involvement in blood-brain barrier dysfunction. Acta Physiol Scand 1979; 107:227.
33. Light RV: Hemostasis in neurosurgery. J Neurosurg 1945; 2:414.

# CARDIAC SURGERY

*Robert Paulissian and Fawzy G. Estafanous*

## INTRODUCTION

About 280,000 coronary artery surgery (CAS) procedures are performed annually in the United States,[1] and the number continues to rise. The majority of these patients receive blood transfusion, although blood usage statistics vary widely. In one multiinstitutional study, investigators[2] found 68% of first-time CAS patients received an average of 2.9 units of allogeneic packed red blood cells (RBCs), with a range of 0.4–6.3 units. In addition,

38% received fresh frozen plasma (FFP) (range 0–97%), and 22% of patients received platelet concentrates (range 0–80%). To curtail the ever-increasing need for allogeneic blood transfusion, many avenues have been explored. The goal of blood conservation programs is to transfuse blood and blood products only when necessary and to limit patients' exposure to as few donors as possible when transfusion is indicated. In cardiac surgery, these goals are met by the aggressive use of all appropriate blood conservation techniques (acute normovolemic hemodilution, preoperative autologous blood donation (PABD), asanguinous pump primes, retransfusion of residual oxygenator blood, and salvaging of shed blood) and pharmacological interventions to minimize operative blood loss ($\epsilon$-aminocaproic acid [EACA], aprotinin, tranexamic acid [TA], and desmopressin acetate).[3,4]

## FACTORS INCREASING BLOOD REQUIREMENTS IN CARDIAC SURGERY

Improvements in anesthetic and surgical management have allowed the majority of primary uncomplicated CAS and valvular surgery to be performed without the need for allogeneic blood transfusion.[5,6] However, these improvements must be contrasted with other trends that have resulted in the increased need for blood transfusion. Cardiovascular procedures on patients with higher risks for massive blood loss are being performed. Patients with ascending and transverse aortic aneurysms, multivessel aortic arch disease, anatomic abnormality of the chest wall, and prior mediastinal irradiation and patients presenting for reoperation are at particular risk of catastrophic hemorrhage.[7,8]

Reoperation is associated with an increased oozing and possible massive blood loss, increasing need for blood transfusion, and overall morbidity and mortality.[9,10] Excessive oozing is more common in patients who have their reoperations shortly after the first procedure, because adhesions become less dense and vascular with time. Adhesions, along with the resultant anatomic distortions, can complicate both sternotomy and dissection of the heart and coronary vasculature and increase the incidence of massive hemorrhage.

More complex, complicated, and combined cardiovascular surgical procedures are performed with increased frequency. These include multiple valve procedures, combinations of valve replacement, CAS or aortic aneurysm procedures, and the use of bilateral internal mammary arteries for coronary grafts. These complex procedures result in prolonged operative and cardiopulmonary bypass (CPB) times, which are associated with platelet damage and coagulation defects[11] (see Chapter 2: Coagulation and Hemostasis).

An increased number of critically ill and older patients with multiple medical problems (including anemia) are now being accepted for cardiac surgery. Advanced age, prolonged preoperative bleeding time, and low preoperative hematocrit have been shown to be reliable predictors of increased transfusion requirement.[12,13] The majority of patients undergoing emergency cardiac surgery are commonly on anticoagulant or antiplatelet therapy immediately before surgery. Perioperative blood loss and transfusion requirement have been shown to be increased in these patients.[9,14–18]

The various blood conservation methods in cardiac patients can be divided into three different categories according to chronological order of usage, specifically, during the preoperative, intraoperative, and postoperative periods.

## BLOOD CONSERVATION MEASURES DURING THE PREOPERATIVE PERIOD

Patients scheduled to undergo elective cardiac surgical procedures should be prepared, and coagulation status and hemoglobin and RBC levels should be optimized. Patients at high risk for bleeding should be identified and treated. If surgery cannot be delayed, increased pre-CPB blood loss should be anticipated and blood salvage techniques instituted.

### Preoperative Assessment of Coagulation

The value of preoperative coagulation testing in predicting blood loss and transfusion requirement in the absence of a positive history is controversial.[19–21] Nevertheless, it seems reasonable to routinely obtain complete blood count, prothrombin and activated partial thromboplastin times, and a platelet scan. A history of abnormal bleeding or intake of drugs that cause platelet dysfunction would necessitate the addition of a template bleeding time; a fibrinogen determination and/or transfusion medicine consultation may also be indicated.[21-23]

## Preoperative Medical Therapy and Coagulation System

Drugs that affect the coagulation system, such as aspirin, heparin, coumadin, dipyridamole, clofibrate, antihistamines, nonsteroidal antiinflammatory drugs (NSAIDs), and thrombolytic drugs, should be discontinued and coagulation abnormalities treated before surgery whenever possible[24] (see Chapter 2: Coagulation and Hemostasis).

### ASPIRIN AND OTHER DRUGS AFFECTING PLATELET FUNCTION

Avoidance of aspirin (acetylsalicylic acid) intake is an important measure to preserve platelet function and to decrease blood loss during surgery.[25,26] Aspirin is the most commonly ingested drug that impairs platelet function. It irreversibly inactivates a fatty acid cyclooxygenase that converts arachidonic acid to prostaglandin endoperoxides $G_2$ and $H_2$ and thereby inhibiting thromboxane $A_2$ synthesis. Low-dose aspirin (2 mg/kg) inhibits the platelet secretory process and diminishes collagen-induced aggregation and the second phase of adenosine diphosphate (ADP) and epinephrine-induced aggregation.[27,28] Aspirin is commonly used in cardiac patients as an adjunct to thrombolytic therapy[16] and in the prevention and treatment of acute myocardial ischemia[29,30] or infarction.[14] It has also been considered effective in the prevention of myocardial infarction.[29] Preoperative aspirin therapy improves the long-term patency of coronary vessels treated with percutaneous transluminal angioplasty[31] and vein-graft patency after CAS.[32,33] Thus, patients on aspirin therapy may present for urgent or emergency cardiac surgical procedures.[34]

The preoperative administration of aspirin, even a single dose of 325 mg on the day before surgery, appears to have an adverse effect on the hemostatic mechanisms. In patients treated with aspirin, intraoperative and post-operative blood loss and transfusion requirements for RBCs, FFP, and platelets are significantly increased as is the incidence of reexploration for excessive postoperative bleeding.[17,26] However, aspirin therapy instituted 6 hours postoperatively does not increase the extent of postoperative bleeding. Because the beneficial effects of aspirin therapy on vein-graft patency are similar whether aspirin therapy is initiated before or after surgery, avoidance of aspirin preoperatively will decrease the perioperative bleeding without compromising vein-graft patency after CAS.[17] Finally, intensive care unit and total hospital stays are significantly longer in patients receiving preoperative aspirin therapy.[18]

If time allows, aspirin administration should be discontinued at least 5–7 days before operation. Because the inhibitory effects of aspirin on platelet aggregation persists for the life span of platelets (about 7 days), this interval allows permanently inhibited platelets to be replaced by fully functional new platelets. If not hospitalized before surgery, the patient should be given a list of aspirin-containing drugs to be avoided.[35] Because avoidance or termination of aspirin therapy and delaying of surgery are not always viable options, desmopressin acetate administration,[36] platelet transfusion, and aprotinin[37] have been used to reduce perioperative blood loss in these patients.[8,27]

Dipyridamole is a pyridopyrimidine compound with antithrombotic and vasodilating properties. It has been widely used for many years in different cardiac conditions to prevent thromboembolism. Frequently, it was administered in conjunction with aspirin for their synergistic effect to inhibit platelet function. The current recommended use of dipyridamole is in combination with warfarin to prevent thromboemboli in patients with prosthetic cardiac valves, because dipyridamole is most effective against thrombus formation on prosthetic material.[38] The mechanisms of action of dipyridamole are most probably due to the increase in circulating adenosine levels by inhibition of adenosine uptake by RBCs and vascular endothelium and phosphodiesterase inhibition in platelets resulting in an increase in platelet 3′,5′-cyclic adenosine monophosphate to reduce platelet adhesion as well as aggregation and prolongation of platelet life span.

Dipyridamole, administered preoperatively to patients undergoing cardiac procedures, reduces platelet activation by the prosthetic material in the extracorporeal pump circuit, maintains the platelet count, and reduces myocardial platelet deposition and cardiac thromboxane release without increasing the risk of bleeding during cardiac surgery.[38-42] Teoh and coworkers[43] established that preoperative (oral or intravenous) dipyridamole therapy, in patients undergoing elective CAS, resulted in considerably less blood loss (42–46% less) than patients who did not receive dipyridamole. Postoperative platelet counts were highest in patients receiving intravenous dipyridamole, intermediate in orally treated patients, and lowest in patients not treated with dipyridamole. Based on these results, further study of preoperative dipyridamole administration seems warranted.

Calcium channel antagonists are widely used for the treatment of angina pectoris and systemic hypertension (diltiazem, nicardipine, nifedipine, verapamil) and cardiac arrhythmias (verapamil). Consequently, many patients appearing in the operating room for cardiac surgery have been receiving a calcium channel antagonist preoperatively. Calcium channel antagonists have been shown to inhibit in vitro platelet aggregation by decreasing nucleotide release and thromboxane $A_2$ generation. It is theorized that the resulting vasodilation may also contribute to increased blood loss. In animals preoperatively treated with calcium channel antagonists, bleeding from the incision site and measured bleeding time were increased. However, their effect on blood loss and hemorrhagic complications in humans undergoing CAS is not known.[15]

Numerous other commonly used drugs may affect platelet function or cause thrombocytopenia. NSAIDs exhibit, to a somewhat lesser degree, similar antiplatelet properties as aspirin. NSAIDs only inhibit platelet cyclooxygenase temporarily, and platelet function returns to normal after their elimination from the body. High doses of antibiotics (particularly the penicillins) interfere with ADP receptors on the platelet membrane and thus interfere with platelet aggregation. Sodium nitroprusside and nitroglycerin, both commonly used during and after cardiac surgery for reduction of preload, afterload, and blood pressure, can also significantly alter platelet function. Other drugs that affect platelet function or count include bronchodilators, $\beta$-adrenergic blockers, adenosine, diuretics, heparin, protamine, hydralazine, and quinidine.

## FIBRINOLYTIC THERAPY

Heparin is an anticoagulant that accelerates the formation of a molecular complex between antithrombin III and serine proteases of the coagulation system, thereby blocking the enzymatic activity of coagulation factors. The treatment of choice in the first 6 hours after acute myocardial infarction is intravenous thrombolysis, using heparin and/or aspirin, to improve ventricular performance and survival.[44] Heparin (and/or aspirin) have also been used after angiography or percutaneous transluminal coronary angioplasty to prevent reocclusion after successful dilation. Thus, patients arriving in the operating room with evolving or acute myocardial infarction or directly from angiography or unsuccessful angioplasty may be receiving an intravenous heparin infusion. Preoperative heparinization may cause increased bleeding in the pre-CPB period. A delay in surgery of even 12 hours after discontinuation of fibrinolytic therapy can result in a significantly lower requirement for blood components.[45] Unfortunately, delaying surgery is not always a viable option. However, with meticulous surgical and blood salvage technique, a high proportion of blood shed during the pre-CPB period can be retrieved and autotransfused.

# Preoperative Autologous Blood Donation

PABD should be discussed with the patient and if possible implemented in procedures in which blood transfusion is anticipated. A program should be instituted for PABD from patients scheduled to undergo cardiac surgery. Although patients who might not tolerate changes in intravascular volume or oxygen-carrying capacity, including those suffering from congestive heart failure, idiopathic hypertrophic subaortic stenosis, congenital cyanotic heart disease, recent myocardial infarction, and patients with unstable angina and left main coronary artery disease, have been traditionally contraindicated or discouraged from predonating, these views are now being challenged.[46–50] PABD in high-risk patients is often possible but may necessitate a change in venue from the traditional blood bank to one where more aggressive monitoring capabilities, nursing and physician care, and resuscitation equipment are available. The recovery room has been suggested as a potential site for predonation by high-risk patients.[50] Currently, PABD is underused and accounts for only about 2% of blood transfusions in the United States.[51] The reasons include inconvenience to participating patients and blood banks, the high costs involved, and concern over safety factors involved in phlebotomizing patients with cardiac disease.

Clinical studies have shown that the availability of autologous blood significantly reduces the need for allogeneic blood transfusion. Before CAS, the predonation of 3–4 units of blood is ideal. In patients who are able to donate 3–4 units of autologous blood, allogeneic blood usage may be completely eliminated up to 33% of patients and significantly reduced in the remainder.[48,49,52] To stimulate erythropoiesis and maximize the collection, oral iron supplementation should be started at least 1 week before the first donation and continued for several months, or as necessary, after surgery (see Chapter 6: Preoperative Autologous Blood Donation).

The efficacy of recombinant human erythropoietin to increase RBC volume for PABD before the elective surgery is now unquestionable. Hillman and Finch[53] showed that the administration of recombinant human erythropoietin increased erythropoiesis three- to fourfold after 7–10 days of therapy. Goodnough and coworkers[54] demonstrated that patients receiving recombinant human erythropoietin were able to donate more blood than patients receiving placebo. Recombinant human erythropoietin therapy may not only be important preoperatively but also postoperatively to improve recovery of RBC mass.[55] This improvement is limited to the period of therapy; after discontinuation of therapy, the hemoglobin levels rapidly decrease. Levine and colleagues[56] suggested that after CAS, there is a deficiency of endogenous erythropoietin and that the administration of recombinant human erythropoietin may correct this deficiency and accelerate postoperative erythropoiesis.

Recombinant human erythropoietin is available as epoetin alfa (Epogen, Amgen Inc.) for subcutaneous or intravenous administration. The hematopoietic response to recombinant human erythropoietin requires an adequate supply of iron to the bone marrow, and thus therapy should be accompanied by supplemental oral iron administration or iron dextran injection. However, it should be noted that each vial of epoetin alfa contains 2.5 mg of human albumin, which may not be acceptable to some Jehovah's Witnesses.[57,58] There is a possibility that a formulation of recombinant human erythropoietin without human albumin will soon be available that presumably should be acceptable to Jehovah's Witnesses (see Chapter 11: Blood Conservation in Jehovah's Witnesses).

## BLOOD CONSERVATION TECHNIQUES IN THE INTRAOPERATIVE PERIOD

Blood conservation methods during cardiac surgery routinely are used with some degree of variation in major medical centers. These techniques include intraoperative blood withdrawal before CPB, normovolemic hemodilution by priming the oxygenator with crystalloids, salvage of shed blood, reinfusion of remaining blood in oxygenator and tubings back to patient, and accepting some degree of postoperative anemia in the hemodynamically stable patient. Intraoperative bleeding can be minimized by meticulous attention to surgical hemostasis, which includes the use of various hemostatic substances such as bone wax, absorbable gelatin sponge, thrombin, absorbable microfibrillar collagen (Ativene®), oxidized regenerated cellulose (Surgicel®), and fibrin glue (see Chapter 13: Surgical Hemostasis and Blood Conservation: Cardiac and Thoracic Surgery).

## Withdrawal of Blood Before Cardiopulmonary Bypass

The concept of withdrawal of blood in the pre-CPB period was originally introduced by Dodrill and colleagues[59] by removing a portion of the patients own blood and replacing it by allogeneic banked blood. This partial exchange transfusion was aimed at obtaining several units of the patient's own fresh whole blood for transfusion postoperatively while maintaining the intraoperative hematocrit with allogeneic blood. Today, the acceptance of a lower perioperative hemoglobin has enabled the replacement of withdrawn blood with an asanguineous solution rather than allogeneic blood (i.e., acute normovolemic hemodilution).

By avoiding the damaging effects of the pump oxygenator, autologous blood withdrawn before CPB is rich in hemoglobin, functional platelets, and a full complement of coagulation factors. Various investigators have demonstrated that the hemostatic effect of 1 unit of fresh whole blood is roughly the equivalent of 6–10 platelet units.[60,61] Because this blood is autologous, the risks of transfusion-transmitted disease or transfusion reaction are greatly reduced or eliminated. Other advantages include an immediate source of blood in case of acute hemorrhage, no typing and compatibility testing required, and an alternative for patients unable to predonate blood. Finally, this technique with some alterations can be used in patients whose religious beliefs prevent the infusion of extravasated blood that does not remain in continuous contact and motion with their circulating blood (see Chapter 11: Blood Conservation in Jehovah's Witnesses).

The technique of pre-CPB blood withdrawal has been shown to be a safe and effective technique in most patients undergoing elective cardiac surgery. Possible contraindications to the use of pre-CPB blood withdrawal may include a preoperative hemoglobin below 14 g/dL or the presence of unstable angina, abnormal left ventricular function (ejection fraction below 0.5 or cardiac index below 2.5 L/min/m$^2$), left main coronary stenosis, resting ischemic electrocardiographic changes, and impaired lung function.[62]

The collection and reinfusion of autologous blood should be in compliance with standards recommended by the American Association of Blood Banks. It should be safe, aseptic, and assured of adequate identification. Ideally, approximately 15–20% of the patient's estimated blood volume is withdrawn from a central venous access site after the induction of anesthesia and preferably before systemic heparinization. The blood is collected into citrate (citrate-phosphate-dextrose [CPD] or acid-citrate-dextrose [ACD]) anticoagulated blood bags and stored in the operating room. Blood can also be collected after

heparinization, although this method is less desirable and may lead to platelet dysfunction or reheparinization.[63]

In less hemodynamically stable patients and in patients with severe coronary artery disease or aortic stenosis, blood collection should be delayed until after aortic and venous cannulations. This sequence would enable the immediate initiation of CPD should patient condition deteriorate during blood withdrawal. This blood is collected into blood bags without anticoagulants.

The choice of replacement fluid to maintain adequate intravascular volume includes crystalloids, colloids, or combinations of both. In our institution, crystalloid (usually lactated Ringer's solution) is the preferred solution and is administered simultaneously with the removal of blood. The actual volume of blood withdrawal and fluid replacement should be guided by close monitoring of the electrocardiogram and heart rate and arterial central venous pressures, pulmonary artery pressures, and cardiac output.

The autologous blood could be stored in the operating room at room temperature for up to 8 hours or refrigerated at 1–6°C for up to 24 hours. If the blood collected is removed from the presence of the patient, each unit should be labeled with the patient's name, hospital identification number, date and time of collection and expiration, and the statement "For Autologous Use Only."

With the initiation of CPB with a crystalloid prime, a further and more profound hemodilution will develop, especially if the patient is anemic preoperatively. This substantial decrease in oxygen-carrying capacity of the blood may result in ischemia and acidosis. Consequently, patients with severe anemia, unstable angina, left main coronary artery stenosis, and severe aortic stenosis are sometimes excluded from this technique.[64]

After discontinuation of CPB and the reversal of systemic heparinization with protamine, blood transfusion is used to attenuate severe post-CPB anemia. The intraoperatively collected blood is reinfused before the use of any predonated autologous or allogeneic blood.

Various authors have demonstrated significant reductions in blood and blood product usage as well as better postoperative hemostasis. The reduction in blood or blood product usage has been estimated at between 20 and 58%.[62,63,65,66]

## Sequestration of Platelet-Rich Plasma

Thrombocytopenia and platelet dysfunction are common occurrences after CPB[27,61,67-75] (see "Pathophysiology of Platelet Dysfunction during Cardiopulmonary Bypass"). Although the consensus development conference[76] deemed routine platelet administration in cardiac surgery as unwarranted, there remains a significant and continued use of platelets necessitated by clinical bleeding.[77] In an attempt to eliminate or reduce the increased risks associated with the transfusion of pooled blood products, there has been great interest in an autologous source of platelets to promote postoperative hemostasis after cardiac surgery.

Sequestration of platelet-rich plasma by plasmapheresis has been used to reduce perioperative allogeneic blood transfusion and promote postoperative hemostasis.[72,77,78] A modification of the cell processor can enable the pre-CPB sequestration of platelet-rich plasma, which can then be reinfused after the discontinuation of CPB. Before the institution of extracorporeal circulation, blood is withdrawn, through a central venous access site, at a rate of 50–70 mL/min. After anticoagulation with either ACD or CPD, this blood is drawn into the centrifuge bowl, where centrifical force separates cellular components by density from plasma. A needle continuously aspirates platelets, suspending them in the plasma. The plasma, rich in platelets, is transferred into a transfusion bag for storage at room temperature, whereas the RBCs can either be added to the CPB priming solutions or immediately reinfused to the patient. Twenty to 25 mL of platelet-rich plasma can be accumulated per 225- to 250-mL centrifuged blood. In this manner, a mean 337–1000 mL of platelet-rich autologous plasma can be made available for use after bypass.[74,78-82] Both colloid and crystalloid are acceptable for replacement of the lost plasma volume, although the use of colloid has been shown to be superior.[80]

The main advantage of sequestration of platelet-rich plasma is the elimination in risk of transmitting bloodborne disease. FFP is in-variably a pooled blood product, with a dramatically increased risk of transfusion reaction or disease transmission. The use of autologous platelet-rich plasma has been shown to be effective in reducing allogeneic blood requirement in cardiac surgery patients.[75,77,78,82]

## Intraoperative Blood Salvage

Cardiac surgeons were the first to routinely integrate intraoperative blood salvage techniques into their comprehensive program of blood conservation.[83] Intraoperatively, blood salvage is most often accomplished with a centrifuge-based cell processor, yielding packed RBCs suspended in 0.9% NaCl. The cell processor is used primarily before the initiation of CPB to collect blood shed during sternotomy, dissection, and cannulation and after discontinuation of CPB to concentrate residual oxygenator blood and collect blood lost during decannulation and closure. The use of blood salvage techniques is associated with an overall significant reduction in allogeneic blood usage.[84-87] The major indication for the use of blood salvage during cardiac surgery is an anticipated blood loss in excess of 1500 mL, which may include both uncomplicated and complicated CAS, valvular and combination procedures, reoperation, and complex repair of congenital heart defects.[83,87,88] As blood conservation techniques have been successful in significantly reducing or eliminating the need for both autologous and allogeneic blood transfusion in uncomplicated primary CAS, often only collection reservoir, suction tubing and wand, and anticoagulant are routinely set up. This collection apparatus may be a filtration-based blood salvage system or simply a cardiotomy reservoir. If blood loss exceeds expectations, the blood collected in the canister can be reinfused or transferred to a cell processor to salvage RBCs (see Chapter 9: Blood Salvage Techniques).

## Hemoconcentrator as a Blood Conservation Device

The management of excessive hemodilution during extracorporeal circulation has traditionally been accomplished by pharmacological-induced diuresis. However, certain situations arise when diuresis is impractical or too inefficient. In such situations, blood volume adjustments have also been achieved by diverting dilute oxygenator blood to a cell processor for centrifugation into packed cells. This diverted blood can either be stored for postoperative infusion or immediately returned to the oxygenator.[89] However, this method is laborious, time-consuming, and results in loss of platelets and plasma constituents. Furthermore, occasionally when venous return vastly exceeds cardiotomy reservoir and oxygenator capacities, the inefficiency of cell processors in handling large volumes of fluid often necessitates discarding of large amounts of dilute blood. Hemoconcentration by hemofiltration (ultrafiltration) has emerged as the superior method of control of intravascular volume during CPB.

The hemofilter is either a hollow fiber filter or a parallel plate with designated membrane pore size. The hollow fiber filter appears to be more popular because of its ease of use and larger surface-area-to-volume perfusate. Hemofiltration is based on a process that imitates physiological glomerular filtration by applying a hydrostatic pressure gradient across a porous membrane (Fig. 12–3). This efficient method of removing excess circulating blood volume can be achieved without significant alteration in serum electrolyte concentrations or acid-base status. Ultrafiltrate removal at rates greater than 100 mL/min of plasma water are possible. Because the composition of the ultrafiltrate is similar to glomerular filtrate with concentrations of solute the same as plasma water, electrolyte and acid-base status remain stable. The technique of hemoconcentration is a convective process with plasma and dissolved solutes filtering at the same rate, limited only by the pore size of the device. Transmembrane pressure (gradient) is the driving force and is calculated by the formula

$$TMP = \frac{P_A + P_V}{2} + |P_N|$$

where TMP is the transmembrane pressure (mm Hg), $P_A$ is the arterial (inlet) pressure (mm Hg), $P_V$ is the venous (outlet) pressure (mm Hg), and $|P_N|$ is the absolute value of the negative pressure at the ultrafiltrate outlet (mm Hg). To avoid RBC lysis, the transmembrane pressure should remain below 600 mm Hg.[84] Ultrafiltrate flux is determined by several factors, including properties of the membrane, pump flow rate, transmembrane pressure, hematocrit, and plasma protein concentration.[90] Membrane pore size varies among manufacturers (16,000–60,000 d). Depending on pore size, heparin with a molecular weight of less than 20,000 d can be filtered.[91] Thus, anticoagulation status should be closely monitored during intraoperative use and for post-CPB concentration of residual oxygenator blood.[84,91]

Originally developed for the treatment of renal failure, hemofiltration was first used during cardiac surgery to concentrate residual oxygenator blood after CPB. The hemofilter is now commonly incorporated into the extra-

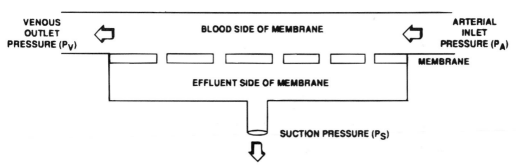

**Fig. 12–3.** Hemofiltration of free water and solutes across a semipermeable membrane occurs because of a combination of the blood pressure differential across the filter—the mean of the arterial inlet pressure ($P_A$) and the venous outlet pressure ($P_V$)—and any vacuum pressure placed on the effluent side of the membrane ($P_N$). The combination of these pressures is equal to the transmembrane pressure, which is the primary factor determining filtration rate. Modified from Moore RA, Laub GW: Hemofiltration, dialysis, and blood salvage techniques during cardiopulmonary bypass. In: Gravlee GP, Davis RF, Utley JR, eds, Cardiopulmonary Bypass: Principles and Practice. Baltimore, 1993, Williams & Wilkins, pp. 93–123, with permission.

corporeal circuit to regulate the extracorporeal volume during CPB while preserving platelets, coagulation factors, and plasma proteins.[90,92,93] The placement of the hemofilter with the extracorporeal circuit depends on when the decision to use hemofiltration was made (before or after institution of CPB) and depending on type of oxygenator (bubble or membrane). When incorporated before CPB in both bubble and membrane oxygenator systems, the hemofilter can serve as a branch from the arterial line filter, with outflow returned to the cardiotomy reservoir (Fig. 12–4). After the institution of CPB, hemofil-

tration can be accomplished by diversion of blood directly from the bubble oxygenator through the hemofilter and draining into the cardiotomy reservoir (Fig. 12–5). When using a membrane oxygenator, the ultrafilter can branch off the recirculation line and drain into the cardiotomy reservoir (Fig. 12–3).[94]

Currently, the main use of the hemofilter in cardiac surgery is for the purpose of hemoconcentration of hemodiluted blood during CPB. Hemoconcentration offers many advantages over cell processing, including the ability to precisely control hematocrit and preservation plasma electrolytes, proteins (albumin),

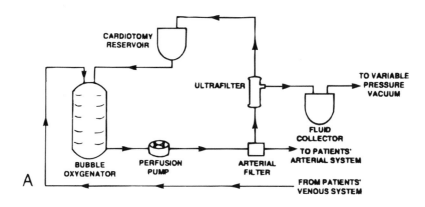

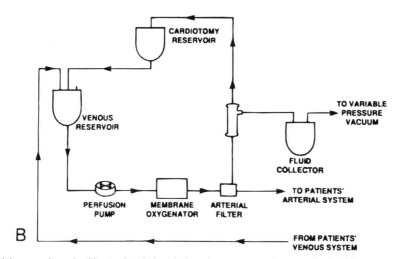

**Fig. 12–4.** If the use of an ultrafilter is decided on before the initiation of CPB and a bubble oxygenator is used, a branch connector from the arterial line filter is the easiest method for establishing hemofiltration (A). With the use of a membrane oxygenator, a branch connection from the arterial line filter can also be used effectively, with return of the filtered blood to the cardiotomy reservoir (B). The effluent outlet in both cases is connected to a variable pressure vacuum. From Moore RA, Laub GW: Hemofiltration, dialysis, and blood salvage techniques during cardiopulmonary bypass. In: Gravlee GP, Davis RF, Utley JR, eds, Cardiopulmonary Bypass: Principles and Practice. Baltimore, 1993, Williams & Wilkins, pp. 93–123, with permission.

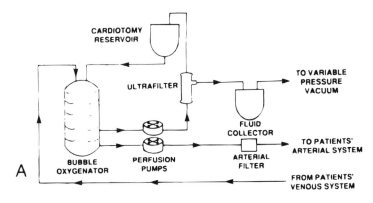

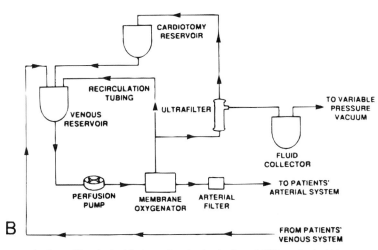

**Fig. 12–5.** If the use of a hemofilter is decided on after the institution of CPB and a bubble oxygenator is used, a separate dedicated pump head can be used to direct blood from the coronary arterial port of the oxygenator into the hemofilter (A). In the case of a membrane oxygenator (B), blood flow to the hemofilter can be established by using a branch connector from the recirculation tubing. In this situation, the perfusion pump flow will have to be increased to compensate for perfusion that is redirected from the patient into the hemofilter. From Moore RA, Laub GW: Hemofiltration, dialysis, and blood salvage techniques during cardiopulmonary bypass. In: Gravlee GP, Davis RF, Utley JR, eds, Cardiopulmonary Bypass: Principles and Practice. Baltimore, 1993, Williams & Wilkins, pp. 93–123, with permission.

colloid osmotic pressure, platelets, and fibrinogen.[95–100] Other advantages of the hemoconcentrator are speed, lower cost, and single pass hemofiltration at rates of 500 mL/min.[101] The downside of the hemofilter over a cell processor are higher concentrations of plasma free hemoglobin and proteolytic enzymes. However, plasma free hemoglobin values are rarely in excess of 10.0 $\mu$g/dL, and evidence of leukocyte activation is also seen in blood recycled by cell processing.[100] The clinical implications of these negative aspects are not fully understood.

There are no absolute contraindications for the use of hemoconcentration during or after cardiac surgery. Although passage of blood through a filter system should lead to RBC damage, significant increases in serum free hemoglobin concentrations have not been observed during use of the hemoconcentrator.[99,102] Other potential concerns include activation of the complement cascade and leukocyte sequestration in the pulmonary circulation. Immunological reactions to ultrafilter materials also have been reported.[103]

## Reinfusion of Residual Oxygenator Blood

After the discontinuation of CPB, several hundred milliliters of blood remain in the oxygenator. Previously, this dilute blood-prime mixture was slowly infused through the aortic canulae until acceptable left and right heart filling pressures were achieved. In many patients, however, it was impossible to infuse the total oxygenator contents without producing hypervolemia and ventricular failure.[104-106] Furthermore, objections about the safety of infusing oxygenator blood have been raised. These objections included an extremely low hematocrit,[105] damaged RBCs by mechanical trauma of the pump oxygenator,[107] acidotic infusate, and the heparin content.[108] Upon the introduction of cell-processing devices, it was recognized that many of the drawbacks to reinfusion of residual oxygenator blood could be avoided by hemoconcentration of this blood by centrifugation and washing, yielding concentrated RBCs.[104,105,108-113]

## Antifibrinolytics

### APROTININ

Aprotinin, a natural polypeptide serine protease inhibitor currently isolated from bovine lung tissue, has been used in Europe for more than three decades for treatment in pancreatitis, fibrinolysis, and shock. Since Royston and coworkers[114] and Van Oeveren and coworkers[115] reported decreased bleeding after CPB in patients treated with aprotinin, interest in this drug has increased. Although the drug has been intensively studied over the last several years, the exact mechanism of action is still not well understood.[116-118]

A major source of blood loss after CPB, postperfusion syndrome has been attributed to complement activation when blood contacts the foreign surfaces of the extracorporeal circuit. The resulting whole-body inflammatory reaction affects platelets and hemostatic mechanisms through release of proteolytic enzymes (proteases), such as plasmin and kallikrein. These proteases block two main receptors in platelets, the von Willebrand and fibrinogen receptors. The von Willebrand receptor, important in platelet adhesion, can be blocked by plasmin. The fibrinogen receptor, important for platelet aggregation, is affected by adenosine, thromboxane $A_2$, and proteolytic enzymes. The administration of aprotinin seems to have a protective effect on platelet receptors by blocking plasmin activity and maintaining normal platelets function and hemostatic mechanisms, thus reducing postoperative bleeding and blood loss.[119] Marx and coworkers[120] demonstrated a suppression of systemic and local fibrinolysis and thus fibrin and fibrinogen degradation products. Their study did not, however, demonstrate a protective effect on platelets, suggesting the hemostatic effects of aprotinin are related to its antifibrinolytic action rather than its action on platelets.

The use of aprotinin has made a considerable contribution to blood conservation in cardiac surgery. The need for allogeneic blood is greatly reduced, and postoperative anemia is avoided. Intraoperative aprotinin administration has resulted in an approximate threefold decrease in postoperative blood loss after CAS, with a significant reduction in blood transfusion requirements.[37,115,121,122] The bleeding time stays within the normal range with aprotinin, although the platelet count is reduced. In patients at higher risk of bleeding postoperatively (reoperation, valve replacement in acute stage of endocarditis), the benefits of aprotinin is greater. Because a majority of patients receiving aprotinin have not required allogeneic blood transfusion, patients who for religious or other reasons cannot or will not accept blood transfusion will benefit from its use.[114,122-126]

The prophylactic use of aprotinin is indicated for reducing perioperative blood loss and transfusion requirements of blood and blood products for patients undergoing repeat CAS and for selected primary CAS where the risk of bleeding is especially high (impaired hemostasis) or when transfusion is unavailable or unacceptable (Jehovah's Witnesses).[114,127] The use of aprotinin in low-risk primary CAS and valvular repair or replacement procedures is probably unwarranted. Not only are these procedures associated with less blood loss, but clinical studies in these patients have failed to demonstrate statistically significant decreases in blood loss or transfusion requirement.

The drug is water soluble and is supplied as a clear colorless sterile isotonic solution containing 10,000 kallikrein inhibitor units (KIU)/mL (1.4 mg/mL) at a pH of

4.5–6.5.[128] Aprotinin is supplied in 100- or 200-mL vials containing 140 (1 million KIU) and 280 (2 million KIU) mg, respectively. The recommended dosage regimen is as follows. A test dose of 1 mL (1.4 mg or 10,000 KIU) is administered at least 10 minutes before the loading dose. After induction of anesthesia, but before sternotomy, and in the absence of allergic reaction, a loading dose of 200 mL (280 mg = 2.0 million KIU) is given intravenously over 20–30 minutes with the patient in supine position. After infusion of the loading dose, a constant infusion of aprotinin 50 mL/h (70 mg/h = 500,000 KIU/h) is begun and continues until surgery is complete. Finally, 200 mL of aprotinin is added to the pump priming solution.[121,124,126,129] All intravenous doses of aprotinin should be administered through a dedicated central line, avoiding contact with other drugs or solutions. Anaphylaxis to aprotinin has occurred in less than 0.5% of cases but is greater in patients repeatedly exposed to the drug. Despite an uneventful test dose, or without previous exposure to aprotinin, the full therapeutic dose may cause anaphylaxis.

The addition of aprotinin to the prime is associated with an increased activated clotting time during CPB ($834 \pm 30$ versus $495 \pm 29$ seconds). Furthermore, the activated clotting time remained above 400 seconds throughout the period of CPB without the necessity for additional doses of heparin and responded appropriately to the administration of protamine.[125] Wang and colleagues[130] demonstrated that the increase in activated coagulation time (ACT) is caused by the interaction of aprotinin with celite used as surface activator in the ACT test and not from inhibition of the coagulation system, whereas the use of kaolin-ACT reflected ACT more accurately. Therefore, it has been recommended that ACT be maintained above 750 seconds,[131–133] or a fixed regimen of heparin should be used,[134] usually 3–4 mg/kg before CPB followed by 1 mg/kg/hr during CPB should be used. Alternatively, the use of a whole-blood high-dose thrombin time assay (Hemochron, International Technidyne Corp., Edison, NJ), which is unaffected by aprotinin, has been described.

## SYNTHETIC ANTIFIBRINOLYTICS

The synthetic lysine analogs EACA and TA (AMCA; Cyklokapron, KabiVitrum, Ala-meda, CA) have antifibrinolytic properties because of their reversible complex formation with plasminogen and with the active protease, plasmin. They bind to plasminogen or plasmin at the lysine binding sites, displacing plasminogen from the fibrin molecule surface. Even if plasminogen is converted to active plasmin, this drug's binding to plasmin will prevent binding of plasmin to fibrin and hence inhibit its proteolytic activity.[135] It is postulated that these drugs prevent the premature dissolution of normal fibrin clots. Both EACA and TA undergo minimal metabolism, mostly excreted in urine unchanged within a few hours. Because of their short half-lives, they are administered as a bolus followed by intravenous infusion. Antifibrinolytic therapy is contraindicated in the presence of disseminating intravascular coagulation and can theoretically be associated with an increased risk of systemic thrombosis.[135]

The use of EACA and TA have been effective in reducing bleeding in various clinical situations.[135–141] However, its use in cardiac surgery is controversial. EACA was widely used in the 1960s and 1970s for the prevention and treatment of bleeding during cardiac valvular surgery and correction of congenital heart defects, with generally favorable results.[142–144] However, these early studies were uncontrolled, nonrandomized, and retrospective, ignoring possible preexisting coagulation defects associated with congenital heart disease and the various types of CPB equipment used. Prospective studies revealed that EACA was somewhat effective in reducing blood loss in patients with cyanotic congenital heart defects on CPB for over 60 minutes[145] and in reducing transfusion requirement but not overall blood loss in adults undergoing CAS.[138,139] These minimal beneficial effects of EACA in regard to bleeding and the uncertainty of possible increased thrombotic events have generally discouraged it clinical use. The prophylactic use of EACA in patients undergoing primary combined CAS and valve surgery or any reoperation has been recommended.[146] To achieve a therapeutic plasma concentration of EACA (13 mg/dL) requires an intravenous loading dose of 100–150 mg/kg followed by an infusion at 10–15 mg/kg/h.

The prophylactic TA administration has been shown to be safe and effective in reducing blood loss and transfusion requirement after cardiac surgery.[140,147,148] TA has approximately 10 times the potency and provides more intense and longer fibrinolytic activity than EACA, requiring a loading dose of 10 mg/kg and an infusion at 0.5–1 mg/kg/ h.[135]

Although both EACA and TA have been shown to be effective in selected situations, their efficacy in cardiac surgery has not been clearly established, and thus their routine use cannot be recommended.

## Measures to Decrease Blood Loss after Cardiopulmonary Bypass

### PERIOPERATIVE MONITORING OF HEMOSTASIS

After termination of CPB, heparin should be neutralized by protamine sulfate. ACT, used to monitor the adequacy of heparinization during CPB, is the most practical and widely used instrument to monitor the heparin neutralization. Heparinization is fully reversed when the ACT is within the normal range of 90–110 seconds. However, the ACT is subject to inaccuracies under various conditions, such as excess protamine sulfate, hypofibrinogenemia, hypothermia, and hemodilution.[134] Thrombocytopenia and platelet dysfunction also prolong the ACT. Alternatives to the use of ACT include the Hepcon (Medtronic-HemoTec, Inc., Parker, CO) and Rx-Dx (International Technidyne, Inc., Edison, NJ) systems, which use protamine and heparin titration to monitor hemostasis.

After CPB, coagulation tests are usually abnormal, platelet count is low, platelet function impaired, and bleeding time prolonged. Therefore, trends in laboratory values are more important than the individual values. Treatment of postoperative nonsurgical bleeding is determined by laboratory evaluation of platelet count, prothrombin and activated partial thromboplastin time, bleeding time, thrombin time, and fibrinogen levels. An approach to the management of diffuse bleeding is presented in Figure 12–6.[21]

### DESMOPRESSIN

Desmopressin acetate is a synthetic vasopressin analog. It's hemostatic properties are derived from increase in plasma levels of factor VIII, von Willebrand factor, and enhanced platelet adhesiveness to vascular subendothelium. The infusion of desmopressin (0.3 μg/ kg) in patients with von Willebrand's disease, mild hemophiliacs, and uremic patients results in a shortening of bleeding time and a reduction in surgical blood loss.

The effect of desmopressin, administered after CPB and reversal of heparin, in reducing blood loss and transfusion requirements in patients undergoing complicated cardiac procedures has been studied. Desmopressin significantly reduced both intraoperative and postoperative blood loss without apparent adverse effects.[73,149] However, the use of desmopressin was not found to be beneficial in cardiac surgery for children,[150–152] in primary CAS,[153,154] in CAS patients on antiplatelet therapy, nor in adults with valvular and congenital heart anomolies[155] and was associated with hypotension and decreased systemic vascular resistance.[156,157]

The beneficial effects of desmopressin in decreasing blood loss in the post-CPB period was reviewed by Morgan and Hosking.[158] In patients with abnormal platelet function (diagnosed by thromboelastography), desmopressin significantly reduced mediastinal chest drainage and requirements for blood transfusion. However, the conflicting results indicate that the routine use of desmopressin in uncomplicated cardiac surgical cases cannot be recommended until further controlled studies determine the role of desmopressin in cardiac surgery.[159]

### BLOOD COMPONENT THERAPY

#### Platelet Therapy

***Pathophysiology of Platelet Disfunction During Cardiopulmonary Bypass.*** Hemodilution is a major cause of decrease in platelet count during CPB.[160] The volume of crystalloid used in prime solution will affect the degree of thrombocytopenia, usually a 50% reduction due to the hemodilution effect,[161] platelet adhesion to synthetic surfaces, and platelet aggregate formation. This reduction in platelet count occurs immediately after the institution of CPB, and further decreases may occur over the next several days. Platelet count usually returns to preoperative values by the 6th or 7th day.

Damage to platelets is multifactorial during

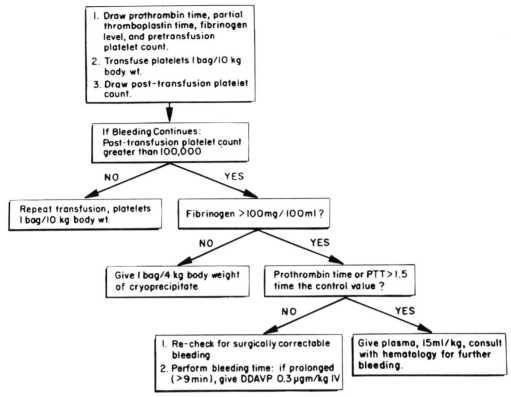

1. Draw prothrombin time, partial thromboplastin time, fibrinogen level, and pretransfusion platelet count.
2. Transfuse platelets I bag/IO kg body wt.
3. Draw post-transfusion platelet count.

If Bleeding Continues:
Post-transfusion platelet count greater than 100,000

NO → Repeat transfusion, platelets I bag/IO kg body wt.

YES → Fibrinogen >100mg/100ml ?

NO → Give I bag/4 kg body weight of cryoprecipitate

YES → Prothrombin time or PTT>1.5 time the control value ?

NO →
1. Re-check for surgically correctable bleeding
2. Perform bleeding time: if prolonged (>9min), give DDAVP 0.3μgm/kg IV

YES → Give plasma, 15ml/kg, consult with hematology for further bleeding.

**Fig. 12–6.** Management of postoperative bleeding in cardiac surgery patients: an algorithm approach. DDAVP, deamino-D-arginine vasopressin; PTT, partial thromboplastin time. From Goodnough LT, Johnston MFM, Ramsey G, et al.: Guidelines for transfusion support in patients undergoing coronary artery bypass grafting. Ann Thorac Surg 1990; 50:675, with permission.

CPB. Turbulent flow and shear stresses are generated during extracorporeal circulation. Cardiotomy suction, which returns blood from the operative field, provides blood-air and blood-tissue interfaces at which platelet activation may occur. The loss of platelets correlates with the amount of blood suctioned from the surgical field.[162] Platelets also adhere to the surfaces of the extracorporeal perfusion apparatus.[22,163,164] Oxygenators and filters provide additional surfaces for platelet activation and destruction.[165] The degree of platelet dysfunction is proportional to the duration of CPB and the degree of hypothermia.[161,164,166,167] Other factors causing qualitative and quantitative platelet abnormality are aggregation of platelets induced by pulmonary artery catheters, heparin, protamine sulfate, heparin-protamine complexes, hemolysis, and disseminated intravascular coagulation.

The intravenous infusion of protamine sulfate after CPB reduces platelet count by one-third, within a few minutes.[168] This effect could be due to temporary sequestration of platelets in the liver and lasts for less than 1 hour. In most patients, platelet dysfunction reverses within a few hours after discontinuation of CPB.[162,164] When platelet dysfunction persists, abnormal bleeding usually occurs. The presence of clinically abnormal bleeding does not correlate with platelet count during the perioperative period because the platelet count is usually not low enough to be an explanation. If platelets are functionally normal with a platelet count over $100,000/\mu L$, abnormal bleeding is unlikely. In this case, the platelet count must drop below $50,000/\mu L$ before bleeding will occur.[169] Thus, platelet dysfunction is a more important factor in causing bleeding in the perioperative period than the platelet count.

*Platelet Transfusion.* Platelets harvested from a single donor by platelet pheresis provides the platelet equivalent of 5–8 units of whole blood. However, these platelets, though having the advantage of minimal exposure, are usually in small supply. The majority of platelets available is separated from whole blood donations from multiple donors and pooled before administration. Each unit of platelets raises the platelet count by 5000–10,000/$\mu$L in the average adult.

After CPB and reversal of heparin, platelet count is reduced, platelet function is impaired, and bleeding time is prolonged. Abnormal post-CPB bleeding may occur with a definable or predictable cause. Coagulation studies may be helpful when surgical bleeding is not the etiology of excessive hemorrhage. Bleeding time after cessation of CPB is prolonged, although most patients do not bleed abnormally. A bleeding time longer than 20 minutes after administration of protamine sulfate and in the presence of abnormal bleeding may indicate the transfusion of platelets, even when the platelet count is adequate ($>$100,000/$\mu$L).[170] Because it is not always practical to check bleeding time intraoperatively, thromboelastography may be useful in determining the need for platelet transfusion. Patients on antiplatelet therapy preoperatively will increase the likelihood of postoperative platelet administration. It should be emphasized that platelets should be given only if necessary and not based on the duration of CPB, amount of autologous or allogeneic transfused, isolated laboratory tests, preoperative drug therapy, or on a protocol basis. There is no justification for prophylactic platelet administration.[21,76,171]

## Coagulation Factors

Hemodilution associated with CPB produces a significant reduction in most coagulation factors.[160] These reductions will persist intraoperatively and gradually return to normal levels within 48 hours. Under normal conditions, reduction in coagulation factor levels will not lead to abnormal bleeding because these levels are still adequate for hemostasis. However, further hemodilution or the presence of preexisting coagulation defects could precipitate abnormal bleeding during and after surgery.

Indications for the use of FFP and cryoprecipitate in cardiac surgery are limited and specific. There is no scientific evidence supporting prophylactic use of either FFP or cryoprecipitate as replacement therapy in massive transfusion or during cardiac surgery.[161,171,172] Whenever possible, or ideally before administration of blood components, measurements of platelet count, prothrombin time, and activated partial thromboplastin times are advisable to validate the clinical decision for transfusion.

### Fresh Frozen Plasma

FFP should not be used for volume expansion, nutritional support, and coagulation factor replacement in patients needing massive transfusion, because coagulation factors rarely decrease to such critically low levels as to be the cause of abnormal bleeding. FFP administration in cardiac surgery should be limited to patients with acquired deficiency of vitamin K-dependant coagulation factors caused by warfarin or congestive hepatic dysfunction. FFP may rarely be required for patients with inherited deficiencies of factors V, VII, X, or XI who are undergoing cardiac surgery.[161,173]

The consensus conference for FFP[174] concluded that indications for FFP are as follows: (*a*) replacement of isolated factor deficiency, which includes factors II, V, VII, IX, X, and XI when specific component therapy is unavailable or inappropriate; (*b*) for the reversal of the effects of sodium warfarin; (*c*) treatment of pathological bleeding in patients who have received massive transfusions of more than one blood volume (In these patients, abnormal coagulation usually is the result of dilutional thrombocytopenia or platelet dysfunction. Platelet transfusion should be attempted first and if ineffective, then FFP should be used.); (*d*) in antithrombin III deficiency; and (*e*) treatment of immunodeficiencies.

### Cryoprecipitate

Cryoprecipitate administration may be needed for patients with von Willebrand's disease who are undergoing cardiac surgery.[161,175–177] Cryoprecipitate also may be indicated for patients who have had unsuccessful thrombolytic therapy and develop excessive bleeding after emergency CAS.[161] Cryoprecipitate provides a more concentrated level of fibrinogen than is present in FFP: 1 unit containing 100 antihemophilic units and

250 mg of fibrinogen. Patients having a massive and rapid transfusion, particularly when intravascular coagulopathy has developed after prolonged shock, may benefit from the additional factor VIII and fibrinogen given as cryoprecipitate.

### Fibrin Glue

In cardiac surgery, local hemostasis may be improved by topical fibrin glues.[178–181] The fibrin is formed by the local application of reconstituted topical thrombin with fibrinogen and factor XIII obtained from cryoprecipitate or autologous plasma.[178,179,181] If a high concentration of fibrinogen (90 mg/mL) is used, local hemostasis may be achieved in more than 95% of patients despite the presence of systemic heparinization.[178] Fibrin glue has been particularly useful in CAS associated with internal mammary grafts,[178] reoperation for bleeding,[181] and vascular prostheses.[179] Potential complications of this material include tamponade due to adhesions, transfusion-transmitted viral infections (although the risks do not exceed that associated with FFP transfusion), and the development of thrombin and factor V inhibitors after exposure to bovine thrombin glue.[179,181,182]

## BLOOD CONSERVATION MEASURES IN THE POSTOPERATIVE PERIOD

Causes of excessive postoperative bleeding after cardiac surgery include hemostatic derangements resulting from CPB (inadequate heparin reversal, thrombocytopenia or platelet dysfunction, complement activation, coagulation factor consumption or dilution, and fibrinolysis), surgical sources (trauma from the surgical incision and dissection, sites of arterial and venous cannulation for CPB or previous cardiac catheterization, sites of saphenous vein harvesting, and bypass graft anastomoses and side branches), and preoperative and early postoperative factors (drugs that interfere with normal hemostasis, postoperative hypertension, preexisting inherited or acquired diseases or disorders affecting coagulation, structural lesions or neoplasms of the gastrointestinal or genitourinary tracts).[11]

Blood conservation techniques in the postoperative period are of little value if surgical bleeding is not controlled. Moreover, excessive mediastinal bleeding after cardiac surgery is associated with increased incidences of heart failure, hypotension, shock, dysrhythmias, infection, and mortality.[11,143] Thus, early return to the operating room for reexploration is beneficial not only from a blood conservation standpoint but also reduces morbidity and mortality. Mediastinal exploration is required in 3–14% of cardiac surgical procedures and is indicated when chest tube drainage exceeds 500 mL/h or over 300 mL/h for 3 consecutive hours.[24]

## Prevention of Postoperative Hypertension

Control of postoperative hypertension is another important aspect of reducing blood loss after cardiac surgery. Other hazards of untreated hypertension in the early postoperative period include bleeding or rupture of fresh vascular anastomoses, depressed left-ventricular function, increased myocardial oxygen consumption, cerebrovascular accidents, myocardial ischemia, and infarction. A hypertensive episode has been defined as an arterial blood pressure above 160/100 mm Hg in previously normotensive patients or an increase of more than 30 mm Hg (systolic or diastolic) above preoperative levels in hypertensive patients.[183] Hypertension occurs after CPB in 15–60% of patients undergoing CAS.[183] The causes of postoperative hypertension are unclear and may involve several mechanisms. Suggested mechanisms include arousal from anesthesia, tracheal or nasopharyngeal manipulations, pain, hypothermia, shivering, inadequate ventilation, and use of pressor agents as well as diminishing effect of antihypertensive medication. In addition, postoperative coronary insufficiency, myocardial infarction, and sympathetic response to hypovolemia may also contribute to hypertension.[183] Control of hypertension may be accomplished by continuation of $\beta$-adrenergic and calcium channel blockade and antihypertensive drugs throughout the perioperative period and by appropriate use of narcotics and benzodiazepines, vasodilator drugs, and muscle relaxants.[184,185] Therapy is aimed at achieving a systolic blood pressure between 110 and 130 mm Hg, although a somewhat higher systemic pressure may be required in patients with cerebral, renal, or intestinal hypoperfusion syndromes.[183]

## Acceptance of Postoperative Anemia

An increasing knowledge of hemodilution and its physiological effects allows lower degrees of anemia to be accepted as safe levels perioperatively.[11,186–188] Available evidence does not support the 10 g/dL hemoglobin (or 30% hematocrit) "transfusion trigger" that has traditionally been used by anesthesiologists and surgeons.[186,189,190] In patients with good ventricular function, blood loss can usually be replaced with appropriate volumes of crystalloid or colloid. Post-CPB hematocrits of 24% (or even lower) are often acceptable in these patients.[189–191] In critically ill patients with fixed cardiac outputs, increased oxygen demand, or dependent on inotropic support, higher hematocrits may be necessary[187] (see Chapter 5: Perioperative Hemoglobin Requirements and Chapter 7: Acute Normovolemic Hemodilution).

## Postoperative Autotransfusion

Mediastinal drainage after cardiac surgery is a major source of blood loss during the perioperative period. However, the collection and reinfusion of mediastinal chest drainage remains a controversial subject. Although studies have indicated that postoperative autotransfusion can reduce allogeneic blood requirement,[12,192–195] the technique is neither universally accepted nor routinely used.[196] Postoperative blood salvage is most commonly accomplished with filtration-based blood salvage devices. Blood draining from mediastinal chest tubes is collected in reservoir drawing at a negative pressure of −20 cm H$_2$O. The addition of an underwater seal prevents communication between the pleural cavity, mediastinum, and the ambient environment.[197] Because mediastinal chest drainage is devoid of fibrinogen, anticoagulation is usually unnecessary unless bleeding is profuse, in which case early reexploration is probably indicated.[70] A detailed discussion of postoperative blood salvage after cardiac surgery can be found in Chapter 9 on Blood Salvage Techniques.

### REFERENCES

1. Killip T: Twenty years of coronary artery bypass surgery. N Engl J Med 1988; 319:366.

2. Goodnough LT, Johnston MF, Toy PTCY: The variability of transfusion practice in coronary artery bypass surgery. JAMA 1991; 265:86.

3. Øvrum E, Åm Holen E, Lindstein-Ringdal M-A: Elective coronary artery bypass surgery without homologous blood transfusion. Early results with an inexpensive blood conservation program. Scand J Thorac Cardiovasc Surg 1991; 25:13.

4. Hynes MS: Whole blood transfusions are useful in patients undergoing cardiac surgery. Pro J Cardiothorac Vasc Anesth 1992; 6:756.

5. Cosgrove DM, Thurer RL, Lytle BW, et al.: Blood conservation during myocardial revascularization. Ann Thorac Surg 1979; 28:184.

6. Weniger J, Shanahan R: Reduction of bank blood requirements in cardiac surgery. Thorac Cardiovasc Surg 1982; 30:142.

7. Loop FD: Catastrophic hemorrhage during sternal reentry. Ann Thorac Surg 1984; 37:271.

8. Estafanous FG: Anesthesia for heart reoperation. In: Estafanous FG, ed, Anesthesia and the Heart Patient. Boston, 1989, Butterworths.

9. Estafanous FG: Management of emergency revascularization and cardiac reoperation. In: Kaplan JA, ed, Cardiac Anesthesia. Philadelphia, 1987, W.B. Saunders, vol. 2, pp. 845–848.

10. Salomon NW, Scott Page U, Bigelow JC, et al.: Reoperative coronary surgery: comparative analysis of 6591 patients undergoing primary bypass and 508 patients undergoing reoperative coronary artery bypass. J Thorac Cardiovasc Surg 1990; 100: 250.

11. Czer LSC: Mediastinal bleeding after cardiac surgery: etiologies, diagnostic considerations, and blood conservation methods. J Cardiothorac Anesth 1989; 3:760.

12. Cosgrove DM, Loop FD, Lytle BW, et al.: Determinants of blood utilization during myocardial revascularization. Ann Thorac Surg 1985; 40:380.

13. Ferraris VA, Gildengorin V: Predictors of excessive blood use after coronary artery bypass grafting: a multivariate analysis. J Thorac Cardiovasc Surg 1989; 98:492.

14. Hennekens CH, Buring JE, Sandercock P, et al.: Aspirin and other antiplatelet agents in the secondary and primary prevention of cardiovascular disease. Circulation 1989; 80:749.

15. Becker RC, Alpert JS: The impact of medical therapy on hemorrhagic complications following coronary artery bypass grafting. Arch Intern Med 1990; 150:2016.

16. Hennekens CH: Role of aspirin with thrombolytic therapy in acute myocardial infarction. Chest 1990; 97:151S.

17. Sethi GK, Copeland JG, Goldman S, et al.: Implications of preoperative administration of aspirin in patients undergoing coronary artery bypass grafting. J Am Coll Cardiol 1990; 15:15.

18. Bashein G, Nessly ML, Rice AL, et al.: Preoperative aspirin therapy and reoperation for bleeding after coronary artery bypass surgery. Arch Intern Med 1991; 151:89.

19. Morengo-Rowe AJ, Lambert CJ, Levenson JE, et al.: The evaluation of hemorrhage in cardiac patients who have undergone extracorporeal circulation. Transfusion 1979; 19:426.

20. Suchman AL, Mushlin AI: How well does the activated partial thromboplastin time predict postoperative hemorrhage? JAMA 1986; 256:750.

21. Goodnough LT, Johnston MF, Ramsey G, et al.: Guidelines for transfusion support in patients undergoing coronary artery bypass grafting. Ann Thorac Surg 1990; 50:675.

22. Bick RL: Hemostasis defects associated with cardiac surgery, prosthetic devices, and other extracorporeal circuits. Semin Thromb Hemost 1985; 11:249.

23. Torosian M, Michelson EL, Morganroth J, et al.: Aspirin and coumadin-related bleeding after coronary artery bypass grafting surgery. Ann Intern Med 1978; 89:325.

24. Yared J-P, Estafanous FG: Blood conservation during cardiac surgery. Curr Opin Anaesthesiol 1992; 5:82.

25. Ferraris VA, Swanson E: Aspirin usage and perioperative blood loss in patients undergoing unexpected operations. Surg Gynecol Obstet 1983; 156:439.

26. Ferraris VA, Ferraris SP, Lough FC, et al.: Preoperative aspirin ingestion increases operative blood loss after coronary artery bypass grafting. Ann Thorac Surg 1988; 45:71.

27. Inada E: Blood coagulation and autologous blood transfusion in cardiac surgery. J Clin Anesth 1990; 2:393.

28. Simon TL: Platelet consumption and dysfunction. In: Rossi EC, Simon TL, Moss GS, eds, Principles of Transfusion Medicine. Baltimore, 1991, Williams & Wilkins, pp. 265–269.

29. Lewis HD, Davis JW, Archibald DG, et al.: Protective effect of aspirin against acute myocardial infarction and death in men with unstable angina. N Engl J Med 1983; 309:396.

30. Carins J, Gent M, Singer J, et al.: Aspirin, sulfinpyrazone, or both in unstable angina. N Engl J Med 1985; 313:1369.

31. Schwartz L, Bourassa MG, Lesperance J, et al.: Aspirin and dipyridamole in the prevention of restenosis after percutaneous transluminal coronary angioplasty. N Engl J Med 1988; 318:1714.

32. Chesebro JH, Clements IP, Fuster V, et al.: A platelet inhibitor drug trial in coronary artery bypass operations. Benefit of perioperative dipyridamole and aspirin therapy on early postoperative vein-graft patency. N Engl J Med 1982; 307:73.

33. Chesebro JH, Fuster V, Elveback LR, et al.: Effect of dipyridamole and aspirin on late vein-graft patency after coronary bypass operations. N Engl J Med 1984; 310:209.

34. Barner HB: Coronary artery bypass surgery with minimal use of homologous blood. Effects of a simple and inexpensive blood conservation programme (Letter). Eur J Cardiothorac Surg 1991; 5:111.

35. Clagett CP: Perioperative assessment of hemostasis. In: Rossi EC, Simon TL, Moss GS, eds, Principles of Transfusion Medicine. Baltimore, 1991, Williams & Wilkins, pp. 453–460.

36. Kobrinsky NL, Isreals ED, Gerrard OM, et al.: Shortening the bleeding time by 1-deamino-8-D-arginine vasopressin in various bleeding disorders. Lancet 1984; 1:1145.

37. Murkin JM, Lux JA, Shannon NA, et al.: Aprotinin significantly decreases bleeding and transfusion requirements in patients receiving aspirin and undergoing cardiac operations. J Thorac Cardiovasc Surg 1994; 107:554.

38. Webster MWI, Chesebro JH, Fuster V: Dipyridamole. In: Messerli FH, ed, Cardiovascular Drug Therapy. Philadelphia, 1990, W.B. Saunders, pp. 1434–1443.

39. Nuntinsen LS, Pihlajaniemi R, Saarela E, et al.: The effect of dipyridamole on the thrombocyte count and bleeding tendency in open-heart surgery. J Thorac Cardiovasc Surg 1977; 74:295.

40. Feinberg H, Rosenbaum DS, Levitsky S, et al.: Platelet deposition after surgically induced myocardial ischemia: an etiologic factor for reperfusion injury. J Thorac Cardiovasc Surg 1982; 84:815.

41. Teoh KH, Christakis CT, Weisel RD, et al.: Prevention of myocardial platelet deposition and thromboxane release with dipyridamole. Circulation 1986; 74(suppl III):III-145.

42. Teoh KH, Christakis CT, Wersel RD, et al.: Blood conservation with membrane oxygenators and dipyridamole. Ann Thorac Surg 1987; 44:40.

43. Teoh KH, Christakis GT, Weisel RD, et al.: Dipyridamole preserved platelets and reduced blood loss during cardiopulmonary bypass. J Thorac Cardiovasc Surg 1988; 96:332.

44. Verstraete M: Heparin. In: Messerli FH, ed, Cardiovascular Drug Therapy. Philadelphia, 1990, W.B. Saunders, pp. 1457–1469.

45. Lee KF, Mandell J, Rankin JS, et al.: Immediate versus delayed coronary grafting after streptokinase treatment. J Thorac Cardiovasc Surg 1988; 95:216.

46. Mann M, Sacks HJ, Goldfinger D: Safety of autologous blood donation prior to elective surgery for a variety of potentially "high-risk" patients. Transfusion 1983; 23:229.

47. Love TR, Hendren WG, O'Keefe DD, et al.: Transfusion of predonated autologous blood in elective cardiac surgery. Ann Thorac Surg 1987; 43:508.

48. Britton LW, Eastlund DT, Dziuban SW, et al.: Predonated autologous blood use in elective cardiac surgery. Ann Thorac Surg 1989; 47:529.

49. Owings DV, Kruskall MS, Thurer RL, et al.: Autologous blood donations in cardiac surgery. JAMA 1989; 262:1963.

50. Spiess BD, Sassetti R, McCarthy RJ, et al.: Autologous blood donation: hemodynamics in a high-risk patient population. Transfusion 1992; 32:17.

51. Toy PTCY, Strauss RG, Stehling LC, et al.: Predeposited autologous blood for elective surgery. N Engl J Med 1987; 316:517.

52. Zussa C, Polesel E, Salvador L, et al.: Efficacy and safety of predeposit blood autodonation in 500 cases of myocardial revascularization. Scand J Thorac Cardiovasc Surg 1990; 24:171.

53. Hillman RS, Finch CA: Erythropoiesis: normal and abnormal. Semin Hematol 1967; 4:327.

54. Goodnough LT, Rudnick S, Price TH, et al.: Increased preoperative collection of autologous blood with recombinant human erythropoietin therapy. N Engl J Med 1989; 321:1163.

55. Watanabe Y, Fuse K, Konishi T, et al.: Autologous blood transfusion with recombinant human erythropoietin in heart operations. Ann Thorac Surg 1991; 51:767.

56. Levine EA, Rosen AL, Sehgal LR, et al.: Erythropoietin deficiency after coronary artery bypass procedures. Ann Thorac Surg 1991; 51:764.

57. Rothstein P, Roye D, Verdisco L, et al.: Preoperative use of erythropoietin in an adolescent Jehovah's Witness. Anesthesiology 1990; 73:568.

58. Gaudiain VA, Mason HD: Preoperative erythropoietin in Jehovah's Witness. Ann Thorac Surg 1991; 51:823.

59. Dodrill FD, Marshall N, Nyboer J, et al.: Use of the heart-lung apparatus in human cardiac surgery. J Thorac Surg 1975; 33:60.

60. Mohr R, Martinowitz U, Lavee J, et al.: The hemostatic effect of transfusing fresh whole blood versus platelet concentrates after cardiac operations. J Thorac Cardiovasc Surg 1988; 96:530.

61. Lavee J, Martinowitz U, Mohr R, et al.: The effect of transfusion of fresh whole blood versus platelet concentrates after cardiac operations—a scanning electron microscope study of platelet aggregation on extracellular matrix. J Thorac Cardiovasc Surg 1989; 97:204.

62. Klovekorn WP, Richter J, Sebening F: Hemodilution in coronary bypass operations. Bibl Haematol 1981; 47:297.

63. Wagstaffe JG, Clarke AD, Jackson PW: Reduction of blood loss by restoration of platelet levels using fresh autologous blood after cardiopulmonary bypass. Thorax 1972; 27:410.

64. Cohn LH, Fosberg AM, Anderson RP, et al.: The effects of phlebotomy, hemodilution and autologous transfusion on systemic oxygenation and whole blood utilization in open heart surgery. Chest 1975; 68:283.

65. Hardesty RL, Bayer WL, Bahnson HT: A technique for the use of autologous fresh blood during open-heart surgery. J Thorac Cardiovasc Surg 1968; 56:683.

66. Hallowell P, Bland JHL, Buckley MJ: Transfusion of fresh autologous blood in open heart surgery. A method for reducing bank blood requirements. J Thorac Cardiovasc Surg 1972; 64:941.

67. Cosgrove DM, Loop FD, Lytle BW: Blood conservation in cardiac surgery. Cardiovasc Clin 1981; 12:165.

68. Grindon AJ, Schmidt PJ: Platelet-poor blood in open-heart surgery. N Engl J Med 1969; 280:1337.

69. McKenzie FN, Heimbecker RO, Wall W, et al.: Intraoperative autotransfusion in elective and emergency vascular surgery. Surgery 1978; 83:470.

70. Cosgrove DM, Loop FD, Lytle BW: Blood conservation in cardiac surgery. Cardiovasc Clin 1981; 12:165.

71. Iyer VS, Russell WJ: Fresh autologous blood transfusion and platelet counts after cardiopulmonary bypass surgery. Anaesth Intensive Care 1982; 10:348.

72. Mohr R, Golan M, Martinowitz U, et al.: Effect of cardiac operation on platelets. J Thorac Cardiovasc Surg 1986; 92:434.

73. Kendell AG, Lowenstein L: Alterations in blood coagulation and hemostasis during extracorporeal circulation. Part 1. Can Med Assoc J 1962; 87:786.

74. Ferrari M, Zia S, Valbonesi M, et al.: A new technique for hemodilution, preparation of autologous platelet-rich plasma and intraoperative blood salvage in cardiac surgery. Int J Artif Organs 1987; 10:47.

75. Giordano GF Sr, Giordano GF Jr, Rivers SL, et al.: Determinants of homologous blood usage utilizing autologous platelet-rich plasma in cardiac operations. Ann Thorac Surg 1989; 47:897.

76. National Institutes of Health: Consensus development conference: platelet transfusion therapy. JAMA 1987; 257:1777.

77. Giordano GF, Rivers SL, Chung GKT, et al.: Autologous platelet-rich plasma in cardiac surgery: effect on intraoperative and postoperative transfusion requirements. Ann Thorac Surg 1988; 46:416.

78. Tawes RL Jr, Sydorak GR, Duvall TB, et al.: The plasma collection system: a new concept in autotransfusion. Ann Vasc Surg 1989; 3:304.

79. Cohn LH, Solomon S, Lee-Son S, et al.: Sequestration of platelet-rich plasma for patients undergoing coronary bypass operations. Proc Blood Conserv Inst, Chicago, Illinois, 1978.

80. Boldt J, Kling D, Zickmann B, et al.: Acute plasmapheresis during cardiac surgery: volume replacement by crystalloids versus colloids. J Cardiothorac Anesth 1990; 4:564.

81. Boldt J, von Baermann B, Kling D, et al.: Preoperative plasmapheresis in patients undergoing cardiac procedures. Anesthesiology 1990; 72:282.

82. Jones JW, McCoy TA, Rawitscher RE, et al.: Effects of intraoperative plasmapheresis on blood loss in cardiac surgery. Ann Thorac Surg 1990; 49:585.

83. Williamson KR, Taswell HF: Indications for intraoperative blood salvage. J Clin Apheresis 1990; 5:100.

84. Vertrees RA, Engelman RM, Johnson JW III, et al.: Blood Conservation during open heart surgery: a literature review. J Extra-Corp Technol 1986; 18:200.

85. McCarthy PM, Popovsky MA, Schaff HV, et al.: Effect of blood conservation efforts in cardiac surgery at the Mayo Clinic. Mayo Clin Proc 1988; 63:225.

86. Øvrum E, Åm Holen E, Lindstein-Ringdal M-A: Coronary artery bypass surgery with minimal use of homologous blood: effects of a simple and inexpensive blood conservation programme. Eur J Cardiothorac Surg 1990; 4:644.

87. Ikeda S, Johnston MFM, Yagi K, et al.: Intraoperative autologous blood salvage with cardiac surgery: an analysis of five years' experience in more than 3,000 patients. J Clin Anesth 1992; 4:359.

88. Giordano GF, Goldman DS, Mammana RB, et al.: Intraoperative autotransfusion in cardiac operations. J Thorac Cardiovasc Surg 1988; 96:382.

89. Messick KD, Gibbons GA, Fosburg RG, et al.: Intraoperative use of the Haemonetics cell saver. Proc Blood Conserv Inst, Chicago, Illinois, 1978.

90. Klineberg PL, Kam CA, Johnson DC, et al.: Hematocrit and blood volume control during cardiopulmonary bypass with the use of hemofiltration. Anesthesiology 1984; 60:478.

91. Nelson RL, Tamari Y, Tortolani AJ, et al.: Ultrafiltration for concentration and salvage of pump blood. In: Utley JR, ed, Pathophysiology and Technique of Cardiopulmonary Bypass. Baltimore, 1983, Williams & Wilkins, vol. II, pp. 229–237.

92. Hopeck JM, Lane RS, Schroeder JW: Oxygenator volume control by parallel ultrafiltration to remove plasma water. J Extra-Corp Technol 1981; 13:267.

93. Holt DW, Landis GH, Dumond DA, et al.: Hemofiltration as an adjunct to cardiopulmonary bypass for total oxygenator volume control. J Extra-Corp Technol 1982; 14:373.

94. Moore RA, Laub GW: Hemofiltration, dialysis, and blood salvage techniques during cardiopulmonary bypass. In: Gravlee GP, Davis RF, Utley JR, eds, Cardiopulmonary Bypass: Principles and Practice. Baltimore, 1993, Williams & Wilkins, pp. 93–123.

95. Breyer RH, Engelman RM, Rousou JA, et al.: A comparison of cell saver versus ultrafilter during

coronary artery bypass operations. J Thorac Cardiovasc Surg 1985; 90:736.

96. Solem JO, Steen S, Olin C: A new method for autotransfusion of shed blood. Acta Chir Scand 1986; 152:421.

97. Solem JO, Tengborn L, Olin C, et al.: Autotransfusion of whole blood in massive bleeding. An experimental study in the pig. Acta Chir Scand 1986; 152: 427.

98. Solem JO, Tengborn L, Steen S, et al.: Cell saver versus hemofilter for concentration of oxygenator blood after cardiopulmonary bypass. Thorac Cardiovasc Surg 1987; 35:42.

99. Nakamura N, Masuda M, Toshima Y, et al.: Comparative study of cell saver and ultrafiltration nontransfusion in cardiac surgery. Ann Thorac Surg 1990; 49:973.

100. Boldt J, Zickmann B, Fedderson B, et al.: Six different hemofiltration devices for blood conservation in cardiac surgery. Ann Thorac Surg 1991; 51:747.

101. Boldt J, Kling D, von Baermann B, et al.: Blood conservation in cardiac operations. Cell separation versus hemofiltration. J Thorac Cardiovasc Surg 1989; 97:832.

102. Karliczek GF, Tigchelaar I, Kijck L, et al.: How much additional blood trauma is caused by haemofiltration during cardiopulmonary bypass? Life Support Syst 1986; 4(suppl 1):167.

103. Craddock PR, Fehr J, Brigham KL: Complement and leukocyte mediated pulmonary dysfunction in hemodialysis. N Engl J Med 1977; 296:769.

104. Moran JM, Babka R, Silberman S, et al.: Role of the Haemonetic cell saver following cardiopulmonary bypass. Proc Adv Comp Sem, Chicago, Illinois, 1977.

105. Moran JM, Babka R, Silberman S, et al.: Immediate centrifugation of oxygenator contents after cardiopulmonary bypass: role in maximum blood conservation. J Thorac Cardiovasc Surg 1978; 76: 510.

106. Mayer ED, Welsch M, Tanzeem A, et al.: Reduction of postoperative donor blood requirement by use of the cell separator. Scand J Thorac Cardiovasc Surg 1985; 19:165.

107. Pruitt KM, Stroud RM, Scott JW: Blood damage in the heart-lung machine (35651). Proc Soc Exp Biol Med 1971; 137:714.

108. Utley JR, Moores WY, Stephens DB: Blood conservation techniques. Ann Thorac Surg 1981; 31:482.

109. Kelly PB, Smelloff EA, Miller GE, et al.: Intraoperative autotransfusion of centrifuged oxygenator perfusate using a disposable blood centrifuge. Proc Haemonetics Res Sem 1975; 6:33.

110. Tucker WY, Cohn LH: Intraoperative use of the haemonetics cell saver in open heart surgery. Proc Haemonetics Res Sem 1976; 7:25.

111. Cordell AR, Lavender SW: An appraisal of blood salvage techniques in vascular and cardiac operations. Ann Thorac Surg 1981; 31:421.

112. Chua PS, Carlos CJ, Gozo FR Jr, et al.: Asanguinous open-heart surgery. Indiana Med 1985; 78: 494.

113. Reid CBA, Graham AR, Lord RSA: Initial experience of intra-operative red cell salvage. Aust N Z J Surg 1990; 60:959.

114. Royston D, Bidstrup BP, Taylor KM, et al.: Effect of aprotinin on need for blood transfusion after repeat open-heart surgery. Lancet 1987; 2:1289.

115. van Oeveren W, Jansen NJG, Bidstrup BP, et al.: Effects of aprotinin on hemostatic mechanisms during cardiopulmonary bypass. Ann Thorac Surg 1987; 44:640.

116. Dietrich W, Spannagl M, Jochum M, et al.: Influence of high-dose aprotinin treatment on blood loss and coagulation pattern in patients undergoing myocardial revascularization. Anesthesiology 1990; 73:1119.

117. Allison PM, Whitten CW: What is the mechanism of action of aprotinin? Anesthesiology 1991; 75: 377.

118. Merle J-P, Lançon JP, Dutrillaux F, et al.: Effects of aprotinin on postoperative bleeding. Anesthesiology 1991; 75:379.

119. van Oeveren W, Harder MP, Roozendaal KJ, et al.: Aprotinin protects platelets against the initial effect of cardiopulmonary bypass. J Thorac Cardiovasc Surg 1990; 99:788.

120. Marx G, Pokar H, Reuter H, et al.: The effects of aprotinin on hemostatic function during cardiac surgery. J Cardiothorac Vasc Anesth 1991; 5:467.

121. Vedrinne C, Girard C, Jegaden O, et al.: Reduction in blood loss and blood use after cardiopulmonary bypass with high-dose aprotinin versus autologous fresh whole blood transfusion. J Cardiothorac Vasc Anesth 1992; 6:319.

122. Lemmer JH, Stanford W, Bonney SL, et al.: Aprotinin for coronary bypass operations: efficacy, safety, and influence on early saphenous vein graft patency. A multicenter, randomized, double blind, placebo-controlled study. J Thorac Cardiovasc Surg 1994; 107:543.

123. Bidstrup BP, Royston D, Sapsford RN, et al.: Reduction in blood loss and blood use after cardiopulmonary bypass with high dose aprotinin (Trasylol). J Thorac Cardiovasc Surg 1989; 97:364.

124. Correl T, Bauer E, Laske A, et al.: Low-dose aprotinin and reduction of blood loss after cardiopulmonary bypass. Lancet 1991; 337:673.

125. Harder MP, Eijsman L, Roozendaal KJ, et al.: Aprotinin reduces intraoperative and postoperative blood loss in membrane oxygenator cardiopulmonary bypass. Ann Thorac Surg 1991; 51:936.

126. Baele PL, Ruiz-Gomez J, Londot C, et al.: Systemic use of aprotinin in cardiac surgery: influence on total homologous exposure and hospital cost. Acta Anaesthesiol Belg 1992; 43:103.

127. Dietrich W, Barankay A, Dilthey G, et al.: Reduction of blood utilization during myocardial revascularization. J Thorac Cardiovasc Surg 1989; 97: 213.

128. Trasylol Package Insert, Miles Inc., Pharmaceutical Division, West Haven, CT, 1994.

129. Covino E, Pepino P, Iorio D, et al.: Low dose aprotinin as blood saver in open heart surgery. Eur J Cardiothorac Surg 1991; 5:414.

130. Wang J-S, Lin C-Y, Hung W-T, et al.: Monitoring of heparin-induced anticoagulation with kaolin-activated clotting time in cardiac surgical patients treated with aprotinin. Anesthesiology 1992; 77: 1080.

131. Hunt BJ, Segal HC, Yacoub M: Guidelines for monitoring heparin by the activated clotting time when aprotinin is used during cardiopulmonary bypass (Letter). J Thorac Cardiovasc Surg 1992; 104: 211.

132. Hunt BJ, Segal HC, Yacoub M: Aprotinin and heparin monitoring during cardiopulmonary bypass. Circulation 1992; 86(suppl II):II-410.

133. Royston D: High-dose aprotinin therapy: a review of the first five years experience. J Cardiothorac Vasc Anesth 1992; 6:76.

134. Culliford AT, Gitel SN, Star N, et al.: Lack of correlation between activated clotting time and plasma heparin during cardiopulmonary bypass. Ann Surg 1981; 193:105.

135. Verstraete M: Clinical application of inhibitors of fibrinolysis. Drugs 1985; 29:236.

136. Sharifi R, Lee M, Ray P, et al.: Safety and efficacy of intervesical aminocaproic acid for bleeding after transurethral resection of the prostate. Urology 1986; 27:214.

137. Kang Y, Lewis JH, Navalgund A, et al.: ε-Aminocaproic acid for treatment of fibrinolysis during liver transplantation. Anesthesiology 1987; 66:766.

138. Vander Salm TJ, Ansell JE, Okike ON, et al.: The role of epsilon-aminocaproic acid in reducing bleeding after cardiac operation: a double blind randomized study. J Thorac Cardiovasc Surg 1988; 95:538.

139. Del Rossi AJ, Cernaianu AC, Botros S, et al.: Prophylactic treatment of postperfusion bleeding using EACA. Chest 1989; 96:27.

140. Harrow JC, Hlacvacek J, Stron MD, et al.: Prophylactic tranexamic acid decreases bleeding after cardiac operations. J Thorac Cardiovasc Surg 1990; 99:70.

141. Yau TM, Carson S, Weisel RD, et al.: The effect of warm heart surgery on postoperative bleeding. J Thorac Cardiovasc Surg 1992; 103:1155.

142. Sterns LP, Lillehei CW: Effect of ε-aminocaproic acid to reduce bleeding during cardiac bypass in children with congenital heart disease. Can J Surg 1967; 10:304.

143. Gomez MMR, McGoon DC: Bleeding patterns after open-heart surgery. J Thorac Cardiovasc Surg 1970; 60:87.

144. Lambert C, Marengo-Rowe A, Levenson J, et al.: The treatment of postperfusion bleeding using ε-aminocaproic acid, cryoprecipitate, fresh frozen plasma, and protamine sulfate. Ann Thorac Surg 1979; 28:440.

145. McClure PD, Izsak J: The use of epsilon-aminocaproic acid to reduce bleeding during cardiac bypass in children with congenital heart disease. Anesthesiology 1974; 40:604.

146. Hardy JF, Desroches J: Natural and synthetic antifibrinolytics in cardiac surgery. Can J Anaesth 1992; 39:353.

147. Tanaka K, Takao M, Yada I, et al.: Alterations in coagulation and fibrinolysis associated with cardiopulmonary bypass during open heart surgery. J Cardiothorac Anesth 1989; 3:181.

148. Harrow JC, Van Riper DF, Strong MD, et al.: Hemostatic effects of tranexamic acid and desmopressin during cardiac surgery. Circulation 1991; 84:2063.

149. Czer LSC, Bateman TM, Gray RJ, et al.: Treatment of severe platelet dysfunction and hemorrhage after cardiopulmonary bypass: reduction in blood product usage with desmopressin. J Am Coll Cardiol 1987; 9:1139.

150. Sarraccino S, Adler E, Gibbons PA, et al.: DDAVP does not decrease post bypass bleeding in acyanotic children (Abstract). Anesthesiology 1989; 70:A1057.

151. Brodsky I, Gill DN, Lusch CJ: Fibrinolysis in congenital heart disease: preoperative treatment with ε-aminocaproic acid. Am J Clin Pathol 1969; 51:51.

152. Seear MD, Wadsworth LD, Rogers PC, et al.: The effect of desmopressin acetate (DDAVP) on postoperative blood loss after cardiac operation in children. J Thorac Cardiovasc Surg 1989; 98:217.

153. Reich DL, Hammerschlag BC, Rand JH, et al.: Desmopressin acetate is a mild vasodilator that does not reduce blood loss in uncomplicated cardiac surgical procedures. J Cardiothorac Vasc Anesth 1991; 5:142.

154. Hackmann T, Gascoyne RD, Naiman SC, et al.: A trial of desmopressin (1-desamino-8-D-arginine vasopressin) to reduce blood loss in uncomplicated cardiac surgery. N Engl J Med 1989; 321:1437.

155. Rocha E, Llorens R, Paramo JA, et al.: Does desmopressin acetate reduce blood loss after surgery in patients on cardiopulmonary bypass? Circulation 1988; 77:1319.

156. D'Alauro FS, Johns RA: Hypotension related to desmopressin administration following cardiopulmonary bypass. Anesthesiology 1988; 69:962.

157. Frankville DD, Harper GB, Lake CL, et al.: Hemodynamic consequences of desmopressin administration after cardiopulmonary bypass. Anesthesiology 1991; 74:988.

158. Morgan PD, Hosking MP: The role of desmopressin acetate in patients undergoing coronary artery bypass surgery. Anesthesiology 1992; 77:38.

159. Marquez J, Koehler S, Strelec SR, et al.: Repeated dose administration of desmopressin acetate in uncomplicated cardiac surgery: a prospective, blinded, randomized study. J Cardiothorac Vasc Anesth 1992; 6:674.

160. Mammen EF, Koets MH, Washington BC, et al.: Hemostasis changes during cardiopulmonary bypass surgery. Semin Thromb Hemost 1985; 11:281.

161. Woodman RC, Harker LA: Bleeding complications associated with cardiopulmonary bypass. Blood 1990; 76:1680.

162. Edmunds LH Jr, Saxena NC, Hilyer P, et al.: Relationship between platelet count and cardiotomy suction. Ann Thorac Surg 1978; 25:306.

163. Addonizio VP, Colman RW: Platelets and extracorporeal circulation. Biomaterials 1982; 3:9.

164. Harker LA: Bleeding after cardiopulmonary bypass. N Engl J Med 1986; 314:1446.

165. Dutton RC, Edmunds LM Jr, Hutchinson JC, et al.: Platelet aggregate emboli produced in patients during cardiopulmonary bypass with membrane and bubble oxygenators and blood filters. J Thorac Cardiovasc Surg 1974; 67:258.

166. Thomas R, Hessel EA III, Harker LA, et al.: Platelet function during and after deep surface hypothermia. J Surg Res 1981; 31:314.

167. Valeri CR, Feingold H, Cassidy G, et al.: Hypothermia-induced reversible platelet dysfunction. Ann Surg 1987; 205:175.

168. Heyns A du P: Kinetics and in vivo redistribution of 111 indium-labeled human platelets after intravenous protamine sulfate. Thromb Haemost 1980; 44:65.

169. Bowie EJW, Owen CA: The clinical and laboratory diagnosis of hemorrhagic disorders. In: Ratnoff OD, Forbes CD, eds, Disorders of Hemostasis. Orlando, FL, 1984, Grune & Stratton, pp. 43–72.

170. Harker LA, Malpass TW, Branson HE, et al.: Mechanism of abnormal bleeding in patients undergoing

cardiopulmonary bypass: acquired transient platelet dysfunction associated with selective $\alpha$-granule release. Blood 1980; 56:824.

171. Simon TL, Akl BF, Murphy W: Controlled trial of routine administration of platelet concentrates in cardiopulmonary bypass surgery. Ann Thorac Surg 1984; 37:359.

172. Oberman HA: Intraoperative use of fresh frozen plasma. JAMA 1985; 253:556.

173. Brunken R, Follette D, Wittig J: Coronary artery bypass in hereditary factor XI deficiency. Ann Thorac Surg 1984; 38:406.

174. National Institutes of Health: Consensus development conference: fresh frozen plasma. Indications and risks. JAMA 1985; 253:551.

175. Young PH, Bouhasin JD, Barner HB: Aortic valve replacement in von Willebrand's disease. J Thorac Cardiovasc Surg 1978; 76:218.

176. Ma DDF, Chang VP, Concannon AJ, et al.: Aortic valve replacement in a patient with von Willebrand's disease. Aust N Z J Surg 1979; 49:247.

177. Roskos RR, Gilchrist GS, Kazmier FJ, et al.: Management of hemophilia A and B during surgical correction of transposition of the great arteries. Mayo Clin Proc 1983; 58:182.

178. Dresdale A, Bowen FO Jr, Malm JR, et al.: Hemostatic effectiveness of fibrin glue derived from single-donor fresh frozen plasma. Ann Thorac Surg 1985; 40:385.

179. Lupinetti FM, Stoney WS, Alford WC Jr, et al.: Cryoprecipitate-topical thrombin glue. Initial experience in patients undergoing cardiac operations. J Thorac Cardiovasc Surg 1985; 90:502.

180. Jessen C, Sharma P: Use of fibrin glue in thoracic surgery. Ann Thorac Surg 1985; 39:521.

181. Garcia-Rinaldi R, Simmons P, Salcedo V, et al.: A technique for spot application of fibrin glue during open heart operations. Ann Thorac Surg 1989; 47:59.

182. Berruyer M, Amiral J, French P, et al.: Immunization by bovine thrombin used with fibrin glue during cardiovascular operations: development of thrombin and factor V inhibitors. J Thorac Cardiovasc Surg 1993; 105:892.

183. Estafanous FG, Tarazi RC: Systemic arterial hypertension associated with cardiac surgery. Am J Cardiol 1980; 46:685.

184. Flaherty JT, Magee PA, Gardner TL, et al.: Comparison of intravenous nitroglycerin and sodium nitroprusside for treatment of acute hypertension developing after coronary artery bypass surgery. Circulation 1982; 65:1072.

185. David D, Dubois C, Loria Y: Comparison of nicardipine and sodium nitroprusside in the treatment of paroxysmal hypertension following aortocoronary bypass surgery. J Cardiothorac Vasc Anesth 1991; 5:357.

186. National Institutes of Health: Consensus development conference: peri-operative red blood cell transfusion. JAMA 1988; 260:2700.

187. Robertie PG, Gravlee GP: Safe limits on isovolemic hemodilution and recommendations for erythrocyte transfusion. Int Anesthesiol Clin 1990; 28:197.

188. Stehling LC, Zauder HL: How low can we go? Is there a way to know (Editorial)? Transfusion 1990; 30:1.

189. Carson JL, Poses RM, Spence RK, et al.: Severity of anaemia and operative mortality and morbidity. Lancet 1988; 1:727.

190. Johnson RG, Thurer RL, Kruskall MS, et al.: Comparison of two transfusion strategies after elective operations for myocardial revascularization. J Thorac Cardiovasc Surg 1992; 104:307.

191. Leone BJ, Spahn DR: Anemia, hemodilution, and oxygen delivery (Editorial). Anesth Analg 1992; 75:651.

192. Schaff HV, Hauer JM, Gardner TJ, et al.: Routine use of autotransfusion following cardiac surgery: experience in 700 patients. Ann Thorac Surg 1979; 27:493.

193. Johnson RG, Rosenkrantz KR, Preston RA, et al.: The efficacy of postoperative autotransfusion in patients undergoing cardiac operations. Ann Thorac Surg 1983; 36:173.

194. Hartz RS, Smith JA, Green DL: Autotransfusion following cardiac surgery: assessment of hemostatic factors. J Thorac Cardiovasc Surg 1988; 96:178.

195. Eng J, Kay PH, Murday AJ, et al.: Postoperative autologous transfusion in cardiac surgery—a prospective, randomized study. Eur J Cardiothorac Surg 1990; 4:595.

196. Roberts SR, Early GL, Brown B, et al.: Autotransfusion of unwashed mediastinal shed blood fails to decrease banked blood requirement in patients undergoing aortocoronary bypass surgery. Am J Surg 1991; 162:477.

197. Voegele LD, Causby G, Utley T, et al.: An improved method for collection of shed mediastinal blood for autotransfusion. Ann Thorac Surg 1982; 34:471.

# PEDIATRIC SURGERY

## *Paul D. Schanbacher and M. Ramez Salem*

Blood conservation strategies have assumed escalating importance in recent years. These strategies have been extended to neonates, infants, and children. Therefore, physicians involved in the care of pediatric patients should be familiar with the principles and practices of blood conservation methods. Almost all techniques of blood conservation have been used in pediatric patients, though some may have a limited application in infants and children. Strategies directed to decrease the recipient's exposure to allogeneic blood in pediatric patients include (*a*) appropriate use of blood and blood products, (*b*) minimal-exposure transfusion (MET), (*c*) decreasing intraoperative blood loss, (*d*) autologous blood transfusion, and (*e*) a combination of techniques. For detailed discussions, the reader is referred to appropriate chapters throughout the text.

## GUIDELINES FOR TRANSFUSION THERAPY

Transfusion therapy may be a life-saving measure. However, in some cases it may be detrimental. Transfusion of viral-tainted blood products, risks of transfusion reactions, and graft versus host disease are all potential lethal complications. Many institutions have established guidelines to monitor and govern the transfusion practices of their physicians. It is imperative that the practitioner have a firm grasp on guidelines for the appropriate use of blood and blood products. We review guidelines for red blood cell (RBC) transfusion and blood component therapy in infants with special emphasis on neonates. In addition, we review cardiopulmonary bypass (CPB)-induced coagulopathy in neonates. The reader is also referred to Chapter 5: Perioperative Hemoglobin Requirements.

## Red Cell Transfusion

RBC transfusion is indicated for patients that require an increase in oxygen-carrying capacity either because of reduction in the hemoglobin (HGB) concentration or abnormally functioning RBCs. Clinically, HGB reduction plus symptoms of cardiorespiratory dysfunction (e.g., tachycardia and tachypnea) due to anemia are generally agreed on as a need for transfusion. The well-established indications include exchange transfusion for hemolytic disease of the newborn, anemia causing cardiorespiratory failure, and anemia from acute blood loss. There are other controversial indicators for RBC transfusion therapy that include poor weight gain, very low birth weight, respiratory distress syndrome, and apnea.[1–6] Unfortunately, there is a paucity of scientific data that unequivocally support transfusion in those conditions. In terms of an HGB value below which the neonate should be transfused, it is generally recommended that a symptomatic neonate with an HGB value less than 10.5 g/dL receives a blood transfusion.[7] On the other hand, when a neonate requires transfusion therapy, it is a practical point to increase the HGB level to the upper limits of normal. This will decrease the further likelihood of a subsequent transfusion.

Exchange transfusion is most frequently performed on neonates with hemolytic disease of the newborn. In this disease process, hemolysis results in anemia and hyperbilirubinemia from maternal antibodies directed against fetal RBCs. Exchange transfusion of one to two blood volumes effectively removes unconjugated bilirubin and antibody coated RBCs. In more severe cases, in utero exchange transfusion via percutaneous intraumbilical cannulation can be performed with good survival rates. RBCs used for exchange transfusion should be fresh washed type O Rh negative, cytomegalovirus seronegative reconstituted with fresh frozen plasma (FFP) to prevent depletion of plasma proteins, or ABO compatible fresh whole blood. In addition, blood used for exchange transfusion should be cross matched against the mother's serum to detect alloantibodies present on donor cells. If the neonate has received intrauterine transfusion or is immunodeficient, it is recommended that the RBCs be irradiated to destroy accompanying lymphocytes to prevent the rare occurrence of posttransfusion graft-versus-host disease.[8] In full-term neonates hyperbilirubinemia exceeding 25 mg/dL is generally an indication for exchange transfusion. In the preterm neonate, because of an immature blood-brain barrier, exchange transfusion is necessary when the total serum bilirubin is in the range of 12–18 mg/dL with lower values set for smaller preterm neonates.[9] Other accompanying factors, such as cardiopulmonary disease, sepsis, and hypoxemia, will hasten the need for exchange transfusion in these affected neonates.

In neonates with cardiopulmonary failure secondary to anemia, blood transfusion will alleviate tissue hypoxia and usually resolve the accompanying tachycardia and tachypnea with improvement in cardiopulmonary function. Because these neonates are anemic but usually euvolemic, care must be taken to avoid a hypervolemic state with transfusion therapy. Neonates are particularly susceptible to volume overload, which may precipitate pulmonary edema and wide oscillations in blood pressure. The following formula will guide transfusion therapy:

$$V_{PRBC} = \frac{EBV \times (HGB_{desired} - HGB_{observed})}{HGB_{PRBC}}$$

where $V_{PRBC}$ is the volume of packed red blood cells, EBV is the estimated blood volume, $HGB_{desired}$ is the desired hemoglobin concentration, $HGB_{observed}$ is the initial hemoglobin concentration, and $HGB_{PRBC}$ is the packed red blood cell hemoglobin concentration.

Transfusion rates of 2–5 mL/kg/h are generally used for neonates, with the lower value recommended for infants in heart failure.[7] If transfusion must be given at a quicker rate, the use of diuretics should also be considered. Because the volume of transfused cells is small, syringe pumps are regarded as safe and convenient. The syringe should be filled with blood drawn through a filter assembly and delivered within 5 hours to reduce the risk of bacterial proliferation in nonrefrigerated blood. As with adult transfusion therapy, microaggregate filters in this situation have not been shown to be necessary.

Acute blood loss in neonates resulting in hypovolemia and anemia is a straightforward indication for RBC transfusion. Whole blood or RBCs reconstituted with crystalloid or colloid should be given at a rate necessary to maintain hemodynamic stability. With whole blood transfusion therapy, the possibility of clinically significant hyperkalemia and hypocalcemia exists, particularly with transfusion rates exceeding 2.0 mL/kg/min.[10] It is important in these situations to monitor the electrocardiogram closely for changes such as widening of the QRS complex, prolonged QT interval, or flattening or peaking of the T waves. Treatment of both hypocalcemia and hyperkalemia consists of exogenous calcium administration. In addition, if RBC replacement is much greater than one blood volume, there may be a need for platelet and plasma transfusion to prevent dilutional thrombocytopenia and dilutional factor coagulopathy, respectively. It is important to maintain body temperature in the neonate during blood transfusion. Depending on the rate and volume of blood administered, warming of transfused blood can be accomplished by a standard fluid warmer or, for smaller volumes, by simply allowing blood-filled syringes to equilibrate with the isolette temperature before infusing.

Repeated laboratory analysis of blood specimens is a well-recognized cause of neonatal anemia and is a very common indication for transfusion in preterm infants. Efforts aimed at decreasing the amount of analyzed blood and the use of other sophisticated monitoring devices, such as transcutaneous monitoring of respiratory gases, has helped minimize these blood losses but has not eliminated the need for blood transfusions.

## Platelet Transfusion

Platelet counts in neonates are normally the same as in the adult population. It is known, however, that thrombocytopenia is more hazardous in the neonate with an increased risk of renal, pulmonary, and intraventricular hemorrhage when platelet counts drop below $100,000/mm^3$.[11,12] The etiology of thrombocytopenia encompasses multiple factors that include decreased production, increased destruction, dilution from massive transfusion, or a combination of factors. Functional abnormalities in neonatal platelets may also increase the risk of bleeding for a given platelet count. In the neonatal population, some of the more common causes of thrombocytopenia include disseminated intravascular coagulation (DIC), sepsis, asphyxia, necrotizing enterocolitis, and indwelling catheters.[12]

The approach to platelet transfusion in the neonate must take into consideration not only the etiology of the underlying thrombocytopenia but also the rate of decrease in the platelet count. With ongoing platelet consumption as in DIC, the platelet requirement is higher than with dilutional thrombocytopenia from blood transfusion. A neonate whose platelet count has gradually decreased from a disease process will tolerate a lower platelet count than a patient whose platelet count has dropped suddenly from acute surgical blood losses. Platelet transfusion therapy in the neonate, as in the adult, is indicated to treat or prevent bleeding from thrombocytopenia. The exact platelet count used to decide whether to transfuse is somewhat empirical and must always take into consideration the entire clinical picture, such as coexisting illness, concurrent drug therapy that may effect platelet function, or a planned surgical procedure. In practice, platelet transfusion to prevent bleeding is indicated in almost all cases when the platelet count has fallen below $30,000–50,000/mm^3$.[13] Higher platelet counts are prophylactically indicated in situations such as DIC, functionally abnormal platelets, or surgical intervention. During active bleeding it is recommended that platelet counts be maintained above $75,000–100,000/mm^3$ for adequate hemostasis.

Platelet transfusion therapy is usually calculated on a kilogram basis. A platelet transfusion of $0.1–0.3$ units/kg of body weight will increase the platelet count $20,000–70,000/mm^3$. Each unit of platelets contains approximately 50 mL of plasma. If volume overload is to be avoided, particularly in the premature neonate or one with cardiovascular instability, the platelets can be concentrated into a volume of 20 mL without functional damage to the platelets. In all cases of platelet transfusion, an attempt should be made to use ABO compatible platelets to increase in vivo platelet survival. Also, platelets should be infused through a standard $170-\mu m$ filter and not a microaggregate filter, which results in large platelet losses.

## Fresh Frozen Plasma and Cryoprecipitate Transfusion

There are relatively few indications for the use of FFP in the neonate. The major indications include replacement of deficient plasma proteins because of consumption coagulopathy, congenital factor deficiency, or lack of protein production by an immature liver. Neonates are developmentally deficient in vitamin K-dependent factors (II, VII, IX, X), yet rarely is this a cause of major bleeding. Hospital-born babies receive $0.5–1.0$ mg phytonadione so that bleeding because of vitamin K factors is seen only with liver disease, malabsorption, gut sterilization, or exclusively breast-fed neonates. FFP may also be indicated as part of exchange transfusion, congenital factor IX deficiency, DIC, and in neonates with protein-losing enteropathies. In the event of anticipated surgery or active bleeding with known factor deficiency, FFP is indicated at a dose of $15–20$ mL/kg. Because FFP contains relatively more citrate than whole blood, it should be administered slowly at a rate less than 1 mL/kg to avoid clinically significant drops in ionized calcium.[10]

The use of cryoprecipitate is infrequent and limited to a few specific indications. It is used in the treatment of quantitative and qualitative deficiencies of fibrinogen, for example, congenital afibrinogenemia. It can also be used to treat deficiencies of factor VIII and von Willebrand's disease. However, desmopressin acetate and commercial concentrates of factor VIII are probably safer alternatives.[12]

## Granulocyte Transfusion

Granulocyte transfusions have decreased significantly over the last several years as new and improved antibiotic therapy has been instituted for the effective treatment of neonatal sepsis. The strongest indication for the use of granulocyte transfusion appears to be in those neonates that have bacterial sepsis not responding to antibiotic therapy and in which a low blood neutrophil count can be demonstrated. In those neonates, transfusion of $0.5-1.0 \times 10^9$ granulocytes has increased survival rates in some studies.[14,15] Granulocyte transfusion may be required twice daily for several days.

In summary, transfusion therapy in the neonatal period deserves the same thoughtful considerations in terms of risks and benefits as in any other time of life, with noted differences in volume, rate, and indications for transfusion therapy. The practitioner must have a firm grasp of guidelines governing appropriate use of blood and blood products. The decision to transfuse should ideally be made in conjunction with a neonatologist who can offer expertise in overall patient management.

## Cardiopulmonary Bypass-Induced Coagulopathy in Neonates

Neonates undergoing CPB are subjected to multiple risk factors that have profound effects on their coagulation systems (Table 12–1).[16] Preoperative factors such as cyanosis, low cardiac output and tissue hypoperfusion, hepatic immaturity, and the use of platelet inhibitors (prostaglandin $E_1$) are recognized factors that contribute to postoperative hemorrhagic diathesis.[16–22] Among these factors, reduced hepatic synthetic capac-

**Table 12–1.  Factors contributing to post-CPB coagulopathy in neonates**

Preoperative factors
  Cyanosis (hypoxemia)
    Low plasma coagulation factors
    Defective clot retraction
    Disseminated intravascular coagulation
    Qualitative platelet dysfunction
  Hypoperfusion
    Ischemic hepatic injury
  Hepatic immaturity
    Antithrombin III deficiency
  Use of platelet inhibitors
    Prostaglandin $E_1$
Intraoperative factors
  Extreme hemodilution
  Deep hypothermia?
  Exposure of blood to large extracorporeal surfaces?
  Total circulatory arrest?
  High pump flow rate and nonpulsatile perfusion?
Post-CPB
  Increased transfusion requirements of blood and blood products causing deficiencies in labile factors V and VII

ity probably plays a major role.[16] In neonates with complex cardiac defects, hepatic maturation, which normally continues throughout the first 3 weeks of life, may be delayed or impaired by poor organ perfusion or severe hypoxemia.[16,23,24] In more than 50% of neonates undergoing CPB, preoperative levels of coagulation factors are lower than that of normal neonates.[16] These neonates experience a greater decrease in their intraoperative factor levels as well. Kern et al.[16] showed the fibrinogen levels were uniformly less than 1 g/L throughout the CPB period for neonates with low preoperative factor levels (Fig. 12–7). The levels of antithrombin III, a plasma protein that binds to heparin and accelerates thrombin and factor II inactivation, are much lower in neonates than in adults.[16,25,26] Nonetheless, heparin resistance does not occur in neonates because thrombin and activated factor II levels are also reduced, thus allowing for an effective anticoagulation when heparin is given.[16,25,26]

Differences in the etiology of post-CPB coagulopathy between neonates and adults are striking. In the adult, coagulopathy is most commonly due to acquired defects in platelet function induced by the passage of blood through the membrane oxygenator.[27–29]

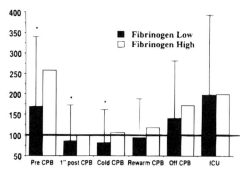

**Fig. 12–7.** Effects of initiation of CPB on patients with normal and low prebypass fibrinogen levels are demonstrated. Fibrinogen levels significantly fell in both groups. In the neonates with a prebypass fibrinogen level less than 200 mg/dL (2 g/L), measured levels of fibrinogen were uniformly less than 100 mg/dL with mean values ranging between 81 and 85 mg/dL. This was significantly less ($P < .05$) than fibrinogen assays obtained from neonates with normal prebypass fibrinogen. Statistical differences between the two groups are designated by an asterisk. ICU, intensive care unit. From Kern FH, Morana NJ, Sears JJ, et al.: Coagulation defects in neonates during cardiopulmonary bypass. Ann Thorac Surg 1992; 54: 541.

Hemodilution, in adult CPB patients, does not cause a significant reduction in coagulation factor levels or platelet number[27] (see Chapter 7: Acute Normovolemic Hemodilution). Although acquired platelet dysfunction also contributes to post-CPB hemorrhage in the neonate, global and severe deficits in factor levels and platelet number do occur.[16] Immediately after the initiation of CPB in neonates, coagulation factor levels and platelet counts are reduced by 50 and 70%, respectively.[16] Neither cooling to deep hypothermic levels nor prolonged exposure of blood to the extracorporeal circuit results in demonstrable changes in coagulation factor levels, platelet count, or antithrombin III levels.[16] This suggests that the predominant factor affecting the coagulation system in neonates undergoing CPB is hemodilution.[16] In comparison with adults, the hemodilution associated with CPB is 5–10 times greater in neonates.[10] This is due to the blood volume of the neonate being diluted by a prime volume that is two to three times larger.

Prophylaxis and therapy for neonatal post-CPB hemorrhage must account for these global coagulation deficiencies. The addition of whole blood to the prime volume, especially fresh blood (less than 48 hours old), may

moderate the dilutional effects of hemodilution by providing additional coagulation factors.[16] In contrast, substituting packed RBCs for whole blood may result in substantially lower levels of coagulation factors and more hemorrhagic diathesis after CPB.[16] Because fresh whole blood contains both coagulation factors and active platelets, its use is ideally suited for the treatment of post-CPB hemorrhage in the neonate.[30,31] Improved platelet function and decreased transfusion requirements have been demonstrated with the use of fresh whole blood as compared with component therapy.[30] The balanced product of whole blood, which contains RBCs, platelets, and coagulation factors, avoids the occurrence of RBC depletion, which tends to occur with either platelet or FFP transfusion.[16,30–32] A significant reduction in postoperative blood loss has been demonstrated when fresh whole blood rather than component therapy is given to children younger than 2 years of age.[31] However, the neonatal population is most likely to achieve the greatest benefit from whole blood therapy after weaning from CPB.[16,31]

In the absence of fresh whole blood, component therapy should be used to normalize coagulation factors, platelets, and RBC levels. Because of the small size of the neonate's blood volume, concentrated plasma products are preferred.[16] Platelet concentrates restore platelet count with a minimal transfusion volume. The marked reduction in fibrinogen levels in neonates undergoing CPB makes cryoprecipitate preferable to FFP.[16] One or two units of cryoprecipitate effectively restore circulating fibrinogen levels without substantially increasing the neonate's blood volume.[16] In contrast, the large volume of one or two units of FFP is more likely to dilute the circulating RBCs and platelets.[16]

## MINIMAL EXPOSURE TRANSFUSION

Because the use of allogeneic blood is sometimes unavoidable, some centers have advocated the use of a minimal number of donors (preferably one committed donor) who contribute all the allogeneic blood and blood components a pediatric patient is expected to need to decrease the recipient's exposure to transfusion-transmitted disease.[33–36] Such a practice has been referred to as MET and has been primarily used in pediatric cardiac surgery.[36] In a broader sense, any strategy used to decrease the recipient's exposure to allogeneic blood or blood products should be thought of as part of the MET program.[36] Brecher et al.[36] reviewed their experience with 50 pediatric cardiac surgical patients on such a program. They found the mean decrease is allogeneic-donor exposure was 57%. Thirteen of these patients received only allogeneic blood products from one committed donor. To implement such a program, it is absolutely necessary to track and access rapidly a particular unit from the committed donor. Extensive computer support is required for successful and consistent implementation of such a MET committed-donor program. Without adequate computer support, available units from the committed donor may be overlooked or may be difficult to locate.

## DECREASING INTRAOPERATIVE BLOOD LOSS

A variety of blood conservation procedures are currently available for use in infants and children. A "flawless" anesthetic technique; proper positioning; and prevention of hypertension, hypercapnia, and systemic or regional increases in venous pressure are essential to avoid unnecessary blood loss during surgery. Infiltration with vasoconstriction solutions can be used in a variety of minor and major surgical procedures, such as cleft lip repair, cleft palate closure, and correction of scoliosis. The use of pneumatic tourniquets after exsanguination of the upper or lower extremity permits a bloodless operative field. When tourniquets are used, certain precautions should be taken to minimize systemic and metabolic effects after tourniquet release (see Chapter 4: Blood Conservation Techniques).

### Deliberate Hypotension

Deliberate hypotension, whether used alone or in conjunction with other measures of blood conservation, can markedly decrease blood loss and the use of allogeneic blood in pediatric patients. Some pertinent points must be considered when deliberate hypotension is selected for pediatric patients: (*a*) children respond to most hypotensive drugs by tachycardia; (*b*) the incidence of failed hypotension may be relatively high unless the heart rate is controlled; (*c*) because of the child's height, tilting may not produce as great a pressure gradient and peripheral venous pooling; (*d*) the physiological dead space does not increase in pediatric patients; (*e*) lower blood pressure may be necessary to achieve the desired bloodless field as compared with adults; and (*f*) cyanide toxicity due to sodium nitroprusside overdose is a preventable complication.

### Pharmacological Enhancement of Hemostatic Activity

The reader is referred to Chapters 2 (Coagulation and Hemostasis) and Chapter 12 (Part IV) (Blood Conservation in Special Situations–*Anesthesiologists' Viewpoints*: Cardiac Surgery).

## AUTOLOGOUS TRANSFUSION
### Preoperative Autologous Blood Donation

Although preoperative autologous blood donation has gained wide acceptance and has been extended to children as young as 4 years of age, technical problems and lack of cooperation usually make young children unlikely candidates. The volume of blood that can be donated may be augmented by iron and recombinant human erythropoietin therapy. The reader is referred to Chapter 6 (Preoperative Autologous Blood Donation) for more information.

### Blood Salvage Techniques

The indications for the use of blood salvage in children weighing more than 10 kg include an anticipated blood loss of 20% or more of their estimated blood volume or procedures in which greater than 10% of patients are transfused with more than 1 unit. This is based on the fact that an average of only 50–70% of shed blood is being salvageable and a minimum 250–350 mL in volume of captured shed blood is necessary to fill a pediatric-sized (125–175 mL) centrifuge bowl with RBCs. Blood salvage in infants and small children (<10 kg) is rarely feasible because current pediatric salvage technology would require a minimum anticipated blood loss equal to

1–1.5 times their estimated blood volume. With allogeneic blood transfusion unavoidable in these patients, many of the advantages of autologous transfusion are negated. Such patients are probably best served through the use of minimal (single) blood donor exposure, that is, the use of "mini" (50 or 100 mL) blood packs derived from a single donor. The reader is referred to Chapter 9 (Blood Salvage Techniques).

## Acute Normovolemic Hemodilution

Patients who are to undergo operations in which major blood losses are expected may be considered candidates for acute normovolemic hemodilution. The technique has been extended to pediatric cardiac surgery, scoliosis correction, and operations for malignant disease. Age is not a contraindication to the use of hemodilution. In fact, it has been used in patients weighing 5 kg. When combined with other blood conservation measures, acute normovolemic hemodilution can substantially minimize intraoperative blood loss and the use of allogeneic blood.

### REFERENCES

1. Stockman JA III, Clark DA: Weight gain: a response to transfusion in selected preterm infants. Am J Dis Child 1984; 138:828.
2. Blank JP, Sheagren TG, Vajaria J, et al.: The role of RBC transfusion in the premature infant. Am J Dis Child 1984; 138:831.
3. Joshi A, Gerhardt T, Shandloff P, et al.: Blood transfusion effect on the respiratory pattern of preterm infants. Pediatrics 1987; 80:79.
4. Brown MS, Berman ER, Luckey D: Prediction of the need for transfusion during anemia of prematurity. J Pediatr 1990; 116:773.
5. Demaio JG, Harris MC, Deuber C, et al.: Effect of blood transfusion on apnea frequency in growing premature infants. J Pediatr 1989; 114:1039.
6. Alverson DC, Isken VH, Cohen RS: Effect of booster blood transfusions on oxygen utilization in infants with bronchopulmonary dysplasia. J Pediatr 1988; 113:722.
7. Voak D, Cann R, Finney RD, et al.: Guidelines for administration of blood products: transfusion of infants and neonates. Transfus Med 1994; 4:63.
8. Leitman SF, Holland PV: Irradiation of blood products: indications and guidelines. Transfusion 1985; 25:293.
9. Avery GB, Fletcher MA, MacDonald MG: Neonatology: Pathophysiology and Management of the Newborn. Philadelphia, 1994, J.B. Lippincott, pp. 687–689.
10. Coté CJ, Ryan JF, Todres DI, et al.: A Practice of Anesthesia for Infants and Children. Philadelphia, 1993, W.B. Saunders, pp. 191–194.
11. Andrew M, Castle V, Saigal S, et al.: Clinical impact of neonatal thrombocytopenia. J Pediatr 1987; 110:457.
12. DePalma L, Luban NLC: Blood component therapy in the perinatal period: guidelines and recommendations. Semin Perinatol 1990; 14:403.
13. Blanchette VS, Hume HA, Levy GJ, et al.: Guidelines for auditing pediatric blood transfusion practices. Am J Dis Child 1991; 145:787.
14. Christensen RD, Rothstein G, Anstall HB, et al.: Granulocyte transfusions in neonates with bacterial infection, neutropenia, and depletion of mature marrow neutrophils. Pediatrics 1982; 70:1.
15. Cairo MS: Neutrophil transfusions in the treatment of neonatal sepsis. J Pediatr 1987; 110:935.
16. Kern FH, Morana NJ, Sears JJ, et al.: Coagulation defects in neonates during cardiopulmonary bypass. Ann Thorac Surg 1992; 54:541.
17. Ekert H, Gilchrist GS: Coagulation studies in congenital heart disease. Lancet 1968; 2:280.
18. Massicotte P, Mitchell L, Andrew M: A comparative study of coagulation systems in newborn animals. Pediatr Res 1986; 20:961.
19. Mauerer H, McCue CM, Caul J, et al.: Impairment in platelet aggregation in congenital heart disease. Blood 1972; 40:207.
20. Gross S, Keefer V, Liebman J: The platelet in cyanotic congenital heart disease. Pediatrics 1968; 42:651.
21. Monada S, Vane JR: Arachidonic acid metabolites and the interactions between platelets and blood-vessel walls. N Engl J Med 1979; 300:1142.
22. Greeley WJ, Kern FH: Anesthesia for pediatric cardiac surgery. In: Miller RD, ed, Anesthesia, 3 ed. New York, 1990, Churchill-Livingstone, pp. 1653–1691.
23. Andrew M, Paes S, Milner R, et al.: Development of the human coagulation system in full-term infants. Blood 1987; 70:175.
24. Greeley WJ, de Bruijn NP: Changes in sufentanil pharmacokinetics within the neonatal period. Anesth Analg 1988; 67:86.
25. Peters M, ten Cate JW, Koo LH, et al.: Persistent antithrombin III deficiency: risk factor for thromboembolic complications in neonates small for gestational age. J Pediatr 1984; 105:310.
26. Barrowcliff TW, Johnson EA, Thomas D: Antithrombin III and heparin. Br Med Bull 1978; 34:143.
27. Harker LA: Bleeding after cardiopulmonary bypass. N Engl J Med 1986; 314:1447.
28. Harker LA, Malpass TW, Branson HE, et al.: Mechanism of abnormal bleeding in patients undergoing cardiopulmonary bypass: acquired transient platelet dysfunction associated with selective-granule release. Blood 1980; 56:824.
29. Mohr R, Golan M, Martinowitz V, et al.: Effect of cardiac operation on platelets. J Thorac Cardiovasc Surg 1986; 92:434.
30. Lavee J, Martinowitz U, Mohr R, et al.: The effect of transfusion of fresh whole blood versus platelet concentrate after cardiac operations. A scanning electron microscope study of platelet aggregation on extracellular matrix. J Thorac Cardiovasc Surg 1989; 97:204.
31. Manno CS, Hedberg KW, Kim HW, et al.: Comparison of the hemostatic effects of fresh whole blood, stored whole blood and components after open heart surgery in children. Blood 1991; 77:930.

32. Mohr R, Martinowitz U, Lavee J, et al.: The hemostatic effect of transfusing fresh whole blood versus platelet concentrates after cardiac operations. J Thorac Cardiovasc Surg 1988; 96:530.

33. McLeod BC, Sassetti RJ, Cole ER, et al.: A high-potency, single-donor cryoprecipitate of known factor VIII content dispensed in vials. Ann Intern Med 1987; 106:35.

34. McLeod BC, Sassetti RJ, Cole ER, et al.: Long-term frequent plasma exchange donation of cryoprecipitate. Transfusion 1988; 28:307.

35. Goldfinger D: Directed blood donations. Pro. Transfusion 1989; 29:70.

36. Brecher ME, Taswell HF, Clare DE, et al.: Minimal-exposure transfusion and the committed donor. Transfusion 1990; 30:599.

# ORTHOPEDIC SURGERY

## *Nabil R. Fahmy*

The last three decades have witnessed tremendous advances in the surgical management of patients with orthopedic problems. New operations have been introduced and improvements of old procedures were developed. The ensuing elaborate and extensive surgical procedures were associated with excessive amounts of blood loss and the need for allogeneic transfusions. Hemolytic reactions, metabolic side effects, and the transmission of infectious diseases may complicate these allogeneic transfusions.[1] Several techniques have been used to decrease the requirements for allogeneic blood and blood products. The recognition of acquired immunodeficiency syndrome as a transfusion-transmissible disease spurred renewed interest in blood conservation techniques. Orthopedic procedures associated with excessive intraoperative blood loss include total hip replacement (especially revision hip operations), scoliosis surgery, and resection of bone tumors with allograft placement. There are three main methods for minimizing or avoiding the need for allogeneic blood transfusion in orthopedic surgery: accepting a lower hematocrit (HCT), decreasing intraoperative blood loss, and transfusion of autologous blood. The present chapter addresses these concepts. The last section deals with the use of the pneumatic tourniquet.

## ACCEPTANCE OF A LOWER HEMATOCRIT

There are no definitive well-controlled studies that evaluate the potential risks or benefits of a specific HCT that is tolerated by surgical patients. An HCT of less than 30% has traditionally been considered an indication for blood transfusion, even in young healthy individuals.[2] Czer and Shoemaker,[3] in a retrospective study, demonstrated little benefit in transfusing critically ill postoperative patients to an HCT of more than 30%.

Currently, there is little consensus among anesthesiologists or surgeons as to the optimal perioperative HCT at which to transfuse.

Studies in baboons showed that these animals could tolerate anemia to an HCT of 10%; below this level cardiac decompensation ensued.[4] A few case reports showed that with careful management patients can survive HCTs of 10% or less.[5,6] In severely traumatized patients,[7] maintaining HCTs near 40% (control group) did not improve cardiopulmonary function, compared with HCTs maintained near 30% (study group). Pulmonary shunt increased at HCTs of 40%. Singbartl et al.[8] studied ST segment changes during extreme hemodilution in patients undergoing elective orthopedic procedures who refused to receive allogeneic blood. These authors found that ST segment changes appeared in 11 of 73 American Society of Anesthesiologists physical status (ASA ps) III patients at HCTs of 30%; there were no changes in ASA ps I or II at this HCT. At HCTs of 24%, ST segment changes were observed in five of ASA ps I or II patients and in eight additional ASA ps III patients. Further reduction of the HCT resulted in the development of ST segment changes in additional ASA ps I, II, and III patients. There was no evidence of perioperative myocardial infarction in any of the patients. Nelson et al.[9] investigated the relationship of postoperative anemia and cardiac morbidity in high-risk vascular patients in the intensive care unit. They found a significant increase in myocardial ischemia and morbid cardiac events in patients whose HCTs were 28% or less (Fig. 12–8). They concluded that the HCT should be maintained above 28% in these high-risk patients.

From the above discussion, it seems that patients with good cardiac function can tolerate HCTs in the mid-20s, whereas those with impaired cardiac function require HCTs of 30%.

## DECREASING BLOOD LOSS

This section discusses deliberate hypotension and pharmacological adjuvants that may be used to decrease blood loss.

### Deliberate Hypotension

Deliberate hypotension, as a means of reducing surgical blood loss, has proved to be beneficial in total hip[10,11] and scoliosis surgery.[12,13] It may be the only option available in Jehovah's Witnesses. Indeed, 100 Jehovah's Witness patients underwent total hip arthroplasty without transfusion.[14]

Rosberg et al.[15] showed that the average blood loss in patients undergoing total hip arthroplasty during sodium nitroprusside-induced hypotension with nitrous oxide-halothane anesthesia was significantly lower (1.3 L) when compared with normotensive tech-

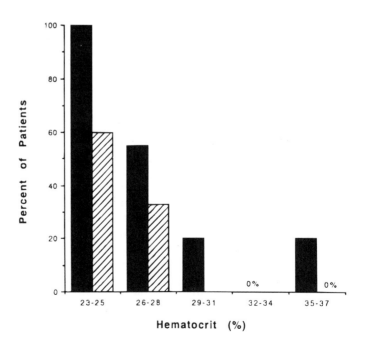

**Fig. 12–8.** Relationship between postoperative myocardial ischemia (solid bars) and cardiac morbidity (hashed bars) and postoperative hematocrit in a group of high-risk patients who underwent vascular surgery. From Nelson AH, Fleisher LA, Rosenbaum SH: Relationship of postoperative anemia and cardiac morbidity in high risk vascular patients in the intensive care unit. Crit Care Med 1993; 21:860, with permission.

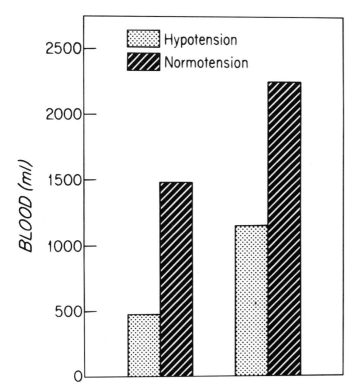

**Fig. 12–9.** *Left:* Lawson et al.[11] measured intraoperative blood loss during total hip replacement in two groups: hypotension (light bars) and normotension (dark bars). *Right:* Davis et al.[10] studied blood replacement during the entire hospitalization period (intraoperative and postoperative) in total hip replacement patients who had either deliberate hypotension (light bars) or normotension (dark bars). From Lawson NW, Thompson DS, Nelson CL, et al.: Sodium nitroprusside-induced hypotension for supine total hip replacement. Anesth Analg 1976; 55:654; and Davis NJ, Jennings J, Harris WH: Induced hypotensive anesthesia for total hip replacement. Clin Orthop Rel Res 1974; 101:93, with permission.

niques using neurolept anesthesia (2.5 L) or nitrous oxide-halothane anesthesia (2 L). Davis et al.[10] found that the blood replacement during the entire hospitalization (intraoperative and postoperative) period was significantly reduced by 50% when intraoperative hypotension was used (Fig. 12–9). Intraoperative blood loss was reduced by 67% (475 versus 1475 mL) when deliberate hypotension was used for total hip arthroplasty.[11] The use of low-dose epinephrine infusion has been reported to support cardiac output (without hypotension or increased bleeding) under hypotensive epidural anesthesia for total hip replacement.[16] Induced hypotension with ganglionic blockade and general anesthesia was associated with attenuation or elimination of the adverse effects of methylmethacrylate and insertion of prostheses during hip arthroplasty.[17]

In a study of scoliosis surgery, deliberate hypotension, achieved with ganglionic blockade (pentolinium or trimethaphan), or deep halothane anesthesia was associated with a blood loss that was 900 mL less than that during normotensive anesthesia.[12] Operative time decreased by 33 minutes in the hypotensive group.[12] Knight et al.,[13] using pentolinium (a ganglion-blocking drug) and propranolol during nitrous oxide-morphine anesthesia, obtained a "dry" operative field with a mean blood pressure of 40–55 mm Hg in patients undergoing scoliosis surgery. Heart rate and cardiac index did not change, and there were no increases in plasma renin activity, angiotensin II, norepinephrine, or dopamine. Induced hypotension is also used in patients undergoing resection of bone tumors with or without an allograft. Intraoperative blood loss decreases by 40–50% in patients in whom deliberate hypotension is used.

Intraoperative hypotension can be induced with sodium nitroprusside, nitroglycerin, trimethaphan, sodium nitroprusside-trimethaphan mixture, labetalol, deep inhalational anesthesia, or epidural anesthesia.[18,19] Hypotension induced with a 10:1 mixture of nitroprusside and trimethaphan is not associated with tachycardia.[18] Because of the synergistic or additive actions of both drugs, the dose of sodium nitroprusside used is much less than when sodium nitroprusside is used alone for a comparable level of hypotension. Furthermore, plasma cyanide levels are significantly lower with use of the mixture compared with sodium nitroprusside alone (see Chapter 8: Deliberate Hypotension).

## Pharmacological Adjuvants

Several drugs have been used in an attempt to reduce a surgical blood loss and consequently limit the need for allogeneic blood transfusion. Desmopressin acetate is a synthetic analog of L-arginine vasopressin (antidiuretic hormone). It increases von Willebrand's factor and factor VIII activity. Desmopressin acetate has been demonstrated to decrease surgical blood loss in patients undergoing spinal fusion[20] and in cardiac surgical patients.[21] It shortens bleeding time in normal subjects receiving aspirin and normalizes the bleeding time in uremic patients by nonspecific enhancement of platelet function. ε-Aminocaproic acid, tranexamic acid, and aprotinin inhibit the fibrinolytic system. They have been used in the treatment of postoperative bleeding disorders associated with cardiac bypass and prostatic surgery.[22,23] Aprotinin reduces blood loss in patients undergoing cardiac reoperations (see Part IV: Cardiac Surgery).[24]

## AUTOLOGOUS TRANSFUSIONS

There are four approaches to acquiring autologous blood for transfusion in orthopedic surgical procedures: preoperative autologous blood donation (PABD), preoperative acute normovolemic hemodilution, intraoperative blood salvage, and postoperative collection of shed blood.

## Preoperative Donation of Autologous Blood

In recent years, PABD has become increasingly popular because of fear of transfusion-transmitted human immunodeficiency virus. The amount of blood donated preoperatively depends on the contemplated procedure. Patients scheduled for an elective hip replacement usually donate 1–3 units of blood. Four to 6 units are usually required for revision hip surgery. The amount of blood collected from scoliosis patients is determined by the patient's weight. A full unit is taken from patients 50 kg or more, and a half-unit is collected from those weighing 25–50 kg. Blood

is usually collected at the hospital where the surgery is scheduled. However, for out-of-town patients, blood is donated at a regional blood bank center and then transferred to the hospital.

Donation of 1 unit of blood lowers the HCT by approximately 3% and the hemoglobin by approximately 1 g/dL. Donation of blood stimulates erythropoiesis approximately 1.5 times the norm in healthy men. Oral iron supplementation is important in maintaining the rate of erythropoiesis. The use of recombinant erythropoietin can accelerate red cell regeneration, increase the amount donated, and diminish transfusion needs in the postoperative period (see Chapter 6: Preoperative Autologous Blood Donation).

### ADVANTAGES

Autologous blood transfusion eliminates the transmissible infectious diseases and prevents the occurrence of transfusion reactions (except those caused by clerical errors) and antigen formation. In addition, the surgical patient is both physiologically and psychologically better prepared for operation.[25] PABD increases the production of red blood cells by the bone marrow, increases the level of 2′,3′-diphosphoglycerate, and improves tissue perfusion (from reduced blood viscosity). Psychologically, autologous blood donation reduces the patients' fear of receiving allogeneic blood and makes them feel involved in their medical care. Autologous blood frees the patient from possible delays of operation caused by the unavailability of banked blood and may be the only option for patients with antibodies for whom a safe cross match is unavailable.

### DISADVANTAGES

Vasovagal reactions occur in 2–5% during donation of blood, especially first-time donors, young donors, and females.[26] Lightheadedness usually occurs due to a transient hypotension and is self-limited. Loss of consciousness (0.3%) and convulsive syncope (0.03%) are rare reactions. Autologous blood donation may cause administrative and scheduling challenges in hospitals. Clerical errors may be responsible for a lethal hemolytic reaction after autologous blood transfusion.[27] Furthermore, the cost per unit of autologous blood may be slightly more expensive than that of allogeneic blood.

PABD obviates the need for allogeneic transfusion in the majority of patients undergoing elective orthopedic procedures. However, allogeneic transfusion may still be needed in 28–39% of patients undergoing hip replacements, knee replacements, and especially scoliosis correction.[28] In these situations, the need for additional allogeneic blood can be reduced by using deliberate hypotension or hemodilution.

## Preoperative Acute Normovolemic Hemodilution

Acute normovolemic hemodilution can be used in elective orthopedic procedures when an intraoperative blood loss of 1000–2000 mL is anticipated. This technique is a possible approach to reduce the use of allogeneic blood products, especially in patients who have not participated in an autologous predonation program.[29] In children having spinal surgery, target HCTs of 22% have been used. Typical target HCTs for adults are between 25 and 30%[30] (see Chapter 7: Acute Normovolemic Hemodilution).

Perioperative normovolemic hemodilution is a safe procedure. It should be an important part of the total strategy to limit the use of allogeneic blood, especially in patients with rare blood groups. Additional advantages include the saving of time required for typing and cross matching, the immediate availability of blood for reinfusion, and substantial savings in the use of bank blood and its products. It can be combined with other methods aimed at diminishing the use of allogeneic blood, such as predonation programs, intraoperative autotransfusion, and deliberate hypotension.

## Combined Use of Hemodilution and Hypotension

Because deliberate hypotension can decrease blood loss significantly and because acute normovolemic hemodilution minimizes the need for homologous blood, it seems logical that the combined use of both techniques should be more advantageous.[31,32] The effects of deliberate hypotension and normovolemic hemodilution on operative blood loss were compared in patients undergoing total hip arthroplasty.[33] Deliberate hypotension was superior to hemodilution in decreasing blood loss. We have pioneered the feasibility of the combined use of these techniques since 1975. Two reports have described the usefulness of this combination.[34,35] The discussion that follows is based on our own experience.

## CLINICAL EXPERIENCE WITH HEMODILUTION AND HYPOTENSION

Our work has been primarily with major orthopedic procedures, including revision of total hip replacement, insertion of Harrington rods for repair of scoliosis, bone transplant operations, and hemipelvectomies. In general, we find that most patients do not require allogeneic blood transfusions, despite the extensiveness of the surgery involved.

In a serious of 104 patients undergoing revision of total hip arthroplasty, intraoperative allogeneic blood replacement was 800 ± 105 mL (mean ± SEM) when both hemodilution and deliberate hypotension were combined. Autologous blood (collected preoperatively) transfused to these patients was 950 ± 85 mL. When deliberate hypotension was used alone in a group of 36 patients undergoing similar operative procedures, mean intraoperative blood replacement was 2450 ± 205 mL of allogeneic blood and blood products. With normotensive anesthesia alone, intraoperative blood requirement was 4500 ± 340 mL in 54 similar patients. The difference between normotension and hemodilution with hypotension was statistically significant ($P < .05$). These figures strongly support the claim for a diminished need for allogeneic blood when combined with moderate hemodilution with hypotension. This is supported further by the finding that no allogeneic blood was required in 47 patients of the Jehovah's Witness faith who underwent (for the first time) total replacement of the hip joint.[19] In all patients there were no complications attributable to the combined use of deliberate hypotension and hemodilution.

Preoperative examination and adequate evaluation of the various organ systems are imperative. In general, patients with no history or clinical evidence of any disease that may compromise the circulation to any major organ are considered good-risk candidates for the combined technique. Contraindications apply equally to the use of either technique separately.

Autologous blood is collected either several days before operation or in the immediate preoperative period. In the latter situation, equal volumes of albumin (5% solution) and lactated Ringer's solution are infused while blood is withdrawn. After induction of anesthesia and with the patient hemodynamically stable, hypotension is induced to a mean arterial pressure of approximately 70 mm Hg. We find that in the hemodiluted patient, cardiac output decreases significantly if mean arterial blood pressure falls below 70 mm Hg.[31] Consequently, we consider that organ blood flow might decrease below acceptable safe levels if it were allowed to fall below this figure, and it is our practice therefore to limit hypotension accordingly. We prefer short-acting (e.g., sodium nitroprusside, nitroglycerin, or trimethaphan) to long-acting hypotensive drugs (e.g., labetalol) because arterial blood pressure can be more quickly and easily restored if there should be hemodynamic instability. It is our clinical experience that blood pressure decreases easily when sodium nitroprusside is used in hemodiluted normovolemic patients. Hemodynamically, they respond by a decrease in systemic vascular resistance, whereas cardiac output increases provided mean arterial pressure remains at or above 70 mm Hg. This is in contrast to the findings in hemodiluted dogs in which the administration of sodium nitroprusside was associated with a hazardous decrease in cardiac output.[36] Continuous monitoring of the arterial, central venous, pulmonary arterial, and capillary wedge pressures; electrocardiograph (leads 2 and $V_5$); arterial and mixed venous blood gases; blood loss; body temperature; and urine output is essential with induced hypotension and hemodilution.

It should be emphasized that the combined use of both techniques requires experience and vigilance. Collaboration between anesthesiologists and surgeons is imperative, and an understanding of the physiology and pharmacology of the various interventions is mandatory.

## Intraoperative Blood Salvage

Transfusion of salvaged blood is undertaken in patients undergoing total hip replace-ment, total knee replacement (when a tourniquet is not used), extensive surgery of the spine, and scoliosis surgery.[37] The combined use of intraoperative blood salvaging and induced hypotension decreased total blood transfusion needs by approximately 50% (from 3.4 to 6.0 units) in patients undergoing spinal surgery.[38] Similarly, the requirements for allogeneic transfusions were decreased in patients undergoing hip replacement.[39] In children undergoing surgical correction of scoliosis, intraoperative salvage was effective in reducing or eliminating allogeneic blood needs when combined with preoperative donation of autologous blood.[40] Some Jehovah's Witnesses may accept autologous transfusions provided the blood is collected and retained through an uninterrupted circuit.

Automated cell scavengers are cost-effective for operations with moderate anticipated blood loss, that is, more than 2 units. Several studies agree that the break-even point for this technique occurs when the allogeneic equivalents of between 2.7 and 3.1 units of blood have been collected.[39,41] However, most of the analyses do not consider some of the hidden costs of allogeneic transfusion that may not be immediately apparent (see Chapter 9: Blood Salvage Techniques).

## Postoperative Collection of Shed Blood

Blood that drains from the surgical site after surgery is filtered and given back to the patient. The blood should be reinfused within 4 hours to prevent the possibility of bacterial colonization because it is at room temperature (See Chapter 9: Blood Salvage Techniques).

## Erythropoietin

Erythropoietin is an obligatory growth factor of erythroid cells.[42,43] It is a single-chain polypeptide composed of 106 amino acids and has a molecular weight of 30,400 d. This hormone is produced by the kidney, but the liver may produce it in response to anemia. Tissue hypoxia is an important trigger for erythropoietin production. Recombinant human erythropoietin has been given to patients who have to donate a large number of units of blood before surgery.[44–47] In 47 adult patients scheduled for elective orthopedic procedures in which 31 underwent hip replacement, the use of erythropoietin and iron increased the number of predonated units. Twenty-two of 23 patients in the erythropoietin-iron group donated 4 or more units compared with 17 of 24 in the placebo-iron group. Furthermore, the red blood cell mass of the predonated units was higher in the erythropoietin-treated group. Birgegard et al.[48] suggested the use of erythropoietin in combination with predonation. Iron must be given when recombinant human erythropoietin is administered, because the acceleration of erythropoietin frequently outstrips the rate of mobilization of storage iron, creating a state of relative iron deficiency.[45,49] Recombinant erythropoietin has no adverse effects on blood pressure or cardiovascular function and does not appear to be antigenic in humans.[42] Side effects may include a "flu-like" syndrome, hypertension, hypertensive encephalopathy and seizures (see Chapter 6: Preoperative Autologous Blood Donation).

## PNEUMATIC TOURNIQUETS

The purpose of a tourniquet is to apply sufficient pressure to the blood vessels of an extremity to occlude the arterial inflow but not enough to harm any of the structures compressed. Use of the pneumatic tourniquet provides a bloodless field for operations on the extremities. If a tourniquet is to be used, it should be both effective and safe.

### Checking the Equipment

The pressure gauge should be accurate, and all connections should be tested for leaks. Daily calibration of the gauge against a mercury manometer is recommended because a gauge that reads low may cause excessively high pressure on the patient's extremity and a gauge that reads high may lead to loss or inadequate control of hemostasis.

### Site and Application of the Tourniquet

A tourniquet is applied only to the proximal part of a limb where muscle provides protective padding for nerves and vessels. After wrapping several layers of padding (to avoid minor trauma to the skin), the cuff is applied closely to achieve effective tissue compression.

### Tourniquet Pressure and Duration of Inflation

It is generally accepted that a reasonable pressure for an upper limb tourniquet is 200–275 mm Hg and for a lower limb 300–350 mm Hg.[50] Some authors apply a pressure that is 50 mm Hg above that patient's systolic blood pressure for the arm and 150 mm Hg for the thigh. The limb is exsanguinated before application of the tourniquet. Inflation should be as rapid as possible to avoid venous congestion; slow inflation briefly blocks venous return while allowing the arterial inflow to persist, thus producing a degree of congestion. The "tourniquet time" should be the shortest time necessary for the planned surgery. A 2-hour limit to a single application of a tourniquet is suggested by the majority of authors. If the operation necessarily goes beyond the suggested time limit, the tourniquet should be deflated for a period of 15–20 minutes to allow the tissues to recover. After the surgery is completed, the tourniquet is deflated rapidly to avoid the risk of venous congestion.

### Effects of Tourniquet Deflation

#### LOCAL EFFECTS

Reactive hyperemia, increased fibrinolytic activity,[51,52] a transient increase in potassium concentration in the venous blood leaving the limb, increased extracellular water content (edema), a fall in $PO_2$, and rise in $PCO_2$ of the ischemic limb have all been reported.[53]

#### SYSTEMIC EFFECTS

A decrease in blood pressure occurs after tourniquet deflation.[54] Metabolic changes include a fall in arterial $PO_2$ and pH and an increase in serum potassium, lactate, and arterial $PCO_2$.[55] These changes are moderate and reversible. Pulmonary vascular changes have recently been reported[56] (see Chapter 4: Blood Conservation Techniques).

### Complications

Nerve injury is probably due to direct pressure of the tourniquet on the nerve. Ischemia and metabolic changes may play a role. The extent of muscle damage is related to the duration of ischemia.[57] Postoperative edema is believed to be multifactorial in origin; tissue ischemia, increased capillary permeability, serotonin, kinins, and disturbance of acetylcholine-esterase system have been postulated as causative factors.

## Contraindications

Peripheral arterial disease, calcification of vessels, deep venous thrombosis, and crushed injuries are contraindications to the use of a tourniquet. A tourniquet should be used with caution in the presence of sickle cell disease.

### REFERENCES

1. Dodd RY: The risk of transfusion transmitted infection. N Engl J Med 1992; 327:14.
2. Kowalyshyn TJ, Prager D, Young J: A review of the present status of preoperative hemoglobin requirements. Anesth Analg 1972; 51:75.
3. Czer LS, Shoemaker WC: Optimal hematocrit value in critically ill postoperative patients. Surg Gynecol Obstet 1978; 147:363.
4. Wilkerson DK, Rosen AL, Lakshman R, et al.: Limits of cardiac compensation in anemic baboons. Surgery 1988; 103:6654.
5. Tremper KK, Freedman AE, Levine EM, et al.: The preoperative treatment of severely anemic patients with perfluorochemical emulsion oxygen transporting fluid, Fluosol-DA. N Engl J Med 1982; 307: 277.
6. Lichtenstein A, Echhart WF, Swanson KJ, et al.: Unplanned intraoperative and postoperative hemodilution: oxygen transport and consumption during severe anemia. Anesthesiology 1988; 69:119.
7. Fortune JB, Feustrel PJ, Saifi J, et al.: Influence of hematocrit on cardiopulmonary function after acute hemorrhage. J Trauma 1987; 27:243.
8. Singbartl G, Becker M, Frankenberger C, et al.: Intraoperative on-line ST segment analysis with extreme normovolemic hemodilution (Abstract). Anesth Analg 1992; 74:S295.
9. Nelson AH, Fleisher LA, Rosenbaum SH: Relationship of postoperative anemia and cardiac morbidity in high risk vascular patients in the intensive care unit. Crit Care Med 1993; 21:860.
10. Davis NJ, Jennings J, Harris WH: Induced hypotensive anesthesia for total hip replacement. Clin Orthop Rel Res 1974; 101:93.
11. Lawson NW, Thompson DS, Nelson CL, et al.: Sodium nitroprusside-induced hypotension for supine total hip replacement. Anesth Analg 1976; 55:654.
12. McNeil TW, DeWald RL, Kuo KN, et al.: Controlled hypotensive anesthesia in scoliosis surgery. J Bone Joint Surg [Am] 1974; 56A:1167.
13. Knight PR, Lane GA, Nicholls GM, et al.: Hormonal and hemodynamic changes induced by pentolinium and propranolol during surgical correction of scoliosis. Anesthesiology 1980; 53:127.
14. Nelson CC, Bowen WS: Total hip arthroplasty in Jehovah's Witnesses without blood transfusion. J Bone Joint Surg [Am] 1986; 68A:350.
15. Rosberg B, Fredin H, Gustafson C: Anesthetic techniques and surgical blood loss in total hip arthroplasty. Acta Anaesthesiol Scand 1982; 26:189.
16. Sharrock NE, Mineo R, Urquhart B: Haemodynamic effects and outcome analysis of hypotensive extradural anaesthesia in controlled hypertensive patients undergoing total hip arthroplasty. Br J Anaesth 1991; 67:17.
17. Fahmy NR, Harris WH, Laver MD: Modification of systemic effects following insertion of bone cement during deliberate hypotension. Abstracts of Scientific Papers, Annual Meeting of the American Society of Anesthesiologists, Washington, D.C., 1974:79.
18. Fahmy NR: Nitroprusside vs. a nitroprusside-trimethaphan mixture for induced hypotension: hemodynamic effects and cyanide release. Clin Pharmacol Ther 1985; 37:264.
19. Fahmy NR: Haemodilution and hypotension. In: Enderby GEH, ed, Hypotensive Anaesthesia. London, 1985, Churchill Livingstone, p. 164.
20. Kobrinsky NL, Letts RM, Patel LR, et al.: 1-Desamino-8-D-arginine vasopressin (Desmopressin) decreases operative blood loss in patients having Harrington rod spinal fusion surgery. Ann Intern Med 1987; 107:446.
21. Salzman EW, Weinstein MJ, Weintraub RM, et al.: Treatment with desmopressin acetate to reduce blood loss after cardiac surgery: a double-blind randomized trial. N Engl J Med 1986; 314:1402.
22. van Oeveren W, Jansen NJG, Bidstrup BP, et al.: Effects of aprotinin on hemostatic mechanisms during cardiopulmonary bypass. Ann Thorac Surg 1987; 44:640.
23. Royston D: High-dose aprotinin therapy: a review of the first five years' experience. J Cardiothorac Vasc Anesth 1992; 6:76.
24. Cosgrove D, Heric B, Lytle BW, et al.: Aprotinin therapy for reoperative myocardial revascularization. A placebo controlled study. Ann Thorac Surg 1992; 54:1031.
25. Yomtovian R, Ceynar J, Kepner JL, et al.: Predeposit autologous blood transfusion: an analysis of donor attitudes and attributes. QRB 1987; 13:45.
26. Ruetz PP, Johnson SA, Collahan R, et al.: Fainting: a review of its mechanism and a study in blood donors. Medicine (Baltimore) 1967; 46:363.
27. Myrhe DA: Fatalities from blood transfusion. JAMA 1980; 244:1333.
28. Bailey TE Jr, Mahoney OM: The use of banked autologous blood in patients undergoing surgery for spinal deformity. J Bone Joint Surg [Am] 1987; 69A: 329.
29. Vela R: Hemodilution in hip surgery. Bibl Haematol 1975; 41:271.
30. Messmer KFW: Acceptable hematocrit levels in surgical patients. World J Surg 1987; 11:41.
31. Fahmy NR, Chandler HP, Patel DG, et al.: Hemodynamics and oxygen availability during acute hemodilution in conscious man (Abstract). Anesthesiology 1980; 53:S84.
32. Fahmy NR: A comparison of three methods for blood conservation for major orthopedic procedures (Abstract). Anesthesiology 1994; 81:A1248.
33. Barbier-Bohm G, Desmonts JM, Couderc E, et al.: Comparative effects of induced hypotension and normovolaemic haemodilution on blood loss in total hip arthroplasty. Br J Anaesth 1980; 52:1039.
34. Eerola R, Eerola M, Kaukinen L, et al.: Controlled hypotension and moderate hemodilution in major hip surgery. Ann Chir Gynaecol 1979; 68:109.
35. Wong KC, Webster LR, Coleman SS, et al.: Hemodilution and induced hypotension for insertion of a

Harrington rod in a Jehovah's Witness patient. Clin Orthop Rel Res 1980; 152:237.

36. Boon JC, Jesch F, Stelter WJ, et al.: Sodium nitro-prusside induced hypotension and isovolemic hemo-dilution in dogs. Chir Forum Exp Klin Forsch (Berlin) 1977; Apr:27.

37. Viviani GR, Sadler JTS, Inghan GK: Autotransfusions in scoliosis surgery. Clin Orthop Rel Res 1978; 135:74.

38. Lennon RL, Hosking MP, Gray JR, et al.: The effects of intraoperative blood salvage and induced hypotension on transfusion requirements during spinal surgical procedures. Mayo Clin Proc 1987; 62:1090.

39. Bovill DJ, Moulton CW, Jackson WST, et al.: The efficacy of intraoperative autologous transfusion in major orthopedic surgery: a regression analysis. Orthopedics 1986; 9:1403.

40. Kruger LM, Colbert JM: Intraoperative autologous transfusion in children undergoing spinal surgery. J Pediatr Orthop 1985; 5:330.

41. Solomon MD, Rutledge ML, Kane LE, et al.: Cost comparison of intraoperative autologous versus homologous transfusion. Transfusion 1988; 28:379.

42. Biesma DH, Kraaijenhagen RJ, Dalmuder J, et al.: Recombinant human erythropoietin in autologous blood donors: a dose-finding study. Br J Haematol 1994; 86:30.

43. Saikawa I, Hotokebuchi T, Arita C, et al.: Autologous blood transfusion with recombinant erythropoietin treatment. 22 arthroplasties for rheumatoid arthritis. Acta Orthop Scand 1994; 65:15.

44. Beris P, Mermillod B, Levy G, et al.: Recombinant human erythropoietin as adjuvant treatment for autologous blood donation. A prospective study. Vox Sang 1993; 65:212.

45. Mercuriali F, Zanella A, Barosi G, et al.: Use of erythropoietin to increase the volume of autologous blood donated by orthopedic patients. Transfusion 1993; 33:55.

46. Mercuriali F, Adamson JW: Recombinant human erythropoietin enhances blood donation for autolo-gous use and reduces exposure to homologous blood during elective surgery. Semin Hematol 1993; 30:17.

47. Mercuriali F, Gualtieri G, Sinigaglia L, et al.: Use of recombinant human erythropoietin to assist autolo-gous blood donation by anemic rheumatoid arthritis patients undergoing major orthopedic surgery. Transfusion 1994; 34:501.

48. Danersund BG, Hogman C, Milbrink J, et al.: Physi-ological response to phlebotomies for autologous transfusion at elective hip-joint surgery. Eur J Haematol 1991; 46:136.

49. Goodnough LT, Verbrugge D, Marcus RE, et al.: The effect of patient size and dose of recombinant human erythropoietin therapy on red blood cell volume expansion in autologous blood donors for elective orthopedic operation. J Am Coll Surg 1994; 179:171.

50. Klenerman L: The tourniquet in surgery. J Bone Joint Surg [Br] 1962; 44B:937.

51. Klenerman L, Chakrabarti R, Mackie I, et al.: Changes in haemostatic system after application of a tourniquet. Lancet 1977; 1:970.

52. Fahmy NR, Patel D: Hemostatic changes and post-operative deep vein thrombosis associated with pneu-matic tourniquet. J Bone Joint Surg [Am] 1981; 63:A461.

53. Wilgis EF: Observations on the effects of tourniquet ischaemia. J Bone Joint Surg [Am] 1971; 53A:1343.

54. Bradford EMW: Hemodynamic changes associated with the application of lower limb tourniquets. An-aesthesia 1969; 24:190.

55. Modig J, Kolstad K, Wigren A: Systemic reactions to tourniquet ischemia. Acta Anaesthesiol Scand 1978; 22:609.

56. Fahmy NR, Patel D, Sunder N: Hemodynamic ef-fects of the pneumatic tourniquet in patients with and without cardiovascular disease (Abstract). Anes-thesiology 1991; 75:A905.

57. Rorabeck GH: Tourniquet-induced nerve ischaemia: an experimental investigation. Trauma 1980; 20:280.

# 13

# SURGICAL HEMOSTASIS AND BLOOD CONSERVATION

## ENDOVASCULAR EMBOLIZATION IN THE MANAGEMENT OF SKULL-BASE TUMORS

### *Fernando Viñuela and Rinaldo F. Canalis*

## INTRODUCTION

The development of a new generation of microcatheters and microwires allows a safer superselective catheterization of extracranial and intracranial vessels, thereby permitting a better identification of the blood supply of vascular malformations and tumors at the skull base. These advances have greatly contributed to our current ability to remove these lesions with increased precision, more rapidly, and with significant reduction of blood loss during surgery. In this chapter we primarily address preoperative embolization methods used to decrease intraoperative blood loss. These embolizations are usually performed immediately before the surgical procedure.

## PREOPERATIVE EMBOLIZATION OF SKULL-BASE HYPERVASCULAR TUMORS

Performance of therapeutic superselective angiography of skull-base tumors requires (*a*) an in-depth knowledge of the normal vascular anatomy, (*b*) identification of unusual vascular anomalies, (*c*) recognition of hemodynamic balances among different vascular territories, and (*d*) awareness of dangerous vascular anastomoses that can be the source of untoward embolization structures (Fig. 13–1).[1] The tumors most frequently embolized are paragangliomas (glomus caroticum glomus jugulare, glomus vagal, glomus tympanicum), juvenile angiofibromas, meningiomas, and schwannomas.

Before embolization it is important to delineate (*a*) anastomoses between branches of the external carotid artery (ascending pharyngeal, middle meningeal, accessory meningeal and internal maxillary arteries) with the intracavernous branches of the carotid artery, (*b*) anastomoses between external carotid artery branches (ascending pharyngeal and occipital arteries) and the vertebral artery (Figure 13–1), and (*c*) ophthalmic artery/external carotid artery anastomoses (middle meningeal, internal maxillary, and facial arteries). Untoward delivery of embolic agents through these anastomoses may be the source of intracranial ischemic complications.[2]

In addition, attention must be given to the neuromeningeal branches of the external carotid artery that contribute to the blood supply of the cranial nerves as they transverse the skull base.[3] Occlusion of these branches will result in the cranial nerve dysfunction. For example, the stylomastoid artery, a branch of the occipital artery, supplies the facial nerve at the

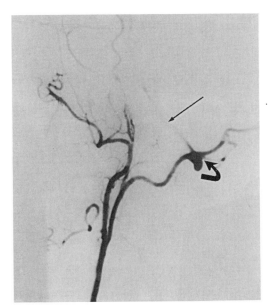

**Fig. 13–1.** Example of dangerous anastomosis. Lateral view of external carotid angiogram shows visualization of the vertebral artery (arrow) through occipital-vertebral anastomosis (curved arrow).

stylomastoid foramen. Accidental emboliza-tion of this branch may produce a facial palsy. Similarly, occlusion of the middle meningeal artery proximal to the foramen spinosum may elicit a facial palsy related to ischemia of the geniculate ganglion or intrapetrous segment of the facial nerve.[4]

## Paragangliomas

These tumors arise from brachiomeric and intravagal paraganglion structures, including the carotid bodies at the bifurcation of the common carotid arteries, the glomus jugulare in the adventitia of the jugular bulb, the glomus tympanicum associated with the glosso-pharyngeal nerve, the vagal body found within the perineurium of the vagus nerve, and the aorticopulmonary ganglia situated at various levels of the aortic arch.[3]

Most cases occur in middle age, with a 2:1 female preponderance.[5] Approximately 7% have been reported to be familial, and it is well known that they may be multiple.[6] Paragan-gliomas are usually benign.[7] They vary in size from 5 to 15 cm in diameter, and they tend to be globular within a fibrous capsule. Be-cause 5% of these tumors are catecholamine and serotonin secretors, angiography and em-

bolization may precipitate a hypertensive cri-sis. However, in clinical practice this is rarely seen.

The evaluation of paragangliomas includes computed tomography, magnetic resonance imaging, and superselective angiography. Ir-respective of their topography, the tumors have a typical angiographic architecture con-sisting of enlarged arterial feeders, early ap-pearance and persistence of an intense blush, and demonstration of drainage through en-larged veins.

The majority of paragangliomas is supplied from the musculospinal branch of the ascend-ing pharyngeal artery and not usually from branches of the occipital artery and posterior auricular artery (Fig. 13–2). Depending on its extension, the tumor may recruit blood supply from meningeal branches of the internal ca-rotid and vertebral artery, as well as pial branches from posterior inferior and anterior inferior cerebellar arteries (intradural compo-nent of the tumor).[8]

It is possible to selectively catheterize the individual feeders of a paraganglioma and identify the different vascular compartments of the tumor.[8] This procedure is performed in the radiology angiography suite, with the patient under neuroleptic analgesia. Preembo-lization injection of 30 mg of lidocaine into the arterial feeders may produce a transient cranial nerve palsy, thereby allowing identifi-cation of blood supply to cranial nerves.[9]

The most frequent embolic agent used for preoperative occlusion of the blood supply of these tumors is polyvinyl alcohol particles (PVA), 300–600 $\mu$m in diameter. The em-bolic material is suspended in nonionic con-trast material and slowly injected into the arte-rial feeder under permanent fluoroscopic control. It is essential to deposit the PVA into the tumor bed to reduce the possibility of tumor recanalization.

Evidence of recruitment of blood supply from the internal carotid artery indicates tumor infiltration of the arterial wall. In these cases, it may be necessary to perform preoper-ative temporary balloon occlusion of the inter-nal carotid artery. This maneuver allows the surgeon to know whether the patient will tol-erate permanent occlusion of the internal ca-rotid artery when total tumor removal is con-sidered. A preoperative permanent occlusion of the internal carotid artery with detachable

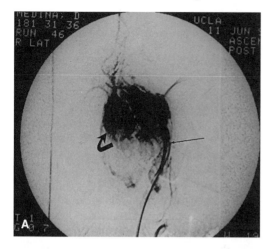

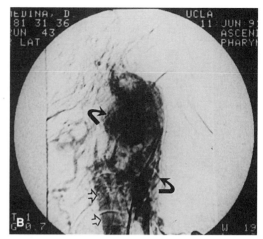

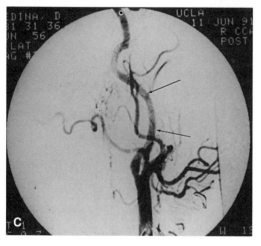

**Fig. 13–2.** Embolization of paraganglioma. Early arterial (*a*) and venous (*b*) phases of ascending pharyngeal angiogram show the feeding artery (straight arrow), classical intense tumor blush (curved arrow), and drainage into the jugular vein (open arrows). *c*: Postembolization external carotid angiogram shows absence of tumor blush and displacement of the internal carotid artery (straight arrow) by the embolized tumor.

balloons may also be performed immediately before surgery in tumors encasing the intrapetrous segment of the internal carotid artery, in paragangliomas infiltrating the cavernous sinus, and in tumors eroding the carotid canal, recruiting blood supply from caroticotympanic and cavernous branches of the internal carotid artery. Complications of this technique that drastically reduces intraoperative blood loss remain rare.[2,10]

## Juvenile Nasopharyngeal Angiofibromas

Juvenile nasopharyngeal angiofibromas constitute 0.5% of head and neck tumors and are predominantly found in adolescent males.[11] They are benign highly vascular tumors that originate in the nasopharynx but may extend into the orbit infratemporal space

and intracranially.[12] Computerized tomography and magnetic resonence imaging give valuable information of the location and extension of these lesions. Superselective angiography determines their blood supply and sets the stage for preoperative embolization to facilitate total surgical removal with reduced blood loss.

The arterial supply to juvenile nasopharyngeal angiofibromas arises primarily from branches of the internal maxillary artery, though not infrequently there is participation of the facial and ascending pharyngeal arteries as well as ethmoidal branches of the ophthalmic artery (Fig. 13–3). The tumor attached to the skull base may also recruit blood supply from the vidiomandibular branch of the internal carotid artery. This artery shares the same vascular territory as the ipsilateral ascending pharyngeal artery.[13]

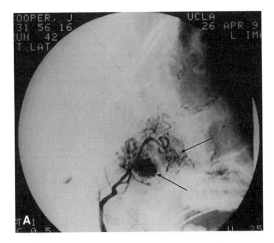

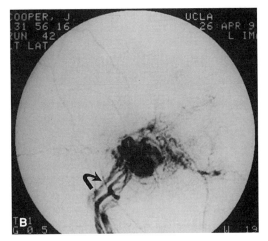

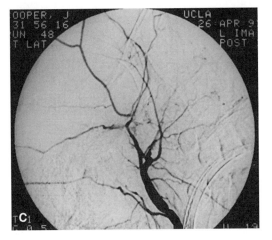

**Fig. 13–3.** Embolization of juvenile angiofibroma. Early (*a*) and late (*b*) phases of internal maxillary arteriogram show the tumor blush (straight arrows) supplied by numerous branches of the internal maxillary artery as well as its venous drainage (curved arrows). *c*: Postembolization external carotid angiogram shows absence of tumor blush, after embolization with PVA, 300–600 $\mu$m in diameter.

The use of small microcatheters allows safe selective catheterization and embolization of all feeders arising from the external carotid artery and sometimes from enlarged feeders arising from the internal carotid artery. Embolization is performed in the angiography suite, with the patient under neuroleptic analgesia and immediately before surgery. PVA, 300–600 $\mu$m in diameter, is the most frequently used embolic agent, and at the end of embolization, the trunk of the arterial feeder is occluded with coils or absorbable gelatin sponge. This last maneuver avoids early tumor recanalization through local arterial collaterals. The injection of embolic material must be gentle and staged to decrease the possibility of untoward delivery of particles into the intracranial circulation through external carotid/internal carotid anastomoses. Not infrequently, it is necessary to embolize both internal maxillary and ascending pharyngeal

arteries if the tumor has extended beyond the midline. Ischemic cranial nerves palsies are rarely seen in the embolization of juvenile nasopharyngeal angiofibromas. The vascular supply to the cranial nerves in the cavernous sinus (III, IV, V, and VI cranial nerves) is mainly from branches of the internal maxillary and intracavernous branches of the internal carotid artery. These include the cavernous branch of the middle meningeal artery, the accessory meningeal artery, and the artery of the foramen rotundum. The use of PVA particles 300–600 $\mu$m in diameter decreases the risk of compromising collaterals to the supply of these cranial nerves. Serious complications occur from the use of improper embolic material or proximal localization of the delivery system. Safe and successful embolization depends on detailed analysis of vascular anatomy and depiction of dangerous external carotid/internal carotid or external carotid/ophthalmic anastomoses with appropriate subtraction techniques.

## Meningiomas

Meningiomas represent 15% of all intracranial tumors. They are most common in middle-aged women.[14] Meningiomas of the skull base may involve anterior, middle, or posterior fossae, and they collect their vascular supply from regional meningeal vessels.[15] Anterior fossa meningiomas are mainly supplied from ethmoidal branches of the ophthalmic artery as well as branches of the anterior division of the middle meningeal artery.

Meningiomas of the middle fossa are supplied from branches of internal maxillary, middle meningeal, and accessory meningeal arteries as well as intracavernous branches of internal carotid artery.

Posterior fossa and foramen magnum meningiomas are supplied from meningeal branches of ascending pharyngeal and occipital arteries as well as meningeal branches of vertebral arteries. The posterior inferior and anterior inferior cerebellar arteries may also supply the deepest portion of these tumors.

Superselective catheterization of most of these arteries identifies the lesion's blood supply and permits preoperative occlusion of significant portions of the tumor. Before embolization, selective injections of the vessels should be performed to depict dangerous anastomoses between extracranial and intracranial circulation as well as potential compromise of blood supply of cranial nerves, where they pierce the dura to become extracranial. For example, the neuromeningeal branch of the ascending pharyngeal artery is commonly involved in the blood supply of posterior fossa meningiomas. It also supplies the 9th–12th cranial nerves, and it has anastomoses with the internal carotid and vertebral arteries.

PVA is usually used as the preferred embolic material and is injected through microcatheters positioned as close as possible to the tumor bed. Postembolization steroids are used to decrease swelling of the tumor and potential compression of cranial nerves or brainstem.

Complications related to preoperative embolization of meningiomas are rare. Lasjuanias and Berenstein[16] report 1.6% of long-term morbidity and no mortality in 185 patients. Larger series have also shown safety and effectiveness of the preoperative embolization of meningiomas.[17]

## Schwannomas

These tumors arise from the sheath of cranial and spinal nerve roots and less often from peripheral nerves[7] and account for 8% of all intracranial tumors and 80% of tumors in the cerebello-pontine angle. They are seen in middle-aged patients and are twice as common in females as in males.[7] Multiple tumors are seen in patients with neurofibromatosis.

The authors have been involved in the embolization of Vth and Xth cranial nerve Schwannomas. These tumors show a pathognomonic angiographical picture characterized by a "leaflet tree" appearance in homogeneous blush and areas of contrast puddling. The tumor blush is not as intense and disappears earlier in the angiogram than the blush observed in paragangliomas.[18]

The main arterial supply from Schwannomas in the neck arise from the ascending pharyngeal artery. Selective catheterization of this artery allows safe preoperative embolization of the tumor with PVA 300–600 $\mu m$ in diameter. The trunk of the ascending pharyngeal artery is permanently occluded with microcoils after the delivery of the particles into the tumor bed to avoid early tumor recanalization. Not unusually, local muscular branches of the occipital artery and ascending cervical arteries are recruited by the tumor. These arteries may also be selectively catheterized and embolized before surgery.

### REFERENCES

1. Lasjuanias P, Berenstein A: Surgical Neuroangiography. Functional Anatomy of Craniofacial Arteries, 1 ed. New York, 1987, Springer-Verlag, vol. 1.
2. Valavanis A: Preoperative embolization of the head and neck: indications, patient selection, goals and precautions. Am J Neuroradiol 1986; 7:943.
3. Glenner GG, Grimley PM: Tumors of the extra-adrenal paraganglion systems (including chemoreceptors). Atlas of Tumor Pathology, 2nd series, fascicle 9. Washington, DC, 1974, Armed Forces Institute of Pathology.
4. Lasjuanias P: Aspect sagiographique de la vascularisation des nerfs craniens. Presented at 4eme. Cong Annuel de la Societe Francaise de Neuroradiologie, Toulouse, 1979.
5. Parry DM, Li FP, Strong L, et al.: Carotid body tumors in humans: genetics and epidemiology. J Natl Cancer Inst 1983; 68:563.
6. Dunn GD, Brown MJ, Sapsford RN, et al.: Functioning middle mediastinal paraganglioma associated with intercarotid paragangliomas. Lancet 1986; 1: 1061.

7. Russell DS, Rubinstein LJ: Pathology of Tumors of the Nervous System, 5 ed. Baltimore, 1989, Williams and Wilkins, p. 961.

8. Moret J, Picard L: Vascular architecture of tympano-jugular glomus tumors: its relevance in therapeutic angiography. Semin Intervent Radiol 1987; 4:291.

9. Horton JA, Kerber CW: Lidocaine injection into the external carotid branches: provocative test to preserve cranial nerve function in therapeutic embolization. Am J Neuroradiol 1986; 7:105.

10. Lacour P, Doyon D, Manelfe C, et al.: Treatment of chemodectomas by arterial embolization. J Neuroradiol 1975; 2:275.

11. Christiansen TA, Duvall AJ, Rosenberg Z, et al.: Juvenile nasopharyngeal angiofibroma. Trans Am Acad Ophthal Otolaryngol 1974; 78:140.

12. Changani DL, Sharma SD, Popli SP: Intracranial extensions in nasopharyngeal fibroma. J Laryngol Otol 1969; 82:1137.

13. Davis KR, Debrun GM: Embolization of juvenile nasopharyngeal angiofibromas. Semin Intervent Radiol 1987; 4:309.

14. Rubinstein LJ: Atlas of tumor pathology: tumors of the central nervous system. Washington, DC, 1972, Armed Forces Institute of Pathology.

15. Lasjuanias P, Berenstein A, Moret J: The significance of dural supply of central nervous system lesions. J Neuroradiol 1983; 10:31.

16. Lasjuanias P, Berenstein A: Surgical Neuroangiography. Endovascular Treatment of Craniofacial Lesions, 1 ed. New York, 1987, Springer Verlag, vol. 11, p. 96.

17. Manelfe C, Lasjuanias P, Ruscalleda J: Preoperative embolization of intracranial meningiomas. Am J Neuroradiol 1986; 5:963.

18. Abramowitz J, Dion J, Jensen M, et al.: Angiographic diagnosis and management of head and neck schwannomas. Am J Neuroradiol 1991; 12:977.

# CARDIAC AND THORACIC SURGERY

## *Renée S. Hartz and Hanafy M. Hanafy*

## INTRODUCTION

A certain amount of blood loss is obviously unavoidable when surgery on thoracic organs or blood vessels is performed. Many patients present to the hospital more concerned with the possibility of blood transfusion than with operative procedure itself. Improvements in myocardial protection, anesthetic techniques, and instrumentation have all effected a marked reduction in the operative mortality of open-heart surgery. Despite these improve-ments, all benefit is lost if a patient acquires a transmissible disease from unnecessary blood transfusion. In no other surgical subspecialty (except perhaps major orthopedic surgery and liver transplantation) is the potential for blood loss greater or the responsibility for avoiding transfusion more consistent than in the cardiac surgical arena. The mean homologous red blood cell use per coronary artery surgery patient, for example, is estimated to be 2.9 units, with an institutional range of 0.4–6.3 units.[1] Efforts to minimize the need for transfusions must be exerted at all stages of care of the cardiac surgery patient (Table 13–1). The application of these methods in cardiothoracic surgery is outlined, and the surgical technical methods of minimizing blood loss are detailed.

## BLOOD CONSERVATION MEASURES
### Preoperative Assessment

The subset of patients who have a bleeding diathesis should be identified by history, particularly if they had a previous surgical procedure, and by the basic coagulation profile that

**Table 13–1. Minimizing blood-component transfusion requirements in cardiac surgery**

Preoperatively
  Identify history of bleeding diathesis
  Obtain history of current medications (platelet function inhibitors, anticoagulants, thrombolytic drugs)
  Identify special risk factors for bleeding (reoperation, endocarditis, cyanotic heart disease)
  Coagulation profile (PT, APTT, bleeding time)
  Correct anemia (iron, erythropoietin)
  Discontinue aspirin (if possible) or dipyridamole
  Preoperative autologous blood donation
  Preoperative collection of blood with acute normovolemic hemodilution
Perioperative pharmacological agents
  Aprotinin
  Iloprost
  Desmopressin (DDAVP)
  ε-Aminocaproic acid
  Tranexamic acid
Intraoperatively
  *Cardiopulmonary bypass technique*
    Asanguineous prime
    Adequate heparinization
  *Operative technique*
    Surgical hemostasis
    Shorten cardiopulmonary bypass time
    Careful conduit (vein or internal mammary) harvest
  *Intraoperative blood salvage techniques*
    Washed cell-saver blood
    Cardiotomy suction
    Reinfusion of residual oxygenator blood (after concentrating and washing)
Postoperatively
  Autotransfusion of unwashed shed blood
  Accept anemia/hemodilution with normovolemia
  Early reoperation for rebleeding when indicated
  Achieve normothermia

includes prothrombin time, activated thromboplastin time, platelet count, and bleeding time. The presence of specific abnormalities may require the involvement of the hematologist. Preoperative red cell mass (as determined by the hematocrit, age, sex, and body size) and age are independent predictors of the need for blood transfusion during coronary artery surgery.[2] Therefore, preoperative correction of anemia should be planned whenever possible. On the other hand, patients admitted for cardiac surgery will more often than not be on medication that affects coagulation or bleeding, for example, aspirin, nonsteroidal antiinflammatory drugs, dipyridamole, coumadin, heparin, and thrombolytic therapy. These agents should be discontinued before

surgery, when possible. There is evidence that aspirin ingestion in the preoperative period is associated with increased perioperative bleeding and transfusion requirements.[3–7] Aspirin irreversibly inhibits cyclooxygenase and ideally should be stopped at least a week before surgery. Certain procedures are known to be associated with higher transfusion requirements (reoperations, valve replacement, endocarditis, repair of cyanotic heart disease). Identification of these patients allows serious consideration and planning for additional pharmacological interventions, for example, aprotinin.

## Preoperative Autologous Blood Donation

Preoperative self-donation of blood in the absence of specific contraindications is a simple, safe, and cost-effective method of reducing homologous blood-component transfusions in cardiac surgery. It resulted in decreasing allogenic transfusion from 64 to 38%.[8] In a recent survey, it was estimated that only 8% of coronary artery surgery patients participated in preoperative autologous blood donation, indicating severe underutilization of the program.[1]

## Collection of Blood Before Sternotomy and Acute Normovolemic Hemodilution

Many surgeons rely on intraoperative phlebotomy before sternotomy. If the patient's hemodynamics permit this approach, it is an ideal procedure because both platelets and factor-enriched blood can be retransfused after the discontinuation of cardiopulmonary bypass (CPB). Often, however, the unstable nature of the patient's hemodynamics prohibit the application of autologous removal of blood in the operating room.

### Platelet Pheresis

Some surgeons have used platelet pheresis as an alternative to the removal of whole blood from the patient. We have found this technique cumbersome and have noted anecdotally that there is a higher incidence of neurological complications postoperatively in this group, especially after valve surgery.

## Pharmacological Agents

Of the pharmacological agents available for reducing blood loss, $\epsilon$-aminocaproic acid has not been useful unless there is obvious fibrinolysis. On the other hand, for reoperations, those that require prolonged cardiopulmonary bypass and for patients who have either been on aspirin therapy or are Jehovah's witnesses, aprotinin is used on a routine basis. We use the low-dose protocol and have been extremely happy with the decreased blood loss in our patients with this drug.

## SURGICAL HEMOSTASIS

Defective hemostasis is a common cause of bleeding after CPB. The current incidence of reoperation for excessive bleeding is estimated to be 5–6%,[7,9] and incomplete surgical hemostasis is found in at least half of these instances.[10] To avoid this problem, the highest degree of surgical dexterity, competence, and commitment to minimizing transfusion is required. Procedures should be performed only by, or with the teaching assistance of, surgeons who are experienced with the procedure to avoid problems that will lead to unnecessary blood transfusion. Attention to detail in surgical technique is crucial.

## General Principles

Good exposure remains the golden rule. In general, dissection should be limited to what is necessary to provide excellent exposure. Dissection that will not contribute to the achievement of the surgical procedure in our opinion is unnecessary. Well-focused light of adequate brightness is indispensable. The fiberoptic headlight is particularly valuable when dissecting in confined spaces, such as during harvesting the internal mammary (thoracic) artery or working to secure hemostasis in the posterior angle of a posterolateral thoracotomy. Magnification with the aid of binocular surgical loops ($2-3.5\times$) is of great help in accurate identification of bleeding from small side branches of vessels or grafts. In vascular surgery, a rule of thumb is to initially secure proximal and distal control of the vessel to be operated on. During vascular anastomoses, atraumatic passage of the needles, proper placement of the sutures, avoidance of calcified areas, preclotted gratfs,[11] and maintenance of proper tension on the suture before tying should ensure a perfect suture line. Pledgeted sutures are advisable in dealing with unusually thin-walled vessels relative to high hemodynamic pressures. During thoracotomy the use of the electrocautery is of paramount importance to minimize blood loss, and injury to the intercostal vessels should be avoidable because they invariably lie in the groove along the inside of the lower edge of the rib. Bleeding from the posterior end of a posterolateral thoracotomy may result from fracture or disarticulation of a rib. Routine disarticulation of a rib is discouraged, and the ribs should be spread gradually. Planned resection of a part or entirety of a rib may be used selectively. There are reports of patients developing paraplegia after attempted hemostasis in this posterolateral angle caused by epidural hematoma[12] or migration of oxidized regenerated cellulose (Surgicel®, Johnson & Johnson Medical Inc., Arlington, TX) in the spinal cord.[13] It is important to appreciate that the posterior end of the intercostal incision may be only millimeters away from the spinal cord, and there should be no place for blind electrocautery in this area.[14]

## Cardiac Surgery

The cardiac surgeon is more challenged in the current era by having to operate on many patients who are inherently at risk of higher requirements for blood transfusion (Table 13–2). Therefore, the importance of meticulous surgical technique cannot be overemphasized. Major amounts of blood can be lost in a few seconds. In routine first-time heart surgery, the incidence of blood transfusion

**Table 13–2. Risk factors for increased need of blood transfusion in cardiac surgery**

Low preoperative hematocrit
Older age
Increased body mass index
Reoperation
Endocarditis
Cyanotic heart disease
Medications: antiplatelet drugs (e.g., aspirin, NSAIDs, dipyridadmole), anticoagulants (heparin, coumadin), thrombolytics (streptokinase, urokinase, tPA)
Diseases causing platelet dysfunction (renal failure)

Preoperative red blood cell mass is determined by the hematocrit, age, sex, and body size.

should be very low in the presence of normal baseline hemoglobin level (only approximately one-third of patients in our practice). However, in those patients who are anemic, those undergoing reoperation, and those on antiplatelet therapy, the surgeon should be prepared for the possibility of exsanguinating hemorrhage at every step of the procedure. In the operating room the surgeon has complete control of all the procedures available to effect significant reduction of blood transfusions. The following is a description of those methods we find most useful in avoiding unnecessary blood transfusions.

## Cardiopulmonary Bypass

Excessive hemodilution can be avoided by paying attention to the patient's body surface area. Down-sizing of the circuitry in the heart-lung machine is desirable in small patients. The perfusionist should be keenly aware that a 40- to 50-kg patient requires smaller oxygenators, reservoirs, and pump tubing than a 70-kg patient. The practice of setting up the same type of equipment on every patient, simply for convenience, is to be condemned.

In patients who are in cardiac or renal failure, the perfusionist should be able to perform intraoperative ultrafiltration, and, in those with renal failure, intraoperative hemodialysis may be used. These are extremely important technical maneuvers that can restore normal blood volume and an acceptable hemoglobin concentration at the end of CPB in the majority of patients.

Although the use of the membrane oxygenator is accompanied with less platelet damage and hemolysis,[15] this difference has not led to a significant reduction in postoperative blood loss in elective coronary artery surgery[16] or aortic valve replacement.[17,18] The advantage of using the membrane oxygenator has been demonstrated, however, in patients with long perfusion times (greater than 2 hours).[19] Cardiotomy suction should be used in preference to the cell saver whenever applicable.

Anticoagulation with heparin should be complete. Inadequate systemic heparinization will allow extensive activation of the coagulation cascade and microthrombosis, resulting not only in organ ischemia but also causeing severe consumptive coagulopathy and fibrinolysis.

## Hemostasis in the Operative Field

Procedures we find to be invaluable in controlling blood loss during cardiac surgery are as follows.

1. Use of pericardial pledget sutures. Most surgeons prefer Teflon felt pledgets on the aorta and other bleeding sites. Over the years we have relied more and more on small pledgets and fashioned from the pericardial edges for bleeding sites on proximal anastomoses, cannulation sites, and elsewhere (Fig. 13–4). Foreign material can therefore be avoided. Pericardium is also easy to tie over as compared with bulky Teflon felt pledgets. Another extremely important adjunct is to decrease the blood flow on the heart-lung machine to a few hundred milliliters when tying down a suture on the aorta. This allows the knot to be tied under no tension. The blood flow is brought slowly back up during completion of the other throws in the knot. Pericardial pledgets are particularly useful when there is bleeding from a proximal anastomosis in which a small vein graft has been used. Coupling a very small pledgeted suture with decreasing the pump flow virtually obviates the problem of compromising flow at the proximal anastomosis.

2. Our favorite topical hemostatic agent is the "Avitene sandwich." This consists of a square of absorbable microfibrillar collagen (Avitene®, Avicon, Inc., Ft. Worth, TX) wrapped in a piece of Surgicel. For minor bleeding points on the myocardium, this "sandwich" is applied to the bleeding site and gentle pressure with a surgical sponge is applied. Once the surgical sponge is removed, if there is persistent bleeding from the edges of the sandwich, the bleeding is excessive and should be readdressed with sutures. However, if there is no oozing from around the Surgicel and Avitene, the hemostasis is adequate. The Avitene sandwich can be left in place, and the chest closed. We have not seen thrombosis of a graft site when this sandwhich is left in place, but we have observed proximal graft occlusion in areas treated with absorbable gelatin sponge (Gelfoam®, UpJohn Laboratory, Kalamazoo, MI) and thrombin.

3. In patients with excessive bleeding from the surface of the myocardium, such as from dissection of an intramyocardial left anterior descending coronary, the use of fibrin glue is

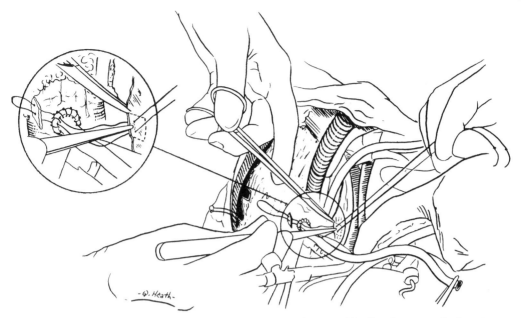

**Fig. 13–4.**   Small pledgets are fashioned from the pericardiol edges for use on bleeding sites on proximal anastamoses, cannulation sites, and elsewhere.

invaluable. This biodegradable agent is prepared from topical bovine thrombin and single-donor source of fibrinogen (fresh frozen plasma or cryoprecipitate). Ideally, the fibrin glue should be placed over the bleeding area while the cross clamp is still in place. Once the cross clamp is removed and there is oozing from the myocardium, it is virtually impossible to control with topical bleeding agents. Significant reductions in chest-tube drainage were reported with the use of topical fibrin glue to anterior mediastinum structures before closure of the sternum.[20] The incorporation of an antibiotic with the glue is an attractive idea and was found experimentally to reduce vascular graft infection and pseudoaneurysm formation.[21] Using single-donor components will reduce the risk of transmission of viral disease,[22] and the risk can be eliminated by using autologous fibrin glue.[23–25] A complication of the use of bovine thrombin is the development of IgC antibodies to thrombin and factor V that may result in erroneous thrombin time values using bovine thrombin reagent[26] and may cause severe bleeding diathesis.[27]

4. To decrease the amount of bleeding from the sternal edges, we use Vancomycin paste in the sternal edges at the end of the case. Two to 3 g of Vancomycin paste or powder, depending on the size of the patient, are mixed with a few drops of saline until a gel the consistency of the bone wax is obtained (Fig. 13–5a). This paste is packed into the sternal edges after the sutures are placed and the sutures are tied over the Vancomycin (Fig. 13–5b). If there is excessive bleeding earlier on, the Vancomycin can be placed sooner to eliminate the sternal edges as a source of ongoing blood loss that is difficult to identify. Other biodegradable alternatives include a paste made with Gelfoam moistened with thrombin[28] or strips of Avitene.[29] Bone wax has the potential to promote infection[30] and delay healing[31] in experimental animals.

5. We routinely open the pleural space widely when the internal mammary artery is being harvested. Before chest closure, a pericardial opening is created posterior to the heart (Fig. 13–6) so that any blood accumulating in the pericardial sac is channeled into the left chest by gravity. A chest tube with a stiff wire can be fashioned to fit in the most dependent portion of the left pleural cavity. The benefits of this technique are that patients virtually never have tamponade and the blood from the chest tubes can be collected in an autotransfusion device and retransfused. Tam-

**Fig. 13–5.** Two to 3 g Vancomycin paste or powder, depending on the size of the patient, are mixed with a few drops of saline until a gel the consistency of the bone wax is obtained (a). This paste is packed into the sternal edges after the sutures are placed, and the sutures are tied over the Vancomycin paste (b).

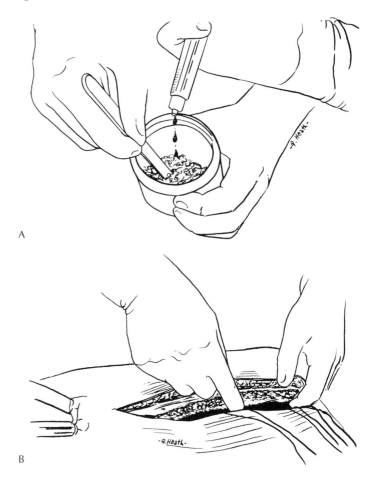

A

B

**Fig. 13–6.** Before chest closure, a pericardial opening is created posterior to the heart so that any blood accumulating in the pericardial sac is channeled into the left chest by gravity.

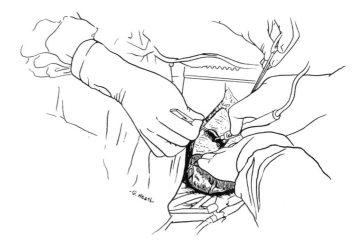

ponade is not an issue in these patients because there is easy access to the left chest both through the widely opened pleural space and to the posterior pericardial vent. We have found this procedure so useful in coronary patients undergoing harvest of the internal mammary artery that we now use it in other patient groups in whom there is a large amount of bleeding during the procedure.

## Reoperations

Reoperations are associated with a significant risk of bleeding and, therefore, increased transfusion requirements.[2] Careful analysis of the preoperative lateral chest roentgenogram or computerized tomography should give a good idea about the retrosternal space. We routinely place femoral artery and vein catheters in the right groin. These catheters should be large enough (16G) to allow the passage of long guide wires. In this fashion, assuming that the heart-lung machine is primed, the patient can be placed on CPB in seconds. We have avoided exsanguination from hemorrhage in at least a half dozen patients in the last few years using this approach. In patients undergoing a second or third resternotomy, we routinely cut down on the femoral vessels, assuming that the incidence of needing emergency CPB will be higher in these patients.

Before reoperation, patients should be typed and cross matched for 4–6 units of packed red blood cells, which should be in the operating room, checked by the anesthesiologist, and ready to administer instantly. We do not routinely type and cross match first-time coronary surgery patients with normal hemoglobins, but we do not begin a reoperation without the blood hanging on the intravenous pole and ready to be transfused.

If all of the above methods are used, hemorrhage encountered during the redo sternotomy can usually be well controlled. The patient can be placed on CPB quickly, the cell saver and cardiotomy suction device can be used immediately, and if the hemodynamics deteriorate, consequences to the myocardium can be avoided.

Most surgeons agree that use of the oscillating saw for resternotomy is safer. For added safety, the divided sternal wires may be left in place while working with the oscillating saw to identify the posterior table of the sternum.[32]

After completing the sternotomy, the edges should not be widely distracted because this may tear the heart or the innominate vein by pulling on fibrous adhesions. As the adhesions are released, the sternal edges can be gradually retracted. We have also found that use of an internal mammary artery retractor can greatly facilitate the dissection of the sternal edges. Once the sternal edges have been dissected, we routinely place two edges of Surgicel on the sternum followed by laparotomy pads and then a sternal retractor with wide blades to compress the bleeding edges of the sternum. We virtually never use bone wax. Bleeding from the marrow can be avoided with the abovementioned measures, and once the procedure is over, reapproximation of the sternal edge stops any unnecessary blood loss from the marrow (see above concerning Vancomycin paste).

Although some surgeons believe that dissecting the entire heart is necessary for all cardiac surgical procedures, our practice has been to perform minimal dissection of the surface of the heart and perform the rest of the dissection while on CPB. The latter can be accomplished in 5–10 minutes on most all reoperation patients. For valve surgery we do not dissect the back of the heart.

Before discontinuing CPB, suture lines should be checked for bleeding. The arterial cannula is used to return as much of the pump blood as possible before its removal. The development of a routine to check on possible bleeding sources, as a final step before closing the sternum, is advisable. This final assessment should be performed while the patient has good hemodynamics. After passing the sternal wires or sutures, it is wise to inspect the back of the sternal and parasternal area for bleeding before tying them.

## Postoperative Care

Clearly, the state of anticoagulation induced by the heart-lung machine is beneficial both in patients having coronary artery surgery and in those having valve surgery. It allows the endothelialization of small caliber grafts in the first 24–48 hours after cardiac surgery and it provides the anticoagulated state necessary to avoid thrombus formation on artificial heart valves until the patient can be suitably anticoagulated postoperatively.

Thus, a delicate balance between a desirable and an excessive state of anticoagulation is the goal in every patient. Infusion of shed blood has been demonstrated to be safe and is used whenever possible.[33] It is our philosophy that blood collected in the first 6–12 hours, depending on the bleeding rate, should be transfused. Blood should not be allowed to collect in the autotransfusion device for more than a few hours. Patients who are bleeding excessively can be retransfused continuously while plans are underway to return the patient expeditiously to the operating room.

It cannot be emphasized strongly enough that early return to the operating room is the key to minimizing blood transfusions. In the absence of evidence of generalized bleeding (e.g., epistaxis or oozing from puncture sites) and grossly abnormal coagulation studies, the chest should be reexplored immediately when the rate of bleeding exceeds preset reentry criteria. Bleeding in excess of 10 mL/kg in the first postoperative hour or an average of 5 mL/kg/h the first 3 postoperative hours is a good guideline.[34] Waiting longer invites the use of more blood products and precipitates a vicious circle of coagulopathy, bleeding, and blood product.

## REFERENCES

1. Goodnough LT, Johnson MFM, Toy PTCY, et al.: The variability of transfusion practice in coronary artery bypass surgery. JAMA 1991; 265:86.
2. Cosgrove DM, Loop FD, Lytle BW, et al.: Determinants of blood utilization during myocardial revascularization. Ann Thorac Surg 1985; 40:380.
3. Ferraris VA, Ferraris SP, Lough FC, et al.: Preoperative aspirin ingestion increases operative blood loss after coronary artery bypass grafting. Ann Thorac Surg 1988; 40:380.
4. Sethi GK, Copeland JG, Goldman S, et al.: Implications of preoperative administration of aspirin in patients undergoing coronary artery bypass grafting. J Am Coll Cardiol 1990; 15:15.
5. Michelson E, Morganroth J, Torosian M, et al.: Relation of perioperative use of aspirin to increased mediastinal blood loss after coronary artery bypass surgery. J Thorac Cardiovasc Surg 1978; 76:694.
6. Taggart DP, Siddiqi A, Wheatley DJ: Low-dose preoperative aspirin therapy, postoperative blood loss, and transfusion requirements. Ann Thorac Surg 1990; 50:425.
7. Bashein G, Nessley ML, Rice AL, et al.: Preoperative aspirin therapy and reoperation for bleeding after coronary artery bypass surgery. Arch Intern Med 1991; 151:89.
8. Love TR, Hendren WG, O'Keefe DD, et al.: Transfusion of predonated autologous blood in elective cardiac surgery. Ann Thorac Surg 1987; 43:508.
9. Taylor GL, Mikell FL, Moses HW, et al.: Determinants of hospital charges for coronary artery bypass surgery: the economic consequences of postoperative complications. Am J Cardiol 1990; 65:309.
10. Woodman RC, Harker LA: Bleeding complications associated with cardiopulmonary bypass. Blood 1990; 76:1680.
11. Thurer RL, Hauer JM, Weintraub RM: A comparison of preclotting techniques for prosthetic aortic replacement. Circulation 1982; 66(suppl 1):143.
12. Perez-Guerra F, Holland JM: Epidural hematoma as a cause of postpneumonectomy paraplegia. Ann Thorac Surg 1990; 4:287.
13. Short HD: Paraplegia associated with the use of oxidized cellulose in posterolateral thoracotomy incisions. Ann Thorac Surg 1990; 50:288.
14. Walker WE: Paraplegia associated with thoracotomy. Ann Thorac Surg 1990; 50:178.
15. Boonstra PW, Vermeulen FEE, Leusink JA, et al.: Hematological advantage of a membrane oxygenator over a bubble oxygenator in long perfusions. Ann Thorac Surg 1986; 41:297.
16. Edmunds LH, Ellison N, Colman RW, et al.: Platelet function during cardiac operation: comparison of membrane and bubble oxygenators. J Thorac Cardiovasc Surg 1982; 83:805.
17. Boers M, van den Dungen JAM, Karliczek GF, et al.: Two membrane oxygenators and a bubbler: a clinical comparison. Ann Thorac Surg 1983; 35:455.
18. Nilsson L. Bagge L, Nystrom SO: Blood cell trauma and postoperative bleeding: comparison of bubble and membrane oxygenators and observations on coronary suction. Scand J Thorac Cardiovasc Surg 1990; 24:65.
19. Clark RE, Beauchamp RA, Magrath RA, et al.: Comparison of bubble and membrane oxygenators in short and long perfusions. J Thorac Cardiovasc Surg 1979; 78:655.
20. Spotnitz WD, Dalton MS, Baker JW, et al.: Reductions of perioperative hemorrhage by anterior mediastinal spray application of fibrin glue during cardiac operations. Ann Thorac Surg 1987; 44:529.
21. Ney AL, Kelly PH, Tsukayama DT, et al.: Fibrin glue-antibiotic suspension in the prevention of prosthetic graft infection. J Trauma 1990; 30:1000.
22. Dresdale A, Bowman FO Jr, Malm JR, et al.: Hemostatic effectiveness of fibrin glue derived from single-donor fresh frozen plasma. Ann Thorac Surg 1985; 40:385
23. Tawes RL Jr, Sydorak GR, Du Vall TB: Autologous fibrin glue: the last step in operative hemostasis. Am J Surg 1994; 168:120.
24. Kjaergard ILK, Weis-Fogh US, Thiis JJ: Preparation of autologous fibrin from pericardial blood. Ann Thorac Surg 1993; 55:543.
25. Hartman AR, Galanakis DK, Honig MP, et al.: Autologous whole plasma fibrin gel: intraoperative procurement. Arch Surg 1992; 127:357.
26. Banninger H, Hardegger T, Tobler A, et al.: Fibrin glue in surgery: frequent development of inhibitors of bovine thrombin and human factor V. Br J Haematol 1993; 85:528.
27. Zehnder J, Leung LLK: Development of antibodies to thrombin and factor V with recurrent bleeding in a patient exposed to topical bovine thrombin. Blood 1990; 76:2011.
28. Jones RH: Invited letter concerning: the promotional effect of bone wax on experimental Staphylococcus aureus osteomyelitis and postoperative medi-

astinitis—a comparison of two electrocautery techniques on presternal soft. J Thorac Cardiovasc Surg 1991; 101:1109.

29. Blanche C, Chaux A: The use of absorbable microfibrillar collagen to control sternal bone marrow bleeding. Int Surg 1988; 73:42.

30. Nelson DR, Buxton TB, Luu QN, et al.: The promotional effect of bone wax on experimental *Staphylococcus aureus* osteomyelitis. J Thorac Cardiovasc Surg 1990; 99:977.

31. Howard TC, Kelley RR: The effect of bone wax on the healing of experimental rat tibial lesions. Clin Orthop Rel Res 1969; 63:226.

32. Lytle BW, Loop FD: Coronary reoperations. Surg Clin North Am 1988; 68:559.

33. Hartz RS, Smith JA, Green DL: Autotransfusion following cardiac surgery: assessment of hemostatic factors. J Thorac Cardiovasc Surg 1988; 96:178.

34. Edmunds LH Jr, Addonizio VP Jr: Extracorporeal circulation. In: Coleman RW, Hirsch J, Marder VJ, Salzman EW, eds, Hemostasis and Thrombosis, 2 ed. Philadelphia, 1987, J.B. Lippincott, p. 901.

# NEUROSURGERY

## Jose L. Salazar

## INTRODUCTION

One of the most important techniques in surgery is hemostasis and blood conservation to avoid blood transfusions. Painstaking hemostasis is part of the neurosurgical technique. The development of the neurosurgical technique is closely related to the technological advancement of hemostasis and the development of instruments and different hemostatic substances that will control not only the superficial bleeding from soft tissues but the deep bleeding from the brain tissue itself.

The techniques developed by the early neurosurgeons varied from the simple ones to the more complicated. Krause in 1905[1] and Horsley in 1906[2] stressed the fact that intracranial bleeding was profuse if the patient's body was horizontal, and both recommended elevation of the head to decrease the venous bleeding. They also recommended the lateral position for posterior fossa operations. Sitting position was used by De Martel in 1931[3] for all intracranial operations because of the marked decrease in bleeding and lack of intracranial complications due to hematoma. Dandy in 1932[4] and Bailey in 1933[5] continued to advocate the elevation of the head for bleeding control. Dawborn (1907)[6] attempted to deal with shock during the operation by placing tourniquets on both thighs perioperatively. When the patient's blood pressure fell, the tourniquets were released, mimicking an autotransfusion. The incisions in the scalp were fashioned to the blood supply and therefore were semilunar with the blood supply in the center of the flap to provide adequate blood supply to the scalp. One of the major problems with early neurosurgery was scalp bleeding, which was initially controlled as early as 1900 with the use of tourniquets, such as one designed by Petit,[7] that were applied around the base of the head for arterial compression. These devices were equipped with a key to regulate tension. This was quite effective in reducing excessive bleeding. Cushing[8] designed an inflatable tourniquet cuff suggested by Riva-Rocci but discarded it in 1908[9] in favor of a simple rubber ring adjustable by a buckle. The ring was prevented from rolling down over the orbits by tape along the midline from the glabella to the inion.

Hacker in 1904[10] used a continuous suture on the convex side of the incision, but others used the suture only across the base of the scalp or along the limbs of the incision. Chipault in 1897[11] introduced the serrated spring clip that compressed the scalp edges. Frazier in 1906[12] found that manual pressure around the margins of the wound was very effective when combined with the use of hemostatic clamps in the galea along both wound edges. The hemostats were then reflected over the edge of the scalp and by their weight controlled scalp bleeding. Cushing also used this technique. It was necessary to fold the galeal edge to occlude all the vessels, and no attempt was made to clamp the individual vessels. The technique permitted an almost bloodless incision in the scalp and was superior to any procedure used before that time.

In 1934, Bailey introduced to the United States the automatic Michael clip applicator that he modified from the instrument used by Vincent in Paris.[1] In 1936, the spring scalp clip of Raney was available, and this was immediately adapted by many surgeons in the United States.[1] This was a plastic clip applied to the scalp edges with an applicator. The clip occluded the bleeding vessels of the scalp. Several new devices and procedures were keystones for the development of neurosurgery. Bone wax was introduced by Horsley (1892)[13] in about 1886. Cotton pledgets with black ligatures to prevent their loss in the wound was an innovation by Cushing in 1911.[1] He used muscle stamps and fragments of partially organized blood clots for hemostasis. Metal clips, small bits of U-shaped silver wire applied to the vessels to control bleeding, were also introduced by Cushing in 1911. In 1942, titanium was substituted for silver because of its greater compatibility with living tissue.

Putnam and colleagues in 1943[14] used thrombin oxidized cellulose. Ingraham and Bailey in 1944[15] used fibrin foam as a hemostatic agent. Prentice in 1945 described the efficacy of gelatin sponge as a carrier in the control of ooze and bleeding in inaccessible areas of the brain.[1] W. T. Bovie in 1926 with the help of Cushing introduced the hemostatic and cutting principles of high-frequency electric currents.[1] The early handmade pistol grip was elaborate and operated by an assistant.[16]

To do proper hemostasis in the brain, the suction apparatus helped Cushing clean tracts of brain wounds in the first World War. The power suction was used in ear, nose, and throat operations in 1914, but its adoption to the neurosurgical needs was reported many years later by Olivecrona in 1927.[17] Frazier and Gardner in 1928 described a specially designed curved metal aspirator that is still in use at the present time.[1] A modification combining suction and coagulator whereby the hemostatic current was available at the tip of the suction instrument was introduced by Heyl in 1940.[18] With the above techniques many neurosurgeons were able to extirpate tumors that previously were inaccessible. Horsley in 1893[19] described the technique of a two-stage operation with the sole purpose of saving the patient from excessive blood loss and operative trauma in one sitting. Sometimes, if the patient's blood pressure remained at acceptable levels, it permitted the tumor extirpation in one single operation. In 1908 the practice of closure of the scalp by suturing the galea aponeurotica with only occasional stitches was expanded into closely placed buried silk sutures. This technique became recognized as the most significant contribution toward hemostasis and resulted in more accurate alignment of the scalp tissue. The above neurosurgical techniques were the background for the development of newer techniques with the sole or primary purpose of improving hemostasis and to foster in the atraumatic incision of the brain tissue and removal of intracranial lesions.

## PREOPERATIVE PREPARATION OF THE NEUROSURGICAL PATIENT

The usual preoperative preparation of the patient for an intracranial or spinal procedure is the clearcut delineation of the intracranial lesion by the neuroradiological procedures that will allow us to identify the boundaries of the lesion and the blood supply to the tumor. All patients undergo blood tests to ensure that there is not a bleeding tendency. Coagulation profile should include prothrombin time, partial thromboplastin time, platelet count, and complete blood count. If the patient has been on aspirin, antiinflammatory medication, and other drugs that will alter coagulation function, these are stopped days or weeks before operation (see Chapter 2: Coagulation and Hemostasis). If the lesion to be operated has a significant blood supply, such as arteriovenous malformation or hemangioma, many of these cases will be treated preoperatively with selective embolization using particulate, such as vinyl alcohol sponge, silastic spheres or silastic material, glue, or absorbable gelatin sponge. The procedures are usually done intravascularly by the neuroradiologist-neurosurgeon to decrease the blood supply to the lesion, allowing the neurosurgeon to extirpate the lesion with less blood loss.

With the new microsurgical techniques using the operative microscope for aneurysms and arteriovenous malformations, there is no need for exposure of the internal or external carotid artery as was done in the 1970s. When blood loss is expected, the patient is typed and cross matched for packed red blood cells (RBCs). The operations for which blood is most frequently typed and cross matched are intracranial aneurysms and arteriovenous malformations. In approximately 80% of these operations, no blood is given unless there is an intraoperative rupture of the aneurysm, and in those instances, rapid transfusion may be necessary. In these cases as well as vascular tumors, blood should be made available before surgery. For most spine surgeries, such as diskectomies and laminectomies, only type and screen is currently performed. The notable exception is when large amounts of bone will be removed and grafted; in these situations blood should be typed and cross matched.

## AUTOTRANSFUSION AND THE CELL PROCESSOR

When bleeding is expected, the patient is usually asked to predonate their own blood. One or 2 units (usually 1 unit per week) are usually obtained. However, the patient's condition before surgery can often preclude predonation. Usually 1 or 1.5 units of blood loss during surgery can be allowed without red cell replacement. It used to be common practice to transfuse the patients when hemoglobin was 10 g/dL or slightly lower. At the present time a hemoglobin of 7.0 g/dL and sometimes less has become the trigger to transfuse. Recent estimates of unnecessary transfusions are up to 50%. Research shows that healthy patients can withstand hemoglobin levels between 5.0 and 7.0 g/dL.[20] When excessive bleeding is expected, the cell processor could be used to salvage blood for reinfusion to the patient. However, this particular technique is rarely used in neurosurgery. When blood transfusion is necessary, only packed RBCs are used, reserving other blood components for specific needs.

## SCALP HEMOSTASIS

At the present time scalp hemostasis is accurately done initially by planning the scalp incision, usually in a linear fashion incorporating the blood supply to the affected area. Linear scalp incisions are preferred because of easy control of bleeding and faster closure.

Two techniques are advantageous for scalp incision. If the incision is small, it is possible to get by without using disposable scalp clips, such as the Raney clip or the newest development, the clip gun, which is faster and easier to use than the single clip applicator of the 1980s. A smaller incision in the scalp, neck, or back can be done without clips by using the scalpel to incise the upper layers of the skin and the electrocautery for deeper dermis and subcutaneous tissue. Larger branch vessels of the scalp, such as the superficial temporal or the occipital artery, can be cauterized with bipolar cautery instead of ligated.

## ELECTROCAUTERY-BIPOLAR CAUTERY

The use of the electrocautery has made a great deal of difference in neurosurgery. There are two types of electrocautery: the unipolar and the bipolar. The unipolar can be used as the cutting current only or a combination of cutting and coagulation at different settings. The bipolar cautery has made possible very sophisticated surgical techniques for removal of arteriovenous malformations in the brain and the spinal cord. The electric current flows across the tips of the forceps only and allows a very small area of electric current to be disseminated to the surrounding tissue, permitting exquisite hemostatic control in sensitive areas such as the spinal cord and the brainstem. The bipolar cautery has been improved and can now be used with or without irrigation. There are several different types of forceps—straight, curved, or bayonet—depending on the surgeons special needs.

## HEMOSTATIC, MALLEABLE, SCREW, AND SPRING ANEURYSM CLIPS

Hemostatic clips for intracranial vessels have been used for many years. The advancement of bipolar cautery technology has allowed the neurosurgeon to cauterize blood vessels of 1 mm or less without the use of hemostatic metal clips. However, the Weck or the titanium clips are available for certain vessels larger than 1 mm. These clips are applied with single clip applicator and rely on hand pressure to close the clip. Therefore, these are used only superficially where good control of the tip of the instrument can be achieved.

Carotid clips, screw clips such as Crutchfield, et al. are not frequently used but are still available for gradual closure of the carotid artery lumen when gradual obliteration of the carotid is desired, such as in giant carotid aneurysms and cavernous sinus fistula. Newer intravascular techniques, such as balloon embolization for carotid artery fistulas and obliteration of the carotid artery at the base of the skull, have made the gradual closure clamps almost obsolete.

### Spring Aneurysm Clips

There has been a gradual development of more sophisticated aneurysm clips since the early 1970s. Initially, spring-loaded clips were used for obliteration of the aneurysms. These were high-closing pressure clips for permanent implantation and treatment of intracranial aneurysms. Over the last 20 years, multiple clips have been developed that are not only of greater closing pressure but have the capacity to vary the angle of the clip itself, such as the Vary Angle Codman Clip and the McFadden. In these particular clips, the angle of the

clip can be modified by rotating the clip on the clip applier. This has a great advantage for the occlusion of complicated aneurysms. In recent years, other aneurysm clips have been made available to the neurosurgeon that are low-closing pressure and can be used as temporary clips. They are very useful in the management of difficult intracranial aneurysms. Examples of this clip are the Yasargil temporary clip and the Sugita clip. In addition, the Sugita clip has a multitude of shapes that can be useful for giant aneurysms or encircling an artery. In recent years, Sugita has devised an applier that moves the tip where the clip rests in different directions up to 360°; this has made the application of different clips easier. Aneurysm surgery techniques are markedly improved with the use of the spring-loaded clips, the bipolar techniques, the self-retaining retractors such as the Leyla, and the operative microscope.

## PRESERVING VESSELS IN NEUROSURGERY

With microsurgical techniques and microinstruments, many intracranial vessels can be preserved by careful dissection of the intracranial vessels, dissection of the feeding vessels, and repair or anastomoses of important intracranial vessels to avoid vascular sequelae from ischemic changes.

## BONE HEMOSTASIS IN NEUROSURGERY

Bleeding bone can be easily controlled with the application of wax to the porous portion of the bone. This bone wax is similar to the one used in the early years with some changes in the formula to make it more pliable to the surgeons fingers for easier application. When bone fusion is needed and bone wax is contraindicated, several other hemostatic agents can be used that will control bleeding and not impair fusion.

## HEMOSTATIC AGENTS IN NEUROSURGERY
### Absorbable Gelatin Sponge

The absorbable gelatin sponge (Gelfoam®, UpJohn Laboratory, Kalamazoo, MI) is intended for the application of bleeding surfaces as a hemostatic agent. It is a water-insoluble, off-white, nonelastic, porous, and pliable product prepared from purified porcine skin gelatin. It is soft and absorbs and holds many times its weight in blood and other fluids. Its mode of action is not fully understood, although its effect appears to be more physical than by chemical alteration of blood clotting mechanisms. Absorbable gelatin sponge is absorbed completely with little tissue reaction when placed in soft tissue. It is usually absorbed completely in 4–6 weeks without inducing excessive scar tissue. Absorbable gelatin sterile powder is also available and is very useful in control of bleeding surfaces of bone and soft tissue and oozing from brain tissue.

## Thrombin

Thrombin (Thrombogen®, Johnson & Johnson Medical, Inc., Arlington, TX) is a protein substance produced through a conversion reaction in which prothrombin of bovine origin is activated by tissue thromboplastin in the presence of calcium chloride. It is supplied as a sterile powder that has been freeze-dried. Also contained in this preparation are calcium chloride, sodium chloride, aminoacetic acid (glycine), and benzalkonium chloride as a preservative. Thrombin requires no intermediate physiological agent for its action. It clots the fibrinogen of the blood directly; the speed with which thrombin clots blood is dependent on its concentration. Thrombin spray is also available and is useful for surface oozing of bone and brain tissue or tumor bed after tumor resection.

## Oxidized Regenerated Cellulose

Oxidized regenerated cellulose (Surgicel®, Johnson & Johnson Medical, Inc.) is a sterile absorbable knitted fabric prepared by the controlled oxidation of regenerated cellulose. The fabric is white with a pale yellow cast. It is strong and can be sutured or cut without fraying. It is stable and can be stored at room temperature. Slight discoloration may occur with age, but this does not affect performance. The mechanisms of action whereby oxidized regenerated cellulose accelerates clotting are not completely understood, but it appears to be a physical rather than any other alteration of normal physiological clotting mechanisms. It is used dry in the brain or other tissue. After

it is saturated with blood, it swells into a brownish black gelatin mass that aids in the formation of a clot, serving as an adjunct in the control of local hemorrhage. It is absorbed with practically no tissue reaction; its absorption depends on the amount used, degree of saturation, and the tissue bed where it is applied. Oxidized regenerated cellulose is bactericidal against a wide range of Gram-positive and Gram-negative organisms, including aerobes and anaerobes.

## Microfibrillar Collagen, Hemostatic Powder

Microfibrillar collagen hemostat (Avitene®, Avicon, Ft. Worth, TX) is a white substance, very sticky to the touch, and is applied to fairly dry surfaces for local control of hemorrhage. At the present time, it is supplied in small sheets to avoid sticking to forceps and other tissues when applied to bleeding or oozing surfaces.

## Cryoprecipitate Coagulum

In 1943, Deez and Falx described properties of a coagulum that could be formed by mixing fibrinogen and clotting globulin.[1] It was successfully used for removal of single or multiple renal calculi but was not widely used because the technique was complex. The use of autologous plasma eliminated these problems and now is available in virtually all blood banks, is stable up to 2 years, and can be thawed in 15 minutes. All packets undergo complete disease screening in the blood bank. Although initially described as a means of removing renal calculi, the coagulating properties of the cryoprecipitate coagulum make it ideal for consideration as a topical hemostatic agent. The cryoprecipitate is mixed in a separate syringe, one for the cryoprecipitate and another syringe for the topical thrombin that already includes calcium, and is poured into the area for bleeding control. Immediate coagulation usually occurs with good adherence of the regular brain surface. The preparation and indication for neurological operations was recently described by Stechison.[21]

## Fibrin Glue or Fibrin Seal

A slight modification of the cryoprecipitate technique is known as fibrin glue or fibrin seal

(Immuno, Vienna, Austria) and consists of a mixture of concentrated frozen cryoprecipitate or lyophilized fibrinogen with bovine thrombin, calcium chloride, and aprotinin, a fibrinolytic inhibitor. This system is applied with two syringes and injected at the same time but separately, allowing the droplets of the two components to be injected separately into a gas jet and to mix as they hit the wound surface, yielding a delicate fibrin film that, in the presence of a high thrombin concentration, clots almost instantly. Thus far, no application of this technique to neurosurgery has been widely done except for few reports, but clearly this method has tremendous potential as a topical hemostatic agent and also for gluing surfaces or doing dural patch for specific purpose. This technique has been frequently used in head and neck procedures and also for cardiovascular procedures among others.

## ε-Aminocaproic Acid

ε-Aminocaproic acid (Amicar®, Lederele Laboratory, Wayne, NJ) is a compound frequently used for the prevention of bleeding from a ruptured aneurysm and can be given intravenously or orally to prevent rebleeding when fibrinolysis contributes to the bleeding. Its fibrinolysis inhibitor effects appear to be exerted principally via inhibition of plasminogen activator and to a lesser degree to antiplasmin activity.

## LASERS IN NEUROSURGERY

The term "laser" is an acronym for *Light Amplification by Stimulated Emission of Radiation*. The possibility of the laser action was first suggested by Albert Einstein in 1917.[22] In 1960, Theodore H. Maiman[23] constructed the first working laser at Hughes Laboratories using a rod of crystalline ruby, excited by a coaxial helical flashlamp. In the 1960s, other lasers were reported: the Helium-Neon by Javan and colleagues,[24] the Gallium Arsenide Diode by Hall and associates in 1962,[25] the liquid by Lempick and Samuelson in 1963,[26] the Argon ion by Bridges in 1964,[27] the Carbon Dioxide by Patel in 1964,[28] and the Neodymium-Yttrium Aluminum Garnet (Nd-YAG) by Geusic and colleagues in 1964.[29] The types of lasers most frequently used are the Nd-YAG, Argon-ion, and $CO_2$ lasers. The

near-infrared lasers, notably the Nd-YAG, has stronger absorption and more scattering at any given distance but is less dependent on the color of the tissue.

The Argon laser works well for coagulating moderate volumes of blood in small vessels; it is better absorbed by hemoglobin than white or yellow tissue. However, if the objective is to destroy a heavily pigmented lesion such as a nevus with minimal damage to proximal vasculature, the ruby laser is the best choice. The dye laser would be about as good.

The laser most frequently used for neurosurgical operations because of its adaptability to either a handheld piece or to the operative microscope is the $CO_2$ laser; it can be used with most of the tumors and other lesions (Table 13–3). The size and depth of the lesions can be controlled by focusing or defocusing the beam. Its wavelength of 10,6000 nm is absorbed by liquids—mostly water so neighboring structures can be protected by wet sponges or small patties soaked in saline, exposing only the lesion to be treated by the laser. Its scattered radiation to heat deep structures is shallow so the radiant power of the laser decreases in depths of only 0.1 mm. This causes a rapid raise of temperature in the impacted volume of tissue and explosive boiling of the intracellular and intercellular water at or near 100°C. The expansion causes a thick smoke due to ultrarapid vaporization of the water and destruction of the soft tissue. It also destroys bacteria and viruses, although recent reports note some dispersement of Papilloma

---

**Table 13–3.  Advantages of the $CO_2$ laser for surgery**

- Excellent hemostasis of vessels of 0.5 mm in diameter or smaller
- Sterilizes the impact site: destroys bacteria
- Seals lymphatics to help prevent spread of viable cells from primary malignancies
- Less postoperative edema and scarring than electrocautery or cryoprobe
- Superior precision of tissue destruction or excision, especially when used with the microscope
- The extent of the vaporization can be controlled by the layers, superficial or deep
- Seals the ends of nerves, thus reducing immediate postoperative pain
- Can be used for coagulation, vaporization, or excision, depending on the technique and power density, focused or unfocused beam

viruses onto the treatment field. It sterilizes badly infected wounds such as decubitus ulcers. It seals the nerve endings cut by the beam, and therefore its uses in neuroectomies and amputations is great, reducing postoperative pain and minimizing scar formation.

Current developments in laser surgery include that of Nagata and associates,[30] who developed a projection system for radiosurgery and computerized axial tomography-directed biopsies, and a clinical evaluation of laser endarterectomy by Eugene and associates.[31]

## RADIOSURGERY

Stereotactic $\gamma$ knife surgery is a radiotherapy-radiosurgery technique for the treatment of small arteriovenous malformations or deep-seated tumors in the brain that may or may not be amenable to the usual neurosurgical techniques.

This is a bloodless operation, consisting of stereotactic localization and volumetric measurements of the lesion and intraoperative cerebral angiographic, computerized tomographic, or magnetic resonance imaging of the area of treatment (such as tumors or arteriovenous malformations). After the computerized radiation dosage planning, coordinates, and angles are chosen, the radiation dose is delivered at the target volume lesion as determined by the surgeon and radiation oncologist.[32]

The $\gamma$ knife itself consists of a permanent 18,000-kg metal shield surrounding a hemispheric array of 201 sources of cobalt-60, with an average activity of 30 Ci each.

Similar results can be obtained with a less-complicated system using a small focal spot for delivery of the cobalt 60 stereotactically without the cumbersome metal shield.

## SUMMARY

The current neurosurgical techniques have been described years ago by the neurosurgical pioneers; few modifications have been made so far. The neuromicroscope and new instrumentation have modified our approach to neurosurgical lesions, but basically our technique could not be performed without a solid understanding and practice of accurate and painstaking hemostasis. Good neurosurgical results and accurate hemostatic techniques go hand in hand.

## REFERENCES

1. Walker AE: A History of Neurological Surgery. New York, 1967, Hafner Publishing Co., p. 42.
2. Horsley V: On the technique of operations on the central nervous system. Br Med J 1906; 2:411.
3. De Martel T: Surgical treatment of cerebral tumors. Technical considerations. Surg Gynecol Obstet 1931; 52:381.
4. Dandy WE: Surgery of the brain. In: Lewis' Practice of Surgery. Hagerstown, 1932, W.F. Prior Co., vol. II, pp. 1–682.
5. Bailey P: Intracranial Tumors. Springfield, IL, 1933, Charles C. Thomas, p. 475.
6. Dawborn R: Sequestration, anemia in the brain and skull surgery. Ann Surg 1907; 45:161.
7. Frazier CH: Problems and procedures in cranial surgery. JAMA 1909; 52:1805.
8. Cushing H: Pneumatic tourniquets: with special reference to their use in craniotomies. Med Newsletter Philadelphia 1904; 84:577.
9. Cushing H: Technical methods of performing certain cranial operations. Surg Gynecol Obstet 1908; 6:227.
10. Hacker V: Zür prophylakitischen blutstillung bei der trepanation. Zentralbl Chir 1904; 31:857.
11. Chipault A: Note sur deux instruments destines a facilities les operations craniennes: une pince a compresses, une pinces hemostatique a demeurer. Trav Neurol Chir 1897; 2:15.
12. Frazier CH: Remarks upon the surgical aspects of operative tumors of the cerebrum. Univ Pennsylvania Med Bull 1906; 19:49.
13. Horsley V: Antiseptic way. Br Med J 1892; 1:1165.
14. Putnam TJ, Benedict EB, Teel HM: Studies in acromegaly. VIII. Experimental canine acromegaly produced by injection of anterior lobe pituitary extract. Arch Surg 1943; 18:1708.
15. Ingraham FD, Bailey OT: The use of products from human fibrinogen and human thrombin in neurosurgery. Fibrin foam as hemostatic agents; fibrin films in repair of dural defects and in prevention of meningocerebral adhesions. J Neurosurg 1944; 1:23.
16. Cushing H: Macewen menional lecture of the meningiomas arising from the olfactory groove and their removal by the aid of electrosurgery. Lancet 1927; 1:1329.
17. Olivecrona H: Die Chirurgische Behandlung Der Gehirntumoren. Eine Klinische Studie. Berlin, 1927, J. Springer, vol. 4, p. 344.
18. Heyl H: A coagulating sucker for use in neurosurgery. Ann Surg 1940; 111:159.
19. Horsley V: Discussion of the treatment of cerebral tumors. Br Med J 1893; 2:1365.
20. Welch GH, Meechan KR, Goodnough LT: Prudent strategies for elective RBC transfusion. Ann Intern Med 1992; 116:393.
21. Stechison MT: Rapid polymerizing fibrin glue from autologous or single donor blood: preparation and indications. J Neurosurg 1992; 76:626.
22. Einstein A: On the quantum theory of radiation. Physikalische Zeitschrift 1917; 18:121.
23. Maiman TH: [Report]. Physical Rev Lett 1960; 4:564.
24. Javan A, Bennett WR, Herriott DR: Population inversion and continuous optical mazer oscillation in gas discharge containing helium-neon mixture. Physical Rev Lett 1961; 6:106.
25. Hall RN, Fenner GE, Kingsley JD, et al.: Coherent

light emission from GaAs junctions. Physical Rev Lett 1962; 9:366.

26. Lempick A, Samuelson H: Optical maseraction in euopium benzrylacetonate. Appl Physics Lett 1963; 4:133.

27. Bridges WB: Laser oscillation in single ionized argon in the visible spectrum. Appl Physics Lett 1964; 4:128.

28. Patel CKN: Selective excitation thru vibrational energy transfer and optical maser actions in $N_2$-$CO_2$. Physical Rev Lett 1964; 13:617.

29. Geusic JE, Marcos HW, Van Vitart LG: Laser oscilla-

tions in neodymium yttrium aluminum, yttrium gallium and gadolinium garnets. Appl Physics Lett 1964; 4:182.

30. Nagata Y, Nishidai T, Abe M, et al.: Laser projection system for radiotherapy and CT-guided biopsy. J Comput Assist Tomogr 1990; 14:1046.

31. Eugene J, Ott RA, Nudelman KL, et al.: Initial clinical evaluation of carotid artery laser endarterectomy. J Vasc Surg 1990; 12:499.

32. Lunsford LD, Flickinger J, Coffey RJ: Stereotactic gamma knife radiosurgery. Initial North American Experience in 207 patients. Arch Neurol 1990; 47:169.

# GASTROENTEROLOGY

## *Frank J. Konicek*

This review emphasizes limiting or preventing blood loss in selected gastroenterological conditions and is not intended to be a comprehensive review of all gastroenterological bleeding problems.

## ACUTE HEMORRHAGE

### Acute Nonvariceal Upper Gastrointestinal Hemorrhage

Peptic ulcer disease is the most common cause of acute nonvariceal upper gastrintestinal (UGI) hemorrhage. Over 80% of patients will stop bleeding spontaneously. Those at increased risk for recurrent bleeding and other complications include patients over 60 years of age; nonsteroidal antiinflammatory drug (NSAID) use, especially within the first month of starting the drug; concomitant corticosteroid use; and a prior history of a "gastrointestinal event."[1]

Early UGI endoscopy is recommended in acute UGI bleeding for prognostic and therapeutic reasons. The endoscopic appearance of an ulcer can provide useful prognostic information concerning the likelihood of continued or recurrent bleeding, need for surgery, and mortality.[2] Endoscopic treatments using laser, thermal-contact devices, and injection therapy do reduce the rate of further bleeding, the total blood required, and the need for surgery in those patients actively bleeding or with visible vessels.[3] Orally or parenterally administered pharmacological agents used for therapy of peptic ulcer disease have failed to demonstrate any benefit in acute nonvariceal UGI hemorrhage.[4]

Emergency or early surgery may be required in patients not responding to endoscopic therapy or in those with recurrent hemorrhage. Rebleeding in a stabilized hospitalized patient carries a greater risk for continued bleeding, and surgical intervention should be considered. The surgical procedure of choice will depend on the severity of the bleeding, concomitant medical problems, and the experience of the surgeon.[5]

Angiographic therapy is an alternative to surgery for severe persistent bleeding in those patients failing endoscopic therapy or in those patients at high risk for surgical intervention.[6]

## Acute Esophageal Variceal Hemorrhage

Endoscopic sclerotherapy and banding are very effective in controlling acute bleeding from esophageal varices, and in most studies are superior to medical management and balloon tamponade.[7] Studies comparing endoscopic banding with sclerotherapy suggest fewer treatment-related complications and improved survival rates with banding versus sclerotherapy.[8]

Medical management with vasopressin given intravenously has been shown to be effective in controlling acute hemorrhage from variceal bleeding. Somatostatin is equally effective with fewer complications.[9] The Sengstaken-Blakemore tube is highly successful in controlling distal esophageal and proximal gastric variceal hemorrhage, but lack of permanent hemostasis and significant complications has limited its use.[9]

Bleeding gastric or duodenal varices have a much poorer response to sclerotherapy. In these patients and in patients with esophageal varices who fail sclerotherapy, surgical or radiological therapy may be necessary. Emergency surgical procedures, including portocaval shunts or direct attack on varices, are associated with high morbidity and mortality in all but the fully compensated cirrhotic and are therefore infrequently recommended.

Transjugular intrahepatic portosystemic shunt has been used to control bleeding in patients awaiting liver transplant[10] and has also been used to control esophageal variceal bleeding not responding to endoscopic measures.[11]

## Acute Lower Gastrointestinal Hemorrhage

Diverticula and vascular ectasias account for the majority of cases of acute bleeding from the colon. Bleeding is usually self-limited and rarely massive. Acute lower gastrointestinal hemorrhage from diverticula usually responds to conservative management, but in those patients who continue to bleed, selective angiography with infusion of a vasoconstrictor or with embolization can control the bleeding. Approximately 75% of patients with a diverticular bleed will not experience a second bleed, but of the 25% that do, the majority have further repeated bleeding episodes.[12] Patients with recurrent massive hemorrhage are best treated surgically with segmental resection of the colon if the bleeding site can be identified. Rarely, subtotal colectomy is necessary in massive bleeding with no identifiable bleeding point.[13]

Vascular ectasias are more frequent in the right colon, increase in frequency with increasing age, and are usually inadvertently discovered during colonoscopy while evaluating for more significant lesions. If identified as the bleeding site, endoscopic cautery can be used to ablate the lesions that are usually multiple and recurrent. For recurrent massive bleeding, hemicolectomy may be required.[14]

## PROPHYLAXIS
## Nonsteroidal Antiinflammatory Drug-Induced Ulcers

NSAID use places the patient at increased risk for duodenal ulcer, gastric ulcer, and hemorrhagic gastritis and is associated with a high risk of life-threatening complications, especially in the elderly. The odds ratios for peptic ulcer bleeding varies with the type of NSAID used, and the risk increases with increasing dose.[15] For those patients not responding to non-NSAID analgesics who require NSAID therapy, attempts should be made to reduce the dosage and select a less-toxic drug.

The risk of NSAID-induced duodenal ulceration can be decreased with histamine$_2$ (H$_2$) blocker therapy. Gastric and duodenal ulcer risk is reduced with prophylactic misoprostol therapy. With continued NSAID use, ulcers will respond to H$_2$ blockers and omeprazole therapy but will take longer to heal. If NSAIDs are discontinued, ulcers will readily respond to antiulcer regimens.[16]

Whether H$_2$ blockers, misoprostol, or omeprazole prophylaxis will reduce rebleeding rates is still unknown, but prophylaxis, especially in high-risk patients, seems warranted but controversial.[17]

## Peptic Ulcer Disease

Recurrence rates are very high for both gastric and duodenal ulcers. Several factors increase the risk of bleeding and include longer duration of disease, older age at onset, and prior bleeding from ulcer. Cigarette smoking will delay healing and increase the risk of recurrence. Surgery reduces the recurrence of peptic ulcer disease significantly with the rate of recurrence depending on the type of ulcer surgery performed. Recurrent ulcers after ulcer surgery seldom bleed and are very responsive to standard $H_2$ blocker therapy.[16]

Maintenance therapy with $H_2$ blockers at one-half the dose for active ulcer significantly reduces the recurrence rates for both duodenal and gastric ulcers. Unfortunately, recurrence rates of 50–90% are reported within 1 year of stopping maintenance therapy. For duodenal ulcer prophylaxis long-term maintenance therapy is required, which usually implies greater than 4 years of medication and should therefore be reserved for high-risk patients, such as those with prior ulcer hemorrhage and the elderly with concomitant diseases. For gastric ulcer, recurrence rates of those on standard maintenance therapy approach the placebo group within 2 years. Rather than the usual maintenance dose of one-half the active ulcer dose, gastric ulcer patients may require full-dose therapy during long-term follow-up.[16] A significant reduction in the rate of rebleeding in patients on maintenance therapy has been confirmed in a prospective double-blind study[18] and in a prospective and retrospective study.[19]

The treatment and prevention of peptic ulcer disease has radically changed with the now well-accepted conclusion that the organism *Helicobacter pylori* is responsible for the vast majority of duodenal ulcer disease and a significant proportion of non-NSAID-induced gastric ulcers. The findings of the National Institutes of Health-sponsored *H. pylori* consensus development conference held in February 1994 confirmed this relationship and concluded that the organism was indeed responsible for most peptic ulcer disease and that antibiotic regimens leading to eradication of the organism would not only result in healing of the acute ulcer but would prevent ulcer recurrences.[20–24]

Whether eradication of *H. pylori* will reduce the incidence of serious complications including bleeding awaits further study, but early reports suggest a reduction in the rate of rebleeding.[25–27]

Treatment strategies for eradication of *H. pylori* are still evolving. Triple drug therapy with bismuth, tetracycline, and metronidazole combined with an $H_2$ blocker or omeprazole appears to give the best response, with cure rates up to 90%.[28] But some studies suggest similar cure rates using amoxicillin plus omeprazole compared with triple therapy plus $H_2$ blockers.[29]

## Stress Ulcer

Stress ulcer or stress-related mucosal damage (SRMD) occurs in the setting of major trauma, sepsis, burns, and severe medical problems requiring intensive care unit (ICU) observation and usually develops in the initial 12–24 hours of admission to an ICU. Typically the lesions are multiple, superficial, and involve the proximal stomach. Approximately 20% of patients with SRMD will bleed overtly and 2–5% massively.[30]

Numerous prospective studies and meta-analysis have demonstrated the effectiveness of therapy with antacids, $H_2$ receptor antagonists, and sucralfate in reducing the incidence of clinically important bleeding, but prophylaxis has not reduced mortality rates.[31]

There has been a decline in the risk of clinically significant bleeding from SRMD over the last decade irrespective of prophylaxis, and, although controversial, recent studies question the need for prophylaxis for all patients admitted to ICUs.[32,33] Factors placing ICU patients at increased risk for significant bleeding included coagulopathy and mechanical ventilation.

There is controversy surrounding the incidence of nosocomial pneumonia in patients on stress ulcer prophylaxis with antacids, $H_2$ receptor antagonists, or sucralfate. For the subset of ICU patients on long-term mechanical ventilation (greater than 48 hours), studies favor the use of sucralfate in decreasing the incidence of late-onset pneumonia.[34]

## Esophageal Variceal Hemorrhage Prophylaxis

### PREVENTION OF FIRST BLEEDING IN CIRRHOTICS WITH ESOPHAGEAL VARICES

Propranolol significantly lowers the rate of first bleeding from esophageal varices and reduces mortality.[35] Endoscopic examination of varices can predict those patients at increased risk for bleeding. Propranolol should be reserved for patients with no contraindication to β-adrenergic blocker use who can be identified as high risk and who are reasonably compliant.[36]

Comparing endoscopic esophageal sclerotherapy with β-adrenergic blockers, two trials reported increased mortality in patients treated with prophylactic sclerotherapy and both studies were terminated early.[37,38] However, a recent metaanalysis suggests that prophylactic sclerotherapy is effective provided the sclerosant used is polidocanol.[39] Until the issue is further resolved with appropriate clinical trials, sclerotherapy cannot be recommended as prophylaxis for first bleed from esophageal varices.

## PREVENTION AFTER FIRST BLEED

Based on controlled trials, portacaval shunt, sclerotherapy, and β-adrenergic blockers will all reduce the incidence of rebleeding. Lower rates of recurrent hemorrhage are obtained after surgical shunt therapy than after sclerotherapy and medical management.[40] Sclerotherapy is superior to β-adrenergic blocker therapy in reducing the incidence of rebleeding.[36] Sclerotherapy with β-adrenergic blockers compared with sclerotherapy alone has produced conflicting results.[41] A recently published study demonstrated lower blood requirements in combined versus the sclerotherapy alone group.[42] The transjugular intrahepatic portosystemic shunt is preferred over surgically constructed portacaval shunts for control of recurrent variceal bleeding in those patients failing medical or sclerosing techniques who are candidates for liver transplant for technical reasons related to liver transplant surgery.[10]

# Angiodysplasia: Gastrointestinal Vascular Malformations

The data are conflicting, but in patients with severe and recurrent bleeding secondary to angiodysplasia of the gastrointestinal tract, especially those with end-stage renal disease and Osler-Weber-Rendu Syndrome, a trial of estrogen-progesterone therapy seems warranted.[43,44]

## REFERENCES

1. Gabriel SE, Jaakkimainen L, Bombardier C: Risk for serious gastrointestinal complications related to use of nonsteroidal anti-inflammatory drugs. Ann Intern Med 1991; 115:787.
2. Laine L, Peterson WL: Bleeding peptic ulcer. N Engl J Med 1994; 331:717.
3. Cook DJ, Guyatt GH, Salena BJ, et al.: Endoscopic therapy for acute nonvariceal upper gastrointestinal hemorrhage: a meta-analysis. Gastroenterology 1992; 102:139.
4. Daneshmend TK, Hawkey CJ, Langman MJS, et al.: Omeprazole versus placebo for acute upper gastrointestinal bleeding: randomized double blind controlled trial. Br Med J 1992; 304:143.
5. Cochran TA: Bleeding peptic ulcer: surgical therapy. Gastroenterol Clin North Am 1993; 22:751.
6. Shapiro MJ: The role of the radiologist in the management of gastrointestinal bleeding. Gastroenterol Clin N Am 1994; 23:123.
7. Matloff DS: Treatment of acute variceal bleeding. Gastroenterol Clin North Am 1992; 21:103.
8. Stiegmann GV, Goff JS, Michaletz-Onody PA, et al.: Endoscopic sclerotherapy as compared with endoscopic ligation for bleeding esophageal varices. N Engl J Med 1992; 326:1527.
9. Goff JS: Gastroesophageal varices: pathogenesis and therapy of acute bleeding. Gastroenterol Clin North Am 1993; 22:779.
10. Ring EJ, Lake JR, Roberts JP, et al.: Using transjugular intrahepatic portosystemic shunts to control variceal bleeding before liver transplantation. Ann Intern Med 1992; 116:304.
11. Rössle M, Haag K, Ochs A, et al.: The transjugular intrahepatic portosystemic stent—shunt procedure for variceal bleeding. N Engl J Med 1994; 330:165.
12. Reinus JF, Brandt LJ: Vascular ectasias and diverticulosis. Common causes of lower intestinal bleeding. Gastroenterol Clin North Am 1994; 23:1
13. Jensen DM, Machicado GA: Diagnosis and treatment of severe hematochezia: the role of urgent colonoscopy after purge. Gastroenterology 1988; 95:1569.
14. Richter JM, Christensen MR, Colditz GA, et al.: Angiodysplasia: natural history and efficacy of therapeutic interventions. Dig Dis Sci 1989; 34:1542.
15. Langman MJS, Weil J, Wainwright P, et al.: Risks of bleeding peptic ulcer associated with individual nonsteroidal anti-inflammatory drugs. Lancet 1994; 343:1075.
16. Egan JV, Jensen DM: Long-term management of patients with bleeding ulcers: rationale, results, and economic impact. Gastrointestinal/Endosc Clin North Am 1991; 1:367.
17. Walt RP: Misoprostol for the treatment of peptic ulcer and anti-inflammatory-drug-induced gastroduodenal ulceration. N Engl J Med 1992; 327:1575.
18. Jensen DM, Cheng S, Kovacs TOG, et al.: A controlled study of ranitidine for the prevention of recurrent hemorrhage from duodenal ulcer. N Engl J Med 1994; 330:382.

19. Penston JG, Wormsley KG: Hemorrhage during long-term maintenance treatment of duodenal ulcers (Abstract). Gastroenterology 1992; 102:A145.

20. National Institutes of Health Consensus Development Panel: *Helicobacter pylori* in Peptic Ulcer Disease. JAMA 1994; 272:65.

21. Peura DA, Graham DY: *Helicobacter pylori*: consensus reached: peptic ulcer is on the way to becoming an historic disease. Am J Gastroenterol 1994; 89:1137.

22. Graham DY, Lew GM, Klein PD, et al.: Effect of treatment of *Helicobacter pylori* infection on the long-term recurrence of gastric and duodenal ulcer. Ann Intern Med 1992; 116:705.

23. Hentschel E, Brandstätter G, Dragosics B, et al.: Effect of ranitidine and amoxicillin plus metronidazole on the eradication of *Helicobacter pylori* and the recurrence of duodenal cancer. N Engl J Med 1993; 328:308.

24. Forbes GM, Glaser ME, Cullen DJE, et al.: Duodenal ulcer treated with *Helicobacter pylori* eradication: seven-year follow-up. Lancet 1994; 343:258.

25. Graham DY, Hepps KS, Ramirez FC, et al.: Treatment of *Helicobacter pylori* reduces the rate of rebleeding in peptic ulcer disease. Scand J Gastroenterol 1993; 28:939.

26. Rokkas T, Karameris A, Mavrogeorgis A, et al.: Eradication of *Helicobacter pylori* reduces the possibility of rebleeding in peptic ulcer disease. Gastrointest Endosc 1995; 41:1.

27. Jaspersen D, Koerner T, Schorr W, et al.: *Helicobacter pylori* eradication reduces the rate of rebleeding in ulcer hemorrhage. Gastrointest Endosc 1995; 41:5.

28. Marshall BJ: Treatment Strategies for *Helicobacter pylori* infection. Gastroenterol Clin North Am 1993; 22:183.

29. Labenz J, Gyenes E, Rühl GH, et al.: Amoxicillin plus omeprazole *versus* triple therapy for eradication of *Helicobacter pylori* in duodenal ulcer disease: a prospective, randomized, and controlled study. Gut 1993; 34:1167.

30. Chamberlain CE: Acute hemorrhagic gastritis. Gastroenterol Clin North Am 1993; 22:843.

31. Cook DJ, Witt LG, Cook RJ, et al.: Stress ulcer prophylaxis in the critically ill: a meta-analysis. Am J Med 1991; 91:519.

32. Cook DJ, Fuller HD, Guyatt GH, et al.: Risk factors for gastrointestinal bleeding in critically ill patients. N Engl J Med 1994; 330:377.

33. Ben-Menachem T, Fogel R, Patel R, et al.: Prophylaxis for stress-related gastric hemorrhage in the medical intensive care unit. A randomized, controlled, single-blind study. Ann Intern Med 1994; 121:568.

34. Prod'hom G, Leuenberger P, Koerfer J, et al.: Nosocomial pneumonia in mechanically ventilated patients receiving antacid, ranitidine, or sucralfate as prophylaxis for stress ulcer. A randomized controlled trial. Ann Intern Med 1994; 120:653.

35. Pagliaro L, D'Amico G, Sörensen TIA, et al.: Prevention of first bleeding in cirrhosis: a meta-analysis of randomized trials of nonsurgical treatment. Ann Intern Med 1992; 117:59.

36. Lopes GM, Grace ND: Gastroesophageal varices: prevention of bleeding and rebleeding. Gastroenterol Clin North Am 1993; 22:801.

37. Gregory PB, Veterans Affairs Cooperative Variceal Sclerotherapy Group: Prophylactic sclerotherapy for esophageal varices in men with alcoholic liver disease: a randomized, single-blind, multicenter trial. N Engl J Med 1991; 324:1779.

38. PROVA Study Group: Prophylaxis of first hemorrhage from esophageal varices by sclerotherapy, propranolol or both in cirrhotic patients: a randomized multi-center trial. Hepatology 1991; 14:1016.

39. Fardy JM, Laupacis A: A meta-analysis of prophylactic endoscopic sclerotherapy for esophageal varices. Am J Gastroenterol 1994; 89:1938.

40. Rikkers LF, Jin G: Variceal hemorrhage: surgical therapy. Gastroenterol Clin North Am 1993; 22:821.

41. Burroughs AK, McCormick PA: Prevention of variceal rebleeding. Gastroenterol Clin North Am 1992; 21:119.

42. Vinel JP Lamouliatte H, Cales P, et al.: Propranolol reduces the rebleeding rate during endoscopic sclerotherapy before variceal obliteration. Gastroenterology 1992; 102:1760.

43. Van Cutsem E, Rutgeerts P, Vantrappen G: Treatment of bleeding gastrointestinal vascular malformations with oestrogen-progesterone. Lancet 1990; 335:953.

44. Lewis BS, Salomon P, Rivera-MacMurray S, et al.: Does hormonal therapy have any benefit for bleeding angiodysplasia? J Clin Gastroenterol 1992; 15:99.

# HEAD AND NECK SURGERY

## *Michael Friedman and Sharon Noble*

## INTRODUCTION

The head and neck region is one of the most vascular areas of the human anatomy. Despite this, surgery in this region can be virtually bloodless with adherence to general preoperative and intraoperative principles. These include complete preoperative definition of the lesion's vascular supply, intraoperative positioning, hypotensive anesthesia, precise surgical technique, and adjunctive tools of laser and electrocautery. Attention to these details will enable the surgeon to perform major reconstructive procedures without transfusions even in the most challenging resections.

## PREOPERATIVE EVALUATION AND PREPARATION

Although most benign and malignant neck masses are not highly vascular, a small percentage of tumors represent vascular neoplasms. With the preoperative use of magnetic resonance (MR) imaging or computed tomography (CT) with infusion, vascular masses are easily detected in the preoperative evaluation. Angiography is essential to define the extent of vascular lesions, such as carotid body tumors, glomus jugulare tumors, or lesions at the base of the skull or the superior mediastinum. It allows precise definition of tissue planes as well as identification of feeding arteries and venous drainage.

Angiography is useful not only for initial evaluation of vascular supply but has therapeutic use as well during preoperative embolization. Angiofibromas, glomus jugulare tumors, and arteriovenous malformations are associated with significant intraoperative blood loss. Murphy and Brackmann[1] showed a 50% reduction in operative blood loss with the use of preoperative embolization as well as reduction in operative time. A large variety of catheter systems and embolic materials are currently available. The catheter assembly consists of an introduction sheath that can be sutured to the skin to prevent arterial injury from repeated removal and reinsertion and a hollow catheter with a balloon at its tip that is used to prevent reflux of embolic material and to control its flow. Detachable balloon catheters are also available. Balloon-tipped catheters can also be used to test patient tolerance to arterial occlusion before embolization.[2] Any potential neurological impairment can then be assessed.

Embolic agents can be divided into groups based on their biodegradability and their form. Absorbable gelatin sponge (Gelfoam®, Upjohn Laboratory, Kalamazoo, MI), bits of autologous blood clot, or small pieces of autogenous muscle are frequently used resorbable materials.[3] Silicone is a nonabsorbable product available in flow-directed pellets or in a fluid form that vulcanizes to form a silicone cast of the vasculature. Polyvinyl alcohol foam is a nonabsorbable sponge-like material that expands to 10–15 times its length shortly after contact with fluid. Polyvinyl alcohol foam and isobutyl 2-cyanoacrylate, another polymerizing agent, are especially suited for medium-sized to large vessels.

Choice of a catheter assembly and embolic material is multifactorial, with consideration given to the site and size of the lesion and the location and number of feeding arteries, as well as the flow characteristics of the lesion.

Further discussion is beyond the scope of this text; however, an extensive examination of catheter delivery systems can be found in a review article by Berenstein and Kricheff.[4]

The most important principle in the preoperative assessment is to be prepared ahead of time. Knowing what to expect before the skin incision is made can ultimately diminish operative blood loss. MR or CT imaging with infusion is an essential component of preoperative evaluation of any unknown neck mass. Masses that represent lymph node metastases from a known primary tumor (salivary gland or thyroid) do not routinely require preoperative CT or MR.[5]

## INTRAOPERATIVE PRINCIPLES

Intraoperative preparation begins with positioning of the patient. Reverse Trendelenburg position with the patient's head elevated 30° reduces arterial pressure by 2 mm Hg per inch of elevation of pressure, but more importantly, this position reduces venous congestion associated with the supine position and reduces backbleeding from cut vessels (see Chapter 4: Blood Conservation Techniques).

With controlled hypotensive anesthesia, the blood pressure is intentionally reduced below the level that is normally associated with anesthesia. It is generally agreed that a gradual reduction of the mean arterial pressure to 50 mm Hg is considered safe.[6] A number of studies comparing normotensive to controlled hypotensive anesthesia have been performed since Gardner[7] described the origins of this technique in 1946. The preponderance of evidence indicates that up to 50% reduction in operative blood loss can be achieved, translating into fewer units of blood transfused and more meticulous tumor resection in a drier surgical field[6,8,9] (see Chapter 8: Deliberate Hypotension).

## Surgical Approach

It is of crucial importance to follow sound surgical principles once the operation commences. The skin incision should be planned so that exposure will be optimal. All dissection should proceed along anatomical planes. Many of the structures of the head and neck are surrounded by a thin vascular adventitial layer, which provides the basis for dissection. Another key surgical principle is identification of important vascular and nervous structures before resection. This greatly decreases the risk of inadvertent injury and unnecessary bleeding that occurs when trying to gain control of an already cut vessel. Major cases should be prepared with vascular clamps. Surgery on tumors that may involve the carotid artery should be prepared with vascular surgeons on standby to shunt the carotid artery if it needs to be clamped. A final surgical axiom is to always identify and ligate the feeding vessels to the lesion early in the procedure. This serves to devascularize the tumor and significantly diminish blood loss.

## Surgical Aids

A number of tools available for use in the operating room serve to reduce blood loss. Local infiltration of tissue with lidocaine with epinephrine, the Shaw hemostatic scalpel, the use of cautery (both monopolar and bipolar), laser use, and hemostatic agents such as absorbable gelatin sponge and thrombin all result in a drier surgical field.

### EPINEPHRINE

Local infiltration of tissue with epinephrine-containing solutions in small open procedures was developed as a method for improved hemostasis. This is due to the vasoconstrictive properties of epinephrine combined with a compression effect on the vascular structures within the infiltrated tissue. It also eases dissection by facilitating identification of the tissue planes. Studies have shown 50–75% reduction in blood loss during tonsillectomy with the use of solutions containing 0.25–0.5% epinephrine.[10–12] We recommend injection of 1% lidocaine with 1:100,000 epinephrine solution into the subcapsular plane of the anterior and posterior tonsillar pillar and behind the tonsil, between the tonsillar capsule and surrounding tissue plane. This displaces the tonsil toward the midline and clarifies the plane of dissection.

Caveats do exist with this technique. Cardiac ectopy can be induced with the use of epinephrine and volatile inhalation anesthetics, and there can be marked elevation of the systolic blood pressure as well as the heart rate after the injection of epinephrine (see Chapter 4: Blood Conservation Techniques).

## HEMOSTATIC SCALPEL

The Shaw hemostatic scalpel uses thermal energy for coagulation of blood vessels while cutting. It has the advantage of coagulating vessels without the electrical energy of cautery that can cause injury to surrounding structures. The heat is not transmitted significantly beyond the plane of incision. Although it is not effective for larger vessels and is not a substitute for other forms of hemostasis, it adds to the ease of identifying planes by keeping the field blood free.

## ELECTROCAUTERY

Bipolar and monopolar electrocautery are both used for thermal coagulation of small bleeding vessels. In bipolar cautery, the current travels between the tips of the device and cauterizes only the tissue that is grasped between the tips. Monopolar cautery coagulates tissue at the tip of the electrode but causes more tissue destruction in a pyramid dimension.[13] There is no advantage to cautery use in terms of wound healing or tissue destruction when compared with the use of free ties.[14,15] However, there is some reduction in blood loss.[16,17] Monopolar cautery can be used if no nerves are in the proximity of the vessels to be coagulated. It therefore has limited usefulness in head and neck surgery. Bipolar cautery is essentially useful in controlling small vessels with minimal injury to surrounding tissues.

## LASERS

Lasers have different effects on different tissues based on the specific wavelength and rate of energy delivered. The benefits of laser use are a decrease in blood loss and more precise tissue destruction. However, caution must be taken with lasers to adequately protect both the patient and operating room personnel from unsafe exposure. Eye protection is imperative for all present during laser use, laser-safe anesthetic techniques must be used to prevent endotracheal tube combustion, and care must be taken to ensure that incandescent particles are not sucked into the nasopharyngeal airway, as may occur during the laser ablation of respiratory papillomatosis.[18]

The three types of lasers most commonly used in surgery are the carbon dioxide ($CO_2$) laser, the argon beam coagulator (ABC), and the neodymium:yttrium-aluminum-garnet (Nd:YAG) laser.

The $CO_2$ laser produces infrared light that causes tissue destruction by vaporization. This form of laser is absorbed by water, and the patient's head should be draped with a gauze towel to absorb the laser energy if the target is missed. The $CO_2$ laser has adjustable spot size from 0.1 to 1.5 mm. The power density and rate of energy delivery (continuous versus pulsed) also are adjusted to provide the optimal combination because the hemostatic ability of the laser declines as the speed of tissue destruction increases. Because of the low temperature of 100°C at which vaporization of the cells occurs with the use of the $CO_2$ laser, there is little damage to adjacent normal tissue.[18]

The recently developed ABC uses an invisible noncombustible odorless beam of ionized argon gas to conduct current to the tissues. The ABC causes coagulation within the vessel walls when held at a distance of 1 cm from the tissue at a 60° angle. A thin eschar is formed over the surface 1–2 mm thick that remains firmly attached. Although there are no published data that quantitate the reduction in blood loss, Ward and associates[19] showed a qualitative decrease in blood loss as well as a decrease in the need for transfusion in their review of the ABC.

The Nd:YAG laser is a contact coagulating laser that, in contrast to the $CO_2$ laser, is especially suited for treating vascular lesions. Contact probes made from synthetic sapphires are optically shaped to focus the energy at the probe's tip. One drawback of the Nd:YAG laser is that there is a high degree of backscatter that leads to high energy and subsequent higher risk of thermal damage to adjacent normal tissue.[20] The Nd:YAG laser is ideal for use as a hemostatic tool.

Photodynamic therapy is a technique currently in developmental stages whereby a photosensitive substance given to a patient is selectively absorbed or retained by specific cells. The tissue cells are then treated with a certain wavelength of light that destroys only the cells containing the photosensitive substance.[21]

A variety of hemostatic absorbable agents can be used to control oozing at the end of a procedure. These agents cause no tissue destruction and generally control multiple tiny vessel bleeding within minutes.

In extreme cases where bleeding from small vessels becomes excessive, but not due to a coagulopathic state, packing the operative site and returning in 24–48 hours for delayed removal is an option. This is rarely needed in cases of bleeding from the bone or skull.

## SUMMARY

Head and neck surgery can be relatively bloodless in the vast majority of cases. Preoperative assessment of tumor vascularity is the first step in guaranteeing a bloodless field. Although many surgical tools are helpful in minimizing blood loss, the key is surgical technique that respects planes and identifies all vessels before resection.

### REFERENCES

1. Murphy TP, Brackmann DE: Effects of preoperative embolization of glomus jugulare tumors. Laryngoscope 1989; 99:1244.
2. Valavanis A: Preoperative embolization of the head and neck: indications, patient selection, goals and precautions. Am J Neuroradiol 1986; 7:943.
3. Thompson JN, Fierstien SB, Kohut RI: Embolization techniques in vascular tumors of the head and neck. Head Neck Surg 1979; 2:25.
4. Berenstein A, Kricheff II: Catheter and material selection for transarterial embolization: technical considerations. Parts I and II. Radiology 1979; 132:619.
5. Mafee MF, Campos M, Raju S, et al.: Head and neck: high field magnetic resonance imaging versus computed tomography. Otolaryngol Clin North Am 1988; 21:513.
6. Ward CF, Alfery DD, Saidman LO, et al.: Deliberate hypotension in head and neck surgery. Head Neck Surg 1980; 2:185.
7. Gardner WJ: The control of bleeding during operation by induced hypotension. JAMA 1946; 132:572.
8. Salem MR: Therapeutic uses of ganglionic blocking drugs. Int Anesthesiol Clin 1978; 16:171.
9. Sataloff RT, Brown ACD, Sheets EE, et al.: A controlled study of hypotensive anesthesia in head and neck surgery. Ear Nose Throat J 1987; 66:479.
10. Boliston TA, Upton JJM: Infiltration with lignocaine and adrenaline in adult tonsillectomy. J Laryngol Otol 1980; 94:1257.
11. Broadman LM, Patel RI, Feldman BA, et al.: The effects of peritonsillar infiltration on the reduction of intraoperative blood loss and post-tonsillectomy pain in children. Laryngoscope 1989; 99:578.
12. Rasgon BM, Cruz RM, Hilsinger RL, et al.: Infiltration of epinephrine in tonsillectomy: a randomized, prospective double-blind study. Laryngoscope 1991; 101:114.
13. Bell AF, Shagets FW, Barrs DM: Principle and hazards of electrocautery in otolaryngology. Otolaryngol Head Neck Surg 1986; 94:504.
14. Mann DG, St. George C, Scheiner E, et al.: Tonsillectomy—some like it hot. Laryngoscope 1984; 94:677.
15. Ritter EF, Demas CP, Thompson DA, et al.: Effects of method of hemostasis on wound-infection rate. Am Surg 1990; 10:648.
16. Weber RS, Byers RM, Robbins KT, et al.: Electrosurgical dissection to reduce blood loss in head and neck surgery. Head Neck 1989; 11:318.
17. Weimert TA, Babyak JW, Richter HJ: Electrodissection tonsillectomy. Arch Otolaryngol Head Neck Surg 1990; 116:186.
18. Carruth JAS: The role of lasers in otolaryngology. Ann Chir Gynaecol 1990; 79:216.
19. Ward PH, Castro DJ, Ward S: A significant new contribution to radical head and neck surgery. Arch Otolaryngol Head Neck Surg 1989; 115:921.
20. Midgley HC: Nd:YAG contact laser surgery. Otolaryngol Clin North Am 1990; 23:99.
21. Castro DJ, Saxton RE, Fetterman HR, et al.: Bioinhibition of human fibroblast cultures sensitized to Q-switch II dye and treated with the Nd:YAG: a new technique of photodynamic therapy with lasers. Laryngoscope 1989; 99:421.

# ORTHOPEDIC SURGERY

## *John P. Lubicky*

Orthopedic surgery involves procedures both on soft and hard (bone) tissue. The anatomic site and the type of tissue being operated on have implications on the expected blood loss and the surgeon's ability to minimize it. As a general statement, it is obvious that good surgical technique that minimizes unnecessary tissue trauma will help decrease the blood loss throughout a given case. Additionally, various pharmacological maneuvers to decrease the blood loss (e.g., induced hypotension, the use of desmopression acetate, and so on) can be used to reduce unavoidable blood loss. Intraoperative wound blood recovery and reprocessing (e.g., the Cell Saver, Haemonetics, Braintree, MA) and postoperative wound drainage recovery[1] (see Chapter 9: Blood Salvage Techniques) help to avoid the use of anything but autologous blood products in situations where significant blood loss cannot be otherwise avoided. All of these methods are thoroughly discussed elsewhere in the text but bear mentioning here to emphasize the need for the surgeon, the anesthesiologist, and the nursing staff to plan effective plans of managing blood loss and its replacement. The effects of positioning of the patient during surgery are important and are discussed elsewhere in this text as well (see Chapter 4: Blood Conservation Techniques). Spinal anesthesia has also been found to reduce blood loss in certain situations.[2]

There are maneuvers that the surgeon can use to minimize blood loss. If surgery is to be done on an extremity, the use of a tourniquet should be considered. The tourniquet provides a completely dry field for the surgeon, making dissection safe, allowing meticulous control of vessels, and eliminating the need for rapid maneuvers to decrease the blood loss. Typically, the extremity is exsanguinated with an elastic wrap before inflating the tourniquet (except in cases of tumor or infection, where simple elevation for a minute or so at least partially empties the extremity of blood). There are certain potential problems associated with tourniquet use. The systemic effects include hypothermia and acidosis after tourniquet release (particularly if tourniquets are used and released simultaneously on multiple extremities).[3] Local effects include muscle damage and nerve compression, which are both related to the amount of pressure and the duration of tourniquet use[4] (see Chapter 4: Blood Conservation Techniques).

In other anatomic areas where a tourniquet cannot be used, other methods of controlling blood loss must be applied. These start with the skin incision. Several techniques can be used. Once the epidermis is divided with a knife, further dissection through the dermis and the subcutaneous tissue can be done with electrocautery. This maneuver not only can make this part of the case nearly bloodless (especially if done with coagulation rather than cutting mode) but also saves time compared with the situation in which the same tissues are cut with a knife and then hemostasis is attempted with multiple bleeding sites present. However, a short duration of wound edge compression with sponges or the insertion of a self-retaining retractor that produces tension

on the skin edges and their blood vessels also helps control the bleeding. A local infiltration of dilute epinephrine solution in the proposed site of the skin incision can also help.[5] However, for optimal effect, the epinephrine needs to be in place for several minutes before the incision.

Once deeper dissection is performed, the surgeon must deal with both soft tissue and bony bleeding. Certain soft tissue ooze can be handled by packing with sponges with or without epinephrine.[2] Direct control vessels, of course, should be handled with the electrocautery, ligatures, or vessel clips.

The control of bone bleeding is a much more difficult problem because once the bone is cut, bleeding will ensue, and the usual methods of hemostasis are not possible. One way of decreasing blood loss from the osteotomy or decortication is to postpone these maneuvers until all other parts of the procedure have been completed and the final bone work has been thoroughly prepared. If and when bony bleeding occurs and cannot be further avoided, techniques such as using absorbable gelatin sponge (Gelfoam®, Upjohn, Kalamazoo, MI) soaked in thrombin (Parke-Davis, Morris Plains, NJ), microfibrillar collagen hemostat (Avitine®, Alcon, Ft. Worth, TX), or bone wax may be used. All of these substances may be left in place at the end of the surgery, but in the case of bone wax, it may hinder bone healing if present over a large area. The use of microfibrillar collagen hemostat may be contraindicated if blood salvage techniques are being used.[6] Methylmethacrylate may be used to control bleeding from a bone biopsy site by packing it through the cortical defect into the medullary cavity and sealing off the cortical defect.[7]

Preoperative embolization of lesions known to be particularly vascular also helps with intraoperative blood loss.[8-11] These maneuvers are especially useful when treating aneurysmal bone cyst,[11] metastases from renal cell carcinoma,[12] hemangiomas of the spine, and pelvic fractures. The embolization may also have a therapeutic effect of its own.[11] Extreme care must be exercised by the interventional radiologist so as not to jeopardize the circulation to critical tissues (e.g., the spinal cord) in the area of the lesion. Many substances have been used, including absorbable gelatin sponge, autologous clot, lyophilized human dura matter, steel coils, plastic and glass beads, and rapid-setting polymers.[9] Each of these substances has advantages and disadvantages, and one may be more appropriate for a particular situation than another. The use of lesion embolization of the spine is very helpful, not only in decreasing the blood loss but also in making the surgery technically easier in a dry field and consequently safer (see Chapter 13 (Part I): Endovascular Embolization in the Management of Skull-Base Tumors).

Finally, a factor that is sometimes forgotten is the speed with which the operation is performed. This is not to suggest the surgeon should race through an operation. Rather, it means that if things are going well and the surgeon has a well-thought-out preoperative plan, the procedure should proceed deliberately from one step to the next without delay. This ability to proceed quickly is related to the surgeon's experience, confidence, and ability but also may be affected by the presence of residents who are assisting and/or performing the surgery under the surgeon's supervision. As a good example, Brodsky and associates[13] reported on a series of patients undergoing scoliosis surgery with hypotensive anesthesia. They found that the decreased blood loss was related more to decreased operating time than the presence of the induced hypotension. Bostman and coworkers[14] made a similar observation (see Chapter 8: Deliberate Hypotension).

In summary, there are various ways the surgeon can help to decrease blood loss. Those plus anesthetic maneuvers and patient posi-tioning add to the overall effect of decreasing blood loss during orthopedic surgery.

## REFERENCES

1. Flynn JC, Price CT: The third step of total autologous blood in scoliosis surgery: harvesting blood from the postoperative wound. Proc Scoliosis Res Soc Ann Meet, Honolulu, Hawaii, September, 1990.
2. Nelson CL, Nelson RL, Cone J: Blood conservation techniques in orthopaedic surgery. AAOS Instructional Course Lectures 1990; 39:425.
3. Goodarzi M, Shier N-H, Ogden JA: Physiologic changes during tourniquet use in children. Proc Ann Shrine Surg Meet, Spokane, Washington, September, 1991.
4. Crenshaw AH: Surgical techniques. In: Crenshaw AH, ed, Campbell's Operative Orthopaedics, 7 ed. St. Louis, 1987, C.V. Mosby Co.
5. Phillips WA, Hensinger RN: Control of blood loss during scoliosis surgery. Clin Orthop Rel Res 1988; 229:88.
6. Robiczek F, Duncan GD, Born GVR: Inherent dangers of simultaneous application of microfibrillar collagen hemostat and blood saving devices. J Thorac Cardiovasc Surg 1986; 92:766.
7. Enneking WF: Clinical Musculoskeletal Pathology. Gainesville, FL, 1977, Storter Printing Co.
8. Dick HM, Bigliani LU, Michelsen WJ, et al.: Adjuvant arterial embolization in the treatment of benign primary bone tumors in children. Clin Orthop Rel Res 1979; 139:133.
9. Allison DJ: Therapeutic embolization. J Bone Joint Surg [Br] 1982; 64B:151.
10. Graham JJ, Yang WC: Vertebral hemangioma with compression fracture and paraparesis treated with preoperative embolization and vertebral resection. Spine 1984; 9:97.
11. DeRosa GP, Graziano GP, Scott J: Arterial embolization of aneurysmal bone cyst of the lumbar spine. J Bone Joint Surg [Am] 1990; 72A:777.
12. Bowers TA, Murray JA, Charnsangavej C, et al.: Bone metastasis in renal carcinoma. J Bone Joint Surg [Am] 1982; 64A:749.
13. Brodsky JW, Dickson JH, Erwin WD, et al.: Hypotensive anesthesia for scoliosis surgery in Jehovah's Witnesses. Spine 1991; 16:304.
14. Bostman O, Hyrkas J, Hirvensalo E, et al.: Blood loss, operating time and positioning of the patient in lumbar disc surgery. Spine 1990; 15:360.

# TRAUMA SURGERY

*Sheldon B. Maltz, Michele M. Mellett, and*
*Richard J. Fantus*

## INTRODUCTION

To be faced with a patient suffering from relentless refractory bleeding is both challenging and frustrating for the trauma surgeon. The rapid application of surgical principles and techniques can be lifesaving in many of these situations. It must be recognized that the successful use of blood conserving techniques will be for naught if coagulopathic states are left untreated. The current concern is the acute treatment of massive hemorrhage, and this discussion is focused on preoperative and intraoperative techniques of blood conservation in the trauma patient.

## NONOPERATIVE TECHNIQUES

Specific techniques used to stop bleeding that occurs outside the operating room are manual compression, pneumatic antishock garment (PASG), external pelvic fixators, and autotransfusion devices.

The control of external hemorrhage is best accomplished by direct compression rather than tourniquet. Application of a tourniquet can occlude important collateral vessels and lead to severe ischemia in the distal extremity. Vascular clamps should not be applied into the depths of a wound without adequate exposure. This maneuver can cause additional damage to adjacent neurovascular structures or further damage the already injured vessel.

PASGs were initially developed by the United States Air Force in an attempt to prevent the pooling of blood in the extremities and decreased cerebral circulation during high-speed aircraft flight. This device was adapted by the medical community to augment the management of patients in hemorrhagic shock secondary to abdominal, pelvic, or lower extremity injuries. The physiological effects of PASGs were initially thought to be secondary to the shunting or relocation of blood from the lower extremities and abdomen into the central circulation. Further investigation revealed that the application of PASGs causes an increase in peripheral vascular resistance and therefore increases the blood pressure in the hypovolemic patient.[1]

PASGs may be used in three situations: patients in whom the systolic blood pressure is <80 mm Hg and there is an associated tachycardia; patients who require an indirect mechanism to reduce or control bleeding from the abdomen, pelvis, or thigh; and patients who require stabilization of fractures of the pelvis or femur.

As previously noted, PASGs can be used for the treatment of life-threatening hemorrhage from closed pelvic fractures. The PASG can be maximally inflated for 2 hours in an attempt to tamponade bleeding. During this time, resuscitation with fluid and blood products is continued in the hope that compartmental inflation pressures can be lowered to 40–50 mm Hg. If hemodynamic instability recurs with deflation or the pelvic fracture is severely displaced and/or unstable, reduction and stabilization with an external pelvic fixation device (EPFD) is indicated. The EPFD is a device used to stabilize and, more importantly, to reapproximate the broken and displaced bones of the pelvis. Application of the device increases the tamponade of venous bleeding from cancellous bone and the pelvic venous plexus. Failure to control bleeding with both PASGs and EPFDs indicates a major vascular laceration that may be detected and controlled angiographically. Methods of angiographic control may be autologous clot, metal coils, or topical hemostatic agents such as absorbable gelatin sponge (Gelfoam®, UpJohn Laboratory, Kalamazoo, MI).

The presence of pulmonary edema or intrathoracic hemorrhage are absolute contraindications to the application of PASGs. The relative contraindications for application are patients with impaled objects, pregnant patients, and patients with diaphragmatic injuries or hernias. Complications such as anterior compartment syndrome in the lower extremities have developed when PASGs are left inflated at 100 mm Hg for more than 4 hours.[2,3] The PASG may remain inflated for up to 48 hours if the pressure does not exceed 40–50 mm Hg. The deflation of the PASG must be done gradually and with frequent blood pressure monitoring. The abdominal compartment and individual extremities are deflated sequentially, the abdominal compartment being deflated first. A decrease in blood pressure by 5 mm Hg indicates that further fluid resuscitation is required and deflation should be stopped.

Blood salvage procedures have been extended to trauma patients, especially in thoracic trauma. Another technique for blood conservation is used in thoracic trauma. It is not unusual for a patient to present with thoracic trauma and associated hemothorax requiring tube thoracostomy in the emergency department. In this situation, blood can be retrieved from the pleural cavity through a collection-suction device, mixed with citrate anticoagulants, and returned to the patient. The unwashed blood is then transfused via filtered blood tubing. The successful use of this technique was originally reported at the Ben Taub General Hospital (Houston, TX)[4] and Maryland Institute for Emergency Medical Services.[5] It is now commonly used in trauma centers throughout America. The reinfusion of salvaged blood should be limited to 3000 mL or less and should be performed within 1–4 hours of preparation.[6] If the blood is promptly refrigerated after collection, it can be safely stored for up to 24 hours. Analysis of the blood collected from traumatic hemothoraces reveals low platelet and fibrinogen levels, a normal hemoglobin, and a hematocrit approximating half that of the patient's blood. Clinical trials of the efficacy of this technique

have shown no untoward effects[7] (see Chapter 9: Blood Salvage Techniques).

## INTRAOPERATIVE TECHNIQUES

A significant number of patients who present in hemorrhagic shock require acute operative intervention for the control of ongoing blood loss. Basic surgical principles and techniques must be applied to arrest the hemorrhage and prevent further exsanguination. For instance, a traumatized extremity with vascular injury and external blood loss requires the application of direct compression followed by emergent surgical intervention. In the operating room, an assistant's gloved hand should maintain direct pressure on the wound, be prepped into the sterile field, and only be removed after proximal and distal vascular control is achieved. This technique facilitates vascular control and exploration with minimal further blood loss.

Proximal and distal vascular control should always be attained before exploration of hematomas or attempts at direct visualization of vascular injuries. The importance of this basic principle cannot be overemphasized, particularly in cases of intraabdominal injury. Major vessels within the abdominal cavity include the aorta and inferior vena cava, the celiac axis and superior mesenteric artery and vein, the renal arteries and veins, the iliac arteries and veins, the hepatic artery, the portal vein, and, finally, the retrohepatic inferior vena cava. Without adequate vascular control, exploration of hematomas overlying these vessels can result in acute exsanguinating hemorrhage and death.

The approach to intraabdominal hemorrhage must be rapid, precise, and controlled. After the abdominal cavity is opened, the four quadrants of the abdomen are immediately packed with laparotomy packs to assist in the tamponade of hemorrhage. Active arterial bleeding is treated with direct, continuous, manual compression until vascular control is achieved. Hemorrhage from major venous structures can be controlled with sponge-stick compression, and at times a side-biting vascular clamp can be applied. Various techniques using the principle of proximal and distal control are described[8] and allow adequate exploration of retroperitoneal hematomas safely without the threat of unrelenting blood loss.

Occasionally, patients with apparent abdominal vascular injury present profoundly hypotensive and moribund. Proximal control of abdominal arterial inflow in this situation is achieved via emergent left thoracotomy and cross-clamping of the distal thoracic aorta, thereby enabling the tamponade effect of the abdominal cavity to remain undisturbed. After control of abdominal arterial inflow is attained, exploration of the abdominal cavity is performed. Those patients who are more hemodynamically stable can have proximal aortic control achieved within the abdominal cavity by performing a Mattox maneuver.[9] This technique allows visualization of the entire abdominal aorta from the diaphragmatic hiatus to the aorta bifurcation.

Significant liver injury presents a major challenge to the trauma surgeon, and various blood conserving techniques must be applied in an expeditious fashion. Assessment of the extent of the liver injury must be made as soon as the patient is resuscitated with fluid and blood products. If significant bleeding continues after manual compression of the injury, the portal triad should be occluded (Pringle maneuver) to obstruct liver inflow.[10] If bleeding does not stop or slow significantly, then a retrohepatic caval injury must be considered.

A successful Pringle maneuver enables improved visualization of vascular injuries. Specific techniques to repair hepatic injuries are numerous: (*a*) suture point ligation of lacerated parenchyma vessels; (*b*) application of various hemostatic agents such as thrombin, absorbable gelatin sponge, oxidized regenerated cellulose (Surgicel®, Johnson & Johnson Medical Inc., Arlington, TX), and fibrin glue (all of these agents can be applied to control parenchymal bleeding, but fibrin glue has been shown to be a most valuable adjunctive hemostatic agent in deep hepatic injuries because it can be sprayed onto or injected directly into deep tracks)[11]; and (*c*) specific injuries will at times require liver debridement or even hepatic resection to control parenchyma hemorrhage.

If standard techniques do not control hemorrhage from the liver parenchyma, packing of the injury and closure of the abdomen with planned reexploration in 24–72 hours is indicated.[12] This allows time for adequate resuscitation warming and control of coagulopathy. Primary indications for liver packing are bilateral complex liver injuries, rapidly expanding or ruptured subcapsular hematomas, coagulopathy, and hemodynamic instability. Contraindications to the use of perihepatic packing include large intrahepatic vessels that are actively bleeding or active bleeding from the hepatic veins or the retrohepatic vena cava.[13]

Injuries to the hepatic veins and retrohepatic inferior vena are often fatal. After a Pringle maneuver is performed and dark bleeding is noted from the liver parenchyma or welling up from beneath a liver lobe, these types of injuries must be considered. The two methods commonly used to handle juxtahepatic venous injuries are atrial caval shunt or sequential vascular clamping. The majority of reported experience has been with the atrial-caval shunt technique, proving to have very poor survival rates, with mortality rates of 72–75%.[14] The second technique uses vascular clamps applied to the suprarenal abdominal aorta, portis hepatic, suprarenal inferior vena cava, and suprahepatic inferior vena cava.[15] The high mortality rate associated with these procedures exists because the juxtahepatic venous injury is not recognized until after a significant blood loss and subsequent coagulopathy has occurred. Early recognition of these injuries and expeditious performance of these two techniques can be lifesaving.

Autotransfusion of shed blood has been a valuable adjunct in trauma surgery. Currently, two autotransfusion devices are commonly used. The cell processor is a system that collects the blood in heparin or citrate anticoagulant and washes the red cells. The second technique collects the shed blood with a suction device into citrate anticoagulants. The blood is then directly reinfused through a filter into the patient without washing.

The advantages of autotransfusion are many. Blood is available immediately without performing cross-match analysis. Other advantages include a decreased risk of transmitted diseases and no risk of hemodynamic, febrile, or autotransfusion reactions. The most important advantage is that the transfusing blood is already warm, which prevents or lessens hypothermia. Complications occur infrequently and include air embolism, disseminated intravascular coagulation, and thrombocytopenia. The most controversial question is whether shed blood, contaminated with gastrointestinal contents, can be reinfused. Reinfusing contaminated blood is justified in life-threatening situations.[16] Whenever possible, the use of washed autotransfusion techniques should be applied because this will reduce the bacterial inoculum and remove any small bits of gastrointestinal contents that are contained in the shed blood[16] (see Chapter 9: Blood Salvage Techniques).

Adjuncts to operative therapy include interventions that prevent hypothermia, metabolic acidosis, and ensuing coagulation derangements. A large volume of packed red blood cell transfusion (10 units or more) is associated with coagulation defects secondary to hypothermia, dilution, deficiencies of clotting factors, and metabolic acidosis. To correct a coagulopathy, the previous conditions must be prevented or reversed rapidly by maintaining adequate temperature with blood warming devices, giving platelets and fresh frozen plasma and maintaining arterial pH above 7.25. The combination of coagulopathy, hypothermia, and metabolic acidosis accounts for 80% of all deaths associated with massive hemorrhage. Finally, if the coagulopathy is so severe that the patient remains in shock after all major arterial and venous injuries are controlled, the operation should be aborted, the abdomen rapidly closed with towel clips, and the patient immediately transferred to the intensive care unit for continued resuscitation and correction of coagulopathy.[13]

## REFERENCES

1. Ferrario CM, Nadzam G, Fernandez LA, et al.: Effects of pneumatic impression of the cardiovascular dynamics in the dog after hemorrhage. Aerosp Med 1970; 41:411.
2. Maull KI, Capehart JE, Cardea JA, et al.: Limb loss following military antishock trousers (MAST) application. J Trauma 1981; 21:60.
3. Bass RR, Allison EJ Jr, Reines HD, et al.: Tight compartment syndrome without lower extremity trauma following application of pneumatic antishock trousers. Ann Emerg Med 1983; 12:382.
4. Mattox KL: Autotransfusion in the emergency department. J Am Coll Emerg Physic 1975; 4:218.
5. Hauer JM, Dawson BR: Autotransfusion: an evaluation of it's value in reducing homologous blood use in trauma surgery. Clin Res 1981; 29:583A.
6. Jacobs LM, Hsieh JW: A clinical review of autotransfusion and it's role in trauma. JAMA 1984; 251:3283.
7. Symbas PN, Levin JM, Ferrier FL, et al.: A study on autotransfusion from hemothorax. South Med J 1969; 62:671.
8. Feliciano DV: Management of retroperitoneal hematomas. Am Surg 1990; 211:109.
9. Mattox KL, McCollum WB, Beall AC Jr, et al.: Management of penetrating injuries of supra-renal aorta. J Trauma 1975; 15:808.
10. Pringle JH: Notes on the arrest of hepatic hemorrhage due to trauma. Am J Surg 1908; 48:541.
11. Kram HB, Nathan RC, Mackabee JR, et al.: Clinical use of non-autologous fibrin glue. Am Surg 1988; 54:570.
12. Feliciano DV, Mattox KL, Murch JM, et al.: Packing for control of hepatic hemorrhage: 58 consecutive patients. J Trauma 1986; 26:738.
13. Feliciano DV, Pachter HL: Hepatic trauma revisited. Curr Probl Surg 1989; 26:453.
14. Burch JM, Feliciano DV, Mattox KL: The atriocaval shunt. Facts and fiction. Ann Surg 1988; 207:555.
15. Yellin AE, Chaffee CB, Donovan AJ: Vascular isolation in treatment of juxtahepatic venous injuries. Arch Surg 1971; 102:566.
16. Timberlake GA, McSwain NE Jr: Autotransfusion of blood contaminated by enteric contents: a potentially life saving measure in massively hemorrhage trauma patients. J Trauma 1988; 28:855.

## SUGGESTED READINGS

Current Problems in Surgery: Autotransfusion and Blood Conservation. Vol. 29, #3 March, 1982.
Moore EE, Mattox KL, Feliciano DV: Trauma, 2 ed. Norwalk, CT, 1991, Appleton & Lange.

# PLASTIC SURGERY AND BURNS

## *Raymond L. Warpeha*

Proper surgical technique and knowledge of anatomy are the primary means of reducing blood loss during surgery. Adjuncts in the control of blood loss can be instructed before or after incision or excision for a given surgical procedure by the following methods:

Before incision/excision:
1. tourniquet
2. vasoconstriction (epinephrine, vasopressin)

After incision/excision:
1. pressure and/or packing
2. suture ligation
3. electrical coagulation (electrocautery)
4. augmented coagulation
    (a) blood components
        thrombin
        fibrin "glue"
    (b) synthetic vehicles
        gelatin sponge
        oxidized cellulose
        collagen sponge

## USE OF TOURNIQUET

Complete cessation of bleeding is achieved by tourniquet on the extremities and is most often used to help visualize the small and intricate anatomy rather than a means of reducing blood loss. Where diffuse small vessel bleeding is encountered, such as in tangential excision of burn eschar, little blood is to be saved by the use of the tourniquet because the post-tourniquet bleeding and hyperemia must be dealt with as though the tourniquet was not used. However, when excision of burn eschar is carried to the fascial level, significant saving of blood can be achieved because of the opportunity to close the fewer and larger blood vessels at this level before the release of the tourniquet (see "Burn Wound Excision").

## SUBCUTANEOUS AND DERMAL INJECTION OF EPINEPHRINE

Epinephrine injection into the skin and underlying tissues is the most frequent and efficient method of minimizing blood loss during a surgical procedure. As with a tourniquet, its value lies more in visualization of dissected structure than conservation of blood, although vasoconstriction exerts a profound reduction of blood flow in the skin, mucosa, and underlying tissues. In tangential excision of the burn wound, this effect contributes to substantial reduction in blood loss.

Epinephrine is used in concentrations ranging from $1:100,000$ to $1:800,000$ with decreasing effect with increasing dilution. A waiting period of $5-10$ minutes postinjection is necessary to obtain maximum vasoconstriction. Small pulsatile vessels are obscured by vasoconstriction and can cause postoperative hematoma formation after resorption of the epinephrine. With a more dilute solution, it is theoretically possible to detect the larger of the small pulsatile vessels and coagulate them before wound closure. Epinephrine is resorbed over a few hours and may result in high serum levels. When large volumes are used, it is wise to monitor patients for cardiac arrhythmias and blood pressure elevation, particularly in patients with a history of hypertension, those with known cardiac disease, and the elderly.

## USE OF PRESSURE AND PACKING

Complete hemostasis is desireable and generally attainable before wound closure. Occasionally, this cannot be attained, and some form of temporary low-pressure dressing or packing is required to obtain hemostasis, often in conjunction with a substance that augments or accelerates clotting (vide infra). This approach is only effective with low-pressure capillary or venous bleeding (i.e., bleeding from a torn pterygoid plexus of veins in an infratemporal space resection) and cannot be applied to pulsatile vessels that must be controlled individually. The dressing or pack is either released after clotting has occurred or left in place at the termination of the procedure to be removed at a later time. This approach is often used when dealing with the oozing associated with nasal mucosa.

## SUTURE LIGATION

Bleeding of larger blood vessels is controlled by absorbable or nonabsorbable suture ligation. All suture material acts as foreign bodies, with the nonabsorbable suture causing less tissue reaction. Metallic clips applied with a special forceps can be used for vessel occlusion in difficult recesses but are not as reliable as ligature on larger blood vessels. A properly applied suture ligature should create less necrosis than electrocautery and is preferred in the control of medium and larger vessels.

## ELECTRICAL COAGULATION

Because of ease of operation and reduction in time, electrocautery is the most common method of bleeding control of small blood vessels up to 3–4 mm in diameter. This method involves the necrosis of the vessel wall and a variable amount of the surrounding tissue. Bipolar and unipolar electrical coagulation systems are available and should be adjusted to accomplish electrocoagulation with the least energy necessary so as to minimize tissue necrosis.

Disposable battery-operated cautery units are available for the coagulation of very small blood vessels. These instruments rely on the heat generated through a resistant wire tip. Caution must be used to avoid flaming and skin burns when using these instruments (and electrocautery as well) near an oxygen source, such as a nasal cannula that might be in use during a facial surgery procedure requiring sedation for local anesthesia.

## AUGMENTED COAGULATIONS
### Bovine Thrombin

Thrombin is available as a crystalline powder obtained from a bovine source and standardized as U.S. units, whereby 2 units will clinically clot 1 mL of oxalated blood in 15 seconds. Solutions may be prepared at any concentration from 100 to 2000 units/mL. Thrombin must be used immediately after being placed in solution and is applied in nonadherent dressing or may be combined with a gelatin sponge. Thrombin solution has also been combined with a topical epinephrine solution in the excision of burn wounds. Alternately, thrombin crystal powder sprinkled on the oozing surface, followed by temporary pressure dressing, has been used instead of the solution.

### Fibrin Glue

The use of an autologous fibrin preparation has shown promise in wound hemostasis as well as acting as an adhesive for skin grafts.[1] Fibrinogen concentrate obtained from autologous blood is added to bovine thrombin and a calcium chloride solution. When mixed, the thrombin activates the fibrinogen and creates an adhesive fibrin compound in approximately 2–3 minutes. The adhesive property of this material has made it possible to apply skin grafts to difficult anatomic areas without dressings or suture fixation. The advantages of this approach to hemostasis over other less complex topical approaches to hemostasis remains to be seen.

## SYNTHETIC VEHICLES
### Gelatin Sponge or Powder

A sterile gelatin sponge or powder of porcine skin origin is available as an adjunct to hemostasis, apparently acting as a scaffold for coagulation. Gelatin sponge can be used wet or dry, and as previously noted, this material is commonly combined with thrombin solution before application. It is absorbed with time but is a foreign substance that can increase the possibility of infection when left buried in the tissues. Therefore, only the quantity necessary to obtain surface clotting should be used and not as a cavity filler or packing.

## Oxidized Cellulose

As the name implies, this fabric is produced by a controlled oxidation of cellulose. This material is applied dry, and its hemostatic properties appear to be that of an artificial clot, forming a sticky mass when wetted with blood. As with gelatin sponge, oxidized cellulose is absorbed and carries with it the same general precautions regarding infection.

## Collagen Sponges

Collagen pads are produced from bovine dermal collagen. Collagen produces platelet aggregation and forms the basis of clot formation. Application of this product to an oozing surface will usually cause hemostasis in 3–5 minutes. Unlike oxidized cellulose, collagen pads are readily removed from the surface to which it is applied. It is absorbed by the body when left in place and carries with it the same precautions as gelatin sponge and oxidized cellulose regarding infection.

## BURN WOUND EXCISION

Aside from the superficial self-healing partial thickness burns, full thickness and intermediate partial thickness burns are most frequently excised and covered with autogenous skin grafts or donor homograft. Except for the smallest wounds, blood loss is significant and can be spectacular. Excision is usually carried out tangential to the skin surface and is referred to as a tangential or laminar excision. The procedure is performed with a calibrated handheld knife or oscillating dermatome, usually with excisions of 10–20/one-thousandth inch in thickness. This is carried to a viable bleeding surface, sequentially where necessary, the total depth of excision depending on the depth of the burn and possibly into subcutaneous fat or muscle. The level of excision, which varies with the depth of the burn, will determine the rate of bleeding, but all excisions beyond the most superficial (of approximately 8–10/one-thousandth of an inch) are met with significant bleeding. As noted previously, excision to fascia with tourniquet control is met with less blood loss, although this can be considerable when involving a large portion of an extremity. Excision to fascia creates a considerable esthetic deformity and is used only under exceptional circumstances. Blood loss is controlled by various means, depending on the nature of the bleeding and the personal preference of the surgeon. Larger vessels and pulsatile vessels are best controlled by electrocoagulation. Reduction of low-pressure blood loss can be obtained topically with the application of epinephrine soaks of 1:10,000 concentration[2] and/or with the application of thrombin solution or powder to the excised surface. Blood loss also can be reduced by the subcutaneous injection with epinephrine similar to that of burn wound excision. Skin graft donor sites also can be treated like a burn excision with either topical applications or by epinephrine injection before removal.

An investigative pilot study by Achauer and coworkers[3] reported on the infusion of low-dose vasopressin initiated before burn wound excision and for 1–2 hours after the procedure. Blood loss was cut in half, and the need for postoperative blood transfusion was significantly reduced by the vasoconstriction in the skin vessels. Further studies should determine the efficacy of this approach to blood conservation in burn excision.

The amount of blood loss varies with the depth of the excision, and the amount cannot be predicted with great accuracy but can be approximated before operation knowing the area to be excised. Timing (days postburn) also may affect blood loss with lesser loss when excisions are carried out within the first 24 hours and after 16 days in burns of over 30% of body surface area.[4]

Although actual losses vary from individual to individual, studies by Warden and coworkers[5] established that burn excision blood loss averages approximately 1 mL of blood per cm$^2$ area excised when using topical thrombin and epinephrine to the excision site. Skin graft donor site bleeding is considerable and represents approximately one third of the total operated blood loss. This donor site loss amounts to approximately two thirds of a milliliter per centimeter squared. An average skin graft donor site of $6 \times 25$ cm ($150$ cm$^2$) would produce an approximate 100-mL blood loss. As burn wound excision is often expressed in percent of body surface involved or excised, an average adult of 1.7 m$^2$ would expect a blood loss of approximately 170 mL per percent body area excised. An estimate of additional blood loss due to skin graft donor site bleeding could be predicted on the anticipated area of harvest. As blood losses with burn excision can be rapid, anticipation of the magnitude of the loss is necessary for appropriate concomitant restoration of blood volume. Because of their great variation in size, Housinger and coworkers[6] suggested that blood loss in burn excision in children can be expressed as a percent loss of circulating blood volume rather than a fixed volume as in adults. Their studies report a blood loss of approximately 2.5% of the red blood cell (RBC) mass per 1% body surface excised and approximately 2% reduction for each 1% body surface donor harvest. These figures are based on the use of subcutaneous epinephrine injection before excision. Therefore, a 10% body area excision in a child with a 5% body area skin graft donor site (commonly skin grafts are mechanically expanded at 2:1 ratio) could yield a circulatory RBC reduction of approximately 35% $[(2.5 \times 10) + (2 \times 5)]$. Facial burn excision

doubles the blood loss per given area, and this holds true for adult facial burn excision as well.

Blood losses are replaced by appropriate replacement of RBCs. Although not having an oxygen-carrying capacity of the RBC, synthetic polysaccharides such as hetastarch[7] and pentastarch[8] have been successfully used as a colloid substitute in burn resuscitation and reduce the risks inherent in the use of blood products.

## REFERENCES

1. Saltz R, Dimick A, Harris C, et al.: Application of autologous fibrin glue in burn wounds. J Burn Care Rehabil 1989; 10:504.
2. Heimbach DM, Engrav LH: Surgical Management of the Burn Wound. New York, 1984, Raven Press.
3. Achauer RM, Hernandez BS, Parker A: Burn excision with intraoperative vasopressin. J Burn Care Rehabil 1989; 10:375.
4. Desai MH, Herndon DN, Broemeling L, et al.: Early burn wound excision reduces blood loss. Ann Surg 1990; 211:753.
5. Warden GD, Saffle JR, Kravitz M: Two stage technique for excision and grafting of burn wounds. J Trauma 1982; 22:98.
6. Housinger TA, Lang D, Warden GD: A prospective study of blood loss with excisional therapy in pediatric burn patients (Abstract). Proc Am Burn Assoc, New Orleans, 1989.
7. Waters LM, Christensen MA, Sato RM: Hetastarch: an alternative colloid in burn shock management. J Burn Care Rehabil 1989; 10:1.
8. Waxman K, Holmes R, Tominaga G, et al.: Hemodynamic and oxygen transport effects of pentastarch in burn resuscitation. Ann Surg 1989; 209:341.

# Index

Page numbers in *italics* indicate figures; those followed by "t" indicate tables.

425